VIRAL INFECTIONS IN OBSTETRICS AND GYNAECOLOGY

Edited by

D.J. Jeffries

Professor and Head of the Department of Virology St Bartholomew's Hospital London

and

C.N. Hudson

Emeritus Professor of Obstetrics and Gynaecology St Bartholomew's Hospital London

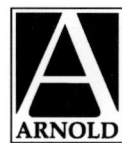

A member of the Hodder Headline Group
LONDON • SYDNEY • AUCKLAND
Co-published in the United States of America by Oxford University Press Inc., New York

First published in Great Britain in 1999 by
Arnold, a member of the Hodder Headline Group,
338 Euston Road, London NW1 3BH

http://www.arnoldpublishers.com

Co-published in the United States of America by
Oxford University Press Inc.,
198 Madison Avenue, New York, NY10016
Oxford is a registered trademark of Oxford University Press

Whilst the advice and information in this book are believed to be true and
accurate at the date of going to press, neither the authors nor the publisher
can accept any legal responsibility or liability for any errors or omissions
that may be made. In particular (but without limiting the generality of the
preceding disclaimer) every effort has been made to check drug dosages;
however, it is still possible that errors have been missed. Furthermore,
dosage schedules are constantly being revised and new side-effects
recognized. For these reasons the reader is strongly urged to consult the
drug companies' printed instructions before administering any of the drugs
recommended in this book.

British Library Cataloguing in Publication Data
A catalogue record for this book is available from the British Library

Library of Congress Cataloging-in-Publication Data
A catalog record for this book is available from the Library of Congress

ISBN 0 340 74095 7

1 2 3 4 5 6 7 8 9 10

Composition by Genesis Typesetting, Laser Quay, Rochester, Kent
Printed and bound in Great Britain by The Bath Press, Bath

What do you think about this book? Or any other Arnold title?
Please send your comments to feedback.arnold@hodder.co.uk

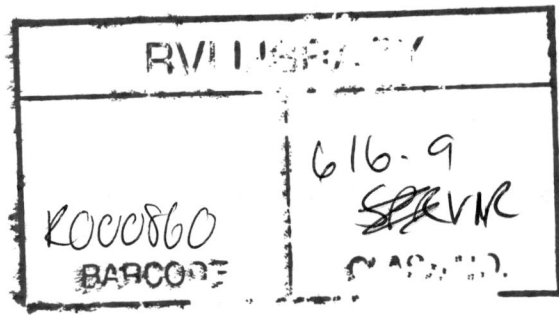

CONTENTS

CONTRIBUTORS

J.E. Banatvala,
Professor of Clinical Virology,
United Medical and Dental Schools of
Guy's and St Thomas's Hospitals,
St Thomas's Campus, Lambeth Palace Road,
London SE1 7EH, UK

K. Birthistle,
Smith Kline Beecham Pharmaceuticals,
Mundells,
Welwyn Garden City,
Hertfordshire AL7 1EY, UK

S. Boppana,
University of Alabama at Birmingham,
Department of Pediatrics,
Division of Infectious Diseases,
1600 7th Avenue South, Suite 752,
Birmingham, Alabama 35233, USA

N.S. Brink,
Department of Virology,
University College London Medical School,
Windeyer Building, 46 Cleveland Street,
London WIP 6DB, UK

D.W.G. Brown,
Central Public Health Laboratory,
Virus Reference Division,
61 Colindale Avenue,
London NW9 5HT, UK

J. Brownlie,
Professor of Veterinary Pathology,
Royal Veterinary College,
University of London,
Hawkshead, North Mimms, Hatfield,
Hertfordshire AL9 7TA, UK

D. Carrington,
Public Health Laboratories,
Myrtle Road,
Bristol BS2 8EL, UK

D. Casalaz,
Consultant and Senior Lecturer,
Peter Dunn Intensive Care Nursery,
St Michael's Hospital,
Bristol BS2 8EG, UK

I.L. Chrystie,
Lecturer in Virology,
United Medical and Dental Schools of
Guy's and St Thomas's Hospitals,
St Thomas's Campus, Lambeth Palace Road,
London SE1 7EH, UK

S. Conway,
Consultant Physician,
Seacroft Hospital,
York Road,
Leeds LS14 6UQ, UK

A. Cunningham,
Professor of Virology,
Institute of Clinical Pathology
and Medical Research,
Westmead Hospital,
New South Wales 2145, Australia

G.C.W. England,
Senior Lecturer of Veterinary Reproduction,
Royal Veterinary College,
University of London,
Hawkshead, North Mimms, Hatfield,
Hertfordshire AL9 7TA, UK

C.N. Hudson,
Emeritus Professor of Obstetrics and
Gynaecology,
2nd Floor, KGV,
St Bartholomew's Hospital,
West Smithfield, London EC1A 7BE, UK

D.J. Jeffries,
Head, Department of Virology,
St Bartholomew's Hospital,
48–53 Bartholomew Close,
West Smithfield, London EC1A 7BE, UK

C.E. Jensen,
Consultant Obstetrician and Gynaecologist,
Department of Obstetrics and Gynaecology,
University Hospital Lewisham,
Lewisham High Street,
London SE13 6LH, UK

S. Locarnini,
Victorian Infectious Diseases
Reference Laboratory,
10 Wreckyn Street,
North Melbourne,
Victoria 3051, Australia

A. MacLean,
Professor, University Department of
Obstetrics and Gynaecology,
Royal Free Hospital School of Medicine,
Pond Street, London NW3 2QG, UK

N. Marlow,
Professor of Neonatal Medicine,
Division of Child Health,
School of Human Development,
University of Nottingham,
Queens Medical Centre,
Nottingham NG7 2UH, UK

D.J. McCance,
Professor, Microbiology and Immunology
and Oncology,
Head of Virology Unit,
School of Medicine and Dentistry,
University of Rochester Medical Center,
New York, USA

J. McIntyre,
Consultant Obstetrician and Gynaecologist,
Co-Director, Perinatal HIV Research Unit,
Chris Hani Baragwanath Hospital,
P.O. Bertsham, Johannesburg 2013,
South Africa

A. Mindel,
Head, Academic Unit of Sexual Health
Medicine, Sydney Hospital, P.O. Box 1614,
Sydney, New South Wales 2001, Australia

P. Morgan-Capner,
Group Director PHLS North West and
Honorary Professor of Clinical Virology,
PHLS North West, Vicarage Lane, Fulwood,
Preston, Lancashire PR2 8DW, UK

D. Nathwani,
Consultant Physician,
Infection and Immunodeficiency Service,
Kings Cross Hospital,
Clepington Road, Dundee DD3 3EA, UK

M.-L. Newell,
Senior Lecturer,
Department of Epidemiology and Public
Health,
Institute of Child Health,
30 Guilford Street,
London WC1N 1EH, UK

R.F. Pass,
University of Alabama at Birmingham,
Department of Pediatrics,
Division of Infectious Diseases,
1600 7th Avenue South, Suite 752,
Birmingham, Alabama 35233, USA

C. Peckham,
Professor of Paediatric Epidemiology,
Department of Epidemiology and Public
Health,
Institute of Child Health,
30 Guilford Street,
London WC1N 1EH, UK

C.E. Roth,
Central Public Health Laboratory,
Virus Reference Division,
61 Colindale Avenue, London NW9 5HT, UK

D. Siebert,
Victorian Infectious Diseases Reference
Laboratory, 10 Wreckyn Street,
North Melbourne,
Victoria 3051, Australia

P. Walker,
Consultant Gynaecologist,
Royal Free Hospital,
Pond Street,
London NW3 2QG, UK

Introduction

D.J. Jeffries and C.N. Hudson

PATHOGENESIS AND IMMUNOLOGY OF FETAL AND NEONATAL INFECTION

The fetus and neonate are potentially vulnerable to a range of viruses which may infect the mother during pregnancy. While most of these infections are prevalent in the community, the fact that pregnant women are often in close contact with small children in the home means that the risk of exposure to common infections is amplified. While many common viral infections are restricted to the mucous membranes of the respiratory and gastrointestinal tracts, those that enter the circulation, e.g. rubella and parvovirus B19, may infect the fetus by transplacental spread.

TRANSPLACENTAL INFECTION

The effects of transplacentally acquired viral infection on the fetus include death and resorption of the embryo, abortion and stillbirth and the live birth of a premature or full-term baby who may have developmental abnormalities or congenital disease, or who may be normal. A viral infection acquired *in utero* may persist in postnatal life and clinical effects may not be apparent for months or even years after birth. Systemic viral infections which produce severe illness in the mother are likely to cause intrauterine death and viruses acquired in later pregnancy, e.g. chickenpox, may precipitate premature labour. In the case of certain viral infections, e.g. cytomegalovirus, herpes simplex virus and rubella, a primary infection is likely to present a more serious threat to the fetus than is a recurrence or secondary infection. Developmental abnormalities have been associated with specific infections including rubella, cytomegalovirus and varicella-zoster virus. The pathogenesis of these abnormalities is not clearly defined, but histological studies, clinical observation, cell culture and animal experiments indicate the involvement of multiple processes which include cytocidal effects of the virus, effects on cell growth, induction of chromosome damage and inflammatory and immunopathogenetic responses to the infection. In addition to (or in place of) the structural changes indicative of developmental disturbances, there may be evidence of active disease, at or soon after, the time of delivery. Thus, intrauterine cytomegalovirus infection may be suggested in the neonate by the presence of jaundice, hepatosplenomegaly, pneumonitis or petechial haemorrhages, all of which indicate continuing organ damage due to the infection. The absence of apparent disease in the neonate may be misleading and careful follow-up of infected neonates may reveal abnormality in the following months or years. This is particularly the case with the development of sensorineural deafness and/or cerebral dysfunction in babies who have

Viral Infections in Obstetrics and Gynaecology. Edited by D.J. Jeffries and C.N. Hudson. Published in 1999 by Arnold, ISBN 0 340 74095 7.

been infected *in utero* with rubella or cytomegalovirus. The immunosuppressive effects of a chronic viral infection, such as cytomegalovirus, may manifest as frequent, recurrent bacterial infections in the first few months of postnatal life. The incidence of transplacental infection, as judged by the infection of the fetus, varies among viruses and may also depend on the stage of pregnancy. Similarly, the incidence of congenital abnormalities may depend on the gestational age at which infection of the fetus occurs; the best example of this is congenital rubella in which the majority of abnormalities result from infection during the first trimester.

INTRAPARTUM INFECTIONS

A number of viruses may be present in the female genital tract, including herpes simplex virus, cytomegalovirus, hepatitis B virus and HIV. While the fetal membranes are intact, the fetus is protected from the microbial flora of the maternal genital tract and from any viruses that may be present on the mucosal surfaces or in the maternal circulation. If delivery is delayed after rupture of the membranes, viruses and microorganisms present in the vagina may ascend into the uterus and infect the baby *in situ*. Passage through the birth canal may also expose the baby to viruses present in mucous membranes (e.g. herpes simplex, cytomegalovirus) or the maternal circulation (e.g. hepatitis B, HIV). Abrasions in the baby's skin caused by birth trauma may provide the portal of entry for viral infections and the risks may be enhanced by the application of invasive techniques such as the use of scalp electrodes (Plate H).

POSTNATAL INFECTIONS

The baby may be exposed to particular risks of infection in the postpartum period and the obstetrician and perinatologist should be aware of these risks. The newborn, particularly if premature, may be vulnerable to a number of common infections (e.g. herpes simplex virus, enteroviruses) which, if acquired later in postnatal life, would not normally cause severe disease. Thus, staff in contact with the newborn baby (and other contacts such as visiting relatives) may present a risk of infection which should be avoided if possible. Any staff or visitors with obvious herpesvirus lesions, such as cold sores or shingles, or febrile illness should avoid contact with neonates until the symptoms and signs have resolved. Human milk presents a risk of infection with several viruses including cytomegalovirus, HIV, HTLV-1 and HTLV-2. While cytomegalovirus infection acquired by breastfeeding is normally benign, advice to avoid breastfeeding may be appropriate to prevent HIV and HTLV infection of babies born to carrier mothers. However, as discussed in Chapters 5, 8 and 9, because of the nutritional benefit to be gained from breastfeeding in developing countries, together with inherent dangers from reconstituting artificial milk with contaminated water, World Health Organization (WHO) guidelines suggest that breastfeeding may still be appropriate in many areas even for mothers known to be HIV infected[1].

HOST DEFENCES IN THE FETUS AND THE NEONATE

The facts that the fetus may be severely damaged by transplacentally acquired virus infection (e.g. rubella, cytomegalovirus) and that the neonate may suffer serious disease from viruses such as herpes simplex virus and enteroviruses, that are normally less severe in later life, raise the question of the competence of the developing immune system to cope with these infections. Viruses are obligate intracellular parasites and therefore cellular immune mechanisms, that control or block infection within cells or spread of virus between cells, are critical for effective host defence. Although this is a difficult area to study, it is possible, on the basis of observations from human medicine and cautious extrapolation from studies in animals, to review the development of the key elements of the immune system of relevance to the control of virus infections.

ANTIGEN PRESENTATION

Expression of MHC molecules (class I and class II) is present by 12 weeks of gestation[2,3] and, at that stage, all the major antigen-presenting cells (macrophages, Langerhans cells and dendritic cells) have differentiated. Expression of class II MHC molecules on these cells appears comparable to that of the adult[4,5].

THE FETAL THYMUS AND T-LYMPHOCYTE DEVELOPMENT

At seven weeks' gestation, before the stage of differentiation of thymic tissue, lymphoid cells with a prethymocyte phenotype (CD7+) are present in the yolk sac and liver[6]. At approximately 8.5 weeks' gestation, the developing thymus becomes colonized with CD7+ cells and expression of different T-cell lineages (CD2, CD4, CD8) becomes evident[6]. By 14 weeks, the organization of the fetal thymus (cortex, medulla and presence of Hassall's corpuscles) and the cellular localization of the major thymocyte subsets are similar to those of the postnatal thymus[7,8]. At this time, CD4 and CD8 cells are also present in the liver and spleen. The cellularity of the thymus increases markedly in the last trimester and this continues into postnatal life, until the age of 10 years, after which the gland atrophies. The number of T-lymphocytes in the fetal circulation increases during the second and third trimesters and continues to increase for about six months after birth[9–11]. The CD4:CD8 ratio is higher in the fetus (c.3.5) than the adult (c.2.0) and the adult ratio is normally reached by the age of four years[9,10]. Fetal and neonatal circulating T-lymphocytes differ from adult T-cells in that

they express the CD38 molecule, which is found on most thymocytes[12]. This suggests that they represent an immature cell population. They also express a surface phenotype similar to that of virgin adult T-cells (CD29^{lo}, CD45RA+CD45RO) which implies a limited degree of exposure to foreign antigens[13]. Neonatal T-cells proliferate less well than adult T-cells after activation by anti-CD2 or anti-CD3 antibodies[14,15], but this phenomenon, which is similar to that observed with adult virgin T-cells[16], probably reflects antigenic naivety rather than immaturity. On exposure to mitogens or allogeneic cells, neonatal T-cells proliferate as well as adult cells and they are able to synthesize IL-2 and express high-affinity IL-2 receptors[17–19]. The capacity of neonatal T-cells to produce other cytokines is variable. IL-3, IL-4, IL-5, interferon-γ and GM-CSF production is markedly deficient[20–22] while TNF-α production may be slightly impaired[23]. Here again, similar impairment of cytokine production is seen with virgin adult T-cells and this probably further reflects antigenic naivety. Neonatal T-cells activated and cultured *in vitro* acquire a memory cell phenotype and develop the capacity to produce cytokines such as IL-4 and interferon-γ to the same level as adult cells[20,24]. There is evidence, however, from *ex vivo* experiments that antigen-specific memory and interferon-γ production is markedly delayed in neonates, compared to adults, after primary herpes simplex infection[25].

Cytotoxic T-lymphocyte (CTL) activity by neonatal T-cells against allogeneic targets has been found to vary from 50% to 100% of adult activity[26,27]. Infants who had had vertically transmitted HIV infection were found to have reduced MHC-restricted CTL activity compared to those who had acquired the infection by blood transfusion in postnatal life[28]. The obvious drawback with these studies is the likely complicating effect of HIV itself and its potential for widespread effects on antigen-specific immunity.

Delayed-type hypersensitivity (DTH) may be assessed by skin-test reactivity. The fact that neonates fail to react to common antigens such as candida, tetanus toxoid and streptokinase-streptodornase[29] may be attributed to lack of prior sensitization. When presumed antigen-specific CD4+ T-cells, from sensitized adults, are transferred to neonates, children or adults, however, only neonates fail to respond on skin testing with the appropriate antigens[30]. This indicates that the neonate may be deficient in other components of the immune system necessary for DTH, e.g. monocyte chemotaxis. DTH anergy persists for approximately one year of postnatal life[31].

Specific cellular immunity, as indicated by lymphocyte proliferation or cytokine production, is usually not detectable at birth and for the first few months of life, in babies infected *in utero* with rubella[32] and cytomegalovirus[33–35]. As both viruses can infect lymphocytes and monocytes, this may indicate a direct immunosuppressive effect of the infections. As stated earlier, lymphocyte proliferation in neonates exposed to primary herpes simplex virus infection has been shown to be very delayed compared to that in adults[25]. This delay may contribute to the severity of neonatal herpes infection.

Thus, in summary, T-lymphocyte function in the fetus and neonate is impaired when compared to that of older children and adults. This impairment includes CTL activity, DTH and T-cell help for B-cell differentiation. In addition, there is evidence of selective impairment in the capacity to produce cytokines. The development of T-cell dependent antigen-specific responses after intrauterine and neonatal virus infections is markedly delayed.

B CELLS AND IMMUNOGLOBULIN PRODUCTION

The B-cell repertoire and the inherent capacity to produce antibodies to a wide range of antigens are limited in the fetus when compared to the adult. This repertoire increases during gestation[36]. At birth, the potential diversity for producing IgM and IgA is well developed but the capacity to produce IgG is impaired[37]. This is probably due to reduced production of cytokines, such as IL-4, which are responsible for IgM/IgG switching[38]. While cultured neonatal B-cells can differentiate into IgM-producing plasma cells as efficiently as adult cells, no IgG- or IgA producing plasma cells are detectable until the age of two years (IgG) or five years (IgA)[39].

There is evidence that production of antibodies by the fetus in response to specific antigens may be absent or delayed. Specific IgM antibody was undetectable in 34% of infants with congenital rubella[40] and 11% of infants with congenital CMV infection[41]. Neonatal immunization with live or inactivated poliovirus vaccine elicits a protective immune response[42] but other vaccines, such as influenza, have failed to induce levels of antibody comparable to those of older children and adults[43]. In one study of the use of hepatitis B vaccine in premature infants, responses were markedly reduced when compared to those of term infants[44].

Maternal IgG is transported across the placenta and provides protection for the fetus and the neonate against those infectious agents against which the mother has circulating antibodies. Circulating IgG can be detected from eight weeks of gestation and the level increases to reach approximately half the term concentration by 30 weeks' gestation. The neonatal IgG concentration is usually 105–110% of the maternal concentration[45]. Premature babies have correspondingly lower concentrations of maternally derived IgG. The other immunoglobulins, IgM, IgA, IgD and IgE, do not cross the placenta.

The amount of IgG synthesized by the infant equals that of maternal origin by about two months of age and by one year almost all the IgG has been synthesized by the child (762±209 ng/dl)[39]. The nadir for circulating IgG (400 mg/dl) occurs at 3–4 months of age.

The transfer of maternal IgG to the fetus may inhibit production of specific antibody if vaccine is given early in life[46]. For this reason, measles and rubella vaccine administration is delayed until after the first year of life.

Serum IgM at birth (c.11 mg/dl) is approximately 10% of the adult level[39]. In premature neonates born at <28 weeks' gestation, the mean level is 6 mg/dl[47]. However, some of this IgM may be in monomeric form and therefore non-functional. After birth, presumably in response to antigenic stimulation, IgM levels rise steeply and by one year are approximately 60% of adult levels[39]. Elevated IgM levels in cord blood samples may suggest intrauterine infection[48] but many infants with confirmed congenital infection have a normal level[41].

IgA is the major immunoglobulin produced on mucosal surfaces, where it is present as a dimer of two IgA molecules joined by a J segment. There are two subclasses of IgA: IgA1 comprises 90% of the immunoglobulin found in serum, while IgA2 makes up 60% of that present in secretions. At birth IgA1- and IgA2-bearing B-cells are present in equivalent numbers. As a result of exposure to antigenic stimuli, the IgA1-producing cells undergo preferential expansion and serum concentrations rise progressively through childhood and adolescence (20% adult level at one year)[39]. As with IgM, some, but not all, babies with intrauterine viral infection have an elevated IgA level in cord blood[48]. Secretory IgA is undetectable at birth but appears in tears, nasopharyngeal secretions and saliva after a few weeks; adult levels are achieved by 6–8 years of age[49,50]. Breast-feeding provides secretory IgA which may offer local gastrointestinal tract protection to the infant[51].

NATURAL KILLER CELLS

Natural killer cells (NK cells) are identified morphologically as large, granular lympho-cytes. They have the capacity to lyse target cells without MHC restriction and without the need for prior sensitization. Thus, they are likely to play an important role early in the course of viral infections. The cytotoxic activity of NK cells is mediated through binding of the cells to targets recognized as 'non-self' or by engagement of antigen–IgG complexes through the CD16 Fc receptor (antibody-dependent cellular cytotoxicity – ADCC). Their importance in the defence against viral infections has been demonstrated with herpes simplex virus[52,53] and cytomegalovirus infection[54] in mice and confirmed by reports of severe herpesvirus infections in patients with selective immunodeficiency syndromes[55]. NK cells are important producers of interferon-γ, TNF-α and GM-CSF in the early phases of the immune response[56]. Cytokine production is triggered by combination with the Fc receptor of IgG or by exposure to IL-2 or IL-12. Proliferation of NK cells is promoted by IL-2 and this is amplified by IL-12, IL-7 and interferon-γ[56].

NK cells can be identified by the expression of the CD16 and/or CD56 surface antigens and by the absence of the CD3 complex[57]. Most cells in the adult express CD57 and many express CD2. Cells expressing the CD16 phenotype make up a considerable percentage of mononuclear cells in the fetal liver and they are present from as early as six weeks of gestation[57]. At term, neonatal blood contains the same relative proportion (15% of total lymphocytes) as that found in the adult and the absolute number is twofold greater than that in adults[57,58]. There are, however, phenotypic differences between neonatal and adult NK cells. Both CD56 and CD57 expression is less, by 50% or more, in the neonatal cells compared with the adult and cytolytic activity appears to be impaired until at least the end of infancy (c.50% of adult activity at term)[57–59]. The cytolytic activity of NK cells is enhanced by IL-2 and interferons. In mice infected with herpes simplex virus, the development of resistance to the virus has been shown to be correlated with age-related maturation of NK cell function[53]. The NK cell cytotoxic activity of human cord blood mononuclear cells against herpes simplex virus in infected cells *in vitro* is markedly diminished, even after addition of IL-2. Antibody-dependent cellular cytotoxicity against herpes simplex virus-infected cells is also diminished, as is NK cell activity against cytomegalovirus-infected cells[69]. Thus, the immaturity of NK cells appears to correlate with reduced activity against herpesvirus-infected cells and this may be important in the pathogenesis of intrauterine or neonatal herpesvirus infections.

MONONUCLEAR PHAGOCYTES

In addition to their roles as antigen-presenting cells, monocytes and macrophages produce a range of cytokines including IL-1, IL-8, IL-6, IL-10, TNF-α, interferon-α and GM-CSF. In the fetus, macrophages are present in the yolk sac as early as four weeks' gestation and slightly later in the liver and bone marrow[61]. The concentration of monocytes in neonatal blood is at least equal to that of the adult[62]. Less is known about the presence of tissue macrophages in intrauterine life. The lung appears to contain very few macrophages until shortly before term[63]. In healthy monkeys, the number of alveolar macrophages increases to adult levels by 24–48 h after birth[64].

The migration of monocytes into sites of inflammation and immunological reaction is very delayed in infants compared to adults. Indeed, monocyte chemotaxis appears to be less active than that of adults until 6–10 years of age[65]. This deficiency may be responsible for the absent or reduced delayed-type hypersensitivity of neonates, described earlier.

COMPLEMENT

There is no significant transfer of complement components from the maternal circulation to the fetus. The fetus synthesizes complement components from as early as six weeks' gestation and, at term, most components are within the adult range apart from the terminal component (C9) which is important for lytic activity against Gram-negative bacteria[66,67]. Most components increase postnatally and reach adult values between the ages of six and 18 months, depending on the protein concerned[68].

SUMMARY

It is clear from the above account that immaturity and/or naivety of the non-specific and specific immune system produces problems for the fetus and the neonate in combating viral infections. In the early containment phase of infection the important mediators of resistance appear to be mononuclear phagocytes, NK cells and the production of interferons by these cells. Other cytokines such as TNF-α may impede viral replication. The important role of mononuclear phagocytes in controlling herpes simplex virus in mice is illustrated by studies using monocyte/macrophage-blocking agents, which enhance the virulence of the infection. NK cells are capable of lysing virus-infected cells and they are also important producers of cytokines, particularly interferon-γ and TNF-α, which augment other immune responses and impede viral replication.

The later phases of viral infection are antigen specific and are mediated by T- and B-cells. These specific responses are detectable approximately one week after infection and reach a peak at 2–3 weeks. The CD4+ subset of T-lymphocytes, acting through cell-to-cell interactions and lymphokine production, stimulates the amplification of antibody-producing B-lymphocytes and MHC class I-restricted cytotoxic CD8 lymphocytes. In animals and humans, herpesvirus infections are particularly severe and prolonged in those with combined T- and B-cell immunodeficiency.

Control of these viruses is not usually problematic in pure B-cell deficiency. It should be noted that this comment applies to most viral infections and, indeed, individuals with agammaglobulinaemia usually have few problems in controlling viral infections. A notable exception to this is enteroviral infection which is controlled predominantly by circulating neutralizing antibody production. Immaturity in neonatal B-cell responses probably accounts for the severe enteroviral infections occasionally encountered in neonates. Although the evidence points strongly towards the T-lymphocyte as the important cell in controlling herpesvirus infections (at any age), antibody may contribute, either by neutralizing extracellular virus or by enhancing the cytocidal effects of NK cells and phagocytes through ADCC. The apparent attenuation of the effects of intrauterine or neonatal viral infection by preexisting IgG in the mother may be an example of the contributory effect of antibody.

The major methods of control exerted by T-lymphocytes appear to be cytolysis of virus-infected cells and the production of cytokines.

MATERNAL AND OTHER ADULT CONSIDERATIONS IN OBSTETRICS AND GYNAECOLOGY

ALTERED IMMUNE STATUS

In the field of obstetrics and gynaecology immunocompetence may be affected by pregnancy, severe intercurrent illness and immunosuppressive therapy. The level of pathogenicity of viral infections will undoubtedly reflect changes in immunocompetence, some of which may have been mediated by pregnancy itself. Other sexually transmitted diseases which may have been acquired at the same time as a viral infection can modulate the immune response[69]. Women on immunosuppressive drugs after organ transplantation may become pregnant and may also be subject to genital tract viral infections (e.g. human papilloma virus – see Chapter 12)[70]. There may be a secondary increase in the risk

of malignancy. Cytotoxic chemotherapy is widely used in the treatment of gynaecological malignancy and the occurrence of herpes-zoster infection is a recognized complication (see Chapter 4)[71].

The concept that a woman is at greater risk from infections in pregnancy is widely held[72] but it is not securely 'evidence based'[73]. There are, however, inconsistencies which are not readily explained. In areas which are holoendemic for malaria, most of the indigenous population has developed immunity to malaria in childhood. This immunity tends to be lost in pregnancy, so much so that malaria-associated deaths are a very important cause of maternal mortality[74]. This altered susceptibility, however, does not seem to apply to typhoid fever, although a first attack in pregnancy, in common with some other bacterial infections, tends to be more severe.

Certain viral infections (e.g. hepatitis E and varicella) may be more severe in pregnancy, although other types of hepatitis may not be[75].

Viral warts of the vagina and vulva may grow during pregnancy in an exuberant and florid fashion, only to regress in the puerperium.

There is, at present, little evidence of enhanced progression of HIV infection in pregnancy, but data suggest an increased susceptibility to secondary infection[76].

IMMUNOCOMPETENCE IN PREGNANCY

Workers have studied the effect of pregnancy on general immunocompetence, principally hoping to solve the immunological puzzle posed by viviparity throughout the mammalian kingdom[77]. These studies have also collected data on the immunological basis for the essentially human disorder of pre-eclampsia and eclampsia. Although Weinberg[78] has claimed that there is a pregnancy-associated immunodeficiency syndrome, it is clear that this is a relative phenomenon which, on its own, will not account for the immunotolerance of viviparity. The uterus itself is not an 'immunologically privileged' site and the main mechanism for non-reactivity towards the fetus must lie in the placenta and, in particular, at its maternal interface with the uterine decidua. These considerations are not, however, specifically relevant to the viral infections which are the topic of this book. The placenta is not a barrier to the transmission of a viral infection and may itself be colonized by microorganisms (e.g. *Myobacterium tuberculosis* and protozoa including *Toxoplasma gondii* and plasmodium species)[79]. Immunoglobulin G can pass freely, conferring passive immunity in some situations (e.g. herpes simplex – see Chapter 7) whereas larger immunoglobulin molecules cannot pass readily. Free passage of IgG into the fetal circulation may account for some lowering of the maternal IgG levels of pregnancy in contrast to those of IgM and IgA which are sustained. The term immunological 'sink' has been coined for the trapping of maternal immunoglobulins by Fc receptors in the placenta.

There is hardly a system in the body whose physiology is not altered in pregnancy. This includes most of the endocrine organs, including the adrenal cortex. Historically, the tendency towards improvement in rheumatoid arthritis in pregnancy triggered the discovery of glucocorticoids. The metabolism of these and other antiinflammatory agents can be expected to modulate the host response to infection, but not necessarily to alter susceptibility[80]. In pregnancy a large number of pregnancy-associated plasma proteins are also produced, some of which may be expected to act in an immunomodulatory manner[81]. Smaller proteins classed as cytokines and growth factors are legion and are secreted by all cell types, particularly by T-cells and macrophages. In tissues they are associated with an equally widespread system of receptors; the latter are a complex of a private ligand-specific receptor with a public 'class-specific' signal transducer. Virtually all maternal and fetal tissues can secrete cytokines and contain cytokine receptors. Cytokines may therefore be involved in many aspects of the physiology and pathophysiology of pregnancy, but there is no general change in the tissue or circulating levels of cytokines during human pregnancy. Local changes in levels, especially in tissues, are associated with the processes of implantation and of labour and may have a secondary effect on the acquisition of infections in the genital tract.

During normal labour commencing at term and in preterm labour, there is an increase in most cytokines in amniotic fluid and in the surrounding membranes[81]. It is believed that these changes are secondary to other events, including uterine contractions, and are not a primary factor in the initiation of normal labour. However, the cytokines may play a significant role in increasing and maintaining established uterine activity. As many cases of preterm labour are believed to be due to infection, in this situation it has been suggested that the release of inflammatory cytokines could be the proximate event which leads to premature uterine contractions. Microorganisms of relatively low pathogenicity have been found in association with chorioamnionitis and this includes some nonspecific viral infections, which have also been implicated in intrauterine fetal growth retardation[82].

CELL-MEDIATED IMMUNITY

Data on changes in cell-mediated immunity are conflicting[83], but where evidence of diminished response in pregnancy has been reported, this is of a minor degree.

Although '*in vitro*' studies have been carried out using lymphocyte blastogenesis assays, more precision has been introduced by the ability to study T-cell subsets in maternal peripheral blood samples. As with many other tests in pregnancy, the effect of haemodilution has to be taken into consideration[84].

LOCAL IMMUNE RESPONSES

The status of the lower genital tract, in particular the cervix, is of particular interest in infection. The vagina is lined by stratified squamous epithelium interspersed with some dendritic cells which may be the vehicle for the passage of viral infections, e.g. HIV (see Chapters 8, 9, 11) and CMV (see Chapter 3).

The condition of the cervix and the transformation zone (squamocolumnar junction) is particularly important. Introduction of antigens will produce a response which is largely of IgA. An inflammatory cell infiltrate is commonly found in this area of the cervix[85]. The epithelium of the transformation zone is itself unstable and the native glandular epithelium undergoes squamous metaplasia after exposure to the antigenic stimulus of semen and this is subsequently enhanced by the first pregnancy[86]. At such times there is increased susceptibility in this area to viral infection, particularly with the human papillomavirus, which has long-term implications for the risk of developing cervical carcinoma (see Chapter 12).

CONSIDERATIONS FOR OBSTETRICIANS AND GYNAECOLOGISTS

Viral genital infections with overt lesions

- *Herpes simplex*. Acute vulvitis with severe pain sometimes provoking acute retention of urine is characteristic of a primary infection (see Chapter 7). The differential diagnosis includes Behçet's disease.
- *Human papillomavirus*. Condylomata acuminata need to be distinguished from the condylomata lata due to *Treponema pallidum*. Malignant transformation can rarely occur and the condition of verrucous carcinoma needs to be distinguished; it may well have a viral aetiology. Non-condylomatous lesions on the cervix may be detected by colposcopy. These have an important relationship with cervical intra-

epithelial neoplasia and with the development of squamous cell carcinoma, principally of the cervix, but actually anywhere in the lower genital tract and even in the anal canal.
- *Herpes-zoster* (varicella) can affect dermatomes at any site in the body and can therefore encroach on the external genitalia.
- *Epstein–Barr virus*. Although not primarily a genital infection, Burkitt's lymphoma can present with ovarian tumours.

Any of the first three viral infections above can be a complication of immunosuppression, particularly iatrogenic.

Asymptomatic genital infection; bloodborne viruses

In such cases there is likely to be no demonstrable lesion within the lower genital tract. In this context the most important viruses are human immunodeficiency virus (HIV) and the hepatitis viruses B and C, which are transmissible in blood and blood-stained body fluids[87].

The risks of nosocomial transmission of these three viruses necessitate a high level of universal clinical precautions when handling body fluids, especially when blood-stained (see Chapter 11). Full personal protection is strongly recommended and should be mandatory when carrying out tasks with a high risk of unexpected and uncontrolled dissemination of blood or blood-stained fluid. *This should include eye and face protection* and avoidance of secondary contamination of distal clothing and footwear when blood is spilled at, or on, floor level[88].

These situations occur so commonly in both obstetric and gynaecological practice that their significance and the need for adequate precautions are commonly overlooked. Operations and procedures in the lithotomy position are especially risky as the operator's face is at the same level as the manoeuvres.

Blood and/or amniotic fluid splashing on the face is a common event, as inspection of spectacles or mask will frequently demonstrate. Furthermore, blood is commonly shed on to the lap and lower drapes with an obvious risk of contamination of the operator's lower garments below any apron, if protective footwear is not worn.

Precisely the same considerations apply to obstetric procedures and delivery as to gynaecological perineal surgery. This is the case for any delivery, operative or spontaneous, in the dorsal, left lateral or lithotomy positions, especially if the membranes have not previously ruptured and if episiotomy is performed. Delivery and handling of the placenta is such a commonplace event that its risky nature is frequently overlooked and one of the manoeuvres most associated with a risk of needlestick is the attempted aspiration of cord blood from the umbilical vessels. Manual removal of the placenta and, indeed, caesarean section cause significant contamination of the operator's forearms if impervious gowns and/or elbow-length gloves are not provided [89].

There is historical reluctance on the part of managers to supply the wherewithal for midwives and obstetricians to use universal precautions or even to appreciate their significance. This is particularly to be regretted because the obstetric attachment is probably the first in which all medical students get exposed to blood and body fluid dissemination and the need to demonstrate and adhere to safe clinical practice at such a time cannot be too strongly emphasized.

Asymptomatic and subclinical viral infections in pregnancy

In the present state of knowledge, antenatal screening for a number of viral infections should be strongly recommended in both the maternal and the fetal interest. Obstetricians and midwives should be aware of interventions which are now available in positive cases to reduce the risk of vertical transmission (mother to fetus) [90] and of neonatal prophylaxis such as vaccination and/or use of immunoglobulin.

Obstetricians should also be aware of the risks of neonatal infection being transferred in breast milk. They should, however, be prepared and able to offer counselling on an individual basis, as in certain situations and environments avoidance of breastfeeding may be contraindicated.

Acute systemic maternal viral infections

The importance of such infections, and indeed the need to include them in the differential diagnosis whenever the history is not typical, must be emphasized. The use of antiviral chemotherapy may warrant consideration. Furthermore, invasive measures (such as amniocentesis) to detect fetal infection may be justified, as may specialized tests in consultation with a virologist.

Obstetricians also need to be alert, with a high index of suspicion, to the significance of apparently trivial febrile episodes. Maternal infection with rubella, parvovirus and herpes simplex virus may be of little maternal importance but may have a very considerable impact on the fetus or newborn.

CONCLUSION

In the early part of the 20th century bacterial infection was probably the greatest cause of maternal morbidity and mortality. In the second half of the century viruses have usurped this position. It therefore behoves all who work in maternity care and in gynaecology to be aware of the range of viral infections and to understand the principles of spread and of safe practice and especially of the hazards both to mother and to her infant before, during and after birth. There is no place for complacency.

ACKNOWLEDGEMENTS

The authors wish to acknowledge valuable contributions to this chapter by Professor T. Chard and Professor Vikhlyaeva.

REFERENCES

1. World Health Organization (1992) Global Programme on AIDS. Consensus statement from the WHO/UNICEF consultation on HIV transmission and breast feeding. *Wkly Epidemiol. Rec.*, **67**, 177–179.
2. Hofman, F.M., Danilovs, J.A. and Taylor, C.R. (1984) HLA-DR (Ia)-positive dendritic-like cells in human fetal nonlymphoid tissues. *Transplantation*, **27**, 590–594.
3. Oliver, A.M., Sewell, H.F., Abramovich, D.R. and Thomson, A.W. (1989) The distribution and differential expression of MHC class II antigens (HLA-DR, DP and DQ) in human fetal adrenal, pancreas, thyroid and gut. *Transplant. Proc.*, **21**, 651–652.
4. Foster, C.A. and Holbrook, K.A. (1989) Ontogeny of Langerhans cells in human embryonic and fetal skin: cell densities and phenotypic expression relative to epidermal growth. *Am. J. Anat.*, **184**, 157–164.
5. Harvey, J., Jones D.B. and Wright, D.H. (1990) Differential expression of MHC- and macrophage-associated antigens in human fetal and postnatal small intestine. *Immunology*, **69**, 409–415.
6. Haynes, B.F., Martin M.E., Kay, H.H. and Kurtzberg, J. (1988) Early events in human T cell ontogeny. Phenotypic characterization and immunohistologic localization of T cell precursors in early human fetal tissues. *J. Exp. Med.*, **168**, 1061–1080.
7. Horst, E., Meijer, C.J.L.M., Duijvestijn, A.M. *et al.* (1990) The ontogeny of human lymphocyte recirculation: high endothelial cell antigen (HECA-452) and CD44 homing receptor expression in the development of the immune system. *Eur. J. Immunol.*, **20**, 1483–1489.
8. Gilhus, N.E., Matre, R. and Tonder, O. (1985) Hassall's corpuscles in the thymus of fetuses, infants and children: immunological and histochemical aspects. *Thymus*, **7**, 123–135.
9. Hohlfeld, P., Forestier F., Marion, S. *et al.* (1990) *Toxoplasma gondii* infection during pregnancy: T lymphocyte subpopulations in mothers and fetuses. *Pediatr. Infect. Dis.*, **9**, 878–881.
10. The European Collaborative Study (1992) Age-related standards for T lymphocyte subsets based on uninfected children born to human immunodeficiency virus 1-infected women. *Pediatr. Infect. Dis.*, **11**, 1018–1026.
11. Erkeller-Yeksel, F.M., Deneys V., Yuksel, B. *et al.* (1992) Age-related changes in human blood lymphocyte subpopulations. *J. Pediatr.*, **112**, 216–222.
12. Wilson, M. (1985) Immunology of the fetus and newborn: lymphocyte phenotype and function. *Clin. Immunol. Allergy*, **5**, 271–286.
13. Gerli, R., Rambotti P., Cernetti, C. *et al.* (1984) A mature thymocyte-like phenotypic pattern on human cord circulating T-lymphoid cells. *J. Clin. Immunol.*, **4**, 461–468.
14. Gerli, R., Bertotto, A., Crupi, S. *et al.* (1989) Activation of cord T lymphocytes. I. Evidence for a defective T cell mitogenesis induced through the CD2 molecule. *J. Immunol.*, **142**, 2583–2589.
15. Pirenne, H., Aujard, Y., Eljaafari, A. *et al.* (1992) Comparison of T cell functional changes during childhood with the ontogeny of CDw29 and CD45RA expression on CD4+ T cells. *Pediatr. Res.*, **32**, 81–86.
16. Byrne, J.A., Butler, J.L. and Cooper, M.D. (1988) Differential activation requirements for virgin and memory T cells. *J. Immunol.*, **141**, 3249–3257.
17. Olding, L.B., Murgita, R.A. and Wigzell, H. (1977) Mitogen-stimulated lymphoid cells from human newborns suppress the proliferation of maternal lymphocytes across a cell-impermeable membrane. *J. Immunol.*, **119**, 1109–1114.
18. Hayward, A.R. and Kurnick, J. (1981) Newborn T cell suppression: early appearance, maintenance in culture, and lack of growth factor suppression. *J. Immunol.*, **126**, 50–53.
19. Wilson, C.B., Westall, J., Johnstone, L *et al.* (1986) Decreased production of interferon-gamma by human neonatal cells. *J. Clin. Invest.*, **77**, 860–867.
20. Ehlers, S. and Smith, K.A. (1991) Differentiation of T cell lymphokine gene expression. The in vitro acquisition of T cell memory. *J. Exp. Med.*, **173**, 25–36.
21. Lewis, D.B., Yu C.C., Meyer, J. *et al.* (1991) Cellular and molecular mechanisms for reduced interleukin 4 and interferon-γ production by neonatal T cells. *J. Clin. Invest.*, **87**, 194–202.

22. English, B.K., Hammond, W.P., Lewis, D.B. *et al.* (1992) Decreased granulocyte-macrophage colony-stimulating factor production by human neonatal blood mononuclear cells and T cells. *Pediatr. Res.*, **31**, 211–216.

23. English, B.K., Burchett, S.K., English, J.D. *et al.* (1988) Production of lymphotoxin and tumour necrosis factor by human neonatal mononuclear cells. *Pediatr. Res.*, **24**, 717–722.

24. Sanders, M.E., Makgoba, M.W., June, C.H. *et al.* (1989) Enhanced responsiveness of human memory T cells to CD2 and CD3 receptor-mediated activation. *Eur. J. Immunol.*, **19**, 803–808.

25. Burchett, S.K., Corey, L., Mohan, K.M. *et al.* (1992) Diminished interferon-γ and lymphocyte proliferation in neonatal and postpartum primary herpes simplex virus infection. *J. Infect. Dis.*, **165**, 813–818.

26. Granberg, C., Hirvonen, T. and Toivanen, P. (1979) Cell-mediated lympholysis by human maternal and neonatal lymphocytes: mother's reactivity against neonatal cells and vice versa. *J. Immunol.*, **123**, 2563–2567.

27. Rayfield, L.S., Brent, L. and Rodeck, C.H. (1980) Development of cell-mediated lympholysis in human fetal blood lymphocytes. *Clin. Exp. Immunol.*, **42**, 561–570.

28. Luzuriaga, K., Koup, R.A., Pikora, C.A. *et al.* (1991) Deficient human immunodeficiency virus type 1-specific cytotoxic T cell responses in vertically infected children. *J. Pediatr.*, **119**, 230–236.

29. Munoz, A.I. and Limbert, D. (1977) Skin reactivity to Candida and streptokinase-streptodornase antigens in normal paediatric subjects: influence of age and acute illness. *J. Pediatr.*, **91**, 565–568.

30. Warwick, W.J., Good, R.A. and Smith, R.T. (1960) Failure of passive transfer of delayed hypersensitivity in the newborn human infant. *J. Lab. Clin. Med.*, **56**, 139–147.

31. Kniker, W.T., Lesourd, B.M., McBryde, J.L. *et al.* (1985) Cell-mediated immunity assessed by multitest CMI skin testing in infants and preschool children. *Am. J. Dis. Child.*, **139**, 840–845.

32. Buimovici-Klein, E., Lang, P.B., Ziring, P.R. *et al.* (1979) Impaired cell-mediated immune responses in patients with congenital rubella: correlation with gestational age at time of infection. *Pediatrics*, **64**, 620–626.

33. Gehrz, R.C., Knorr, S.O., Marker, S.C. *et al.* (1977) Specific cell-mediated immune defect in active cytomegalovirus infection of young children and their mothers. *Lancet*, **2**, 844–847.

34. Reynolds, D.W., Dean, P.H., Pass, R.F. *et al.* (1979) Specific cell-mediated immunity in children with congenital and neonatal cytomegalovirus infection and their mothers. *J. Infect. Dis.*, **140**, 493–499.

35. Starr, S.E., Tolpin, M.D., Friedman, H.M. *et al.* (1979) Impaired cellular immunity to cytomegalovirus in congenitally infected children and their mothers. *J. Infect. Dis.*, **140**, 500–505.

36. Cuisinier, A.M., Fumoux, F., Moinier, D. *et al.* (1990) Rapid expansion of human immunoglobulin repertoire (V_H V_K V_λ) expressed in early fetal bone marrow. *New Biol.*, **2**, 689–699.

37. Mortari, F., Wang, J-Y. and Schroeder, H.W. (1993) Human cord blood antibody repertoire. Mixed population of V_H gene segments and CDR3 distribution in the expressed Cα and Cγ repertoires. *J. Immunol.*, **150**, 1348–1357.

38. Lewis, D.B., Yu C.C., Meyer, J. *et al.* (1991) Cellular and molecular mechanisms for reduced interleukin 4 and interferon-γ production by neonatal T cells. *J. Clin. Invest.*, **87**, 194–202.

39. Stiehm, E.R. and Fudenberg, H.H. (1966) Serum levels of immune globulins in health and disease: a survey. *Pediatrics*, **37**, 715–727.

40. Enders, G. (1985) Serologic test combinations for safe detection of rubella infections. *Rev. Infect. Dis.*, **7**, 5113–5122.

41. Griffiths, P.D., Stagno, S., Pass, R.F. *et al.* (1982) Congenital cytomegalovirus infection: diagnostic and prognostic significance of the detection of specific immunoglobulin M antibodies in cord serum. *Pediatrics*, **69**, 544–550.

42. Smolen, P., Bland, R., Heiligenstein, E. *et al.* (1983) Antibody response to oral polio vaccine in premature infants. *J. Pediatr.*, **103**, 917–920.

43. Yarchoan, R. and Nelson, D.L. (1983) A study of the functional capabilities of human neonatal lymphocytes for in vitro specific antibody production. *J. Immunol.*, **131**, 1222–1228.

44. Lau, Y-L., Tam, A.Y.C. and Ng K.W. (1992) Clinical and laboratory observations. Response of preterm infants to hepatitis B vaccine. *J. Pediatr.*, **121**, 962–965.

45. Kohler, P.F. and Farr, R.S. (1966) Elevation of cord over maternal IgG immunoglobulin – evidence for an active placental IgG transport. *Nature*, **210**, 1070–1071.

46. Sato, H., Albrecht, P., Reynolds, D.W. *et al.* (1979) Transfer of measles, mumps, rubella antibodies from mother to infant. *Am. J. Dis. Child.*, **133**, 1240–1243.

47. Cederqvist, L.L., Dwool, L.C. and Litwin, S.D. (1978) The effect of fetal age, birth weight and sex on cord blood immunoglobulin levels. *Am. J. Obstet. Gynecol.*, **131**, 520–525.

48. Alford, C.A., Stagno, S. and Reynolds, D.W. (1975) Diagnosis of chronic perinatal infections. *Am. J. Dis. Child.*, **129**, 455–463.

49. McKay, E. and Thom, H. (1969) Observations on neonatal tears. *J. Pediatr.*, **75**, 1245–1246.

50. Haworth, J.C. and Dilling, L. (1966) Concentration of gamma A-globulin in serum, saliva and nasopharyngeal secretions of infants and children. *J. Lab. Clin. Med.*, **67**, 922–933.

51. Yap, P.L., Pryde, A., Latham, A.J. *et al.* (1979) Serum IgA in the neonate. *Acta. Paediatr. Scand.*, **68**, 695–700.

52. Kohl, S. (1985) Herpes simplex virus immunology: problems, progress and promises. *J. Infect. Dis.*, **152**, 435–440.

53. Kohl, S. (1989) The neonatal human's immune response to herpes simplex virus infection: a critical review. *Pediatr. Infect. Dis.*, **8**, 67–74.

54. Scalzo, A.A., Fitzgerald, N.A., Wallace, C.R. *et al.* (1992) The effect of CMV-1 resistance gene, which is linked to the natural killer cell gene complex, is mediated by natural killer cells. *J. Immunol.*, **149**, 581–589.

55. Biron, C.A., Byron, K.S. and Sullivan, J.L. (1989) Severe herpesvirus infections in an adolescent without natural killer cells. *N. Engl. J. Med.*, **320**, 1731–1735.

56. Perussia, B. (1991) Lymphokine-activated killer cells, natural killer cells and cytokines. *Curr. Opin. Immunol.*, **3**, 49–55.

57. Phillips, J.H., Hori, T., Nagler, A. *et al.* (1992) Ontogeny of human natural killer (NK) cells: fetal NK cells mediate cytolytic function and express $CD3_E$ δ proteins. *J. Exp. Med.*, **175**, 1055–1066.

58. Sancho, L., de la Hera, A., Casas J. *et al.* (1991) Two different maturational stages of natural killer lymphocytes in human newborn infants. *J. Pediatr.*, **119**, 446–454.

59. Kaplan, J., Shope, T.C., Bollinger, R.O. *et al.* (1982) Human newborns are deficient in natural killer cell activity. *J. Clin. Immunol.*, **2**, 350–355.

60. Harrison, C.J. and Wander, J.L. (1985) Natural killer cell activity in infants and children excreting cytomegalovirus. *J. Infect. Dis.*, **151**, 301–307.

61. Kelemen, E. and Janossa, M. (1980) Macrophages are the first differentiated blood cells formed in human embryonic liver. *Exp. Haematol.*, **8**, 996–1000.

62. Ueno, Y., Koizumi, S., Yamagami, M. *et al.* (1981) Characterisation of hemopoietic stem cells (CFUc) in cord blood. *Exp. Haematol.*, **9**, 716–722.

63. Alenghat, E. and Esterly, J.R. (1984) Alveolar macrophages in perinatal infants. *Pediatrics*, **74**, 221–224.

64. Jacobs, R.F., Wilson, C.B., Smith, A.L. *et al.* (1983) Age-dependent effects of aminobutyryl muramyl dipeptide on alveolar macrophage function in infant and adult macaca monkeys. *Am. Rev. Respir. Dis.*, **128**, 862–867.

65. Klein, R.B., Fischer, T.J., Gard, S.E. *et al.* (1977) Decreased mononuclear and polymorphonuclear chemotaxis in human newborns, infants and young children. *Pediatrics*, **60**, 467–472.

66. Kohler, P.F. (1973) Maturation of the human complement system. I. Onset time and sites of fetal C19, C4, C3 and C5 synthesis. *J. Clin. Invest.*, **52**, 671–678.

67. Lassiter, H.A., Watson, S.W., Seifring, M.L. and Tanner, J.E. (1992) Complement factor 9 deficiency in serum of human neonates. *J. Infect. Dis.*, **166**, 53–57.

68. Davis, C.A., Vallota, E.H. and Forristal, J. (1979) Serum complement levels in infancy: age related changes. *Pediatr. Res.*, **13**, 1043–1046.

69. Laga, M., Manoka, A., Kwuvu, M. *et al.* (1993) Non ulcerative sexually transmitted diseases as risk factors for HIV 1 transmission in women. *AIDS*, **7**, 95–102.

70. Heybourne, V. and Silver, R.M. Immunology of post implantation pregnancy. In *Reproductive Immunology*, (eds R.A. Bronson, N.J. Alexander, D.J. Anderson *et al.*), Blackwell, Oxford, pp. 399–417.

71. Hudson, C.N. (1979) A review of immunological aspects of gynaecological malignancy. *Br. J. Obstet. Gynaecol.*, **86**, 154–158.

72. Brabin, B.J. (1985) Epidemiology of infection in pregnancy. *Rev. Infect. Dis.*, **6**, 814–831.

73. Stirrat, G.M. and Scott, J.R. (1992) *Reproductive Immunopathology.* Clinical Obstetrics and Gynaecology. Baillière, London, pp. 2147.

74. Bruce-Chwatt, L.J. (1983) Malaria and pregnancy. *Br. Med. J.*, **286**, 1457–1458.

75. Floreani, A., Paternoster, D., Zappala, F. *et al.* (1996) Hepatitis C virus infection in pregnancy. *Br. J. Obstet. Gynaecol.*, **103**, 325–329.

76. Semprini, A.E., Cartanga, C., Ravizza, A. *et al.* (1995) The incidence of complications after Caesarean section in 156 HIV positive women. *AIDS*, **9**, 913–917.

77. Stirrat, G.M. (1994) Pregnancy and immunity (editorial). *Br. Med. J.*, **308**, 1385–1386.

78. Weinberg, E.D. (1984) Pregnancy-associated depression of cell-mediated immunity. *Rev. Infect. Dis.*, **6**, 814–831.

79. Hart, C.A. (1988) Pregnancy and host resistance. *Clin. Immunol. Allergy*, **2**, 735–757.

80. Chard, T. and Grudzinskas, J.G. (1992) Placental proteins and steroids and the immune relationship between mother and fetus. In *Immunological Obstetrics*, (eds C.B. Coulam, W.P. Faulk and J.A. McIntyre), Norton, New York, pp. 282–289.

81. Greig, P.C., Herbert, W.N., Robinelte, B.L. *et al.* (1995) Amniotic fluid interleukin concentrations through pregnancy in term and pre-term labour. *Am. J. Obstet. Gynecol.*, **173**, 1223–1227.

82. Vikhlyaeva, E., Barashneu, J. and Paukov, S. (1993) Viral infections in the severe IUGR syndrome. Third World Congress for Infectious Diseases in Obstetrics and Gynaecology, p. 71.

83. Alanen, A. and Lassila, O. (1982) Cell mediated immunity in normal pregnancy and pre-eclampsia. *J. Reprod. Immunol.*, **4**, 349–354.

84. Johnstone, F.D., Thong, K.J., Bird, A.G. *et al.* (1994) Lymphocyte sub-populations in early human pregnancy. *Obstet. Gynecol.*, **83**, 941–946.

85. Edwards, N.T. and Morris, H.B. (1985) Langerhans cells and lymphocyte subsets in the female genital tract. *Br. J. Obstet. Gynecol.*, **92**, 974–982.

86. Reid, B.L. (1992) Carcinogenesis. In *Gynecologic Oncology*, (ed M. Coppleson), Churchill Livingstone, Edinburgh, pp. 71–105.

87. Department of Health, Advisory Committee on Dangerous Pathogens (1995) *Protection against Bloodborne Infection in the Work place. HIV and Hepatitis*, HMSO, London.

88. Department of Health (1997) *Guidance For Clinical Health Care Workers. Protection against Infection with HIV and Hepatitis Virus.* HMSO, London.

89. Royal College of Obstetricians and Gynaecologists (1997) *HIV Infection in Maternity Care and Gynaecology*, 3rd edn. RCOG, London.

90. Royal College of Paediatrics and Child Health (1998) *Prevention of Vertical Transmission. Report of an Inter-collegiate Working Party.* RCPCH.

P. Morgan-Capner

INTRODUCTION

Rubella (German measles) was identified as a distinct illness in the mid-18th century by German physicians and during the earlier part of the 20th century a range of complications was identified. These included arthralgia, purpura and postinfectious encephalomyelitis, but rubella was still considered an essentially benign illness, particularly in childhood, with full recovery assured. Such perceptions changed in 1941 with the sentinel observations of Sir Norman Gregg, an Australian ophthalmologist[1,2]. In spring/summer 1940 a major epidemic of rubella occurred in Australia. The following year Gregg noted an unusually high prevalence of congenital cataracts in Sydney (Plate A). Despite his interest in this 'epidemic', the breakthrough did not come until two mothers made the association in his waiting room, in that both had had rubella in early pregnancy[3]. The association was confirmed when of 71 infants with cataract born in Australia in the first half of 1941, 68 mothers admitted rubella in the first trimester. Congenital heart disease and intra-uterine growth retardation were also noted and so became established the disastrous consequences for the fetus of maternal rubella in early pregnancy.

The following years saw this observation confirmed around the world and the range of congenital abnormalities widened to include almost every organ and system. Thus rubella was recognized as a microbial agent which can cross the placenta from the infected mother to the fetus. A number of other agents including human immunodeficiency virus, cytomegalovirus, *Toxoplasma gondii*, parvovirus B19 and varicella-zoster virus are now known to infect the fetus transplacentally.

It was not until 1961 that the rubella virus was successfully cultured[4,5]. This immediately preceded the worldwide 1962–4 epidemic, when it has been estimated that more than 20 000 cases of congenital rubella occurred in the USA alone. The availability of virus isolation together with such a large number of cases enabled an extended spectrum of neonatal and childhood consequences to be identified and it was demonstrated that babies with congenital rubella were persistently infected with the virus.

The isolation of the virus led to strenuous efforts to develop vaccines and this was accomplished by 1969 when the first live attenuated vaccines were licensed[6]. Rubella vaccine was the essential tool required to control congenital rubella and its widespread use in many countries has had a dramatic effect on the incidence of rubella in pregnancy. It is a remarkably safe vaccine with high efficacy but in the last 25 years concerns have been not so much about the vaccine itself, but how to ensure adequate protection for both

Viral Infections in Obstetrics and Gynaecology. Edited by D.J. Jeffries and C.N. Hudson. Published in 1999 by Arnold, ISBN 0 340 74095 7.

the individual and community by vaccine delivery programmes.

VIRUS

Rubella virus is enveloped so it does not persist in the environment and is inactivated by many chemical agents. It is a single-stranded RNA virus with three major virion polypeptides; C, E1 and E2. No major antigenic variation has been seen and this is not an explanation for reinfections (see below).

POSTNATAL RUBELLA

The characteristic feature of rubella is the widespread maculopapular rash (Plate B). Approximately 50% of children infected with rubella are asymptomatic. With increasing age the proportion with subclinical infection falls, so that by adulthood totally asymptomatic rubella is remarkably uncommon in the experience of most investigators. Subclinical infection, however, still makes an important contribution to the incidence of congenital rubella, as serological investigation may not be performed, infection not identified and termination of pregnancy not offered. Although the rash of symptomatic rubella may be obvious in those of Caucasian origin or with a light skin, it may not be so apparent in those with darker skin.

The incubation period from contact to the development of the rash is some 14–21 days (usually 15–17 days). The pinkish-red maculopapular rash usually starts on the face and neck, but rapidly spreads over the body and limbs. Individual spots may coalesce, but the rash usually clears after 3–4 days, with itching being uncommon. The rash may be preceded and accompanied by non-specific symptoms such as malaise, fever, upper respiratory tract symptoms and even conjunctivitis which rarely may be as severe as that seen in measles. Lymphadenopathy commonly occurs, with suboccipital nodes being those most frequently involved. Rubella in children is usually far milder than in adults and although usually considered a mild disease, recent experience with young adult males in university outbreaks has shown that a significant proportion (estimated at 5–10%) suffer a severe illness necessitating exclusion from studies for two weeks or more.

Rubella in children is rarely complicated but in adults, 30% or more suffer arthralgia and this is particularly common in females. The most frequently involved joints are those of the hands and wrists, with resolution usually occurring within a month, but occasionally persisting for much longer, possibly years[7]. Postinfectious encephalitis[8] and thrombocytopenia are rare, probably occurring in fewer than one in 5–10 000 cases. A fatal outcome is virtually unknown. Even in immunocompromised patients rubella seems to carry no additional complications although the serological response may be abnormal[9]. Rubella is not associated with recurrent abortion, although it may be occasionally associated with spontaneous abortion after primary infection (see below).

The clinical diagnosis of rubella has proved notoriously unreliable, with experienced clinicians only being 50% correct even during an epidemic. A wide range of other infectious agents, and indeed non-infectious causes such as allergy, can present with an essentially identical rubelliform illness. Such infections include measles, enteroviruses such as echoviruses, parvovirus B19 and probably the more recently described human herpesviruses (HHV) such as HHV6 (the causative virus of exanthem subitum) and HHV7. Infection with parvovirus B19 is a particular problem as it is associated not only with a rubelliform rash but also with arthralgia and clinical distinction from rubella is impossible[10]. Parvovirus B19 infection in adults is rarely accompanied by the malar erythema seen in erythema infectiosum (Fifth disease) of children[11]. As some 50% of adult women are susceptible to parvovirus B19, it is likely that adult infection with B19 is more common than rubella in countries where rubella has been largely controlled by extensive use of rubella vaccine. Although parvovirus B19 can cross the placenta and infect the fetus, the outcome for the fetus is markedly different from that seen after intrauterine rubella (see Chapter 6).

Experience has shown, however, that in the majority of rash illnesses in pregnancy, no cause can be identified. One concern is that as rubella becomes controlled by vaccination programmes and becomes a rare illness in the community, physicians may no longer think of the possibility when presented with a patient with a rash illness. A personal experience has been that rubella was not considered as the cause of an outbreak of rash illness in university students until a month after its onset, as the rash was thought to be a reaction to plasticizers in the water after a new water tank was installed!

CONGENITAL RUBELLA

Primary rubella (i.e. the first infection with rubella virus; reinfections will be considered later) in the first 16 weeks of pregnancy constitutes a major risk to the fetus. The consequences for the pregnancy and the fetus may be sufficiently severe to result in abortion or stillbirth. If the pregnancy continues to term a wide range of abnormalities may be seen (Table 2.1), some of which may be apparent at birth while others may take many years to manifest. The classic congenital rubella triad comprises cardiac, ophthalmic and auditory lesions, but neurological problems, purpura and intrauterine growth retardation are also frequent. Cardiac abnormalities include patent ductus arteriosus and pulmonary artery stenosis; ophthalmic manifestations include cataract (bilateral or unilateral) (Plate A), glaucoma (Plate C), microphthalmia and choroidoretinitis, and sensorineural deafness is a common manifestation. Some of these abnormalities are surgically correctable, but many are not. There are usually severe

Table 2.1 Features of congenital rubella

Ocular defects
   Cataracts (uni-/bilateral)
   Pigmentary retinopathy
   Microphthalmia
   Glaucoma
   Iris hypoplasia
Auditory defects
   Sensorineural deafness (uni-/bilateral)
Cardiovascular defects
   Persistent ductus arteriosus
   Pulmonary artery stenosis
   Myocarditis
Central nervous system
   Microcephaly
   Psychomotor retardation
   Meningoencephalitis
   Behavioural disorders
   Speech disorders
Intrauterine growth retardation
Thrombocytopenia, with purpura
Hepatitis/hepatosplenomegaly
Bone 'lesions'
Pneumonitis
Lymphadenopathy
Diabetes mellitus
Thyroid disorders
Progressive rubella panencephalitis

consequences for neurological functions, with mental handicap being common.

In a review of 763 children reported to the UK National Congenital Rubella Surveillance Programme between 1971 and 1984, 47% of the mothers gave a history of a rash illness and 15% had a history of contact[12]. Some of the mothers may not have recalled their illness, but the figures demonstrate that although asymptomatic rubella in adults is uncommon, it can contribute significantly to the incidence of congenital rubella. This is likely to be accentuated by the fact that many women with diagnosed rubella in early pregnancy have a termination[13]. Of the babies in whom the birthweight was known, 54% fell below the 10th percentile. Defects were present in 618 of the children and of these, 47% were multiple and 53% single[12].

At birth, but usually resolving over a short period, there may be thrombocytopenia with a purpuric rash. Hepatosplenomegaly is commonly found. Radiological translucencies may be apparent in the metaphyses of the long bones.

The child is persistently infected and a range of problems may become apparent. A pneumonitis, which may be fatal and is thought to be due to the immune response to the infection, may develop later in the first year of life. Persistence of the virus may also be responsible for a worsening of the deafness. At a few years of age progressive rubella panencephalitis may develop, an illness comparable to the subacute sclerosing panencephalitis seen with persistent measles infection. Later in life, usually the third decade, diabetes mellitus develops in approximately 20% of individuals and growth hormone deficiency can occur during infancy.

Rubella virus, having crossed the placenta and infected the fetus, probably exerts its effects by a number of mechanisms, although the balance of significance between these has not been established. It is known from *in vitro* studies that cell lines infected with rubella virus show inhibition of cell mitosis – a tempting explanation for intrauterine growth retardation[14]. This may also lead to disordered differentiation during organogenesis, with another likely contributing factor being intimal damage to small blood vessels. Manifestations developing after birth presumably result from persistent virus infection with consequent cytolytic damage and in some cases, e.g. pneumonitis, due to the developing immune response.

Onset of clinical illness in the mother prior to conception appears to carry no risk, with no evidence of intrauterine infection being found in 38 pregnancies in which the maternal rash appeared between five weeks before to 11 days after the last menstrual period (LMP). The shortest interval resulting in fetal infection was the onset of rash 12 days after the LMP, with all 10 pregnancies in which the rash appeared 3–6 weeks after the LMP resulting in fetal infection[15].

The stage of gestation at which maternal rubella occurs is critical[13]. Over 1000 pregnancies in which rubella was serologically proven between 1976 and 1978 in the UK were followed up[13]; 95% of women had had a rash and in the 11 asymptomatic women reinfection was proven in four, primary infection in four and in the remaining three there was uncertainty. Of 966 women with known outcome, 54% had termination of pregnancy and 4% had spontaneous abortions. Among the 407 pregnancies continuing to term there were nine stillbirths (2%) – about twice the normal rate. Serological investigation was performed on 269 infants, which demonstrated that overall some 45% were infected *in utero*, with higher rates in early and later pregnancy. Follow-up was achieved for 273 children and defects compatible with congenital rubella were found in 20; all mothers had had rubella in the first 16 weeks of pregnancy; none of the asymptomatic mothers had infected children. When rubella occurred in the first eight weeks of gestation, defects were multiple and severe; between eight and 16 weeks, sensorineural deafness was the only detectable defect.

Overall, the earlier in pregnancy that maternal rubella occurs, the more likely it is that severe manifestations will ensue (Table 2.2). Between conception and the 12th week of pregnancy the risk of fetal damage or death is approximately 90%, although figures vary in different studies. The risk is greater in the first two months than the third month. Between 12 and 16 weeks' gestation, the risk of abnormality falls to about 20% and the more severe manifestations are unlikely with the main damage being unilateral or bilateral sensorineural deafness. If maternal rubella occurs after the 16th week, the risk to the fetus is negligible, with only rare cases of deafness being attributable to rubella[16] and no statistically increased risk over the non-infected child. Despite the fact that fetal damage is

Table 2.2 Incidence of intrauterine rubella and congenital rubella defects following confirmed rubella in pregnancy (modified from reference[13])

Gestation of infection (weeks)	Proportion of infants infected	Proportion of infected infants also damaged	Overall risk of damage
<11	90%	100%	90%
11–16	55%	35%	18%
17–30	34%	0%	0%
31– >36	70%	0%	0%

limited to the first 16 weeks of gestation, rubella can infect the fetus at any stage as demonstrated by detection of rubella-specific IgM in neonatal serum[16,17].

REINFECTION

After first (primary) infection with rubella, immunity to further infection is usually life-long. However, reinfections do occur. These are rarely symptomatic, although a characteristic rubelliform rash can occur, as can milder manifestations such as a flu-like illness or arthralgia[18–20]. In the absence of illness, such reinfections are identified by demonstrating a serological response in someone who has previously had natural, wild rubella or successful immunization.

When reinfections are diagnosed exposure has usually been prolonged and close and characteristically has been from the patient's own child[21]. When rubella is endemic, it is reasonable to presume that reinfection is far more frequent than is diagnosed, as contacts of rubelliform illness may not be investigated because of previous immunization or demonstration of antibody or because testing after exposure was not done until the peak of the secondary antibody response had been reached. This background of undiagnosed reinfection must be considered when assessing the risk to the fetus.

In two retrospective studies[22,23] 40 pregnancies were followed to term after maternal reinfection and no fetus was infected. Only four of the women definitely had vaccine-induced antibody prior to reinfection, the remainder either not having had vaccine or having had vaccine without prior antibody screening. The first of these studies[22] clearly demonstrated that subclinical primary rubella presents a significant risk to the fetus (three of six infants being infected). Therefore, after contact with rubelliform illness in the asymptomatic woman in early pregnancy, distinguishing between subclinical primary rubella and rubella reinfection becomes critical for appropriate advice and management (see below).

There have been many case reports of rubella reinfection leading to intrauterine infection and congenital damage. The reason for some women being susceptible to reinfection and having a viraemia which may infect the fetus is unknown and is not obviously associated with a lack of neutralizing antibodies or ability to mount a specific T-cell response[24]. Those with 'immunity' resulting from vaccination may be more susceptible, as may women with lower concentrations of rubella-specific antibody, but a number of cases have not had vaccine and have had good concentrations of specific IgG prior to reinfection[21,23]. The early reports were reviewed in 1986 and many did not withstand close scrutiny as they were based on circumspect diagnostic testing or unconfirmed history[25]. In 1989 a series of five cases from the UK was reported which left little doubt that reinfection can result in fetal damage, albeit rarely[21]. In addition, congenital rubella as a result of presumptive reinfection was becoming a major concern in the UK as eight of the 94 cases of congenital rubella reported to the National Congenital Rubella Surveillance Programme during 1987–92 resulted from confirmed reinfection[26]. In the five cases there was a history, with documentation in most cases, of past rubella vaccine and past detection of rubella antibody by highly specific tests[21]. Two of the pregnancies were terminated, with rubella virus being isolated from the products of conception, and three pregnancies went to term. Congenital infection was proven in these three cases and all showed defects characteristic of congenital rubella.

On the basis of these five cases and to avoid infections being classified as reinfections when the serological evidence was circumspect, a more formal definition for confirmed reinfection was suggested. This would require the prior demonstration of rubella antibody by a specific technique on at least two occasions or a documented history of rubella vaccine together with prior antibody detection on at least one occasion. A single previous detection of rubella antibody cannot by itself be considered, as rare laboratory or transcriptional error may have occurred and vaccine failure is well documented. In addition, the serological findings soon after exposure may distinguish primary rubella from reinfection, for instance the failure to detect specific IgM or low avidity-specific IgG (see below). In recent years there has been a number of case reports of rubella reinfection, infecting the fetus, from various parts of the world[27–29].

What is the risk of reinfection to the fetus? First, by analogy with primary rubella, no significant risk would be attached to reinfection after 16 weeks gestation. Second, if symptoms such as rash, arthralgia or flu-like illness accompanied the reinfection, viraemia must be presumed to have occurred and consequently a risk to the fetus must be assumed, although as symptomatic reinfection is such a rare event no precise quantification of risk is possible.

Quantification of the risk to the fetus of asymptomatic reinfection in early pregnancy was attempted in a prospective study in the UK carried out between 1987 and 1991[20]. Forty-seven possible reinfections in pregnancy were identified; some of these cases had been included in previous reports[21]. Confirmed reinfection was diagnosed in 34 and probable reinfection in a further eight; persistent specific IgM reactivity was diagnosed in the remaining five and primary rubella or reinfection in the pregnancy was thought highly unlikely[30] (Table 2.3).

Table 2.3 Outcome of 34 confirmed and eight probable rubella reinfections in pregnancy (from reference[20])

| | Gestation (weeks) | | |
	0–12	13–26	27–term
Termination	7	5	–
Products of conception examined	3	3	–
Products of conception positive for rubella virus	2	0	–
Continued to term	7	20	3
Infants examined	7	20	3
Infants with intrauterine infection	1	0	0

Twelve women elected for termination of pregnancy and of the six products of conception (POC) examined in cell culture, rubella virus was isolated from two (Table 2.3). Congenital rubella was serologically confirmed in one of the 30 infants but no congenital abnormalities were found by one year of age in this infected infant. Of the five women with rashes, two went to term and fetal infection was excluded serologically but their reinfections had been at 17 and 32 weeks gestation; the three other women had a termination, but their POC were not examined virologically. This prospective study came to an end in 1991 when the frequency of diagnosed rubella reinfection became close to zero as the 1988 introduction of mumps, measles and rubella vaccine (MMR) began to have a dramatic impact on the incidence of these infections in childhood, effectively removing the potential for pregnant women to have contact with rubella. In this study the observed risk of congenital infection after rubella reinfection was 30% (three of 10 in the first trimester), but in two cases the diagnosis of intrauterine infection was by isolation of rubella from POC after termination and there is uncertainty whether this would of necessity reflect persistent fetal infection; during studies in the 1960s it was shown that rubella could be isolated from the placenta but not the fetus[31,32]. In the case that went to term fetal infection was presumed by detection of specific IgG at one year of age, but neonatal/cord serum had not been obtained and postnatal infection could not be excluded, although this was unlikely.

Combining the data from this study with those from the earlier studies[22,23], the observed risk in the first trimester is three out of 37 (8%), with 95% confidence intervals of 2–22%. Given the uncertainties over the three cases detailed above, an overview would suggest that the risk is almost certainly less than 10% and probably less than 5%.

EPIDEMIOLOGY AND INFECTIVITY

Serological evidence of rubella has been detected in every country in which appropriate investigations have been performed. Therefore, it is reasonable to assume that congenital rubella occurs worldwide, although the attention it has received will depend on local health priorities. In developed countries, prior to immunization programmes, 10–20% of young adults were susceptible and this is still the case for young males in countries where vaccination has been targeted at females. With rubella still endemic in the community, there would be a continuing incidence of infection in adults such that very few elderly people would have escaped infection, although cases in over-60-year-olds are still diagnosed on occasion.

In temperate countries cases of rubella tend to peak in the spring and early summer, although they occur throughout the year. Without comprehensive immunization programmes including childhood vaccination of males and females, rubella epidemics occur every 5–9 years – major epidemics in the UK occurring in 1972–3, 1978–9 and 1983 – but at somewhat longer intervals in the USA. During such epidemics the risk of maternal rubella may increase 10-fold and susceptible parous women are at particular risk from their own children.

Rubella is usually acquired by droplet spread from the nasopharynx of infected persons. Patients may be infectious for up to seven days before and 4–7 days after the onset of the rash. Infectivity probably peaks just before and at the onset of symptoms. The congenitally infected infant may excrete high titres of virus from the nasopharynx and in urine for up to a year or more and may be highly infectious to those providing care. The titre of virus progressively declines, however, and a pragmatic approach is to consider the infant relatively non-infective from the age of six months.

DIAGNOSIS

POSTNATAL RUBELLA

As clinical diagnosis is unreliable, laboratory investigation is required to make the specific diagnosis. Laboratory investigation of a rash illness or contact is required even if there is a past history of immunization, a previous diagnosis of rubella or even prior documented detection of rubella antibody. Immunization may not have been successful and laboratory and transcriptional errors are well recognized although rare. In addition, some assays used in the past for rubella antibody, such as haemagglutination inhibition (HI), may have given non-specific false-positive reactions. Where possible, the source patient should also be tested to validate the diagnosis in the contact.

Virus isolation has no place in the investigation of postnatal rubella, being unreliable and time consuming. Diagnosis is serological and makes use of the antibody response as detailed in Figure 2.1. The essential attributes of the antibody response in primary rubella are as follows.

- There is an incubation period of at least 10 days after infection has been acquired from the contact.
- At about the time of clinical illness (or subclinical infection) antibody starts to develop (although this may be delayed for 7–10 days).
- Once antibody starts to develop, it rises rapidly in concentration, with a doubling time of some 24 h.
- The antibody response is initially with specific IgM, which persists for three weeks to many months, closely followed by specific IgG.

Many tests for rubella antibody are in use including tests for total rubella antibody, for specific IgG (the antibody class which persists lifelong and is transferred across the placenta from mother to fetus) and for specific IgM (as

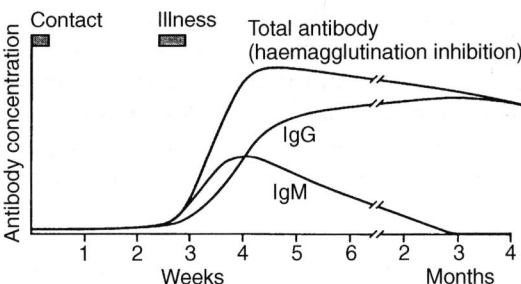

Figure 2.1 Serological response in primary rubella.

an indication of recent infection or fetal infection – maternal IgM does not cross the placenta). HI is a test for total antibody and after its first description in 1967[33] was the mainstay of rubella diagnosis and screening until well into the 1980s and, indeed, is still used by many laboratories. The mechanism of the test is dependent on the ability of rubella antibodies to bind to rubella haemagglutinin, so preventing its ability to agglutinate the erythrocytes of certain species, such as day-old chick cells. It is time consuming and prone to false-positive reactions at low levels. The assays most frequently used are as follows. Latex agglutination (LA) depends on rubella antibody agglutinating rubella antigen-coated latex particles and, although detecting both specific IgM and IgG, is primarily used for antibody screening, being both specific and sensitive. Radial haemolysis (RH) is also sensitive and specific, but detects only specific IgG; this test has achieved widespread use in the UK, being very inexpensive. It depends on rubella antibody in serum placed in wells diffusing through agarose gel and binding to rubella antigen-coated erythrocytes. Complement is also present in the agarose and this leads to lysis of erythrocytes and a clear zone when antibody is present (Plate D). These assays are progressively being replaced by various formats of enzyme-linked immunosorbent assays (EIA; ELISA) where, for specific IgG, a plastic well or bead is coated with rubella antigen and to this, with washing between stages, are added in turn a dilution of the serum being tested, an antibody against human IgG labelled with an enzyme and a chemical substrate which changes colour when acted upon by the enzyme. Hence, sera containing specific IgG will lead to a colour change in the substrate which can be quantified.

For specific IgM the above format can be used, but with replacement of the antibody against human IgG with an antibody against human IgM. An alternative EIA approach is the antibody capture technique with the plastic well or bead being coated with antihuman IgM and progressively adding, with washing between stages, a dilution of the human serum, rubella antigen which will bind to any retained test IgM which is rubella specific, and an antirubella antibody, labelled with an enzyme, which will bind to retained antigen. Bound enzyme is once again detected by changing the colour of a chemical substrate. These EIAs for specific IgM have virtually replaced the techniques of the 1970s and 1980s when serum was fractionated to separate IgM from IgG, with HI being used to identify IgM in the IgM-containing fractions. In recent years tests have been developed which detect rubella-specific IgM in salivary samples[34]. These have been most successful in investigating rash illnesses in children as they are non-invasive, but some unreliability and the inability to perform a range of further tests preclude their use in pregnant women.

An alternative approach to diagnosing recent primary infection is the measurement of rubella-specific IgG avidity. Soon after primary infection the IgG binds weakly to its antigen and hence is of low avidity. The IgG response matures progressively so that, at a later stage, the IgG binds more strongly and is of high avidity. Adaptations of rubella IgG EIA, in which weakly bound specific IgG is washed off or prevented from binding by mild protein denaturants, allow estimates of the presence of low avidity IgG[35].

When investigating a recent or current rubelliform rash or other illness which might suggest rubella, such as acute arthralgia, or contact with rubelliform illness, it is essential to collect a serum sample immediately.

Although some laboratories would test for total antibody-specific IgG in the first instance and then only move to specific IgM testing if total antibody IgG was present in sufficiently high concentration, most laboratories now routinely test for specific IgM as well. An argument for the former approach is that specific IgM testing is not required if specific IgG is detected within 10 days of contact and the patient can be reassured that she had previously had rubella and hence was immune to primary infection on the day of contact. This approach does presume, however, that the contact was limited to the dates stated and this can be most unreliable when investigating individuals after close family contact. In those laboratories which test for both specific IgG/total antibody and specific IgM, the advisory algorithm followed would be that detailed in Figure 2.2. Important aspects are that as the specific IgM may only be detectable for 3–4 weeks, if the first serum is collected more than four weeks after the rash or 6–7 weeks after contact, if rubella IgG is detected (>90% probability in most female populations) but rubella IgM is not, it *cannot* be excluded that rubella occurred some weeks before. Advice has to be based on probabilities, given characteristics of the illness/contact, past vaccination, past rubella antibody testing and perhaps the concentration of specific IgG in the recent test. Also one has to be aware of the problems of specific IgM tests. Although most have appropriate sensitivity, all are beset by problems of specificity[36]. False-positive reactions for specific IgM can occur in any test, either for reasons that are not obvious when this reactivity may persist for years[30], or in other specific infections such as parvovirus B19 and Epstein–Barr virus (infectious mononucleosis), which may have an identical clinical presentation[37]. Hence in pregnancy further confirmation is required from overviewing either the

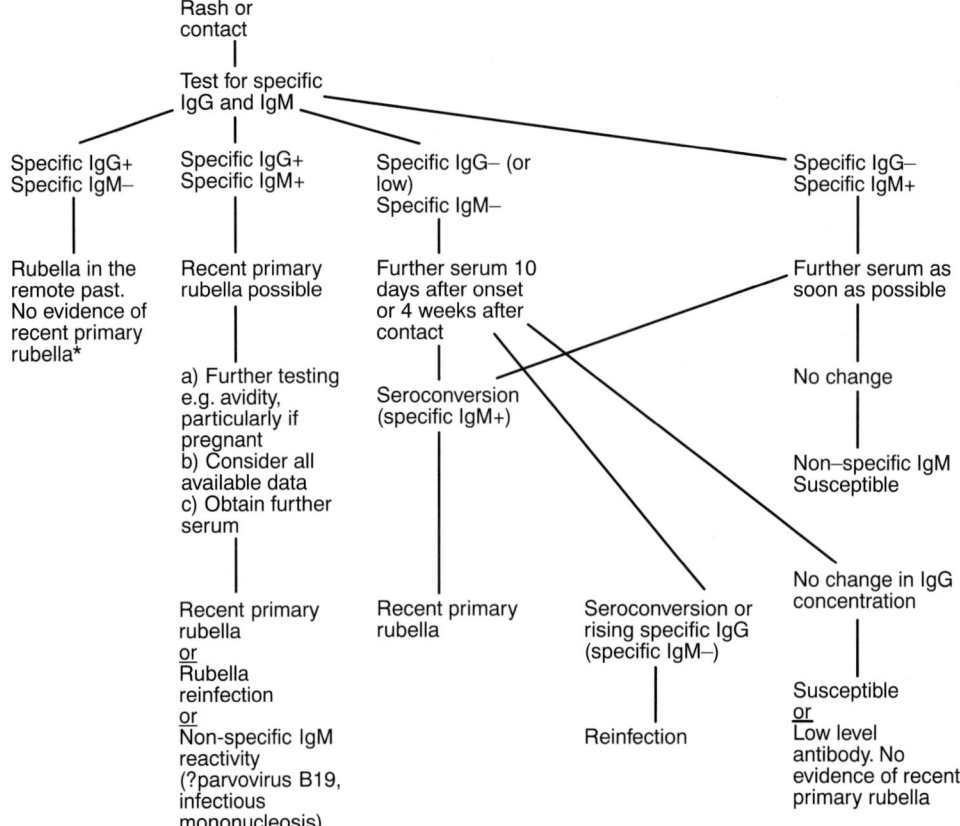

*If onset of rash more than 4 weeks prior or contact 6–7 weeks prior, recent primary rubella cannot safely be excluded.

Figure 2.2 Laboratory investigation of possible contacts or cases of rubella.

complete clinical and serological picture (e.g. seroconversion; proven rubella in contact and rubelliform illness in patient) or preferably by demonstrating low-avidity specific IgG. When the correct diagnosis is so critical for patient management it is also wise to test a further serum sample to exclude typographical or laboratory error. Such retesting is also prudent when a rubelliform rash occurs early in pregnancy but the laboratory results appear to exclude primary rubella. For the laboratory to investigate appropriately and for final management to be decided, it is essential that results are interpreted in relation to all the clinical findings and to the patient's history of immunization and past testing.

REINFECTION

Reinfection will be diagnosed either by demonstrating a rise in specific IgG/total antibody, probably accompanied by an IgM response[23], or by a changing IgM concentration when the peak IgG response has already been achieved in the first serum. The specific IgM response in reinfection is often of lower concentration and shorter duration than that seen in primary infection. The distinction from subclinical primary rubella may be achieved by reviewing the past history of testing and/or vaccination and by showing the IgG avidity to be high. A more common diagnostic problem occurs when IgM reactivity is detected and there is a need to identify whether it is non-specific or indicative of a reinfection. Examination of a further serum sample will usually clarify the situation as in reinfection (and primary rubella) the rubella-specific IgM reactivity will change over time, but if non-specific the reactivity will be unchanging.

An area of current concern is whether evidence of reinfection should be actively sought, and opinions vary. Such an approach would necessitate routinely examining a second serum sample even if the first were clearly positive for specific IgG and negative for specific IgM, so excluding recent primary rubella. The second sample would be examined in duplicate with the first to look for changing specific IgG concentration and/or the development of specific IgM. But this approach will miss reinfections where specific IgM does not develop and the peak specific IgG concentration has been reached in the first serum sample and may well lead to a period of anxiety whilst the second sample is tested. While primary rubella in the community is rare, only a few contacts with rash illness will actually have been in contact with rubella so many unnecessary investigations will be performed. Even if reinfection is identified, the risk to the fetus is low and the management of the pregnancy will vary according to individual maternal circumstances. On occasions the serological findings may be such that even after extensive investigation a definitive diagnosis cannot be reached.

CONGENITAL RUBELLA

A presumptive diagnosis of congenital rubella can often be made on the basis of a combination of characteristic clinical features, but even so a laboratory diagnosis is essential to exclude congenital abnormalities due to unidentified causes or abnormalities, such as mental handicap, which can also be caused by other intrauterine infections such as cytomegalovirus.

Infants with abnormalities due to congenital rubella are persistently infected with the virus. Hence virus isolation is a valid approach to diagnosis, with high titres of virus being found in throat and urine. At birth virus can be isolated from some 80–90% of neonates, with the rate dropping to about 33% at six months of age. Virus can also be recovered from sites such as lens tissue at far older ages. In many laboratories, however, rubella virus isolation techniques have not been well maintained, particularly in those countries which have had a low incidence of congenital rubella for some years.

Diagnosis of congenital rubella is now largely dependent on detection of specific IgM or persistence of specific IgG. Virtually all babies with congenital rubella are positive for specific IgM at birth and for the first three months of life by IgM capture techniques, although those tests which have rubella antigen on the solid, plastic phase tend to be less sensitive [36]. The proportion positive for specific IgM gradually declines with age (Table 2.4). False-positive reactions for specific IgM are exceedingly uncommon in infants and hence in the first three months of life appropriate IgM assays approach 100% sensitivity and specificity.

Table 2.4 Proportion of neonates/infants with congenital rubella positive for rubella-specific IgM

Age	Proportion positive (%)
Birth – 1 month	100
1–3 months	100
3–6 months	75
6–12 months	53

The rubella-specific IgG of maternal origin present in the neonate at birth has a half-life of 21–28 days and hence the concentration will progressively decline over the first year of life. Detection of specific IgG in the last months of the first year of life is very suggestive of congenital rubella, as primary rubella in the first year of life is uncommon although it can undoubtedly occur. In countries which have an infant immunization programme which includes MMR vaccine early in the second year of life, definitive diagnosis of congenital rubella after this age becomes difficult if the patient has been immunized. Even if immunization has not been given, rubella becomes progressively more common as the child ages and antibody detected after wild rubella cannot be distinguished from that found in children with congenital rubella, although occasionally the fact that IgG avidity matures more slowly in babies with congenital rubella is helpful[38].

FETAL INFECTION

On rare occasions when there is diagnostic uncertainty as to whether primary infection has occurred in early pregnancy or whether primary rubella has occurred in the fourth month, it would be helpful at least to ascertain

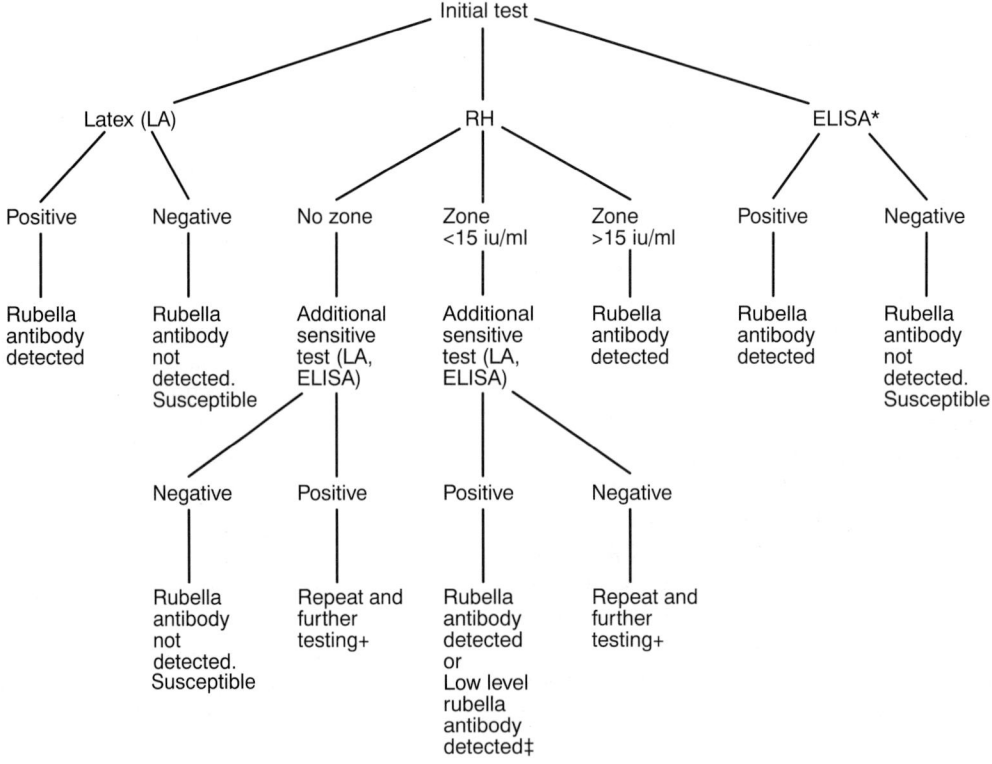

* Assays vary with respect to cut-off concentration of antibody and ability to quantitate
+ Final conclusion will depend on overall assessment of results
‡ See text

Figure 2.3 Approaches to testing for rubella antibody to determine whether immunization is indicated.

whether the fetus has been infected. Even if fetal infection is demonstrated, however, it is impossible to know whether damage has occurred or is likely to occur. It would be most uncommon for even the most modern techniques of fetal imaging to detect any abnormality in the first two trimesters and sensorineural deafness may not even become apparent until some years after birth.

A number of techniques have been described for detecting fetal infection, including virus culture of amniotic fluid[39], detection of specific IgM in fetal blood[40] and detection of viral genome[41,42]. Although the last approach is well validated, it would be available in very few laboratories and the limited demand means that even those with experience of genome detection may well have discontinued the service or have limited ability to test within a short interval.

RUBELLA ANTIBODY SCREENING

The sole reason for rubella antibody screening in pregnancy is to decide whether rubella immunization should be offered after delivery. It does *not* ascertain whether recent primary rubella has occurred and appropriate serological investigations would only be done if specifically requested or recent illness or contact is noted on the request form. The tests used are those that detect total rubella antibody or specific IgG. The 'gold standard' for many years was HI and on the basis of this test the 'cut-off' concentration as indicating 'immunity' of 15 international units (iu)/ml was established. It was set at this concentration to take account of the low non-specific reactivity that can occur in HI, but the tests currently used (LA, RH, ELISA) retain their specificity down to much lower concentrations. Two approaches are used and common algorithms are shown in Figure 2.3. First, there are those who report as positive, and hence immune to primary rubella, any serum which reliably contains specific antibody, whatever the concentration. Second, there are those who

adhere to the 15 iu/ml cut-off and report when a 'low level of rubella antibody (<15 iu/ml)' is detected and advise immunization. The argument for and against these two approaches is finely balanced (Table 2.5) and the approach will vary by laboratory. The USA has recently reduced the 'cut-off' to 10 iu/ml[43].

In the UK, antenatal clinic staff have been advised to test pregnant women for rubella in at least two pregnancies[44] and it may be

Table 2.5 Arguments for and against retaining a cut-off of 15 iu/ml of rubella IgG to indicate desirability of immunization

For	Reinfection is more likely the lower the concentration of antibody
	Reinfection can infect the fetus
	Viraemia reported following vaccine challenge of those with low concentrations of antibody
	A margin of safety for non-specific reactivity in some assays
Against	A concentration of 15 iu/ml was established to compensate for non-specificity of HI at low concentrations of antibody
	Many commercial assays for rubella-specific IgG have a cut-off lower than 15 iu/ml
	Reinfection with intrauterine transmission can occur even if preinfection sera have a concentration greater than 15 iu/ml
	With sera about 15 iu/ml, conflicting advice regarding immunization can be offered on repeated testing
	Reliable detection of rubella antibody precludes susceptibility to primary rubella
	Repeated immunization may occur as antibody concentration may not be boosted by immunization

pragmatic to test in every pregnancy given that most antenatal care includes phlebotomy for treponemal antibody testing and haemoglobin estimation. However, this advice was originally established because of concerns about technical error, the reliability of the assays used and recall of data. As computerized records are now widely established and laboratory procedures and assays have improved, it may be that women need only be tested in one pregnancy. If problems are identified after pregnancy, current advice is that antenatal screening sera should have been retained for at least one year. Indeed, such sera can be of great value in timing rubella undiagnosed during pregnancy or for investigating for other possible intrauterine infections such as cytomegalovirus or *Toxoplasma gondii*.

RUBELLA PREVENTION

HUMAN NORMAL IMMUNOGLOBULIN (HNIG)

Postexposure prophylaxis with HNIG is not recommended for susceptible pregnant women unless they are in the first 16 weeks of pregnancy and also if it is known that termination of pregnancy would not be acceptable if primary rubella were to occur. It does not prevent infection and viraemia, although it may attenuate the illness.

VACCINE

Live rubella vaccines have been available since 1969 and although there were initially a number of varieties attenuated by different procedures, the RA 27/3 strain has become established in the US and UK over the last two decades. This vaccine is produced in human diploid cells and has produced a higher seroconversion rate, a lower rate of reactions and more resistance to reinfection than other strains used in the 1970s.

More than 95% of susceptible individuals seroconvert after RA 27/3 and it seems likely that a significant proportion of non-responders have previously been infected with rubella (either vaccine or natural infection) but have IgG antibody below concentrations easily detectable by routine assays. Indeed, if a woman has had documented immunization at least twice, even if no antibody is detected, immunity to primary rubella can be assured. Also, it is not uncommon for women with detectable but low concentrations of rubella-specific IgG not to boost after reimmunization. As the laboratory will probably not have been informed of past vaccine history, this should be taken into account when rubella IgG is not detected or is present at low concentration and the laboratory advises immunization – it is not unusual for such women to be reimmunized unnecessarily many times (eight times in one personal instance!). Antibody induced by vaccination probably persists for life, with follow-up to date of over 16–18 years showing maintenance of detectable antibodies and protection in over 90% of vaccinees[45]. Vaccination does induce somewhat lower concentrations of antibody than natural infection. With the expected decline of antibody over the years, this may present problems for antibody screening in the future as specific IgG declines below detectable levels in women immunized in childhood. Vaccinees are more prone to reinfection when exposed to natural infection, but whether this is of major significance must be doubted as intrauterine infection can also occur in those having had natural infection and the risk of exposure declines as rubella in children is controlled. Vaccinees may excrete live virus from the throat, but there is no evidence of transmission to susceptible contacts, so exclusion of recently vaccinated health-care care workers from the clinical care environment is not justified. Similarly, recently immunized mothers and children do not present a risk to pregnant contacts. Vaccine rubella virus can be excreted in breast milk and may infect the neonate, but seems to present no risk of significant illness.

Rubella vaccine is a live attenuated virus administered subcutaneously and presumably produces a viraemia. Hence vaccinees can develop attenuated rubella some 1–3 weeks after immunization. Symptoms are rare in children and, indeed, in the 1994 UK measles/rubella vaccine campaign when 8 million children aged 5–16 years were immunized, adverse reactions were reported at one per 6700 children, with no serious consequences being proven[46]. In adults, low-grade fever, rash and lymphadenopathy can occur, but of more significance is the arthralgia which occurs more frequently in women (about 25% of vaccinees). The arthralgia can persist for up to three weeks and, rarely, longer. Such long-term arthralgia and chronic joint symptoms have been reported frequently in some studies, but an overview of available data suggests it is very rare and less common than after natural infection[47].

Rubella vaccine is contraindicated in severely immunocompromised individuals[44] and persistent infection has been demonstrated in a young adult male with acute lymphoblastic leukaemia[48]. Children infected with human immunodeficiency virus do not respond as well as non-infected children[49], although rubella vaccine is not contraindicated in this group. It is contraindicated in those allergic to neomycin and/or polymyxin which are contained in the vaccine – a highly unlikely event. Immunization should be delayed if the patient is suffering from a febrile illness and should either be given simultaneously with other live vaccines or separated by at least three weeks, to avoid the hypothetical risk of interference.

Most concern has been expressed about the risk of fetal infection if the vaccine is given immediately prior to or during pregnancy. There is evidence of fetal infection in about 1% of cases if vaccine is given in early pregnancy, but no evidence of congenital defects characteristic of rubella[50]. Meta-analysis of data from USA, UK and Germany for susceptible women given rubella vaccine shortly before or during pregnancy in 1991 revealed an observed risk of congenital rubella syndrome of 0/492, giving an estimate of overall maximum risk of 0.75%, but some 4.4% for immunization between 14 days before to four weeks after the last menstrual period as only 82 women were immunized between these dates[50]. To date, there are no reports of congenital rubella syndrome following maternal immunization. Administration of rubella vaccine is not an indication for termination of pregnancy, although immunization should not be given during pregnancy and pregnancy should be avoided for at least one month after vaccination[44]. It is advisable to check the rubella antibody status prior to immunization of adult women. Over 95% will have antibody and if the patient later finds she was pregnant or soon became so, anxieties can be discussed on the basis of known susceptibility, rather than the prior rubella antibody status being unknown.

A further anxiety is that the rubella antibodies found in blood products may interfere with successful immunization if given close to the vaccine. Human normal immunoglobulin may interfere although this is unlikely to be used after delivery, but blood transfusion can inhibit the response in some 50% of cases. Immunization should either be given 6–8 weeks later or, if vaccine is given after delivery, the antibody status should be checked eight weeks later, with reimmunization if necessary. It is well established that anti-D immunoglobulin does not interfere with rubella immunization, which should not be delayed.

IMMUNIZATION POLICY

Rubella vaccine is effective and safe and only the problems associated with the correct strategy for use and achieving high uptake have prevented the eradication of congenital rubella. A number of countries are now close to achieving that goal. Essentially, two approaches to effective use of the vaccine are feasible. First, as followed in the UK until 1988, was rubella vaccination targeted at girls and women to attempt to ensure that no woman susceptible to rubella embarked on pregnancy. This was to be achieved by immunizing all girls at 11–13 years, screening all pregnant women and immunizing those susceptible after delivery and *ad hoc* screening and immunization in general practice, occupational health, family planning and well-women clinics. In addition, all health-care workers (male and female) were tested and immunized to reduce the exposure risk of pregnant women in health care. By the mid-1980s, susceptibility in pregnant women was down to 2% in nulliparous women and 1% in the multiparous. It seemed unlikely that this proportion could be further reduced and with rubella still endemic in the community, exposure and infection of pregnant women would continue. In addition, there was the significant problem of reinfections[21]; reexposures were initially thought to be beneficial in boosting immunity when the strategy was first decided in the early 1970s and this was one of the reasons for a programme targeted at females. Consequently a decision was taken to offer immunization (as MMR) to all children in the second year of life from 1988, together with a catch-up campaign targeted at preschool entry at four years of age. This approach was intended to eradicate rubella from the community and augment the continuing screening and immunization of adult women and health-care workers. This second strategy had been used in the USA since the early 1970s with great success[51], although there had been occasional outbreaks associated with particular religious groups, such as the Amish, who refuse immunization[52] or in those of particular ethnic origin. Eradication is the desired objective, but care must be taken that a high (>90%) immunization rate is achieved; at lower rates rubella may be partially controlled, leading to a build-up over the years of susceptible young females and the likelihood of an epidemic some years hence. This may lead to an epidemic of congenital rubella syndrome (CRS) totalling more than a cumulation of an endemic rate of CRS in an unimmunized population or where vaccine has been targeted at women.

Since 1988, remarkable success has been achieved in the UK with the occurrence of rubella-associated terminations of pregnancy down to five in 1994 and congenital rubella down to 19 cases between 1991 and 1995, with 10 cases being associated with infection acquired overseas or recent introduction to the country[53] (Figure 2.4). The success has enabled the UK to discontinue the schoolgirl immunization component of its programme. A continuing problem for countries with successful control will be immigrants from countries with less effective rubella immunization programmes, such as women from South Asia entering the UK[53]. A further problem for countries such as the UK, that had relied on a female immunization programme, is a cohort of young adult males with susceptibility rates up to 20%[53]. Outbreaks will still occur where such young men congregate e.g. university or the military forces, and this may put at risk any susceptible young woman living in the same environment. This problem will gradually resolve itself as males immunized at younger ages reach adulthood and this was helped in the UK by the measles/rubella vaccine campaign of 1994 aimed at all children between five and 16 years of age.

For rubella to be globally eradicated requires the cooperation of all nations, with an immunization rate of at least 90% in infants. Such an objective can be achieved, but perhaps will suffer from the perception in some developing countries that eradication of CRS has less priority than controlling other devastating infectious diseases such as measles, malaria, HIV and tuberculosis. Hence the risk of reintroduction of rubella into developed countries with successful

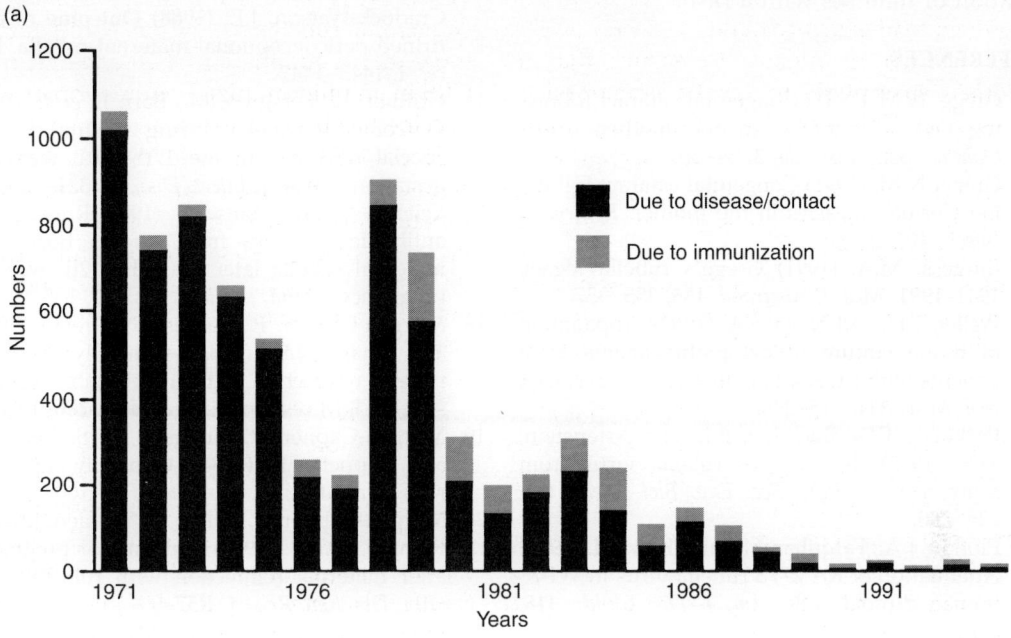

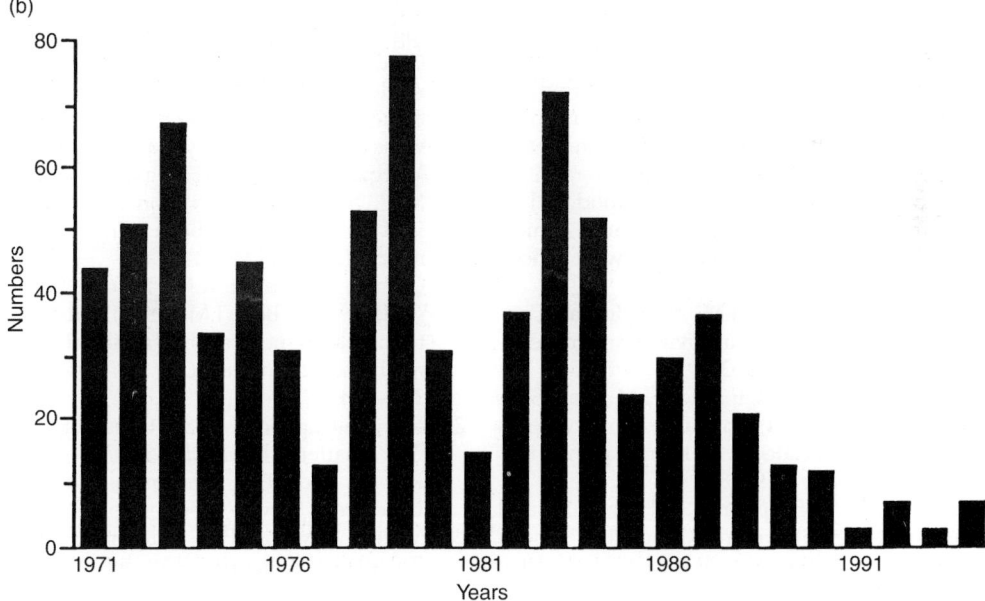

Figure 2.4 (a) Rubella terminations due to disease/contact or immunization. (b) Confirmed cases of congenital rubella syndrome and infection (from reference [44] with permission).

immunization programmes will continue, necessitating vigilance and appropriate investigation of illnesses with a rash.

REFERENCES

1. Gregg, N.M. (1941) Congenital cataract following German measles in the mother. *Trans. Ophthal. Soc. Australia*, **3**, 34–45.
2. Gregg, N.M. (1991) Congenital cataract following German measles in the mother. *Epidemiol. Infect.*, **107**, iii–xiv.
3. Burgess, M.A. (1991) Gregg's rubella legacy 1941–1991. *Med. J. Australia*, **155**, 355–357.
4. Weller, T.H. and Neva, F.A. (1962) Propagation in tissue culture of cytopathic agents from patients with rubella-like illness. *Proc. Soc. Exp. Biol. Med.*, **111**, 215–225.
5. Parkman, P.D., Buescher, E.L. and Artenstein, M.S. (1962) Recovery of rubella virus from army recruits. *Proc. Soc. Exp. Biol. Med.*, **111**, 225–230.
6. Plotkin, J.A., Farquhar, J.D. and Katz, M. (1969) Attenuation of RA 27/3 rubella virus in WI-38 human diploid cells. *Am. J. Dis. Child.*, **118**, 178–185.
7. Cherry, J.D. (1992) Rubella. In *Textbook of Pediatric Infectious Diseases*, 3rd edn, (eds R.D. Feigin and J.D. Cherry), W.B. Saunders, Philadelphia, p. 1792.
8. Dwyer, D.E., Hueston, L., Field, P.R., Cunningham, A.L. and North, K. (1992) Acute encephalitis complicating rubella virus infection. *Pediat. Infect. Dis. J.*, **11**, 238–240.
9. Morris, D.J., Morgan-Capner, P., Wood, D.J. *et al.* (1989) Laboratory diagnosis and clinical significance of rubella in children with cancer. *Epidemiol. Infect.*, **103**, 643–649.
10. Anderson, M.J., Kidd, J.M. and Morgan-Capner, P. (1985) Human parvovirus and rubella-like illness. *Lancet*, **ii**, 663.
11. Anderson, M.J., Lewis, E., Kidd, I.M., Hall, S.M. and Cohen, B.J. (1984) An outbreak of erythema infectiosum associated with human parvovirus infection. *J. Hygiene*, **93**, 85–93.
12. Smithells, R.W., Sheppard, S., Holzel, H. and Dickson, A. (1985) National Congenital Rubella Surveillance Programme 1 July 1971–30 June 1984. *Br. Med. J.*, **291**, 40–41.
13. Miller, E., Cradock-Watson, J.E. and Pollock, T.M. (1982) Consequences of confirmed maternal rubella at successive stages of pregnancy. *Lancet*, **ii**, 781–784.
14. Naeye, R.L. and Blanc, W. (1965) Pathogenesis of congenital rubella. *JAMA*, **194**, 1277–1283.
15. Enders, G., Nickerl-Pacher, U., Miller, E. and Cradock-Watson, J.E. (1988) Outcome of confirmed periconceptional maternal rubella. *Lancet*, **i**, 1445–1447.
16. Grillner, L., Forsgren, M., Barr, B. *et al.* (1983) Outcome of rubella during pregnancy with special reference to the 17th–24th weeks of gestation. *Scand. J. Infect. Dis.*, **15**, 321–325.
17. Vejtorp, M. and Mansa, B. (1980) Rubella IgM antibodies in sera from infants born after maternal rubella later than the 12th week of pregnancy. *Scand. J. Infect. Dis.*, **12**, 1–5.
18. Morgan-Capner, P., Burgess, C., Ireland, R.M. and Sharp, J.S. (1983) Clinically apparent rubella reinfection with a detectable rubella-specific IgM response. *Br. Med. J.*, **286**, 1616.
19. Morgan-Capner, P., Hodgson, J., Sellwood, J. and Tippett, J. (1984) Clinically apparent rubella reinfection. *J. Infect.*, **9**, 97–100.
20. Morgan-Capner, P., Miller, E., Vurdien, J.E. and Ramsay, M.E.B. (1991) Outcome of pregnancy after maternal reinfection with rubella. *Commun. Dis. Rep. Rev.*, **1**, R57–9.
21. Best, J.M., Banatvala, J.E., Morgan-Capner, P. and Miller, E. (1989) Fetal infection after maternal reinfection with rubella: criteria for defining reinfection. *Br. Med. J.*, **299**, 773–775.
22. Cradock-Watson, J.E., Ridehalgh, M.K.S., Anderson, M.J. and Pattison, J.R. (1981) Outcome of asymptomatic infection with rubella virus during pregnancy. *J. Hygiene*, **87**, 147–154.
23. Morgan-Capner, P., Hodgson, J., Hambling, M.H. *et al.* (1985) Detection of rubella-specific IgM in subclinical rubella reinfection in pregnancy. *Lancet*, **i**, 244–246.
24. O'Shea, S., Corbett, K.M., Barrow, S.M., Banatvala, J.E. and Best, J.M. (1994) Rubella reinfection: role of neutralising antibodies and cell-mediated immunity. *Clin. Diagnost. Virol.*, **2**, 349–358.
25. Morgan-Capner, P. (1986) Does rubella reinfection matter? In *Public Health Virology, 12 Reports*, (ed. P.P. Mortimer), Public Health Laboratory Service, London, pp. 50–62.
26. Miller, E., Waight, P.A., Vurdien, J.E. *et al.* (1993) Rubella surveillance to December 1992: second joint report from the PHLS and National Congenital Rubella Surveillance Programme. *Commun. Dis. Rep. Rev.*, **3**, R35–40.
27. Robinson, J., Lemay, M. and Vaudry, W.L. (1994) Congenital rubella after anticipated maternal

immunity: two cases and a review of the literature. *Pediatr. Infect. Dis. J.*, **13**, 812–815.

28. Paludetto, R., van den Heuvel, J., Stagni, A., Grappone, L. and Mansi, G. (1994) Rubella embryopathy after maternal reinfection. *Biol. Neonate*, **65**, 340–341.

29. Weber, B., Enders, G., Schlößer, R. *et al.* (1993) Congenital rubella syndrome after maternal reinfection. *Infection*, **21**, 118–121.

30. Thomas, H.I.J., Morgan-Capner, P., Roberts, A. and Hesketh, L. (1992) Persistent rubella-specific IgM reactivity in the absence of primary rubella and rubella reinfection. *J. Med. Virol.*, **36**, 188–192.

31. Alford, C.A., Neva, F.A. and Weller, T.H. (1964) Virology and serologic studies on human products of conception after maternal rubella. *N. Engl. J. Med.*, **271**, 1275–1281.

32. Cradock-Watson, J.E., Miller, E., Ridehalgh, M.K.S., Terry, G.M. and Ho-Terry, L. (1989) Detection of rubella virus in fetal and placental tissues and in the throats of neonates after serologically confirmed rubella in pregnancy. *Prenatal Diagn.*, **9**, 91–96.

33. Stewart, G.L., Parkman, P.D., Hopps, H.E. *et al.* (1967) Rubella virus haemagglutination-inhibition test. *N. Engl. J. Med.*, **276**, 554–557.

34. Perry, K.R., Brown, D.W., Parry, J.V. *et al.* (1993) The detection of measles, mumps and rubella antibodies in saliva using antibody capture radioimmunoassays. *J. Med. Virol.*, **40**, 235–240.

35. Thomas, H.I.J., Morgan-Capner, P., Enders, G. *et al.* (1992) Persistence of specific IgM and low avidity specific IgG$_1$ following primary rubella. *J. Virological Methods*, **39**, 149–155.

36. Hudson, P. and Morgan-Capner, P. (1996) An evaluation of fifteen commercial rubella IgM assays. *Clin. Diagnost. Virol.*, **5**, 21–26.

37. Kurtz, J.B. and Anderson, M.J. (1985) Cross-reaction in rubella and parvovirus specific IgM tests. *Lancet*, **ii**, 1356.

38. Thomas, H.I.J., Morgan-Capner, P., Cradock-Watson, J.E. *et al.* (1993) Slow maturation of IgG$_1$ avidity in congenital rubella: implications for diagnosis and immunopathology. *J. Med. Virol.*, **41**, 196–200.

39. Skvorc-Ranko, R., Lavoie, H., St-Denis, P. *et al.* (1991) Intrauterine diagnosis of cytomegalovirus and rubella infections by amniocentesis. *J. Can. Med. Assoc.*, **145**, 649–654.

40. Enders, G. and Jonatha, W. (1987) Prenatal diagnosis of intrauterine rubella. *Infection*, **15**, 162–164.

41. Bosma, T.J., Corbett, K.M., Eckstein, M.B. *et al.* (1995) Use of PCR for prenatal and postnatal diagnosis of congenital rubella. *J. Clin. Microbiol.*, **33**, 2881–2887.

42. Tanemura, M., Suzumori, K., Yagami, Y. and Katow, S. (1996) Diagnosis of fetal rubella infection with reverse transcription and nested polymerase chain reaction: a study of 34 cases diagnosed in fetuses. *Am. J. Obstet. Gynecol.*, **1774**, 578–582.

43. Skendzel, L.P. (1996) Rubella immunity. Defining the level of protective antibody. *Am. J. Clin. Pathol.*, **106**, 170–174.

44. Salisbury, D.M. and Begg, T.M. (eds) (1996) *Immunisation Against Infectious Disease*, HMSO, London.

45. Recommendations of the Immunization Practices Advisory Committee (ACIP) (1990) Rubella prevention. *MMWR*, **39**, RR15.

46. Committee on Safety of Medicines (1995) Adverse reactions to measles rubella vaccine. *Curr. Problems Pharmacovigilance*, **21**, 9–10.

47. Howson, C.P., Katz, M., Johnston, R.B. and Fineberg, H.V. (1992) Chronic arthritis after rubella vaccination. *Clin. Infect. Dis.*, **15**, 307–312.

48. Geiger, R., Fink, F.M., Sölder, B., Sailer, M. and Enders, G. (1995) Persistent rubella infection after erroneous vaccination in an immunocompromised patient with acute lymphoblastic leukemia in remission. *J. Med. Virol.*, **47**, 442–444.

49. Breña, A.E., Cooper, E.R., Cabral, H.J. and Pelton, S.I. (1993) Antibody response to measles and rubella vaccine by children with HIV infection. *J. Acq. Immune Defic. Syndr.*, **6**, 1125–1129.

50. Tookey, P.A., Jones, G., Miller, B.H.R. and Peckham, C.S. (1991) Rubella vaccination in pregnancy. *Commun. Dis. Rep. Rev.*, **1**, R86–8.

51. Anonymous (1994) Rubella and congenital rubella syndrome – United States, January 1, 1991–May 7, 1994. *MMWR*, **43**, 391–401.

52. Mellinger, A.K., Cragan, J.D., Atkinson, W.L. *et al.* (1995) High incidence of congenital rubella syndrome after a rubella outbreak. *Pediatr. Infect. Dis. J.*, **14**, 573–578.

53. Miller, E., Waight, P., Gay, N. *et al.* (1997) The epidemiology of rubella in England and Wales before and after the 1994 measles-rubella immunisation campaign: fourth joint report from the PHLS and the National Congenital Rubella Surveillance Programme. *Commun. Dis. Rep. Rev.*, **4**, R26–32.

Cytomegalovirus

3

S. Boppana and R.F. Pass

INTRODUCTION

Cytomegalovirus (CMV) was isolated in tissue culture and associated with congenital infection only a few years after the isolation of rubella virus. However, CMV is now arguably the leading cause of congenital viral infection in the world and congenital rubella has been nearly eliminated in the US by universal childhood immunization.

The public health importance of congenital CMV infection stems from its frequency and the occurrence of central nervous system (CNS) impairments in a significant proportion of cases. Studies that have screened large numbers of newborns for prenatal CMV infection have reported rates of from 0.3 to 1.4%[1,2]. In the US, the overall rate of congenital CMV infection is often estimated at 1% of live births, a rate that equates to around 40 000 new cases per year. Although most infants with congenital CMV infection will not suffer any impairment, studies in Sweden and the US suggest that congenital CMV infection is the leading cause of sensorineural hearing loss in children[3,4]. Considering auditory, visual, cognitive and motor sequelae, congenital CMV infection is probably the leading infectious cause of CNS damage in children in the US. There is no licensed vaccine for cytomegalovirus and there are currently no antiviral agents with demonstrated safety and efficacy for prevention or treatment of disease due to congenital CMV infection. However, knowledge of the epidemiology and biology of CMV infection continues to expand and new antiviral treatments and vaccines are being developed

EPIDEMIOLOGY

PREVALENCE OF CMV INFECTION IN MOTHERS

Numerous cross-sectional, serological studies, dating from the 1960s, have demonstrated that CMV infection is ubiquitous in human populations. Table 3.1 compares the prevalence of CMV infection in women of

Table 3.1 Prevalence of maternal seropositivity to CMV in various populations

Location	% Mothers seropositive	Reference
Aarhus-Viborg, Denmark	52	[160]
Abidjan, Ivory Coast	100	[2]
Birmingham, Alabama, USA		[6]
Low SES	77	
Middle SES	36	
Hamilton, Ontario, Canada	44	[161]
London, UK	56	[1]
São Paulo, Brazil		[162]
Low SES	84	
Middle SES	67	
Seoul, South Korea	96	[163]

SES, socioeconomic status

Viral Infections in Obstetrics and Gynaecology. Edited by D.J. Jeffries and C.N. Hudson. Published in 1999 by Arnold, ISBN 0 340 74095 7.

childbearing age from various populations. Higher rates of infection occur in non-white and low-income populations in developed and developing countries[1,2,5–8]. Because CMV is transmitted by direct contact with body fluids from an infected person, differences in age-related prevalence likely reflect differences in child rearing practices, living circumstances and sexual behaviour. Breastfeeding, group care of children, crowded living conditions and sexual activity have all been associated with high rates of CMV infection[9,10]. The prevalence of maternal CMV infection is an important determinant of the frequency and significance of vertical transmission of CMV in a population. The rates of intrapartum and breast milk transmission vary directly with the rate of maternal seropositivity. The rate of congenital infection is often high in populations with high rates of maternal seropositivity and the prevalence of maternal infection provides a measure of the proportion of the population susceptible to primary infection during pregnancy.

INCIDENCE AND SOURCES OF CMV INFECTION

The overall incidence of CMV infection in adults estimated from large studies of blood donors, hospital workers and pregnant women is around 1–2% per year[6,11–14]. Rates of primary CMV infection for pregnant women are shown in Table 3.2. Higher rates have been observed in women of lower socioeconomic status[6]. On a worldwide basis, most people acquire CMV during childhood.

Potential sources of maternal CMV infections are suggested by Table 3.3 which shows rates of CMV seroconversion in groups with a high incidence of infection; the importance of both sexual activity and daily close contact with a CMV-infected child is apparent. In addition to the cohort studies cited in Table 3.3, evidence for sexual transmission of CMV came from studies that showed higher rates of

Table 3.2 Rates of primary CMV infection during pregnancy

Study	# Seronegative women followed	Seroconversion (%)
Stern, 1973[14]	270	4.1
Griffiths, 1984[13]	4110	0.86
Grant, 1981[164]	1841	0.71
Stagno, 1986[6]		
Low SES	507	3.7
Middle SES	4692	1.6

SES, socioeconomic status

CMV seropositivity in young women with other indicators of sexual activity, such as sexually transmitted infections (*Chlamydia trachomatis*), greater number of sex partners or young age at sexual debut[15–17]. Maternal sexually transmitted disease was found to be an independent risk factor for birth of a newborn with congenital CMV infection in a case control study[18]. The role of young children as a source of CMV infection was revealed by studies in child-care centres. A dramatic rise in age-related prevalence of CMV infection for children in day-care centres compared with those kept at home, high incident rates of infection and molecular evidence of transmission of CMV strains among children showed that child-to-child transmission was common in this setting[19–21]. Serological follow-up studies of parents of children attending day-care centres and child-care workers showed a high rate of seroconversion and a strong association between care of younger, CMV-shedding children and seroconversion[22–24]. DNA fingerprinting of isolates provided further evidence of transmission of CMV from child to caregiver[25,26].

The role of children as a source of CMV infection for their mothers was also supported by the observation that incidence of maternal CMV infection increases with each successive pregnancy, suggesting that with more young

Table 3.3 Settings with observed high incidence of CMV infection among women of childbearing age

Study	Setting	Seroconversion/year
Adler, 1989[23]	Day-care workers	11%
Murph, 1991[165]	Day-care workers	7.9%
Pass, 1990[166]	Day-care workers	20%
Pass, 1986[24]	Day-care parents	15%
Chandler, 1985[15]	STD clinic	37%
Sohn, 1989[17]	Teen contraceptive clinic	34%

Reproduced with permission from Pass, R.F. (1996) Immunization strategy for prevention of congenital CMV infection. *Infect. Agent. Dis.*, **5**, 240–244.

children in the home, the risk of maternal exposure to CMV increases[6]. Further evidence that maternal CMV infection acquired from a child can lead to congenital infection came from studies that showed identity (by DNA restriction fragment profiles) among CMV strains recovered from a first child, the mother and a subsequent child with prenatal infection[27].

VERTICAL TRANSMISSION

Cytomegalovirus can be transmitted from mother to child transplacentally, during birth and via breast milk. Rates of congenital CMV infection from large studies that employed virological screening of newborns are shown in Table 3.4. Rates tend to be higher in populations with a high prevalence of maternal seropositivity (compare Tables 3.4 and 3.1). Whether this consistently observed pattern is due to recurrent maternal infections or to high rates of exposure and primary infection in the portion of the population that is susceptible (or to both) is unknown. Rates of congenital CMV infection are higher in developing countries and in low socioeconomic status groups in developed countries. Two studies of risk factors for congenital CMV infection found that young maternal age was

Table 3.4 Rates of congenital CMV infection in various populations

Location	% Congenital CMV infection	Reference
Aarhus-Viborg, Denmark	0.4	[160]
Abidjan, Ivory Coast	1.4	[2]
Birmingham, Alabama, USA		[7]
Low SES	1.25	
Middle SES	0.53	
Hamilton, Ontario, Canada	0.42	[161]
London, UK	0.3	[1]
Seoul, South Korea	1.2	[163]
São Paulo, Brazil		[162]
Low SES	0.98	
Middle SES	0.46	

SES, socioeconomic status

strongly associated with increased rate of congenital CMV infection[18,28]. Rates of congenital CMV infection by maternal age from a single study in Birmingham, Alabama, are shown in Figure 3.1. Preece *et al.* also found that non-white race and single marital status were independently associated with increased risk of congenital CMV infection in a London population[28]. Fowler and Pass reported that risk of congenital CMV infection was increased in primigravidae, women with sexually transmitted diseases and single mothers as well as those less than 20 years of age[18].

Intrapartum transmission of CMV occurs in around 50% of infants born to mothers shedding CMV from the cervix or vagina at the time of delivery[29]. Genital tract shedding of CMV is more common in younger women, declining from around 15% in young teenagers to less than 1% in women over 30 years of age[30, 31]. Rates of CMV excretion from the cervix and vagina also change during gestation, with low rates early in gestation increasing to rates that equal or exceed those in non-pregnant women late in gestation[16,32–34]. Cervical shedding of CMV has also been associated with other sexually transmitted infections and with greater number of sexual partners[16,35]. In the US approximately 10% of women shed CMV at the time of delivery; rates as high as 40% have been reported in Taiwanese women[34].

Breast milk is the principal route of transmission of CMV from mother to infant. From 27% to 70% of seropositive women shed CMV in milk[36–39]. CMV is more likely to be present in mature milk than in colostrum; Ahlfors and Ivarsson found that 70% of milk samples collected from seropositive women between nine days and three months postpartum yielded CMV[39]. None of the milk samples collected before or after this interval were positive. Dworsky *et al.* reported that transmission of CMV to nursing infants of seropositive mothers was related to duration of breastfeeding and detection of CMV in milk by virus isolation[38]. No infants nursed for less than one month became infected, compared with 39% of those nursed for longer than one month. If CMV was isolated from milk, 69% of infants were infected, compared with 10% of infants nursed by seropositive mothers with negative viral cultures from milk. The proportion of infants acquiring CMV is directly related to the prevalence of maternal seropositivity and the proportion of the population that is breastfed[40]. In some populations, over 50% of infants acquire CMV during the first year of life[37,41].

Vertical transmission of CMV plays a very important role in the epidemiology of human CMV infection. Aside from the medical significance of congenital CMV infection, infants who acquire CMV *in utero*, during delivery or from mother's milk shed virus for years. These infants serve as a source of virus for other children and care givers with whom they have close contact. In countries where a high proportion of infants acquires CMV from a maternal source, the majority of children is infected in early childhood. Even in the US, where approximately 10% of infants acquire CMV from a maternal source, these infants are an important source of virus for other children in day-care centres.

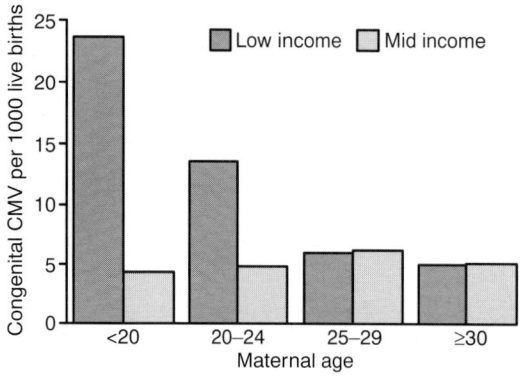

Figure 3.1 Maternal age and rate of congenital CMV infection (adapted from reference [7]).

PRIMARY VERSUS RECURRENT MATERNAL INFECTION

Primary infection is the term used to refer to initial acquisition of CMV. Primary maternal infection is identified by conversion from serum antibody negative to antibody positive or by the detection of circulating IgM antibody to CMV. One must be cautious with the latter investigation as some investigators have found that IgM antibody to CMV appears during pregnancy in women with evidence of past infection[42]. The rate of transplacental transmission of CMV ranges from 20% to 40% as a result of primary maternal infection during pregnancy[6,13,14]. It is extremely difficult to accumulate data on gestational age effects in transplacental transmission of CMV because maternal infection is rarely clinically evident. From the limited data available, there is no clear effect of gestational age at time of maternal primary infection on risk of fetal infection[6], though Griffiths' data showing a 20% rate of transmission with first-trimester infection suggest that the rate may be lower early in pregnancy[13].

Congenital CMV infection can also occur when primary maternal infection occurred in the past[43]. The term 'recurrent' has been used to categorize maternal infection that was present before conception but which leads to congenital infection. The biology of transplacental transmission of CMV in immune women is poorly understood. Recurrent maternal infection could be due to reactivation of endogenous latent CMV, reinfection with new strains or possibly primary infection that occurred in the recent past. Since recurrent maternal infection is only recognized when an infant with congenital CMV infection is born to a mother known to have been immune prior to conception, it is not possible to determine at what time during gestation transmission of virus occurs. It is also not possible to determine what type of maternal event (reactivation, reinfection or preconception primary infection) leads to fetal infection. Case reports of congenital CMV infection in offspring of mothers who were immunocompromised suggest that impaired immunity increases the risk of reactivation of CMV, transplacental transmission and damage to the fetus[44–47].

NOSOCOMIAL TRANSMISSION

Blood products and transplanted organs are the most important vehicles of transmission of CMV in the hospital setting; the latter is unlikely to be a concern during pregnancy. Transmission of CMV through packed red blood cell, leucocyte or platelet transfusions poses a risk of severe disease for seronegative small premature newborns and immunocompromised patients. Transfusion-acquired CMV infection is usually clinically silent, but a small percentage of patients (<5% in most studies) develop a mononucleosis-like postperfusion syndrome[48]. The risk of transmission of CMV with blood products increases with the number of units transfused, the presence of white blood cells and the lack of serum antibody in the recipient[48]. Prevention of blood product transmission of CMV can be achieved by using seronegative donors or by special filters that remove white blood cells[49–51]. Both approaches increase the expense of transfusion and the former also limits the supply of acceptable donors. Many hospitals limit small, premature infants, organ transplant recipients and patients with other immunodeficiencies to blood products from seronegative donors or blood that has been leucocyte-depleted by filtration. Although data on risk to the fetus from maternal transfusion-acquired CMV infection are not available, limiting seronegative pregnant women to blood from seronegative donors or filtered, leucocyte-depleted blood is prudent.

Another potential source of nosocomial CMV infection of particular concern to those in reproductive medicine is semen donated for artificial insemination. Cytomegalovirus persists longer and at higher concentrations in semen than in other body fluids[52,53].

Semen is more likely to be positive after a recent primary infection; young men are also more likely than older men to have CMV in semen[54]. Shedding of CMV in semen is particularly common and persistent in homosexual men, especially those who are HIV positive[53,55]. Although no cases of congenital CMV infection attributed to donor insemination have been reported, the fact that sexual activity is clearly a risk for CMV infection and that the virus can commonly be recovered from semen suggests a need for caution. The American Fertility Society has recommended serological screening of semen donors for antibody to CMV[56]. Limiting seronegative patients to semen from seronegative donors seems advisable. Although it is not known whether congenital CMV infection can result from infection of the oocyte, similar caution and screening should be applied to donor oocyte programmes.

Person-to-person transmission of CMV requires contact with infected body fluids and therefore should be prevented by routine hospital infection control procedures. Studies of neonatal special care nursery nurses, dialysis personnel and patient care personnel in a children's hospital found no evidence of increased risk of CMV infection in these settings in which patients shedding CMV are often encountered[11,12,57]. Cross infection among patients has been demonstrated by isolation of an identical (by restriction endonuclease analysis) CMV strain from more than one patient[58,59]. Although the fact that CMV can remain infective for minutes to hours on surfaces increases opportunities for transfer of virus, patient-to-patient spread appears to be rare and should be preventable by adhering to hospital hygiene protocols[60,61].

NATURAL HISTORY OF CMV INFECTION IN THE NORMAL HOST

Except for an occasional mononucleosis-like illness, CMV infection in normal hosts is most often asymptomatic. Studies of pregnant women found that only around 5% of those with primary infection had any associated symptoms during the interval of seroconversion[6,13,62]. The CMV-induced mononucleosis syndrome is clinically indistinguishable from infectious mononucleosis associated with Epstein–Barr virus (EBV). About 8% of all mononucleosis cases and 20–50% of the heterophil antibody-negative group are due to CMV[63–66]. Protracted fever, myalgia, fatigue and other non-specific constitutional symptoms are seen in most patients. Exudative pharyngitis, lymphadenopathy, splenomegaly and hepatomegaly are less commonly seen in CMV mononucleosis than in that associated with EBV[67,68]. However, there is considerable clinical overlap between the two entities so that virus-specific serological tests are often required for an aetiological diagnosis. Laboratory findings include atypical lymphocytosis, elevated hepatic transaminases and a negative heterophil antibody response[63–66,68,69]. In most patients, the course of CMV mononucleosis is mild and self-limiting. Infrequent complications of CMV mononucleosis include pneumonia, hepatitis and CNS involvement (Guillain–Barré syndrome, encephalitis, aseptic meningitis, neuritis and myelitis)[66,70–77]. A variety of immunological abnormalities suggestive of autoantibody production, including elevated cold agglutinin titres, mixed cryoglobulinaemia, elevated rheumatoid factors, polyclonal hypergammaglobulinaemia, positive direct Coombs test and antinuclear antibodies, are also observed on occasion[63,78–80].

The virological and serological responses following a primary CMV infection in normal adults have been characterized in patients with CMV mononucleosis. Viraemia is detectable for a few weeks to months and reflects the generalized nature of this infection[64,65,67,81]. Virus can be consistently recovered from urine and pharynx at the onset of clinical disease and viral shedding may be persistent or intermittent for a year or more after the resolution of clinical disease[81–83]. CMV antibodies of IgM and IgG classes have all been detected using different serological methods in patients with primary infection and recurrent CMV infections[84,85]. IgM antibodies peak early during the course of infection and tend to disappear 12–16 weeks after the onset in subclinical infection but may persist for longer periods. IgG antibodies peak during the first month or two after onset of infection; these antibodies persist for life and intermittent booster responses are observed[84,86].

CMV mononucleosis can also occur following administration of large volumes of blood or blood products[87–89]. This illness was initially described in patients following cardiac surgery which employed cardiopulmonary bypass and was termed 'postperfusion syndrome'. It is characterized by abrupt onset of fever, atypical lymphocytosis and splenomegaly between three and six weeks following exposure to blood products[88–91]. This illness is self-limiting in most cases and complications are rarely reported.

CLINICAL FINDINGS

NEONATAL FINDINGS

Of the estimated 40 000 children born each year in the US with congenital CMV infection, about 10% exhibit clinical findings suggestive of a congenital infection at birth (symptomatic infection)[6,9,92,93]. Except for a few case reports of symptomatic infection in infants born to immune mothers, clinically apparent congenital CMV infection occurs almost exclusively following primary CMV infection during pregnancy[6,44,93–96]. The typical findings that have been associated with generalized cytomegalic inclusion disease are characterized by multi-organ disease with prominent involvement of the reticuloendothelial and central nervous systems; however, around half of symptomatic infants have mild or atypical findings.

The frequency of various clinical and laboratory findings in 106 neonates with symptomatic congenital CMV infection is shown in Table 3.5. As the initial reports of Weller and Hanshaw suggested, petechiae, jaundice and hepatosplenomegaly are the most frequently noted abnormalities and are present in approximately 75% of symptomatic neonates[92]. In addition, half of the infants are microcephalic (Figure 3.2) and small for gestational age and about a third are born prematurely, suggestive of significant prenatal insult. About two-thirds of symptomatic infants have clinical neurological abnormalities such as microcephaly, lethargy/hypotonia, poor suck and/or seizures. Of the neonates in this series who had ophthalmological and audiological assessments, choroidoretinitis and/or optic atrophy were noted in 20% and an abnormal hearing

Table 3.5 Clinical and laboratory findings in infants with symptomatic congenital CMV infection (modified from reference[92])

Finding	% With abnormality
Clinical abnormality	
Petechiae	76
Jaundice	67
Hepatosplenomegaly	60
Microcephaly	53
Small for gestational age	50
Lethargy/hypotonia	27
Choroidoretinitis/optic atrophy	20
Purpura	13
Seizures	7
Laboratory abnormality	
Elevated transaminases (AST > 80 U/l)	83
Conjugated hyperbilirubinaemia (> 4 mg/dl)	81
Thrombocytopenia (<100 × 10^3/mm^3	77
Elevated CSF protein (>120 mg/dl)	46

AST, aspartate aminotransferase; CSF, cerebrospinal fluid

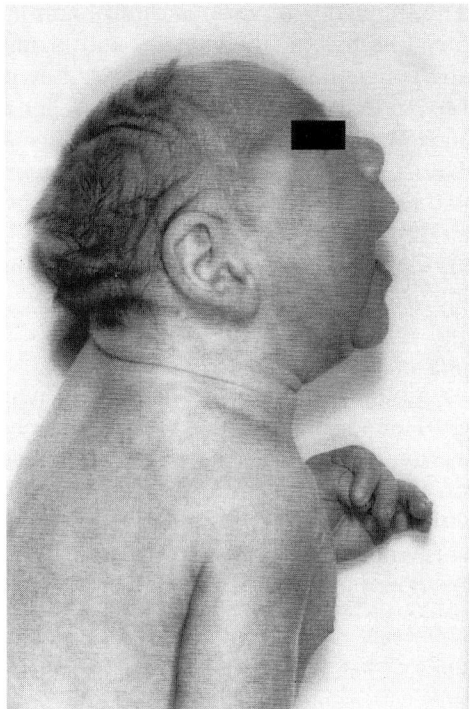 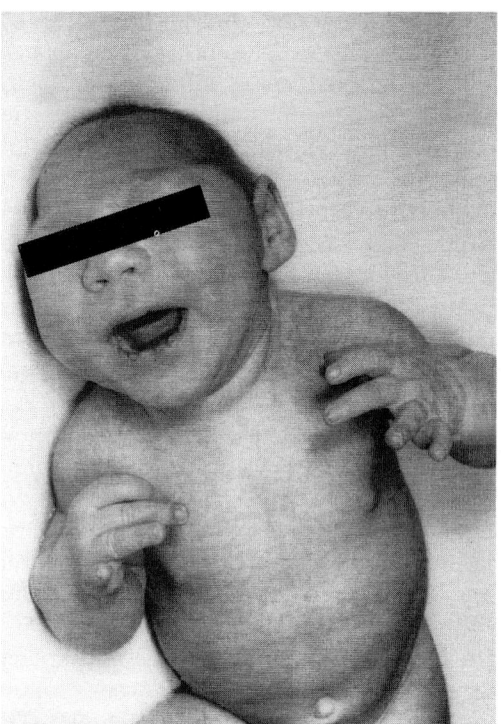

Figure 3.2 Infant with microcephaly due to cytomegalovirus.

screen in 56%[92]. Other less frequent findings include hydrocephalus, inguinal hernia, pneumonitis and haemolytic anaemia. About 10% of infants with symptomatic congenital CMV infection die during early infancy due to multiorgan disease with severe hepatic dysfunction, bleeding diathesis and secondary bacterial infections[92].

The laboratory abnormalities seen in infants with symptomatic congenital CMV infection include (decreasing order of frequency) elevated serum aspartate aminotransferase (AST) (>80 iu/l), conjugated hyperbilirubinaemia (direct bilirubin >2 mg/dl), thrombocytopenia (<100 000/mm^3), atypical lymphocytosis, haemolytic anaemia and elevated cerebrospinal fluid protein (>120 mg/dl)[92]. Elevations of serum transaminases and direct bilirubin are present in the immediate newborn period and peak during the second week

of life (Figures 3.3a and b) However, hyperbilirubinaemia and liver function abnormalities often persist beyond the neonatal period, resolving slowly over a few months[92]. Thus, invasive procedures such as liver biopsy are not justified on the basis of the persistent liver function abnormalities in infants with symptomatic congenital CMV infection. In the majority of infants, thrombocytopenia is noted within the first few days of life: the platelet count reaches a nadir in the second week of life and normalizes in most patients by the third week of life (Figure 3.3c).

CSF abnormalities, especially elevated protein (>120 mg/dl) appear to correlate with clinical indicators of CNS damage[92]. About 70% of infants with symptomatic congenital CMV infection have an abnormal neonatal cranial CT scan; intracerebral calcification is the most frequent finding[97]. Other less

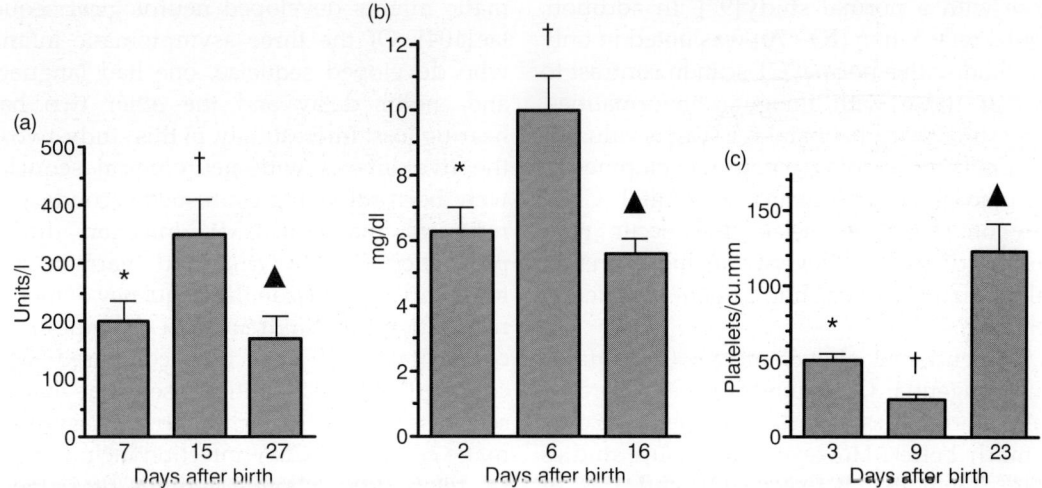

Figure 3.3 The course of hepatobiliary and haematologic manifestations in neonates with symptomatic congenital CMV infection. First (*), peak or trough (†) and prior to discharge (▲) expressed as mean values (columns) with SEM (bars). Serum ALT levels (a), serum conjugated bilirubin levels (b) and platelet concentrations (c) in infants with symptomatic congenital CMV infection with serial measurements (from reference [92] with permission).

frequently noted CT scan findings include ventricular dilatation, cortical atrophy, white matter abnormalities and migration abnormalities.

LONG-TERM OUTCOME

The significance of congenital CMV infection is based primarily on its adverse effects on psychomotor and perceptual function. It is estimated that between 7000 and 8000 children born each year with congenital CMV infection in the US will suffer from significant neurological deficits such as hearing loss, mental retardation and motor disability[93,98]. Symptomatic congenital CMV infection has been identified as a major risk factor for the development of permanent neurological complications and up to 80% of those who survive develop one or more handicaps[5,99–102]. Nearly 70% of children who are symptomatic in the neonatal period later develop psychomotor retardation and sensorineural hearing loss occurs in 58%.

Among patients with hearing loss, bilateral involvement is observed in about half of the children and about 80% exhibit progressive loss during early childhood[103].

Conboy *et al.* examined early clinical findings as possible predictors of mental retardation in a follow-up study of 32 children with symptomatic congenital CMV infection[100]. Microcephaly at birth, choroidoretinitis and an abnormal neurological assessment during the first year of life were associated with adverse intellectual outcome. In a 10-year follow-up study of infants with congenital CMV infection without neurological abnormalities at birth, Ivarsson *et al.* reported that those with a normal developmental assessment at one year of age were not at increased risk for subsequent intellectual impairment[104]. The value of a neonatal cranial CT scan in predicting CNS sequelae was investigated in 56 children with symptomatic congenital CMV infection; 90% of neonates with an abnormal CT scan developed at least one neurological sequel compared with 29% of those with a normal study [97]. In addition, mental retardation (IQ <70) was noted in only one child with a normal CT scan in contrast to 59% of those with imaging abnormalities, suggesting that a neonatal CT scan is valuable as a predictor of adverse neurodevelopmental outcome in symptomatic congenital CMV infection. Other sequelae that occur with varying degrees of severity include cerebral palsy, seizures, visual impairment and dental defects.

As mentioned above, most (90%) infants with congenital CMV infection have no clinical abnormalities at birth and their outcome is much better. However, follow-up studies have shown that between 10% and 15% of these asymptomatic infants will develop auditory or other CNS deficits [1,43,105–109]. The most common sequel in this population is sensorineural hearing loss [43,103,109–111]. In a long-term follow-up study of 307 children with asymptomatic congenital CMV infection, 22 (7.2%) developed hearing loss compared to none of 277 control children [109]. Among those with hearing loss, bilateral loss was noted in 50% and profound hearing deficit in 23%. Furthermore, continued deterioration of hearing was seen in 50% of children; 18% had normal initial auditory evaluations but developed delayed-onset hearing deficit. Based on these results, it is estimated that approximately 2600 children with asymptomatic congenital CMV infection can be expected to develop hearing loss each year in the US. Thus, congenital CMV infection is likely to be a leading cause of sensorineural hearing loss in young children [3,109].

The extent to which more global CNS sequelae such as mental retardation and cerebral palsy are associated with asymptomatic congenital CMV infection remains controversial. In a study of 41 children with asymptomatic congenital CMV who were assessed at two years of age, Pearl *et al.* did not detect mental retardation in any of the study subjects [112]. In a prospective Swedish study, 2/8 (25%) symptomatic and 3/35 (9%) asymptomatic infants developed neurological sequelae [104]. Of the three asymptomatic infants who developed sequelae, one had language and motor delay and the other two had hearing loss. Interestingly, in this study, two of the five infants with neurological sequelae were born following confirmed secondary or recurrent maternal CMV infection during pregnancy. Conboy *et al.* and Ivarrson *et al* found no difference in the frequency of mental retardation in children with asymptomatic congenital CMV infection compared with controls [100,104]. Additional sequelae that are seen less frequently in children with asymptomatic congenital CMV infection include mental retardation, choroidoretinitis and dental defects [103,105–112].

Clinical findings associated with greater risk of CNS sequelae are listed in Table 3.6. In addition to neonatal clinical abnormalities, primary maternal CMV infection during gestation is an important predictor of sequelae in children with congenital CMV infection [2,6,43,98,113]. In a longitudinal follow-up study of 125 infants born following primary infection during pregnancy and 64 infants born to immune mothers (Figure 3.4), Fowler *et al.* reported that one or more sequelae were seen in 25% of the primary infection group compared to 8% of children born to immune

Table 3.6 Predictors of an adverse neurodevelopmental outcome in children with congenital CMV infection

Maternal predictors
    Primary maternal infection
    First-trimester maternal CMV infection
    Low-income, non-white adolescents

Findings at birth
    Microcephaly
    Neurological abnormalities
    Choroidoretinitis
    Abnormal cranial CT scan

Abnormal neurological examination at one year
    of age

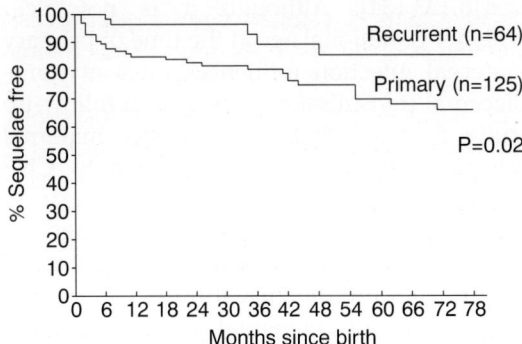

Figure 3.4 Long-term outcome in children with congenital CMV infection according to the type of maternal infection. Percentage of children who remained free of sequelae is shown (from reference [98] with permission).

mothers[98]. None of the children born to immune mothers had mental retardation (IQ <70) compared to 13% of those in the primary infection group. In addition, functionally important bilateral sensorineural hearing loss was only seen in children born following a primary maternal CMV infection. The clinical findings listed in Table 3.6 apply only to neonates who are symptomatic. Except for primary maternal CMV infection, the predictors of adverse long-term outcome in children with asymptomatic infection have not been defined. It has been suggested that the presence of CT scan abnormalities at birth in asymptomatic congenital CMV infection is associated with the development of hearing loss and neurodevelopmental deficits early in life[114,115]. However, this association has not been examined in long-term follow-up studies.

PATHOGENESIS

Although the determinants of intrauterine transmission of CMV have not been clearly identified, the possible mechanisms that could play an important role in the transmission of CMV *in utero* include maternal immune responses, characteristics of the virus and the gestational age at viral infection of the fetus. A direct examination of most of these factors is not possible in humans.

The importance of maternal immune responses is evident by the substantial protection that preconceptional immunity to CMV provides against intrauterine transmission and damaging fetal infection. Although this protection is not complete, the transmission rates decrease by about 25-fold in immune mothers compared to those with primary infection during pregnancy[6,13,14,43,96,116–118]. The nature of those protective maternal immune mechanisms that limit intrauterine transmission has not been clearly defined but could include both cellular and antiviral antibody responses. Decreased or absent lymphoproliferative responses to CMV during pregnancy have been documented by several investigators, suggesting a role for CMV-specific cellular immune response in intrauterine transmission and the virulence of fetal infection[119–121]. Maternal antiviral antibody responses have been characterized in women with primary CMV infection. Higher levels of CMV-specific antibodies were documented in women who transmitted virus to the fetus than in those without transmission[122–124]. However, an examination of the qualitative antibody response revealed lower titres of neutralizing antibodies in transmitters, suggesting an association between virus-neutralizing activity and intrauterine transmission[124]. Furthermore, a significant correlation between neutralizing titres and antibody avidity was demonstrated, indicating that a defect in affinity maturation may play a role in intrauterine transmission.

In a recent study, a replicating Towne strain vaccine failed to prevent infection of immunized women exposed to young CMV-infected children, whereas natural immunity was completely protective[125]. Interestingly, in this study, protective immunity correlated with higher levels of virus-neutralizing antibodies, rather than CMV-specific lymphocyte proliferative responses. In the guinea pig

CMV (gpCMV) model, immunization of animals with recombinant gpCMV glycoprotein B, a major target of virus-neutralizing activity, and with a purified glycoprotein preparation from gpCMV-infected cells reduced both the incidence and severity of congenital CMV disease[126,127].

The mechanisms of severe fetal infection are not clear but could include higher maternal viral load resulting in a more widely disseminated fetal infection, a virulent phenotype of infecting virus and the gestational age at virus acquisition. An association between maternal viraemia and fetal infection was suggested by a study of a limited number of pregnant women using PCR of the leucocytes for the detection of viraemia. The results of this study showed that congenital CMV infection is significantly more frequent in the offspring of viraemic mothers[128]. Interestingly, studies in the gpCMV model also noted a correlation between extended maternal viraemia and fetal infection[129]. In the SCID mouse model of CMV infection, different viral isolates exhibited different *in vivo* behaviour, implying virulence differences between strains of virus[130]. However, the issue of virus strain variation and virulence has not been examined in human CMV infections. A study of CMV immediate-early (IE) enhancer/promoter specificity during embryogenesis in a transgenic mouse model suggested that the expression of IE enhancer/promoter was restricted to neural, epithelial and vascular sites that correlate with known sites of congenital CMV infection in human fetuses[131]. This mechanism could explain the propensity of CMV to infect the developing CNS of the fetus, leading to permanent neurological complications.

Investigations of the gpCMV model have indicated that fetal infection occurred *in utero* regardless of the time of maternal infection[132]. An epidemiological study of human CMV infections also suggested that intrauterine transmission can occur following maternal infection at different stages of gestation[6,133,134]. Although it is not clear whether gestational age at the time of primary maternal infection influences rates of transplacental transmission, a long-term follow-up study revealed that first-trimester maternal infections are more likely to lead to CNS sequelae, especially sensorineural hearing loss[133]. The effect of gestational age on transplacental transmission and fetal damage may be less prominent with CMV than with other causes of congenital infection because active maternal viral infection persists for months. It is possible that transmission to the fetus could occur weeks or even months after primary maternal infection. The role of the placenta in containing CMV. infections during pregnancy is another ill-defined but potentially important area for understanding the pathogenesis of intrauterine infection[132,134,135]. A study of primary CMV infections in the gpCMV model suggested that the placenta not only serves as a reservoir for CMV but also acts to limit transmission of the virus to the fetus[135].

In addition to decreased intrauterine transmission, the presence of maternal immunity to CMV also correlates with outcome of fetal infection both in terms of neonatal findings and long-term neurological outcome. About 10% of infants with congenital CMV infection following a primary maternal CMV infection exhibit clinically apparent congenital CMV infection and up to 80% of these infants will develop permanent neurological sequelae[5,93,98–102]. In contrast, women with preconceptional immunity to CMV rarely, if ever, deliver infants with symptomatic infection[4,44,93–96]. Similarly, the long-term outcome in patients with congenital CMV infection following primary maternal infection is much worse than in the group of children born to immune mothers. Together, these findings strongly suggest that preconceptional immunity to CMV can prevent or modulate fetal CMV infection, as well as reduce the rate of intrauterine transmission of this virus.

LABORATORY DIAGNOSIS

CONGENITAL INFECTION

Congenital CMV infection is proven by isolation of virus from body fluids during the first three weeks of life. Urine and saliva (mouth swab) are equally useful for this purpose, though the latter is more easily collected[136]. It is easy to detect CMV in the saliva and urine of newborns with congenital infection because large amounts of virus are present. Traditional viral isolation in tissue culture is the standard against which other methods are assessed. Centrifugation-enhanced, rapid techniques (shell vial or DEAFF) are similar in sensitivity and specificity to standard viral isolation procedures; however, the rapid methods use monoclonal antibody to CMV immediate/ early antigens to detect infected tissue culture cells and provide results in 24 h, compared with several days to two weeks for tissue culture[62,136–138]. Polymerase chain reaction and other methods for detection of CMV DNA in urine or saliva can also be used, but there is less experience with these methods and less certainty about their sensitivity and specificity[139]. Viraemia is not present in all newborn infants with congenital CMV infection; detection of virus in blood should not be relied on to diagnose congenital infection[128]. Detection of IgM antibody to CMV is not as reliable as viral isolation and is not recommended for diagnosis of congenital infection. The age of the patient when samples are collected for detection of CMV is of some importance. Neonates who acquire CMV during birth or from mother's milk shed virus after three weeks of age. Detection of CMV after three weeks of age is therefore not unequivocal proof of congenital infection.

MATERNAL INFECTION

Questions about maternal CMV infection during pregnancy usually arise because of a maternal mononucleosis-like illness or maternal exposure to CMV. Evaluation of these patients focuses on determination of whether the mother has primary CMV infection. Maternal serum should be tested for IgG and IgM antibody to CMV. If both are negative, the patient does not have CMV infection or has not yet seroconverted; serology should be repeated 1–2 weeks later. If IgG antibody is positive and IgM antibody negative, it suggests past (not primary) maternal CMV infection. However, assays for IgG antibody vary in sensitivity and patients vary in how long IgM antibody persists after primary infection[133,140,141]. If both IgG and IgM antibody are positive, it is likely but not certain that the patient has experienced recent CMV infection. A study employing a commercial ELISA kit found that 2.5% of women who were known to have had CMV for more than a year had serum IgM antibody to CMV[133]. In the same study 83% of women who had seroconverted over an interval of 30 weeks or longer had IgM antibody in their first CMV-IgG positive serum. If the seroconversion interval was 15 weeks or less, 93% of women with primary infection were IgM antibody positive. Many different assays for antibody to CMV are in use by diagnostic laboratories; they may have considerable variability in sensitivity and specificity for detection of IgM antibody. It is essential that clinicians understand the limitations of serological diagnosis of primary maternal CMV infection.

Prenatal screening of expectant mothers for CMV infection is not recommended as a clinical routine. False-positive results with IgM antibody assays are a potential hazard. For example, the rate of maternal primary infection during pregnancy is approximately 2%; a very good IgM antibody assay had a false positivity rate of 2.5% in women with past infection[133]. Thus a positive screening test for IgM antibody is as likely to represent a false-positive test for primary infection as real evidence of recent infection. False-positive laboratory results and erroneous assumptions about the significance of IgG and IgM antibody levels lead to provision of incorrect information regarding risk to the fetus.

TREATMENT

Antiviral agents are commonly used to prevent or treat CMV infections in immunocompromised patients, but none of the available agents has been approved for use during pregnancy and none has been shown to be effective for treatment of congenital CMV infection.

Ganciclovir, a nucleoside analogue of 2'-deoxyguanosine, is used for treatment of cytomegalovirus retinitis in immunocompromised patients, mainly those with AIDS, and for prevention and treatment of CMV disease in transplant patients[142,143]. Foscarnet (phosphonoformic acid) and cidofovir have been shown to be effective in treatment of CMV retinitis in AIDS patients[144–146]. All three of these antiviral agents have significant acute toxicity in humans; studies in animals suggest the potential for late sequelae such as induction of tumours or, in the case of ganciclovir, azoospermia or infertility. These antiviral drugs should not be used in normal hosts. In addition, ganciclovir, foscarnet and cidofovir are classified Category C for use in pregnancy; all three have been teratogenic or embryotoxic in animal studies and they have not been studied in human pregnancy. These agents should not be used during pregnancy or lactation except when the patient is severely immunocompromised and the threat to her from disseminated CMV infection or retinitis is sufficiently grave to justify the risk to the fetus or newborn. With the three agents that are currently licensed for treatment of CMV infection, antiviral treatment during pregnancy with the aim of preventing or treating fetal CMV infection is not recommended.

Neither ganciclovir nor any other antiviral agent is approved for treatment of neonates who are symptomatic from congenital CMV infection. Case reports have described treatment of neonates with symptomatic congenital CMV infection[147–151]. However, it is not possible to determine whether the treatment altered the course of the disease in any of these cases.

Antiviral treatment of the infant with congenital CMV infection could be aimed at control of the neonatal abnormalities such as thrombocytopenia, direct hyperbilirubinaemia or retinitis or at preventing central nervous system sequelae such as hearing loss, cerebral palsy or mental retardation. There is clearly a potential for neonatal treatment with ganciclovir to alter the course of the acute disease, based on experience in immunocompromised patients. However, newborn haematological and hepatic abnormalities resolve spontaneously without treatment in a matter of weeks in almost all cases[92]. The majority of neonates with symptomatic congenital CMV infection have evidence of CNS damage in the newborn period and it is unlikely that antiviral treatment will alter the course of disease that results from prenatal damage. However, hearing loss often appears after the neonatal period or becomes progressively more severe, providing a rationale for evaluation of antiviral treatment for those with symptomatic congenital CMV infection[103]. A collaborative study of ganciclovir in the USA has described the pharmacokinetics of the agent in neonates[152] and reported the results of a phase I/II trial of a six-week intravenous regimen[153]. It is clear that ganciclovir can suppress CMV replication while it is being administered; however, viral shedding resumes after the drug is discontinued. Although there was a suggestion that some patients had improvement in auditory function during the phase I/II trial, results were inconclusive. A randomized trial in newborns with symptomatic congenital CMV infection is under way. Treatment with ganciclovir outside a clinical trial should be approached with caution because there is no evidence that such treatment is beneficial and the drug has the potential for toxicity that may not become apparent for years.

PREVENTION

Limiting exposure is the only approach available for prevention of maternal and congenital CMV infection at this time and it is uncertain whether this approach is effective. Contact with preschool children and sexual contact both appear to be important risks for primary maternal infection (Table 3.3). However, limiting these exposures could prove difficult if not impossible. Altering sexual behaviour is problematic even when it is aimed at preventing infections of more immediate danger to the mother's health. Avoiding contact with preschool children is not practical for women employed in child care and not possible for mothers of young children.

Hygiene, specifically careful attention to handwashing and avoiding direct contact with body fluids, has been recommended for preventing acquisition of CMV from young children[154]. The fact that rates of CMV infection do not appear to be increased for hospital workers who take care of children suggests that handwashing and hygiene are effective. Children in hospitals, day-care centres or schools who are known to have CMV infection should not be singled out for special handling. One should assume that all young children and all body fluids are potential sources of CMV infection.

Cytomegalovirus is shed in semen, cervix/ vaginal fluid, saliva and tears and sexual contact can involve exchange of all of these; the effectiveness of condoms for prevention of CMV transmission has not been defined. However, CMV appears to be shed more persistently in male and female genital fluids than from other body sites and condoms could therefore be at least partially effective. Preventing primary maternal infection during pregnancy is important because most congenital CMV infections that cause central nervous system sequelae result from primary maternal infection. To the extent that congenital CMV infection is due to reactivation of endogenous, latent maternal virus, it may be impossible to prevent. Fortunately, recurrent maternal infection, whether due to reactivation of virus or other mechanisms, is rarely associated with damage to the fetus.

Although no CMV vaccines are currently licensed, candidate vaccines are in preclinical and phase I and II clinical trials. The Towne strain of CMV is the basis for a live attenuated vaccine that has been studied for 20 years. It appears to be safe and immunogenic in normal hosts and protected healthy volunteers challenged with a virulent strain[155,156]. Towne vaccine was effective in reducing the frequency of severe CMV disease in renal transplant patients experiencing primary infection in the immediate post-transplant period[157].

However, a placebo-controlled clinical trial with Towne vaccine in seronegative mothers of young, CMV-shedding children showed no difference in infection rates between vaccine and placebo recipients[125]. In preclinical studies a vaccine comprising a canary pox vector expressing the gene for human CMV glycoprotein B (gB) induced neutralizing antibody and specific cytotoxic T-lymphocytes in both mice and guinea pigs[158]. Phase I trials with a vaccine based on a modified recombinant envelope glycoprotein B from the Towne strain of CMV showed it to be well tolerated and immunogenic, inducing antibody to gB, neutralizing antibody and lymphocyte proliferative responses to gB[159].

Although a vaccine that can be relied on to prevent maternal and congenital CMV infection is not yet available, reports of further trials are likely to be forthcoming.

REFERENCES

1. Peckham, C.S., Chin, K.S., Coleman, J.C. *et al.* (1983) Cytomegalovirus infection in pregnancy: preliminary findings from a prospective study. *Lancet*, **1**, 1352–1355.

2. Schopfer, K., Lauber, E. and Krech, U. (1978) Congenital cytomegalovirus infection in newborn infants of mothers infected before pregnancy. *Arch. Dis. Child.*, **53**, 536–539.

3. Harris, S., Ahlfors, K., Ivarsson, S., Lemmark, B. and Svanberg, L. (1984) Congenital cytomegalovirus infection and sensorineural hearing loss. *Ear Hear.*, **5**, 352–355.

4. Hicks, T., Fowler, K., Richardson, M. *et al.* (1993) Congenital cytomegalovirus infection and neonatal auditory screening. *J. Pediatr.*, **123**, 779–782.

5. Montgomery, J.R., Mason, E.O., Williamson, A.P., Desmond, M.M. and South, M.A. (1980) Prospective study of congenital cytomegalovirus infection. *South. Med. J.*, **73**, 590.

6. Stagno, S., Pass, R.F., Cloud, G. *et al.* (1986) Primary cytomegalovirus infection in pregnancy. Incidence, transmission to fetus, and clinical outcome. *JAMA*, **256**, 1904–1908.

7. Fowler, K.B., Stagno, S. and Pass, R.F. (1993) Maternal age and congenital cytomegalovirus infection: screening of two diverse newborn populations, 1980–1990. *J. Infect. Dis.*, **168**, 552–556.

8. Tookey, P.A., Ades, A.E. and Peckham, C.S. (1992) Cytomegalovirus prevalence in pregnant women: the influence of parity. *Arch. Dis. Child.*, **67**, 779–783.

9. Pass, R.F. (1985) Epidemiology and transmission of cytomegalovirus infection. *J. Infect. Dis.*, **152**, 243–256.

10. Stagno, S. and Cloud, G.A. (1990) Changes in the epidemiology of cytomegalovirus. In *Immunology and Prophylaxis of Human Herpesvirus Infections*, (ed. C. Lopez), Plenum Press, New York, pp. 93–104.

11. Balfour, C.L. and Balfour, H.H. (1986) Cytomegalovirus is not an occupational risk for nurses in renal transplant and neonatal units. *JAMA*, **256**, 1909–1914.

12. Balcarek, K.B., Bagley, R., Cloud, G.A. and Pass, R.F. (1990) Cytomegalovirus infection among employees of a children's hospital: no evidence for increased risk associated with patient care. *JAMA*, **263**, 840–844.

13. Griffiths, P.D. and Baboonian, C. (1984) A prospective study of primary cytomegalovirus infection during pregnancy: final report. *Br. J. Obstet. Gynaecol.*, **91**, 307–315.

14. Stern, H. and Tucker, S.M. (1973) Prospective study of cytomegalovirus infection in pregnancy. *Br. Med. J.*, **2**, 268–270.

15. Chandler, S.H., Holmes, K.K., Wentworth, B.B. *et al.* (1985) The epidemiology of cytomegaloviral infection in women attending a sexually transmitted disease clinic. *J. Infect. Dis.*, **152**, 597–605.

16. Chandler, S.H., Alexander, E.R. and Holmes, K.K. (1985) Epidemiology of cytomegaloviral infection in a heterogeneous population of pregnant women. *J. Infect. Dis.*, **152**, 249–256.

17. Sohn, Y.M., Oh, M.K., Balcarek, K.B., Cloud, G.A. and Pass, R.F. (1991) Cytomegalovirus infection in sexually active adolescents. *J. Infect. Dis.*, **163**, 460–463.

18. Fowler, K.B. and Pass, R.F. (1991) Sexually transmitted diseases in mothers of neonates with congenital cytomegalovirus infection. *J. Infect. Dis.*, **164**, 259–264.

19. Pass, R.F., August, A.M., Dworsky, M.E. and Reynolds, D.W. (1982) Cytomegalovirus infection in a day care center. *N. Engl. J. Med.*, **307**, 477–479.

20. Pass, R.F., Hutto, C., Reynolds, D.W. and Polhill, R.B. (1984) Increased frequency of cytomegalovirus in children in group day care. *Pediatrics*, **74**, 121–126.

21. Adler, S.P. (1985) The molecular epidemiology of cytomegalovirus transmission among children attending a day care center. *J. Infect. Dis.*, **152**, 760–768.

22. Pass, R.F., Hutto, C., Lyon, M.D. and Cloud, G. (1990) Increased rate of cytomegalovirus infection among day care center workers. *Pediatr. Infect. Dis. J.*, **9**, 465–470.

23. Adler, S.P. (1989) Cytomegalovirus and child day care. Evidence for an increased infection rate among day-care workers. *N. Engl. J. Med.*, **321**, 1290–1296.

24. Pass, R.F., Hutto, S.C., Ricks, R. and Cloud, G.A. (1986) Increased rate of cytomegalovirus infection among parents of children attending day care centers. *N. Engl. J. Med.*, **314**, 1414–1418.

25. Murph, J.R., Bale, J.F., Murray, J.C., Stinski, M.F. and Perlman, S. (1986) Cytomegalovirus transmission in a Midwest day care center: possible relationship to child care practices. *J. Pediatr.*, **109**, 35–39.

26. Adler, S.P. (1988) Molecular epidemiology of cytomegalovirus: viral transmission among children attending a day care center, their parents, and caretakers. *J. Pediatr.*, **112**, 366–372.

27. Pass, R.F., Little, E.A., Stagno, S., Britt, W.J. and Alford, C.A. (1987) Young children as a probable source of maternal and congenital cytomegalovirus infection. *N. Engl. J. Med.*, **316**, 1366–1370.

28. Preece, P.M., Tookey, P., Ades, A. and Peckham, C.S. (1986) Congenital cytomegalovirus infection: predisposing maternal factors. *J. Epidemiol. Comm. Health.*, **40**, 205–209.

29. Reynolds, D.W., Stagno, S., Hosty, T.S., Tiller, M. and Alford, C.A. (1973) Maternal cytomegalovirus excretion and perinatal infection. *N. Engl. J. Med.*, **289**, 1–5.

30. Knox, G.E., Pass, R.F., Reynolds, D.W., Stagno, S. and Alford, C.A. (1979) Comparative prevalence of subclinical cytomegalovirus and herpes simplex virus infections in the genital and urinary tracts of low income, urban females. *J. Infect. Dis.*, **140**, 419–422.

31. Pass, R.F., Stagno, S., Dworsky, M.E., Smith, R.J. and Alford, C.A. (1982) Excretion of cytomegalovirus in mothers: observation after delivery of congenitally infected and normal infants. *J. Infect. Dis.*, **146**, 1–6.

32. Numazaki, Y., Yano, N., Morizuka, T., Takai, S. and Ishida, N. (1970) Primary infection with human cytomegalovirus: virus isolation from healthy infants and pregnant women. *Am. J. Epidemiol.*, **91**, 410–417.

33. Stagno, S., Reynolds, D.W., Tsiantos, A. *et al.* (1975) Cervical cytomegalovirus excretion in pregnant and nonpregnant women: suppression in early gestation. *J. Infect. Dis.*, **131**, 522–527.

34. Shen, C.Y., Chang, S.F., Yen, M.S. *et al.* (1993) Cytomegalovirus excretion in pregnant and nonpregnant women. *J. Clin. Microbiol.*, **31**, 1635–1636.

35. Shen, C.Y., Chang, S.F., Chao, M.F. *et al.* (1993) Cytomegalovirus recurrence in seropositive pregnant women attending obstetric clinics. *J. Med. Virol.*, **41**, 24–29.

36. Hayes, D., Danks, M., Givas, H. and Jack, I. (1972) Cytomegalovirus in human milk. *N. Engl. J. Med.*, **287**, 177.

37. Stagno, S., Reynolds, D.W., Pass, R.F. and Alford, C.A. (1980) Breast milk and the risk of cytomegalovirus infection. *N. Engl. J. Med.*, **302**, 1073–1076.

38. Dworsky, M., Yow, M., Stagno, S., Pass, R.F. and Alford, C.A. (1983) Cytomegalovirus infection of breast milk and transmission in infancy. *Pediatrics*, **72**, 295–299.

39. Ahlfors, K. and Ivarsson, S.A. (1985) Cytomegalovirus in breast milk of Swedish milk donors. *Scand. J. Infect. Dis.*, **17**, 11.

40. Pass, R.F. (1986) Transmission of viruses through human milk. In *Role of Human Milk in Infant Nutrition and Health*, (eds R.R. Howell, F.H. Morriss and L.K. Pickering), Charles C. Thomas, Springfield, IL, pp. 205–224.

41. Hirota, K., Muraguchi, K., Watabe, N. *et al.* (1992) Prospective study on maternal, intra-uterine, and perinatal infections with cytomegalovirus in Japan during 1976–1990. *J. Med. Virol.*, **37**, 303–306.

42. McVoy, M.A. and Adler, S.P. (1989) Immunologic evidence for frequent age-related cytomegalovirus reactivation in seropositive immunocompetent individuals. *J. Infect. Dis.*, **160**, 1–10.

43. Stagno, S., Reynolds, D.W., Huang, E.S. *et al.* (1977) Congenital cytomegalovirus infection: occurrence in an immune population. *N. Engl. J. Med.*, **296**, 1254–1258.

44. Schwebke, K., Henry, K., Balfour, H.H. *et al.* (1995) Congenital cytomegalovirus infection as a result of nonprimary cytomegalovirus disease in a mother with acquired immunodeficiency syndrome. *J. Pediatr.*, **126**, 293–295.

45. Morris, D.J., Sims, D., Chiswick, M., Das, V.K. and Newton, V.E. (1994) Symptomatic congenital cytomegalovirus infection after maternal recurrent infection. *Pediatr. Infect. Dis. J.*, **13**, 61–64.

46. Laifer, S.A., Ehrlich, G.D., Huff, D.S., Balsan, M.J. and Scantlebury, V.P. (1995) Congenital cytomegalovirus infection in offspring of liver transplant recipients. *Clin. Infect. Dis.*, **20**, 52–55.

47. Evans, T.J., McCollum, J.P.K. and Valdimarsson, H. (1975) Congenital cytomegalovirus infection after maternal renal transplantation. *Lancet*, **i**, 1359–1360.

48. Ho, M. (1991) *Cytomegalovirus Biology and Infection*. Plenum Press, New York.

49. Yeager, A.S., Grumet, F.C., Hafleigh, E.B. *et al.* (1981) Prevention of transfusion-acquired cytomegalovirus infections in newborn infants. *J. Pediatr.*, **98**, 281–287.

50. de Graan-Hentzen, Y.C.E., Gratama, J.W., Mudde, G.C. *et al.* (1989) Prevention of primary cytomegalovirus infection in patients with hematologic malignancies by intensive white cell depletion of blood products. *Transfusion*, **29**, 757–760.

51. Gilbert, G.L., Hudson, I., Hayes, K. and James, J. (1989) Prevention of transfusion-acquired cytomegalovirus infection in infants by blood filtration to remove leucocytes. *Lancet*, **1**, 1228–1231.

52. Lang, D.J. and Kummer, J.F. (1975) Cytomegalovirus in semen: observations in selected populations. *J. Infect. Dis.*, **132**, 472–473.

53. Collier, A.C., Meyers, J.D., Corey, L. *et al.* (1987) Cytomegalovirus infection in homosexual men. Relationship to sexual practices, antibody to human immunodeficiency virus, and cell-mediated immunity. *Am. J. Med.*, **23**, 593–601.

54. Biggar, R.J., Anderson, H.K., Ebbesen, P. *et al.* (1983) Seminal fluid excretion of cytomegalovirus related to immunosuppression in homosexual men. *Br. Med. J.*, **286**, 2010–2012.

55. Mintz, L., Drew, W.L., Miner, R.C. and Braff, E.H. (1983) Cytomegalovirus infections in homosexual men. *Ann. Intern. Med.*, **99**, 326–329.

56. American Fertility Society (1990) New guidelines for the use of semen donor insemination. *Fertil. Steril.*, **53**(S1), 1–7.

57. Dworsky, M., Welch, K., Cassady, G. and Stagno, S. (1983) Occupational risk for primary cytomegalovirus infection among pediatric health care workers. *N. Engl. J. Med.*, **309**, 950–953.

58. Spector, S.A. (1983) Transmission of cytomegalovirus among infants in hospital documented by restriction endonuclease digestion analyses. *Lancet*, **1**, 378–381.

59. Demmler, G.J., Yow, M.D., Spector, S.A. *et al.* (1987) Nosocomial cytomegalovirus infections within two hospitals caring for infants and children. *J. Infect. Dis.*, **156**, 9–16.

60. Faix, R.G. (1985) Survival of cytomegalovirus on environmental surfaces. *J. Pediatr.*, **106**, 649–652.

61. Hutto, C., Little, E.A., Ricks, R., Lee, J.D. and Pass, R.F. (1986) Isolation of cytomegalovirus from toys and hands in a day care center. *J. Infect. Dis.*, **154**, 527–530.

62. Griffiths, P.D., Panjwani, D.D., Stirk, P.R. *et al.* (1984) Rapid diagnosis of cytomegalovirus infection in immunocompromised patients by detection of early antigen fluorescent foci. *Lancet*, **2**, 1242–1245.

63. Horwitz, C.A., Henle, W. and Henle, G. (1979) Diagnostic aspects of the cytomegalovirus mononucleosis syndrome in previously healthy persons. *Postgrad. Med.*, **66**, 153–158.

64. Klemola, E. and Kaariainen, L. (1965) Cytomegalovirus as a possible cause of a disease resembling infectious mononucleosis. *Br. Med. J.*, **2**, 1099–1102.

65. Klemola, E., Kaariainen, L., von Essen, R. *et al.* (1967) Further studies on cytomegalovirus mononucleosis in previously healthy individuals. *Acta Medica Scand.*, **182**, 311–322.

66. Klemola, E., von Essen, R., Henle, G. and Henle, W. (1970) Infectious mononucleosis-like disease with negative heterophil agglutination test. Clinical features in relation to Epstein–Barr virus and cytomegalovirus antibodies. *J. Infect. Dis.*, **121**, 608–614.

67. Jordan, M.C., Rousseau, W.E., Stewart, J.A., Noble, G.R. and Chin, T.D.Y. (1973) Spontaneous cytomegalovirus mononucleosis: clinical and laboratory observations in nine cases. *Ann. Intern. Med.*, **79**, 153–160.

68. Sterner, G., Agell, B.O., Wahren, B. and Espmark, A. (1970) Acquired cytomegalovirus infection in older children and adults. *Scand. J. Infect. Dis.*, **2**, 95–103.

69. Carlstrom, G., Alden, J., Belfrage, S. *et al.* (1968) Acquired cytomegalovirus infection. *Br. Med. J.*, **2**, 521–552.

70. Arnold, A.G., Lawrence, D.S. and Corbitt, G. (1978) Cytomegalovirus infection and the Guillain–Barré syndrome. *Postgrad. Med. J.*, **54**, 112–114.

71. Browning, J.D., More, I. and Boyd, J.F. (1980) Adult pulmonary cytomegalic inclusion disease: report of a case. *J. Clin. Pathol.*, **33**, 11–18.

72. Kabins, S., Keller, R., Naraqi, S. and Peitchel, R. (1976) Viral ascending radiculomyelitis with severe hypoglycorrachia. *Arch. Intern. Med.*, **136**, 933–935.

73. Leonard, J.C. and Tobin, J.O.H. (1971) Polyneuritis associated with cytomegalovirus infections. *Q. J. Med.*, **40**, 435–442.

74. Back, E., Hoglund, C. and Malmlund, H.O. (1977) Cytomegalovirus infection associated with severe encephalitis. *Scand. J. Infect. Dis.*, **9**, 141–143.

75. Causey, J.Q. (1976) Spontaneous cytomegalovirus mononucleosis-like syndrome and aseptic meningitis. *South. Med. J.*, **69**, 1384–1387.

76. Murray, H.W. (1976) CMV retinitis. *Br. Med. J.*, **2**, 1071.

77. Sahud, M.A. and Bachelor, M.M. (1978) Cytomegalovirus-induced thrombocytopenia. An unusual case report. *Arch. Intern. Med.*, **138**, 1573–1575.

78. Berlin, B.S., Chandler, R. and Green, D. (1977) Anti-'i' antibody and hemolytic anemia associated with spontaneous cytomegalovirus mononucleosis. *Am. J. Clin. Pathol.*, **67**, 459–461.

79. Gadler, H. and Wahren, B. (1978) Increased serum alpha-fetoprotein levels in cytomegalovirus infections. *Scand. J. Infect. Dis.*, **10**, 101–105.

80. Wager, O., Rasanen, J.A., Hagman, A. and Klemola, E. (1968) Mixed cryoimmunoglobulinaemia in infectious mononucleosis and cytomegalovirus mononucleosis. *Int. Arch. Allergy Appl. Immunol.*, **34**, 345–361.

81. Klacsmann, P. (1977) Cytomegalovirus mononucleosis. *Del. Med. J.*, **49**, 499–509.

82. Klemola, E., von Essen, R., Wager, O. *et al.* (1969) Cytomegalovirus mononucleosis in previously healthy individuals. *Ann. Intern. Med.*, **71**, 11–19.

83. Klemola, E. (1973) Cytomegalovirus infection in previously healthy adults. *Ann. Intern. Med.*, **79**, 267–268.

84. Doerr, H.W., Rentschler, M. and Scheifler, G. (1987) Serologic detection of active infections with human herpes viruses (CMV, EBV, HSV, VZV): diagnostic potential of IgA class and IgG subclass-specific antibodies. *Infection*, **15**, 93–98.

85. Linde, G.A., Hammarstrom, L., Persson, M.A.A. *et al.* (1983) Virus-specific antibody activity of different subclasses of immunoglobulins G and A in cytomegalovirus infections. *Infect. Immun.*, **42**, 237–244.

86. Griffiths, P.D., Stagno, S., Pass, R.F., Smith, R.J. and Alford, C.A. (1982) Infection with cytomegalovirus during pregnancy: specific IgM antibodies as a marker of recent primary infection. *J. Infect. Dis.*, **145**, 647–653.

87. Perillie, P.E. and Glenn, W.W.L. (1962) Fever, splenomegaly and eosinophilia: a new post-pericardiotomy syndrome. *Yale J. Biol. Med.*, **34**, 625–628.

88. Reyman, T.A. (1966) Postperfusion syndrome: a review and report of 21 cases. *Am. Heart. J.*, **72**, 116–123.

89. Seaman, A.J. and Starr, A. (1962) Febrile postcardiotomy lymphocytic splenomegaly: a new entity. *Ann. Surg.*, **156**, 956–960.

90. Foster, K.M. (1966) Post-transfusion mononucleosis. *Aust. Ann. Med.*, **15**, 305–310.

91. Holsward, T.R., Engle, M.A., Redo, S.F., Goldsmith, E.I. and Barondess, J.A. (1963) Development of viral diseases and a viral disease-like syndrome after extracorporeal circulation. *Circulation*, **27**, 812–815.

92. Boppana, S.B., Pass, R.F., Britt, W.J., Stagno, S. and Alford, C.A. (1992) Symptomatic congenital cytomegalovirus infection: neonatal morbidity and mortality. *Pediatr. Infect. Dis. J.*, **11**, 93–99.

93. Demmler, G.J. (1991) Infectious Diseases Society of America and Centers for Disease Control. Summary of a workshop on surveillance for congenital cytomegalovirus disease. *Rev. Infect. Dis.*, **13**, 315–329.

94. Ahlfors, K., Harris, S., Ivarsson, S. and Svanberg, L. (1981) Secondary maternal cytomegalovirus infection causing symptomatic congenital infection. *N. Engl. J. Med.*, **305**, 284.

95. Rutter, D., Griffiths, P. and Trompeter, R.S. (1985) Cytomegalic inclusion disease after recurrent maternal infection. *Lancet*, **2**, 1182.

96. Stagno, S., Pass, R.F., Dworsky, M.E. *et al.* (1982) Congenital cytomegalovirus infection: the relative importance of primary and recurrent maternal infection. *N. Engl. J. Med.*, **306**, 945–949.

97. Boppana, S.B., Fowler, K.B., Vaid, Y. *et al.* (1997) Neuroradiographic findings in the newborn period and long-term outcome in children with symptomatic congenital cytomegalovirus infection. *Pediatrics*, **99**, 409–414.

98. Fowler, K.B., Stagno, S., Pass, R.F. *et al.* (1992) The outcome of congenital cytomegalovirus infection in relation to maternal antibody status. *N. Engl. J. Med.*, **326**, 663–667.

99. Pass, R.F., Stagno, S., Myers, G.J. and Alford, C.A. (1980) Outcome of symptomatic congenital CMV infection: results of long-term longitudinal follow-up. *Pediatrics*, **66**, 758–762.

100. Conboy, T.J., Pass, R.F., Stagno, S. *et al.* (1987) Early clinical manifestations and intellectual outcome in children with symptomatic congenital cytomegalovirus infection. *J. Pediatr.*, **111**, 343–348.

101. Bale, J.F., Blackman, J.A. and Sato, Y. (1990) Outcome in children with symptomatic congenital cytomegalovirus infection. *J. Child Neurol.*, **5**, 131–136.

102. Kumar, M.L., Nankervis, G.A., Cooper, A.R. and Gold, E. (1984) Postnatally acquired cytomegalovirus infections in infants of CMV-excreting mothers. *J. Pediatr.*, **104**, 669–673.

103. Fowler, K.B., McCollister, F.P., Dahle, A.J. *et al.* (1997) Progressive and fluctuating sensorineural hearing loss in children with asymptomatic congenital cytomegalovirus infection. *J. Pediatr.*, **130**, 624–630.

104. Ivarsson, S.A., Lernmark, B. and Svanberg, L. (1997) Ten-year clinical, developmental and intellectual follow-up of children with congenital cytomegalovirus infection without neurologic symptoms at one year of age. *Pediatrics*, **99**, 800–803.

105. Stagno, S., Reynolds, D.W., Amos, C.S. *et al.* (1977) Auditory and visual defects resulting from symptomatic and subclinical congenital cytomegaloviral and toxoplasma infections. *Pediatrics*, **59**, 669–678.

106. Melish, M.E. and Hanshaw, J.B. (1973) Congenital cytomegalovirus infection: developmental progress of infants detected by routine screening. *Am. J. Dis. Child.*, **126**, 190–194.

107. Saigal, S., Luynk, O., Larke, B. and Chernesky, M.A. (1982) The outcome in children with congenital cytomegalovirus infection: a longitudinal follow-up study. *Am. J. Dis. Child.*, **136**, 896–901.

108. Kumar, M.L., Nankervis, G.A. and Gold, E. (1973) Inapparent congenital cytomegalovirus infection: a follow-up study. *N. Engl. J. Med.*, **288**, 1370–1377.

109. Reynolds, D.W., Stagno, S., Stubbs, K.G. *et al.* (1974) Inapparent congenital cytomegalovirus infection with elevated cord IgM levels: causal relationship with auditory and mental deficiency. *N. Engl. J. Med.*, **209**, 291–296.

110. Williamson, W.D., Percy, A.K., Yow, M.D. *et al.* (1990) Asymptomatic congenital cytomegalovirus infection. *Am. J. Dis. Child.*, **144**, 1365–1368.

111. Preece, P.M., Pearl, K.N. and Peckham, C.S. (1984) Congenital cytomegalovirus infection. *Arch. Dis. Child.*, **59**, 1120–1126.

112. Pearl, K.N., Preece, P.M., Ades, A. and Peckham, C.S. (1986) Neurodevelopmental assessment after congenital cytomegalovirus infection. *Arch. Dis. Child.*, **62**, 323–326.

113. Ahlfors, K., Ivarsson, S.A., Harris, S. *et al.* (1984) Congenital cytomegalovirus infection and disease in Sweden and the relative importance of primary and secondary maternal infections. *Scand. J. Infect. Dis.*, **16**, 129–137.

114. Williamson, W.D., Demmler, G.J., Percy, A.K. and Catlin, F.I. (1992) Progressive hearing loss in infants with asymptomatic congenital cytomegalovirus infection. *Pediatrics*, **90**, 862–866.

115. Nelson, C.T., Demmler, G.J., Istas, A.S. *et al.* (1996) Neurodevelopmental outcome in asymptomatic congenital cytomegalovirus infection. *Pediatr. Res.*, **39**, 181A.

116. Yow, M.D., Williamson, D.W., Leeds, L.J. *et al.* (1988) Epidemiologic characteristics of cytomegalovirus infection in mothers and their infants. *Am. J. Obstet. Gynecol.*, **158**, 1189–1195.

117. Medearis, D.N. (1982) CMV immunity: imperfect but protective. *N. Engl. J. Med.*, **306**, 985–986.

118. Griffiths, P.D., Campbell-Benzie, A. and Heath, R.B. (1980) A prospective study of primary cytomegalovirus infection in pregnant women. *Br. J. Obstet. Gynaecol.*, **87**, 308–314.

119. Gehrz, R.C., Markers, S.C., Knorr, S.O., Kalis, J.M. and Balfour, H.H. (1977) Specific cell-mediated immune defect in active cytomegalovirus infection of young children and their mothers. *Lancet*, **2**, 844–847.

120. Pass, R.F., Stagno, S., Britt, W.J. and Alford, C.A. (1983) Specific cell mediated immunity and the natural history of congenital infection with cytomegalovirus. *J. Infect. Dis.*, **148**, 953–961.

121. Starr, S.E., Tolpin, M.D., Friedman, H.M., Paucker, K. and Plotkin, S.A. (1979) Impaired cellular immunity to cytomegalovirus in congenitally infected children and their mothers. *J. Infect. Dis.*, **140**, 500–505.

122. Alford, C.A., Hayes, K. and Britt, W.J. (1988) Primary cytomegalovirus infection in pregnancy: comparison of antibody responses to virus encoded proteins between women with and without intrauterine infection. *J. Infect. Dis.*, **158**, 917–924.

123. Britt, W.J. and Vugler, L.G. (1990) Antiviral antibody responses in mothers and their newborn infants with clinical and subclinical congenital cytomegalovirus infections. *J. Infect. Dis.*, **161**, 214–219.

124. Boppana, S.B. and Britt, W.J. (1995) Antiviral antibody responses and intrauterine transmission after primary maternal cytomegalovirus infection. *J. Infect. Dis.*, **171**, 1115–1121.

125. Adler, S.P., Starr, S.E., Plotkin, S.A. *et al.* (1995) Immunity induced by primary human cytomegalovirus infection protects against

secondary infection among women of child-bearing age. *J. Infect. Dis.*, **171**, 26–32.

126. Harrison, C.J., Britt, W.J., Chapan, N.M., Mullican, J. and Tracy, S. (1995) Reduced congenital cytomegalovirus (CMV) infection after maternal immunization with a guinea pig CMV glycoprotein before gestational primary CMV infection in the guinea pig model. *J. Infect. Dis.*, **172**, 1212–1220.

127. Bourne, N., Rosteck, R., Fox, D., Schleiss, M. and Bernstein, D.I. (1996) Immunization with a cytomegalovirus (CMV) glycoprotein vaccine improves pregnancy outcome in an animal model of congenital CMV infection [abstract]. *Program and Abstracts, 36th ICAAC*, p.179.

128. Balcarek, K.B., Oh, M.K. and Pass, R.F. (1993) Maternal viremia and congenital CMV infection. In *Multidisciplinary Approach to Understanding Cytomegalovirus Disease*, (eds S. Michelson and S.A. Plotkin), Excerpta Medica, New York, pp.169–173.

129. Griffith, B.P., Chen, M. and Isom, H.C. (1990) Role of primary and secondary maternal viremia in transplacental guinea pig cytomegalovirus transfer. *J. Virol.*, **64**, 1991–1997.

130. Mocarski, E.S., Bonyhadi, M., Salimi, S. and McCune, J. (1993) Human cytomegalovirus in a SCID-hu mouse: thymic epithelial cells are prominent targets of viral replication. *Proc. Natl Acad. Sci. USA*, **90**, 104–108.

131. Koedood, M., Fichtel, A., Meier, P. and Mitchell, P.J. (1995) Human cytomegalovirus (HCMV) immediate-early enhancer/promoter specificity during embryogenesis defines target tissues of congenital HCMV infection. *J. Virol.*, **69**, 2194–2207.

132. Griffith, B.P. and Hsiung, G.D. (1980) Cytomegalovirus infection in guinea pigs. IV. Maternal infection at different stages of gestation. *J. Infect. Dis.*, **141**, 787–793.

133. Pass, R.F., Fowler, K.B., Boppana, S.B. *et al.* (1997) Congenital cytomegalovirus infection following first trimester maternal infection. *J. Pediatr.*, in press.

134. Preece, P.M., Blount, J.M., Glover, J. *et al.* (1983) The consequences of primary cytomegalovirus infection in pregnancy. *Arch. Dis. Child.*, **58**, 970–975.

135. Griffith, B.P., McCormick, S.R., Fong, C.K. *et al.* (1985) The placenta as a site of cytomegalovirus infection in guinea pigs. *J. Virol.*, **55**, 402–409.

136. Balcarek, K.B., Warren, W., Smith, R.J., Lyon, M.D. and Pass, R.F. (1993) Neonatal screening for congenital cytomegalovirus infection by detection of virus in saliva. *J. Infect. Dis.*, **167**, 1433–1436.

137. Gleaves, C.A., Smith, T.F., Shuster, E.A. and Pearson, G.R. (1984) Rapid detection of cytomegalovirus in MRC-5 cells inoculated with urine specimens by using low-speed centrifugation and monoclonal antibody to an early antigen. *J. Clin. Microbiol.*, **19**, 917–919.

138. Boppana, S.B., Smith, R., Stagno, S. and Britt, W.J. (1992) Evaluation of a microtiter plate fluorescent antibody assay for rapid detection of human cytomegalovirus infections. *J. Clin. Microbiol.*, **30**, 721–723.

139. Pass, R.F., Britt, W.J. and Stagno, S. (1995) Cytomegalovirus. In *Diagnostic Procedures for Viral, Rickettsial and Chlamydial Infections*, 7th edn, (eds E.H. Lennette, D.A. Lennette and E.T. Lennette), APHA, Washington, pp.253–271.

140. Stagno, S., Tinker, M.K., Elrod, C. *et al.* (1985) Immunoglobulin M antibodies detected by enzyme-linked immunosorbent assay and radioimmunoassay in the diagnosis of cytomegalovirus infections in pregnant women and newborn infants. *J. Clin. Microbiol.*, **21**, 930–935.

141. Kangro, H.O., Booth, J.C., Bakir, T.M.F., Tryhorn, Y. and Sutherland, S. (1984) Detection of IgM antibodies against cytomegalovirus: comparison of two radioimmunoassays, enzyme-linked immunosorbent assay and immunofluorescent antibody test. *J. Med. Virol.*, **14**, 73–80.

142. Buhles, W.C., Mastre, B.J., Tinker, A.J. *et al.* (1988) The Syntex Collaborative Ganciclovir Treatment Study Group. Ganciclovir treatment of life- or sight-threatening cytomegalovirus infection: experience in 314 immunocompromised patients. *Rev. Infect. Dis.*, **10**, S495–S506.

143. Collier, A.C. and Corey, L. (1992) Therapy of cytomegalovirus infections with ganciclovir: a critical appraisal. *Curr. Clin. Top. Infect. Dis.*, **12**, 309–328.

144. Polis, M.A., deSmet, M.D., Baird, B.F. *et al.* (1993) Increased survival of a cohort of patients with acquired immunodeficiency syndrome and cytomegalovirus retinitis who received sodium phosphonoformate (foscarnet). *Am. J. Med.*, **94**, 175–180.

145. Chrisp, P. and Clissold, S.P. (1991) Foscarnet. A review of its antiviral activity, pharmacokinetic properties and therapeutic use in immunocompromised patients with cytomegalovirus retinitis. *Drugs*, **41**, 104–129.

146. Rahhal, F.M., Arevalo, J.F., Chavez de la Paz, E., Munguia, D. and Azen, S.P. (1996) Treatment of cytomegalovirus retinitis with intravitreous cidofovir in patients with AIDS. A preliminary report. *Ann. Intern. Med.*, **125**, 98–103.

147. Fukuda, S., Miyachi, M., Sugimoto, S. *et al.* (1995) A female infant successfully treated by ganciclovir for congenital cytomegalovirus infection. *Acta Paediatr. Japon.*, **37**, 206–210.

148. Vallejo, J.G., Englund, J.A., Garcia-Prats, J.A. and Demmler, G.J. (1994) Ganciclovir treatment of steroid-associated cytomegalovirus disease in a congenitally infected neonate. *Pediatr. Infect. Dis. J.*, **13**, 239–241.

149. Nigro, G., Scholz, H. and Bartmann, U. (1994) Ganciclovir therapy for symptomatic congenital cytomegalovirus infection in infants: a two-regimen experience. *J. Pediatr.*, **124**, 318–322.

150. Attard-Montalto, S.P., English, M.C., Stimmler, L. and Snodgrass, G.J. (1993) Ganciclovir treatment of congenital cytomegalovirus infection: a report of two cases. *Scand. J. Infect. Dis.*, **25**, 385–388.

151. Reigstad, H., Bjerknes, R., Markestad, T. and Myrmel, H. (1992) Ganciclovir therapy of congenital cytomegalovirus disease. *Acta Paediatr.*, **81**, 707–708.

152. Trang, J.M., Kidd, L., Gruber, W. *et al.* (1993) Linear single-dose pharmacokinetics of ganciclovir in newborns with congenital cytomegalovirus infections. *Clin. Pharmacol. Ther.*, **53**, 15–21.

153. Whitley, R.J., Cloud, G., Gruber, W. *et al.* (1997) A pharmacokinetic and pharmacodynamic evaluation of ganciclovir for the treatment of symptomatic congenital cytomegalovirus infection: results of a phase II study. *J. Infect. Dis.*, **175**, 1080–1086.

154. Kinney, J.S., Onorato, I.M., Stewart, J.A. *et al.* (1985) Cytomegaloviral infection and disease. *J. Infect. Dis.*, **151**, 772–774.

155. Plotkin, S.A., Farquhar, J. and Hornberger, E. (1976) Clinical trials of immunization with the Towne 125 strain of human cytomegalovirus. *J. Infect. Dis.*, **134**, 470–475.

156. Plotkin, S.A., Starr, S.E., Friedman, H.M. *et al.* (1989) Protective effects of Towne cytomegalovirus vaccine against low-passage cytomegalovirus administered as a challenge. *J. Infect. Dis.*, **159**, 860–865.

157. Plotkin, S.A., Starr, S.E., Friedman, H.M. *et al.* (1991) Effect of Towne live virus vaccine on cytomegalovirus disease after renal transplant. A controlled trial. *Ann. Intern. Med.*, **114**, 525–531.

158. Gonczol, E., Berencsi, K., Kauffman, E. *et al.* (1995) Preclinical evaluation of an ALVAC (canarypox) – human cytomegalovirus glycoprotein B vaccine candidate: immune response elicited in a prime/boost protocol with the glycoprotein B subunit. *Scand. J. Infect. Dis.*, **99**(suppl), 110–112.

159. Pass, R.F., Duliege, A.M., Boppana, S.B. *et al.* (1995) Immunogenicity of a recombinant CMV gB vaccine (abstract). *Pediatr. Res.*, **37**, 185A.

160. Andersen, H.K., Brostrom, K., Hansen, K.B. *et al.* (1979) A prospective study on the incidence and significance of congenital cytomegalovirus infection. *Acta Paediatr. Scand.*, **68**, 329–336.

161. Larke, R.B.P., Wheatley, E., Saigal, S. and Chernesky, M.A. (1980) Congenital cytomegalovirus infection in an urban Canadian community. *J. Infect. Dis.*, **142**, 647–653.

162. Pannuti, C.S., Boas, L.S.V., Angelo, M.J.O. *et al.* (1985) Cytomegalovirus mononucleosis in children and adults: differences in clinical presentation. *Scand. J. Infect. Dis.*, **17**, 153–156.

163. Sohn, Y.M., Park, K.I., Lee, C., Han, D.G. and Lee, W.Y. (1992) Congenital cytomegalovirus infection in Korean population with very high prevalence of maternal immunity. *J. Kor. Med. Sci.*, **7**, 47–51.

164. Grant, S., Edmond, E. and Syme, J. (1981) A prospective study of cytomegalovirus infection in pregnancy. I. Laboratory evidence of congenital infection following maternal primary and reactivated infection. *J. Infect.*, **3**, 24–31.

165. Murph, J.R., Baron, J.C., Brown, K., Ebelhack, C.L. and Bale, J.F. (1991) The occupational risk of cytomegalovirus infection among day care providers. *JAMA*, **265**, 603–608.

166. Pass, R.F., Hutto, C., Lyon, M.D. and Cloud, G. (1990) Increased rate of cytomegalovirus infection among day care center workers. *Pediatr. Infect. Dis. J.*, **9**, 465–470.

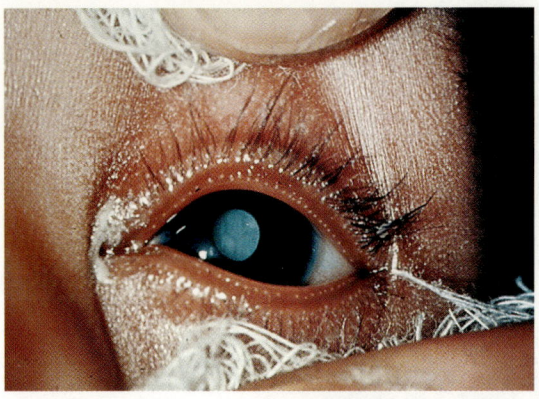

Plate A Cataract caused by intrauterine rubella.

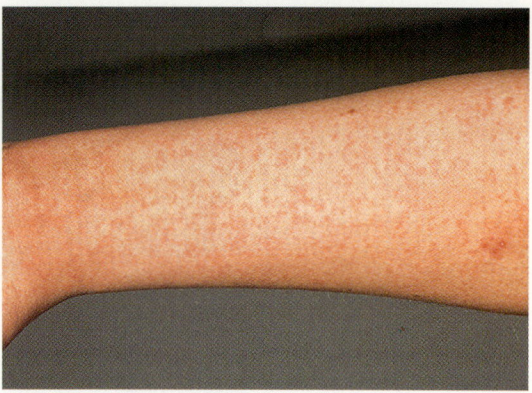

Plate B Rubella rash in adult female.

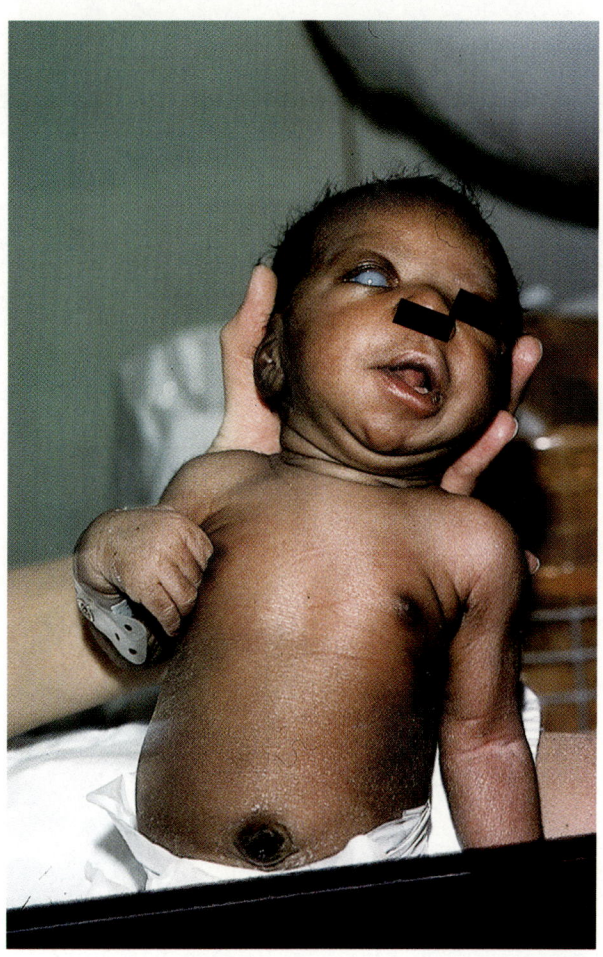

Plate C Glaucoma in infant with congenital rubella (Courtesy of Professor D.J. Jeffries).

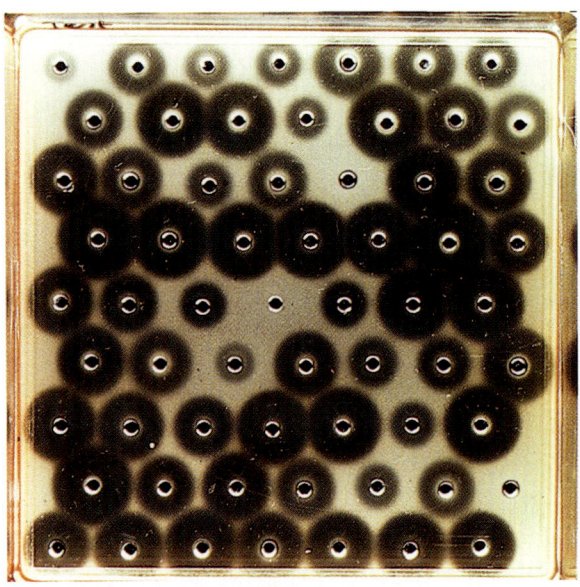

Plate D Radial haemolysis test for rubella antibody: the central well is the negative control and the two wells each side contain control serum at 15iu/ml rubella antibody.

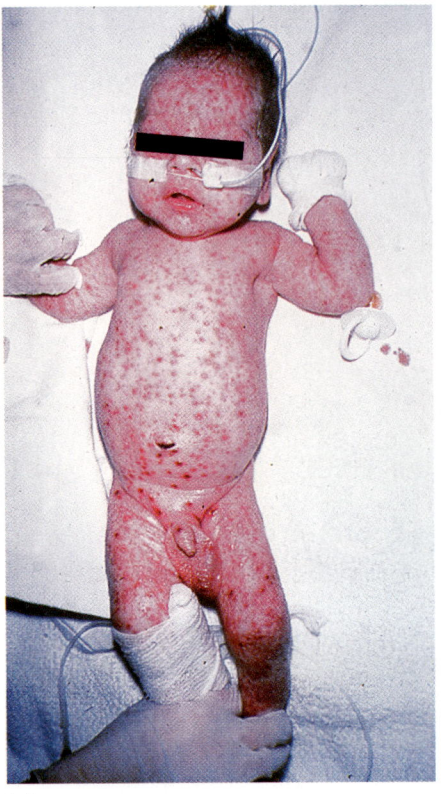

(a)

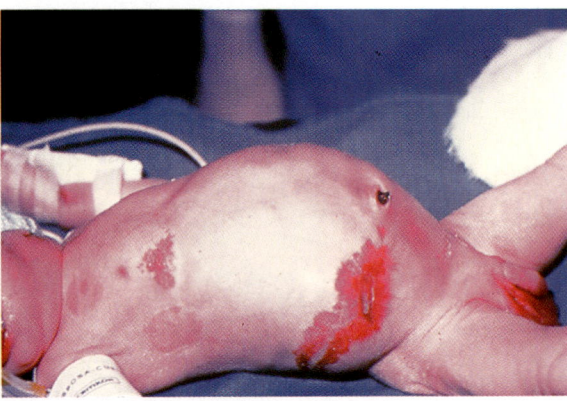

(b)

Plate E (a) Neonatal chickenpox (b) Fetal varicella syndrome.

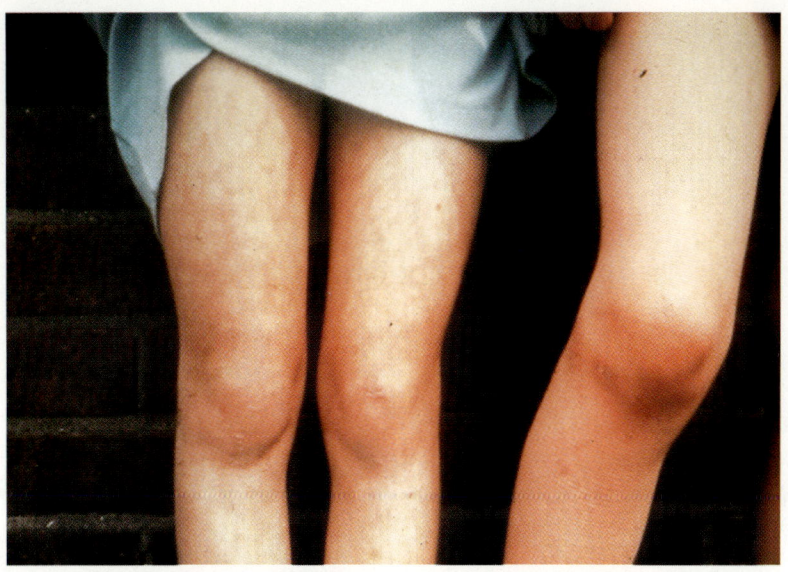

Plate F Parvovirus B19. Rash in a young girl.

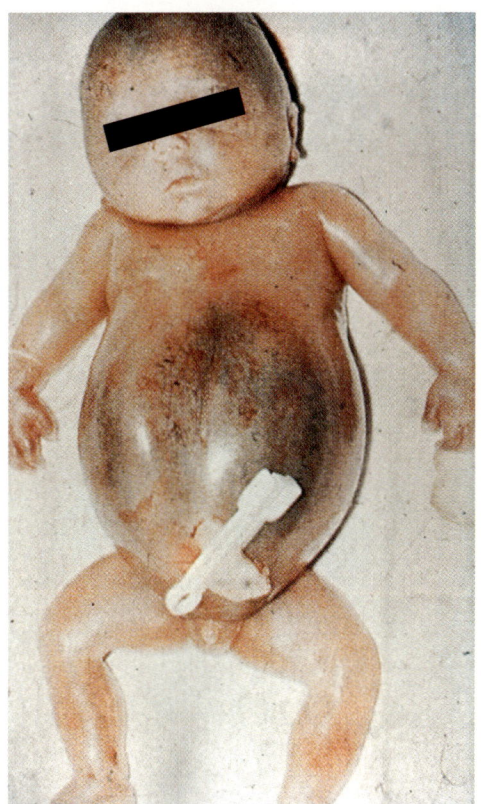

Plate G Hydrops fetalis due to parvovirus B19.

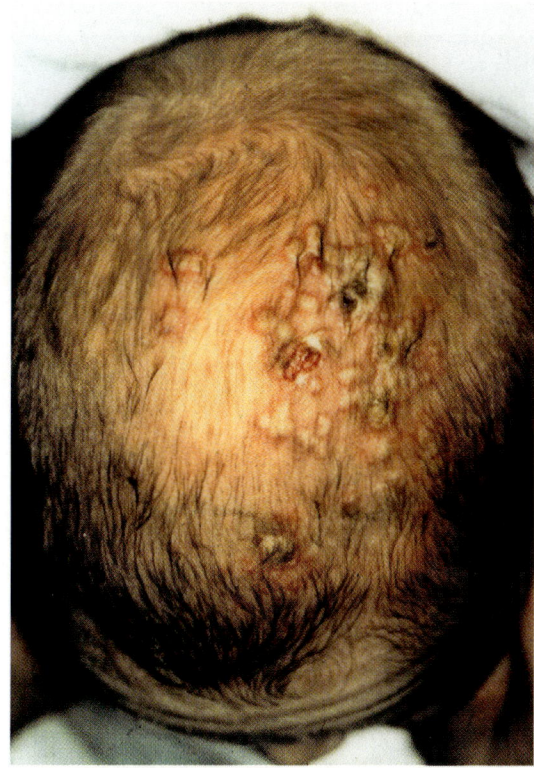

Plate H Herpes simplex vesicles – site of scalp electrode (newborn).

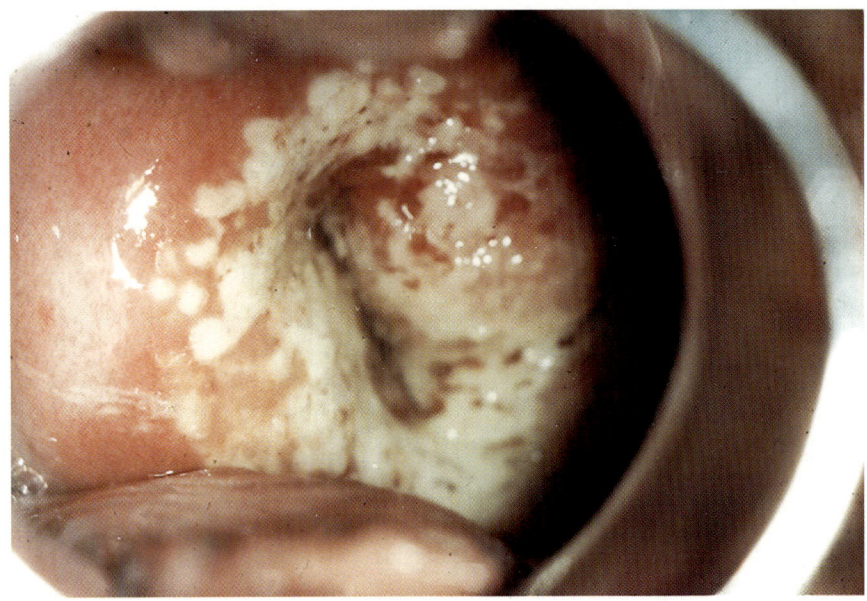

Plate I Primary herpes simplex lesions on the cervix.

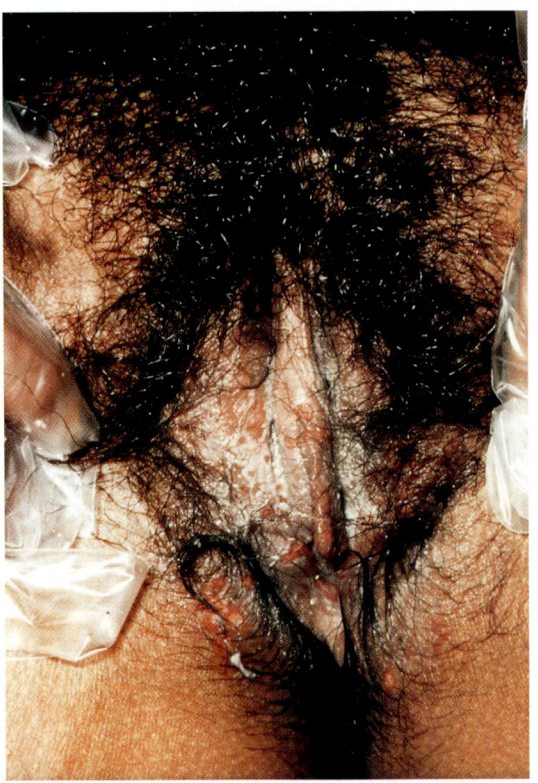

Plate J Primary genital herpes – vulval lesions.

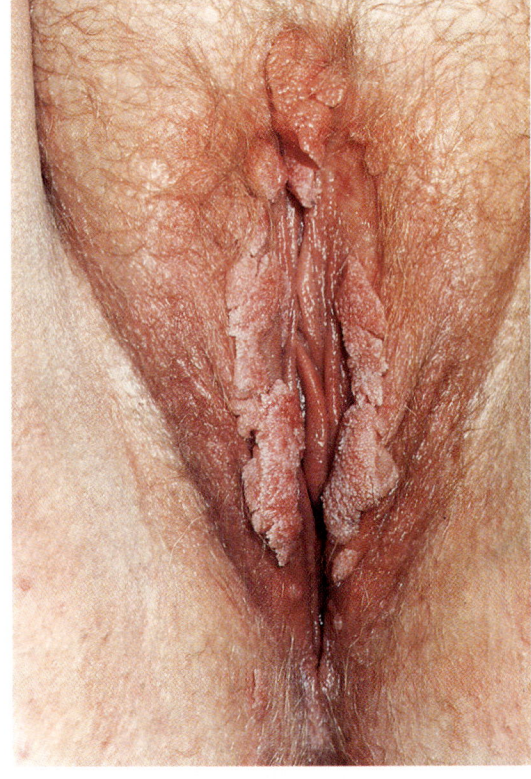

Plate K Vulval condylomata acuminatum.

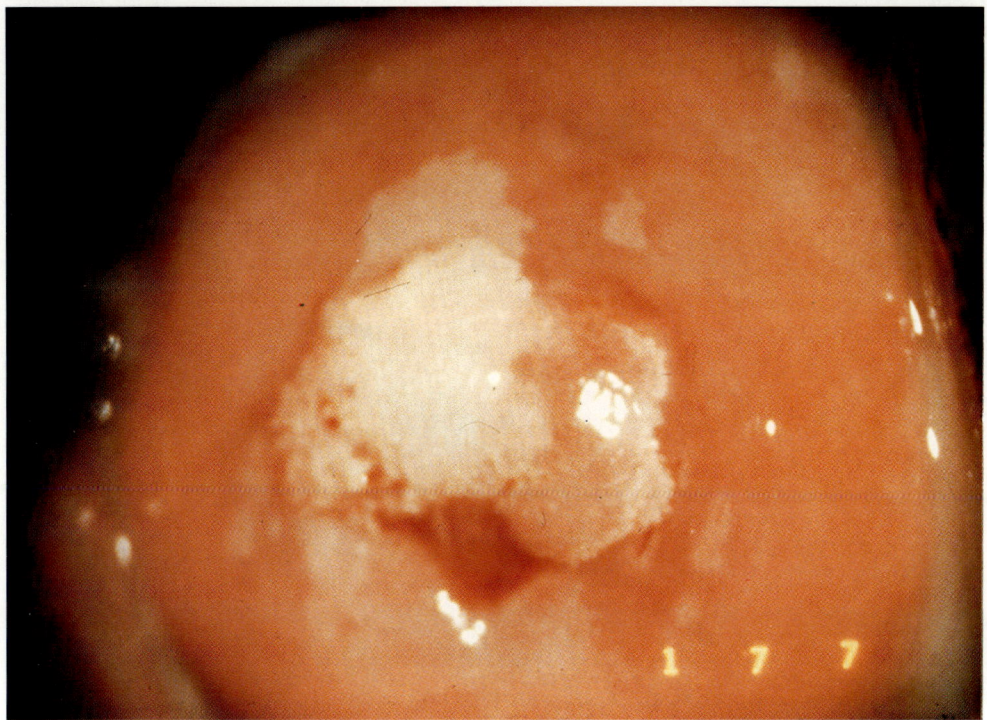

Plate L Colpophotograph of cervical wart viral lesions.

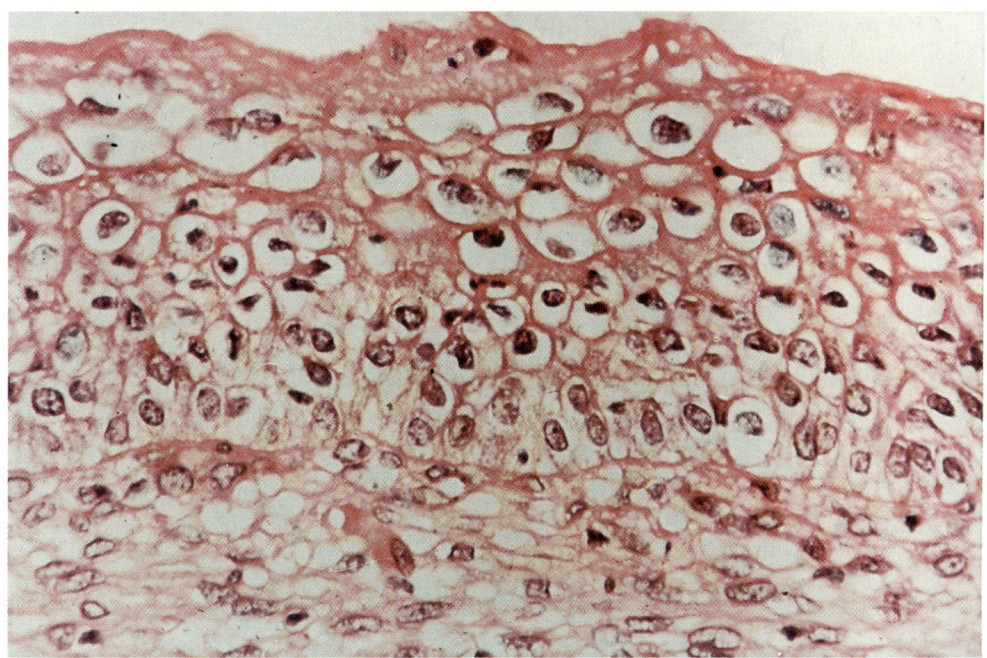

Plate M High-power histopathology of cervical wart viral lesion.

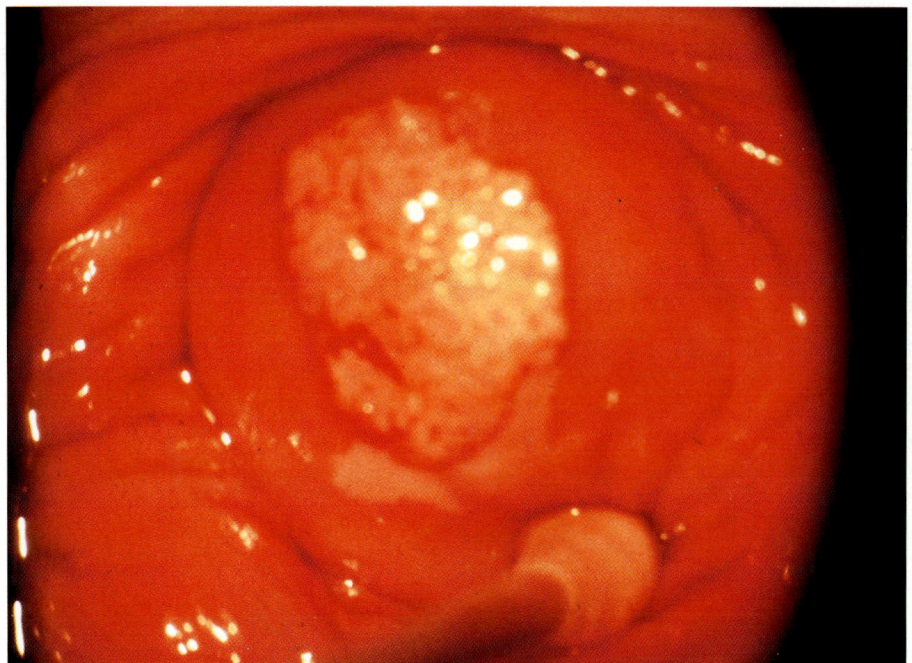

Plate N Low-power colpophotograph of condylomatous carcinoma.

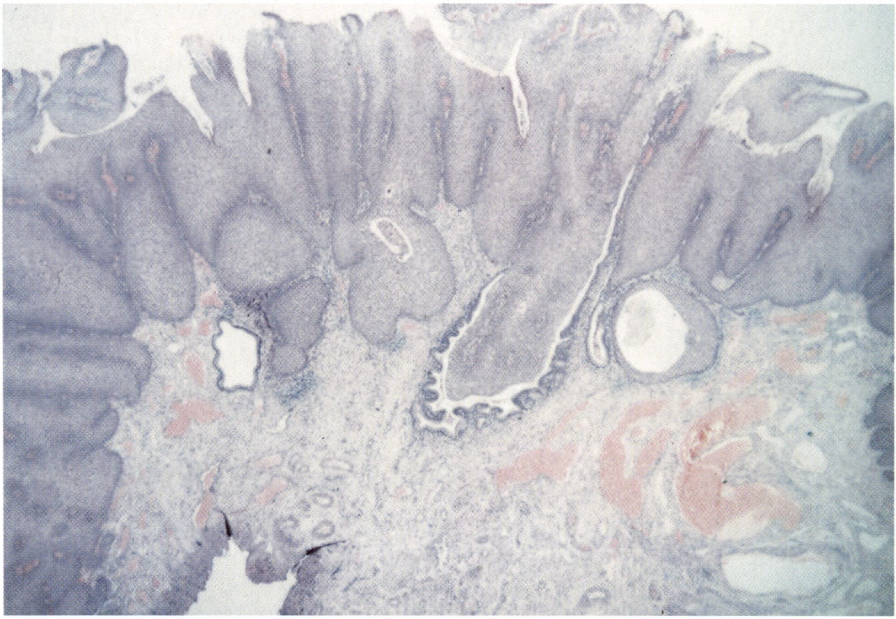

Plate O Low-power histopathology of condylomatous carcinoma.

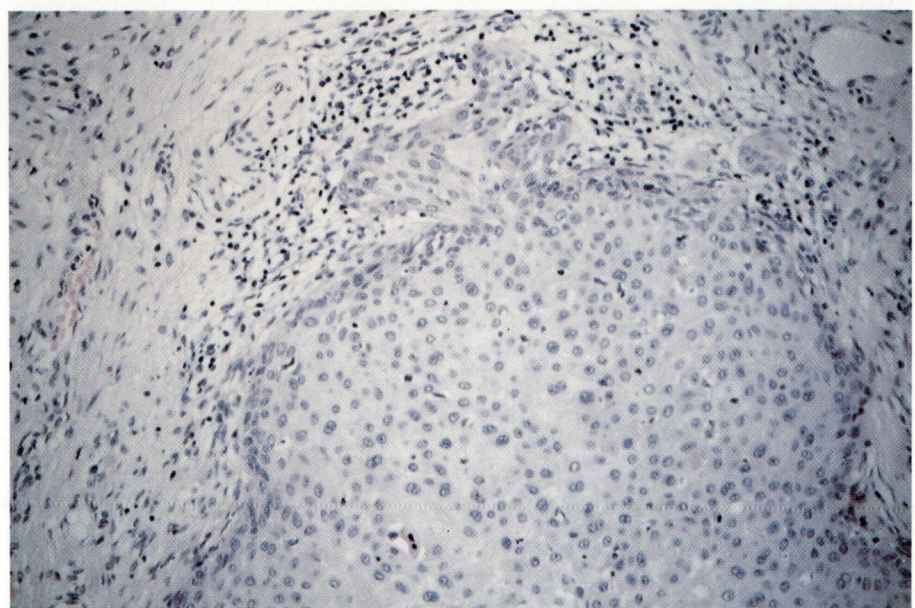

Plate P High power histopathology demonstrating early invasion.

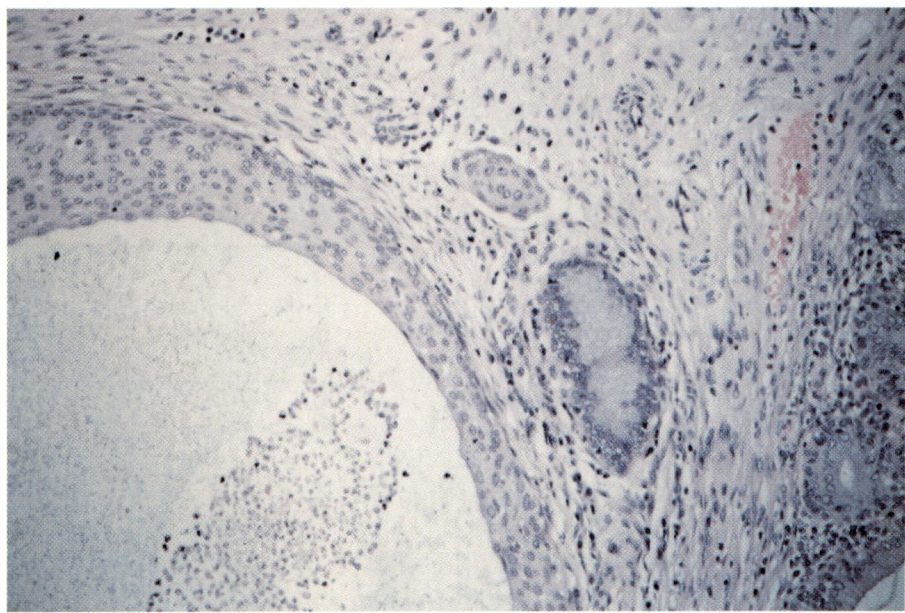

Plate Q Malignant squamous cells in an endothelial space.

Varicella-zoster virus infection in mother and baby

4

D. Carrington, K. Birthistle, D. Nathwani, S. Conway and A. MacLean

Chickenpox (varicella) is the primary infection, characterized by a widespread vesicular rash, seen after exposure to varicella-zoster virus. It is a common infection of childhood but the incidence has been increasing among adults. Complications are uncommon but morbidity and mortality are increased in those patients with an immune response that is impaired by disease and immunosuppressive treatments or compromised by age. Herpes zoster (shingles) is a reactivation of varicella-zoster virus present in a latent form in sensory ganglia and often presents clinically decades after the primary infection. The virus re-emerges as a unilateral rash in the area of the infected sensory dermatome. Complications relate to site affected, the age and immune status of the patient. Although chickenpox and shingles generally lead to uncomplicated disease in childhood, these diseases are not as benign in adults. In addition, primary infection is associated with increased morbidity and mortality for the pregnant woman, especially when varicella pneumonitis is present. A well-described but rare congenital infection is associated with varicella-zoster virus when a fetus is infected during the first 20 weeks of gestation and infection around the time of delivery can lead to neonatal varicella which has a high fatality rate if untreated. The age shift in the incidence of varicella infection presents a worrying trend, as more women will embark on pregnancy with no immunity to varicella-zoster virus.

THE VIRUS OF CHICKENPOX AND HERPES ZOSTER

Varicella-zoster virus (VZV) is member of the alphaherpesvirus group of the Herpesvirus family. The virion consists of a nucleocapsid surrounding a core of double-stranded DNA, a protein tegument which separates the inner from the outer structures of the virus and an envelope made up of human-derived membrane fragments and major viral glycoproteins. It is the smallest of the human herpesviruses but resembles herpes simplex virus (HSV) type 1 in its method of attachment and replication within human cells. VZV is an exclusive human virus and does not cause a natural infection in other mammals or invertebrate animals[1,2].

The complete VZV DNA genome has been sequenced and consists of approximately 125 000 base pairs with at least 69 open reading frames arranged in long and short unique segments with terminal repeats[3]. The infectivity of intact VZV DNA has been demonstrated and infectious virus has been produced from cosmids spanning the entire genome[4]. The major viral glycopeptides are

Viral Infections in Obstetrics and Gynaecology. Edited by D.J. Jeffries and C.N. Hudson. Published in 1999 by Arnold, ISBN 0 340 74095 7.

gB, gC, gE, gH and gL which are all expressed on the infected cell[5]. gB is highly conserved, appears to be the target of neutralizing antibodies and plays a role in virus entry. gH is essential for cell fusion and facilitates the spread of the virus from cell to cell. The latter is an essential function of the virus as VZV is highly cell-associated and there is very little virus released directly from the cell during replication. Virus is subsequently released during cell death. Replication within epidermal cells and destruction of these cells within the skin results in the formation of vesicles and the characteristic rash of chickenpox. The virus is highly contagious from vesicular fluid and easily transmitted to those susceptible individuals who have close contact with the primary or secondary source.

In common with other herpesviruses, VZV establishes latency after primary infection. The process is not as clearly understood as for HSV but does involve LAT (latency associated transcripts) genes[2,6–9]. The latency process takes place in neuronal tissue within dorsal root ganglia and involves both sensory neurones and non-neuronal satellite cells within the dorsal root ganglia (usually multiple). Reactivation of the viral genome from these cells results in reinfection of the sensory neurone and subsequently the development of shingles, usually externally (although internal rashes are seen) at a single dermatomal site (herpes zoster). It is this phenomenon of reactivation which allows the virus to persist and re-emerge to infect susceptible populations as varicella.

There is very little information on the genetic variability of varicella-zoster virus. Only a single antigenic strain is recognized but genomic differences between viruses have been reported in epidemiologically distinct strains. The significance of these changes on virus virulence is currently unknown but is under intense scrutiny.

Takahashi developed the first live attenuated vaccine containing the Oka strain of VZV[10]. This is the first human herpesvirus vaccine to be licensed in Japan and USA. Where licensed, the vaccine is used in immunocompetent children and adults, including acute lymphocytic leukaemic patients in remission, but is contraindicated in pregnancy and in severely immunosuppressed patients including those with symptomatic HIV. In open clinical trials, through sequential annual epidemics, the protective efficacy of the vaccine against varicella was demonstrated in both children and adults including household exposures where the risk of infection was >95%[11–15].

EPIDEMIOLOGY

Varicella-zoster virus is seen worldwide but variation in the epidemic spread of chickenpox is apparent. In tropical countries outbreaks of infection appear somewhat limited in scale so that significant numbers of adults remain susceptible to VZV infection. In temperate climates annual epidemics are more common, occurring mostly in late winter and early springtime[16,17]. Varicella spreads by contact with oropharyngeal secretions during the early symptomatic stage[18,19] but in the later stages transmission is predominantly by contact with vesicular fluid from the skin rash. The varicella attack rate in household contacts is ~90% and ~35% in children at school[20]. In temperate climates almost all children acquire VZV infection before 10 years of age. The susceptibility rates for adults is ~5% in temperate climates but as high as 50% in tropical countries[21]. After chickenpox, immunity to further VZV infection (as chickenpox) is solid and clinically apparent reinfection is very rare[22].

Herpes zoster (shingles) occurs only in those with a history of primary VZV infection. The only exceptions to this are in children born to mothers who had chickenpox during pregnancy. Occasionally these infants present with zoster in the first few years of life without an episode of chickenpox since birth. Studies of shingles in the UK have revealed an incidence rate of 3.4/1000/year in the general population[23] and this rate has been subsequently confirmed by a number of authors elsewhere. The rate for women of childbearing years (20–49) is 2.60/1000/year. The incidence of herpes zoster is constant throughout the year and is not subject to epidemics or case clustering other than by chance. Studies comparing the incidence of varicella and herpes zoster have shown that shingles cases do not increase during epidemics of varicella and clearly shingles has an independent and unrelated epidemiology. Although most cases of shingles occur after the age of 50 years, herpes zoster occurs in all age groups. Shingles under the age of 10 years is uncommon, with an incidence of 0.74/1000/years[24].

PATHOGENESIS OF VARICELLA AND HERPES ZOSTER

Varicella-zoster virus is acquired through inhalation of infected secretions, either by droplet or hand-to-mouth transmission. A history of contact with a known case of varicella is not always given, as VZV is transmissible 24–48 h before the rash appears. Whether from infectious droplets or secretions, the virus infects mucous membranes in the oropharynx and spreads to regional lymph nodes. This results in a primary viraemia that carries the virus to widely disseminated sites including the liver and the mononuclear-macrophagic system[25,26] during the incubation period when virus amplification occurs. This results in a secondary viraemia, at the end of a 10–14 day period from contact, lasting a further 4–5 days[27–30]. The virus is present in blood in infected lymphocytes rather than as free virus and these cells, moving into tissues, deliver the virus to epidermal cell targets. Vesicles containing varicella-zoster virus evolve from a ballooning degeneration of infected epidermal cells through macular and papular stages before bursting. Crops of vesicles appear in waves and rapidly heal through a process of ulceration, crusting and scabbing. During the early stages, infection of capillary endothelial cells occurs and a vasculitis may lead to bleeding into the vesicles. Varicella ulcers do not usually scar because the infected cells are relatively superficial and do not damage the germinal layer of the epithelium. Occasionally deep ulceration does occur following a process of skin thickness necrosis. The latter is often associated with bacterial superinfection.

The process of vesiculation is significantly different in the case of herpes zoster. VZV, during varicella, is carried to the ganglia either by ascending transneuronal flow to cell bodies in the dorsal root or by infected mononuclear cells during the viraemic phase[31,32]. The virus appears to be present in both neuronal and non-neuronal cells but is not as easily reactivated from human explanted ganglion tissue as is the case for herpes simplex virus. This suggests that there are differences in the mechanism of reactivation that pertain for VZV when compared to HSV[33]. Whichever mechanism operates to infect and reactivate virus from ganglion tissue, reactivation of VZV involves the reinfection of sensory neurones. This is followed by movement of virus down the axon to the dermatomal site and infection of epithelial cells in contact with neuronal fibres. From here the mechanism of epithelial infection and vesicle maturation is the same as in varicella. However, the vesiculation is limited to the dermatomal area supplied by the infected sensory neurone and further skin and tissue involvement is limited by humoral and cell-mediated immunity that was generated many years earlier during the previous exposure to chickenpox.

CLINICAL FEATURES

VARICELLA

An incubation period of 10–21 days, and prodromal symptoms of fever, malaise, headache and abdominal pain lasting 24–48 h, precede chickenpox. This is followed by cutaneous vesiculation, initially on the face, scalp and upper trunk, and an increase in fever to 41°C, lethargy and malaise. The skin lesions are pruritic and blisters appear in crops which extend towards the extremities and internally, involving the squamous epithelium of the mouth, conjunctivae and vagina. The number of lesions is very variable ranging from 10 to 1500 with an average of 200–300 lesions. The older the individual, the more lesions are seen. Secondary contracts to a household case are usually more severely affected and have more lesions. This may be the consequence of contact with a heavier inoculum compared to the index case where contact may have been more fleeting. Cutaneous vesiculation continues for 1–7 days and is followed by clouding of the vesicular fluid and crusting of the lesions. Although the crusts appear within 48 h of vesicle development, formation of the scab with healing of the lesions (new epithelial cells form at the base of the lesion) may take a further 7–14 days before detachment. Hypopigmentation of the new skin is common during healing. During this acute phase there may be lymphopenia and a mild elevation of liver transaminases in serum. The most common complication during varicella is secondary bacterial infection[34,35,36], usually due to *Staphylococcus aureus* and *Streptococcus pyogenes*, resulting in septicaemia which may be fatal. Appropriate antimicrobial prophylaxis significantly reduces the risk of life-threatening bacterial infection. Secondary bacterial infection of vesicular lesions results in bullous formation with surrounding cellulitis[37]. Necrotizing fasciitis[36] and varicella gangrenosa[38] are the most serious soft tissue complications resulting from bacterial superinfection. At internal sites streptococcal or staphylococcal infection during varicella may result in pneumonia, arthritis or osteomyelitis. Viral dissemination may result in transient hepatitis[39], pneumonitis[40,41], meningoencephalitis and cerebellar ataxia[42–45].

Varicella in adults is associated with pneumonitis which is evident radiologically in 10% of cases[46]. Most patients with pneumonitis present with cough and shortness of breath towards the end of the first week of the rash and improve without specific therapy. In a few cases, particularly those with high-risk features, e.g. smoking, pregnancy and immunosuppression, progression to hypoxaemia and tachypnoea is seen, as a result of the bilateral interstitial thickening of the alveolar wall with impairment of gaseous exchange. Respiratory failure is seen in severe cases and is one of the commonest causes of death in varicella.

Neurological features are seen in 13% of hospitalized cases of varicella in the US[47], not only in very young children but also in adults[47,48,49]. Encephalitis begins in the second week of the illness with a sudden change in the level of consciousness and/or generalized seizures. Cerebellar involvement is common, with ataxia, nystagmus and speech disturbances. Encephalitis usually resolves within 2–3 days although cerebellar involvement results in delayed convalescence. During the acute episode, cerebrospinal fluid examination reveals a mild lymphocytic pleocytosis, raised CSF protein levels and normal glucose levels. Fatal neurological complications are rare but usually follow encephalitis rather than cerebellitis[43,44]. Persistent seizures, transverse myelitis and paraplegia have been reported but are rare.

Haemorrhagic manifestations are seen in children and adults[49]. These follow thrombocytopenia and may result in disseminated intravascular coagulation. Bleeding into the skin, with petechiae and purpura, haematuria and melaena, epistaxis and vaginal haemorrhage may occur in complicated cases. The most serious bleeding manifestation is purpura fulminans which is the result of arterial thrombosis.

Other rare complications that are particularly serious in adults and pregnant women include nephritis, hypertension, myocarditis and pericarditis. Immunosuppressed patients, particularly those with bone marrow transplants, leukaemia or other disorders associated with depressed cell-mediated immunity, are perceived to be at high risk of the complications described above[50].

HERPES-ZOSTER

Shingles is a recognized complication of cytotoxic chemotherapy; it is therefore important in the field of gynaecological oncology.

The rash of herpes-zoster is a unilateral vesicular eruption limited to the area of the infected sensory dermatome. It may be preceded by prodromal symptoms characterized by tingling, itching and sharp pains in a superficial area of skin or deep tissue. Prodromal pain is rare in children, occasionally seen in young adults, but more consistently seen in individuals over 50 years. The difficulty for physicians is that the pain is not easily identifiable as zoster pain and is often confused with pleurisy, appendicitis or acute nerve compression. VZV-associated unilateral neuropathic pain without a rash[51] is referred to as 'zoster sine herpete' and although very difficult to substantiate, it may be suggested by rising serum antibody titres[51] and polymerase chain reaction (PCR) studies of circulating white blood cells[52].

A typical unilateral vesicular rash provides definitive evidence of herpes zoster. It can appear on any part of the body[23] although in 50% of cases it is seen in the thoracic dermatomes. Other dermatomes are affected in the following proportions: 35% of cases involving cervical and lumbar dermatomes, 15% of cases involving the ophthalmic branch of the trigeminal nerve, and 5% involving the sacral area. The rash starts as an erythematous maculopapular eruption which vesiculates within 12–24 h, ulcerates and crusts within the next three days and scabs over the following 1–3 weeks. Herpes zoster is associated with both acute neuritis and postherpetic neuralgia[53]. The acute neuralgia is often intense, sharp, tender, stabbing, shooting and throbbing in pain quality. This often lasts throughout the cutaneous eruptive stage and may persist after the rash has healed. The zoster episode is usually self-limiting, particularly in young patients, although some patients can be very distressed by sleep disturbance and a slower than expected return to normal activity levels. Shingles is usually confined to a single affected dermatome although some overlapping with adjacent dermatomes is sometimes seen. It is seen with increased frequency in patients with impaired immunity. In these patients, dissemination of varicella-zoster virus can take place with internal spread to all organs. Varicella pneumonitis and encephalitis are serious manifestations of disseminated zoster requiring early clinical recognition and prompt treatment with intravenous antiviral therapy.

The two most important complications of herpes zoster in the immunocompetent patient relate to ophthalmic zoster and postherpetic neuralgia. Ophthalmic zoster involves infection of the ophthalmic branch of the trigeminal nerve. Apart from the acute disfigurement of the rash, the development of ocular complications can be very serious. Anterior uveitis, keratitis and iridocyclitis are common (accounting for 50% of cases) while panophthalmitis, sclerokeratitis and neuropathic keratitis are the most serious complications. Blindness, however, is rare[54,55]. Loss of vision is usually associated with retrobulbar neuritis and optic atrophy[56,57].

Postherpetic neuralgia (PHN) is the most common of all zoster complications and is seen predominantly in older patients although PHN can occur at all ages. This is defined as pain persisting after the rash has healed and is usually considered of significance when pain persists for more than three months after acute symptoms. PHN lasting three months follows in 33–50% of cases, while PHN lasting for more than one year has been reported in 22–33% of patients[58]. The pain of PHN is described as tender, burning, nagging and aching and is a neuropathic pain rather than a neuritis. It is notoriously difficult to treat and best left to pain specialists.

Neurological complications associated with herpes zoster are not infrequent. Forty percent of zoster patients exhibit a raised leucocyte count and protein levels in the cerebrospinal fluid although meningism is rare. Encephalitis is seen in 0.2–0.5% of patients[59] but this complication is reportedly more common in older patients. In these cases, headache, photophobia, delirium and nystagmus are seen during the acute phase, 1–6 weeks after onset of the rash[43,59,60]. More commonly seen is motor paresis, particularly involving cranial nerves[59]. In most patients, the course of the encephalitis is benign[43], as in varicella encephalitis, but occasionally vasculitis, thrombosis and cerebral angiitis cause cerebral infarction, with a resulting mortality of 20%.

LABORATORY DIAGNOSIS OF VARICELLA-ZOSTER VIRUS INFECTIONS

Laboratory methods for the detection of VZV include virus culture, electron microscopy, immunofluorescence tests for virus antigen and nucleic acid tests for virus DNA, e.g. polymerase chain reaction (PCR), all of which can be used on material obtained from respiratory secretions or vesicular fluid. Vesicular fluid provides the optimal chance of detection by electron microscopy since the concentration of virus is greater here than in other biological fluids or tissue. As vesicles are present throughout the period of clinical concern the ability of the laboratory to provide a rapid diagnosis from clinical samples can enable early and appropriate antiviral chemotherapy and prompt infection control management.

Alternatively, serological tests for the detection of VZV-specific IgG and IgM can be performed providing circumstantial evidence of recent exposure. For the detection of antibody, sufficient time must have elapsed between exposure and antibody production. This is also dependent on the host's ability to mount a humoral response which may be compromised by immunosuppressive disease or treatment. The detection of VZV-specific IgG may indicate recent exposure when there is a significant rise in antibody titre between acute and convalescent blood samples, whereas the detection of VZV-specific IgM in a single sample is usually sufficient to indicate recent infection. Serological methods for the detection of antibodies to varicella-zoster virus include the fluorescent antibody membrane antigen assay (FAMA), latex agglutination, enzyme-linked immunoassay (EIA), complement fixation tests and neutralization antibody tests.

These methods vary in their complexity and this is reflected in the turnaround time of a meaningful laboratory result. Virus laboratories that are geared towards rapid diagnostic methods are usually able to offer most of the above tests. It is advisable to contact the virus laboratory before taking samples to ascertain which tests are most suited to the clinical case and when results will be forthcoming.

VZV culture is best obtained from human cell lines, e.g. human fetal embryo lung fibroblasts. Vesicular fluid is used to inoculate tubes of cells which are maintained for several days or weeks depending on the ability of the virus to show a virus cytopathic effect (CPE) which is characteristic of the varicella-zoster virus. This CPE is seen as a ballooning of fibroblasts, in a linear cell-to-cell progression along the fibroblast sheath, occurring after 2–7 days. Because of the similarity in the CPE between herpesviruses, the cultures are often harvested and the cells stained with virus-specific monoclonal antibodies to confirm the virus involved. The method can be accelerated by the use of shell vials, centrifuging the inoculum and staining the culture after 2–3 days with a fluorescein-conjugated monoclonal antibody to VZV, to detect VZV-specific proteins before the CPE is typical.

These methods are highly specific and the definitive standard for diagnosis, but are becoming less common as laboratories become reliant on rapid immunofluorescence tests performed on cells recovered from the base of the vesicle. The cells are obtained by scraping the ulcer with a sterile swab after lifting the roof of the vesicle with a needle. The test using polyclonal or monoclonal antibodies specific to VZV can make results available in 2–3h and is highly specific[61–65]. A further advantage of the direct immunofluorescence test is that the sample can be tested up to three days later if posted to the laboratory and it does not rely on the viability of the virus which rapidly inactivates at room temperature.

Detection of VZV by DNA PCR is becoming available in the specialist virus laboratory and is highly sensitive and specific[66]. In this test total DNA is extracted from the sample. Conserved sequences of specific VZV DNA are recognized by unique nucleic acid primer sets and act on these templates in concert with heat-stable nucleic acid polymerases to produce additional VZV DNA replicons so that amplification of specific VZV DNA is effected. These DNA products are easily characterized by size and can be detected by conventional hybridization or immunological tests. The value of these tests is evident when tissue samples with minute quantities of virus are taken for diagnostic and research purposes. The molecular characterization of isolates by restriction enzyme assays is not routinely available, but can give valuable information on the similarity between isolates. Its use in the primary characterization of chickenpox or zoster is restricted to specialized cases or outbreaks and is more of epidemiological than clinical value.

Antibody assays for VZV IgG are used to identify prior infection (previous exposure) or disease susceptibility, i.e. immune status. Knowledge of the immune status is necessary in those recently exposed because those found to be susceptible can be offered appropriate antiviral prophylaxis by the use of varicella-zoster immune globulin (VZIG/ZIG). In many cases a reliable history of chickenpox can be obtained. In others the history is vague or doubtful. It is in those patients at risk of serious disease that routine screening or post-exposure investigations can be undertaken. The presence of VZV IgG can be taken as evidence of prior exposure to varicella (despite no history of chickenpox) unless the patient has recently received passive antibodies through transfusion of certain blood products or the receipt of VZIG.

The fluorescent antibody membrane antigen assay test detects VZV antibodies in serum by the binding of these antibodies to unfixed VZV-infected cells, and the assay has been widely used in seroepidemiologcal studies and in the clinical laboratory for the determination of VZV-specific immunity. It is being replaced by commercial enzyme-linked immunoassays, which are also highly sensitive and specific now that VZV immunity screens have become widely requested and large batches of tests are done routinely. There are a number of concerns that commercial EIA tests under-detect the presence of VZV antibody in a minority of patients when compared to FAMA[67] but false-positive reactions by EIA appear to be rare. Latex agglutination tests for the detection of VZV IgG are also becoming commercially available[68] and may be useful alternatives to FAMA and EIA for occasional tests and for out-of-hours work. The complement fixation test (CFT) is a useful diagnostic test during primary infection (chickenpox) and reactivation episodes (shingles) during the acute stages, but antibody produced to the CFT antigens used is not sustained and may disappear after 2–3 years. Consequently, CFT antibody tests cannot be used for the determination of VZV immunity unless chickenpox or shingles was a recent occurrence. Neutralization antibody tests are not routinely performed for diagnosis although they can measure the ability of the serum to neutralize a standard virus challenge. Occasionally there is a need to define the quality of a serological response when there has been a loss of immune competence, e.g. after bone marrow transplantation, and residual antibody is of uncertain efficacy.

HOW COMMON IS VARICELLA IN PREGNANCY?

Chickenpox is an uncommon disease in women during their childbearing years. Recent reports from the UK[69] and USA[70] show a significant upward trend in the absolute number, and in the proportion of cases occurring in adults aged 15–44 years over the last 20 years.

In the US, varicella during pregnancy is estimated to occur in ~7.5/10 000 pregnancies[71–74]. This estimate implies approximately 7000 cases of chickenpox in pregnancy/year in the USA[75]. In the UK[69] the reported annual incidence in all adults aged 15–44 years is currently about three per 1000. Based on this figure, the estimated number of chickenpox cases in pregnancy in England and Wales is about 2000 a year. Adults from tropical or subtropical areas with varicella are likely to be over-represented in these national figures as susceptibility rates are higher in these populations.

Data available in temperate countries suggest that 85–90% of pregnant women have been exposed to varicella during childhood and therefore have immunity to VZV. There are concerns that the 10–15% who are susceptible should be identified and there is enthusiasm for serological testing at the initial pregnancy booking visit. This would identify susceptible patients who could be advised on the steps to be taken following exposure to varicella-zoster virus infection. A history of chickenpox or shingles is a good indication of immunity to VZV, while up to 80% of pregnant women who give a negative

or doubtful history of chickenpox are immune. Consequently serological testing need only be offered to the 15–25% who cannot recall having had chickenpox or where there is doubt about their childhood exposure.

IS CHICKENPOX MORE SEVERE IN PREGNANCY?

There is evidence that primary VZV infection in adults leads to increased morbidity and mortality compared with that seen in children[76]. Varicella infection for any adult may range from a trivial illness with a few skin lesions to a major life-threatening episode. The natural history of chickenpox in pregnancy is poorly defined. There is a common perception that chickenpox is generally more severe in pregnant women than in others of the same age. This stems from anecdotal data indicating an increased incidence of complications during primary infections in these women.

In an analysis of death certificates of 100 fatal chickenpox cases during 1985–90[69], immunosuppression contributed 30 cases while pregnancy was complicated by fatal varicella in only one case. The other cases were seen in immunocompetent children and adults. However, adults are 40 times more likely to have a complication during varicella than a child. A report on Confidential Enquiries into Maternal Death in the United Kingdom, 1985–7, includes 84 indirect deaths (death resulting from either a previous existing disease or from a disease which developed during pregnancy and which did not have a direct obstetric cause and which was aggravated by pregnancy), representing 30% of all direct and indirect deaths. There were 10 deaths which were considered to be related to infectious diseases and four of these were related to the respiratory complications of chickenpox. All presented between 27 and 38 weeks' gestation. In the subsequent report for the years 1988–90 (published 1994) there were three chickenpox deaths, all presenting in the second half of pregnancy. The relatively low mortality rate in these UK data is in keeping with other prospective studies which revealed only two deaths among nearly 200 patients[72,77,78].

MANAGEMENT OF VARICELLA CASES

The management of uncomplicated chickenpox in adults is primarily directed towards symptomatic treatment and hygiene to prevent secondary bacterial infection associated with the pruritic skin lesions. Antiviral therapy has traditionally been used in those with complications or severe disease. However, open and controlled trials have shown that, in immunocompetent non-pregnant adults and children, starting oral acyclovir within 24 h of the onset of the rash decreases the time to cutaneous healing and lessens symptoms and fever[79,80]. In view of the concerns related to increased severity of varicella pneumonitis, the balance of risks is in favour of giving oral acyclovir to women in the second half of pregnancy presenting within 24 h of the onset of the rash. Nevertheless, the importance of treating only with full informed consent and of entering all patients on to the Acyclovir in Pregnancy Register is stressed. The register is kept by GlaxoWellcome plc, who should be contacted with the details of the case, recording any adverse features to mother or baby. The patient's clinical progress should be closely monitored, with a full reassessment and immediate referral to hospital if respiratory or other constitutional symptoms develop. There is no evidence that starting antiviral therapy after 24 h of the onset of the rash has any effect on the natural history of chickenpox[79,80]. Pregnant women who present more than 24 h after the onset of varicella should be managed symptomatically with a medical reassessment within 48 h or earlier if there is clinical deterioration, e.g. persistent fever or continued cropping at six days.

Although acyclovir given to women with varicella at term readily crosses the placenta, and has been detectable in cord blood and neonatal urine after delivery, there is no evidence that treating pregnant women with this antiviral drug affects the course of fetal infection or reduces associated embryopathy.

MANAGEMENT OF A PREGNANT WOMAN WITH VARICELLA IN A HOSPITAL SETTING

Ideally, the pregnant woman should be managed in a specialist isolation facility with the combined expertise of obstetrician, infectious diseases physician and paediatrician[81,82]. In one study[81], women with overt varicella, or those who were believed to be incubating the disease, were managed in separately ventilated delivery rooms or ordinary isolated delivery (ID) rooms. Following delivery, the mother and newborn were transferred to an isolated ward room, if possible in an infectious disease unit. These measures led to a significant reduction in nosocomial infection among other pregnant women and newborn children, some of whom were immunocompromised. For a woman in the third trimester of pregnancy, management should ideally be in an obstetric setting or in an ID ward adjacent to an obstetric unit, whereas in the first or second trimester of pregnancy the patient should ideally be in an infectious disease unit or equivalent with close input from the obstetricians.

CRITERIA FOR HOSPITALIZATION FOR CHICKENPOX IN PREGNANCY

It is important to ensure that pregnant women are encouraged to contact their general practitioner at the first sign of chickenpox. The main decision is whether the pregnant woman can be managed in the community or requires hospitalization. This assessment involves knowledge of the risk factors which predispose to the potential complications of varicella infection. The question as to whether the fetus has been affected is frequently paramount. There appears to be no merit in performing amniocentesis or cordocentesis because the presence of virus in the amniotic fluid or fetal blood does not necessarily correlate with damage to the fetus. Scanning for limb abnormalities during the weeks after convalescence is probably the only means of monitoring for this complication, but there are clearly limits to the sensitivity of this technique. Currently it seems inappropriate to recommend termination of pregnancy, but such a decision would depend on the individual patient.

The criteria for hospitalization relate to chest symptoms, neurological symptoms other than headache, haemorrhagic rash or bleeding, disease severity, e.g. dense rash/ numerous mucosal lesions, and significant immunosuppression. Other contributory features are pregnancy approaching term, bad obstetric history, smoking history, chronic lung disease, poor social circumstances, excessive patient/family anxiety and lack of close medical supervision.

VARICELLA PNEUMONITIS

The clinical features of varicella pneumonitis can be divided into early and late manifestations. Early features include: onset of respiratory symptoms 1–6 days after onset of rash, dry cough, exertional dyspnoea, absence of lung signs, absence of cyanosis, normal or abnormal chest X-ray and mild hypoxaemia. Late features include progress of respiratory symptoms, productive cough/haemoptysis, increasing dyspnoea at rest, diminished air entry, basal lung crepitations, cyanosis, abnormal chest X-ray and moderate to severe hypoxaemia. Some patients progress rapidly to respiratory failure and early death, often as a consequence of pulmonary haemorrhage, and in these patients, antiviral therapy may not have sufficient time to limit the extent of the viraemia if there has been a delay in referral. Early referral is therefore vital to effective management of the case.

SEVERITY IN PREGNANCY

While some data suggest that varicella in pregnancy is no more severe than in the non-pregnant adult, other data suggest mortality among pregnant women with pneumonitis is significantly higher. Pneumonitis has been reported to occur in 5–14% of all adults with chickenpox[83]. It is cited as the most common cause of death in adults with varicella, with reported death rates of up to 15–40%[84,85]. Furthermore, 10% of adults with this complication require intubation and ventilation[84,86]. Whether this condition is more common or severe in pregnancy remains uncertain. Without treatment, varicella pneumonia was fatal in approximately 11% of otherwise healthy adults[84] and in 2–41% of pregnant women[78,84–88]. These retrospective data suggest a higher than expected mortality, but there is a strong possibility of a reporting bias towards the most severe cases admitted to hospital.

One prospective study[78] followed 43 pregnancies. Pneumonia occurred in 9%, premature labour in 10%, premature delivery in 5%, and maternal death in 2%. The rates of pneumonia in this study are between those expected for normal and immunocompromised hosts[89]. In a similar study, data indicate that chickenpox was benign in 86% of cases (25 of 29 women) and resulted in pneumonia in 14%, with an overall mortality of 3%[90]. These data are not that different from an analysis of 236 non-pregnant adults, among whom 11% acquired pneumonia[86]. Another large prospective study of 150 pregnancies complicated by varicella reported no cases of pneumonitis[91].

IDENTIFIED RISK FACTORS FOR VARICELLA PNEUMONITIS IN PREGNANCY

Certain risk factors have been put forward as contributory features to the severity of pneumonitis during chickenpox in pregnancy. These are smoking history, pre-existing lung disease, the severity of the rash, particularly haemorrhage, immunocompromising diseases, including use of systemic steroids, and the later stages of pregnancy. Smoking may predispose to varicella pneumonitis by inhibiting mucociliary clearance and/or phagocytosis of the virus by alveolar macrophages. The relative risk of developing pneumonia during varicella is 15 times higher in smokers than non-smokers[92,93]. Pneumonia occurred in 42–47% of smokers with primary varicella.

Adults with chronic obstructive lung disease seem to develop more severe pulmonary complications than previously healthy adults[94]. There is a positive correlation between the degree of cutaneous rash as well as the haemorrhagic character of the cutaneous lesions and the severity of the pneumonia[95].

A recent retrospective case-control study of children reported that systemic corticosteroids substantially increased the risk of severe chickenpox (178-fold), defined as disseminated disease including pneumonia[96]. Despite the problems and limitations of this study[97], the UK Committee for the Safety of Medicines has recommended that when systemic steroids are being received, or have been given within the last three months, chickenpox should be considered in any patient who presents with fever and systemic illness. If suspected or confirmed, the illness warrants specialist care and urgent treatment (e.g. systemic acyclovir). Corticosteroids should not be stopped as the dose may need to be increased[98]. There are no data available in pregnant women regarding an increased susceptibility to chickenpox while on systemic steroids and individual decisions will need to be taken. There is little evidence that cell-mediated immunity is impaired or that pregnancy results in clinically significant immunodeficiency[99] (see Chapter 1). Furthermore, there is little scientific evidence to suggest that pregnant women are more susceptible to communicable diseases[100]. However, varicella acquired later in pregnancy[86,101], particularly in the third trimester[102], appears to be associated with increased morbidity, with a greater severity of pneumonia, a higher incidence of hospitalization and an increased requirement for mechanical ventilation compared to that acquired earlier in pregnancy[75].

CLINICAL AND RADIOGRAPHIC FEATURES OF VARICELLA PNEUMONITIS

In 1942 Waring *et al.* first described the pulmonary manifestation of chickenpox[94]. In adults it can vary substantially in severity[103] but usually occurs in those most severely affected by chickenpox, and the pneumonia is most severe at the time of maximum skin involvement. Pneumonia without a rash has not been reported. At one extreme it can be a catastrophic illness characterized by severe dyspnoea, cyanosis, haemoptysis and prostration; at the other, it is a mild subclinical condition that can only be detected by routine radiography[76] or abnormal pulmonary function tests[104].

In a typical attack the patient has a heavy rash, which may have been present for up to six days, and the spread of disease to the lungs is heralded by a dry cough followed by increasing shortness of breath, initially only on effort, and cyanosis. Abnormal physical signs are seldom present initially and correlate poorly with the degree of pneumonia[94,104]. A chest X-ray typically reveals diffuse infiltrates that may be nodular, the severity correlating with the diffuseness of the rash[105]. The cough may become productive of scanty mucoid sputum which may be streaked with blood and on examination, as air entry diminishes, crackles may be heard. The classical signs of consolidation are not found. After a week the patient's condition begins to improve and towards the end of the second week the cough and abnormal chest signs disappear. Breathlessness may persist for several weeks. In most patients resolution of the radiographic findings occurs within eight weeks[106] but occasionally a coarse reticular pattern of small, very soft, calcified nodules develops which persists for years[106].

MANAGEMENT OF VARICELLA PNEUMONITIS

In the pregnant adult with varicella who demonstrates any respiratory signs or symptoms, arterial blood gases are the 'gold standard' for documenting pulmonary oxygenation. Pulse oximetry, which is widely used, should not be relied upon to document severe hypoxaemia without a baseline blood gas analysis. Most oximeters used on patients with oxygen saturations less than 70% result in imprecise readings and underestimate saturation[107]. They are also adversely affected by a number of parameters which affect accuracy[108]. However, they are effective in monitoring the patient's response to oxygenation and in detecting episodes of desaturation. Measurement of blood gases will give an assessment of the severity of the pneumonia and allow monitoring of response to appropriate therapy.

SPECIFIC MEASURES

The role of supportive ventilation therapy in pneumonia is crucial since antimicrobials may not alter outcome during the first 24 h of treatment. During acute varicella pneumonitis, arterial blood gas measurements typically reveal moderate hypoxaemia and mild hypercapnia (PaCO$_2$ 4.65 kPa = 35 mmHg). Therefore, one should administer 100% oxygen, preferably through a humidifier, aimed at reducing sputum viscosity and promoting mucociliary clearance. Arterial oxygenation should be closely monitored to assess progress. In varicella pneumonia the nature of the pulmonary injury is rather non-specific and the course of the illness unpredictable. The initial event appears to be a diffuse interstitial pneumonitis which leads to impairment of gas exchange[104]. In most cases the condition slowly improves with full return of pulmonary function although subclinical abnormalities of pulmonary function, such as a suboptimal carbon monoxide diffusion capacity, may remain in some patients for over a year[104]. In others the course of the pneumonia is rather more unpredictable, with development of fulminating pulmonary oedema, diffuse pulmonary capillary leakage and arteriovenous shunting.

The antiviral agent acyclovir is an established therapy for serious herpes simplex and varicella infections but is not currently approved for use in pregnancy because of the lack of direct evidence regarding therapeutic efficacy in this patient population and its potential, as a nucleoside-blocking agent, for fetal toxicity. However, reviews of cumulative cases of its use in treating a range of herpes simplex and varicella-zoster virus infections at all stages of pregnancy have reported no untoward adverse effects on the fetus or mother[109,110,111]. It is logical to use antiviral drugs and other supportive therapies early in the development of pneumonitis before the onset of serious hypoxaemia, but the benefits of antiviral therapy have never been proven in a randomized prospective trial in otherwise healthy non-pregnant adults with varicella pneumonia, let alone in a pregnant population. This is largely due to the relative paucity of cases and the inherent difficulties in organizing such a large multicentre trial.

Van der Meer *et al.*[112] in 1980, first used acyclovir to treat successfully a 25-year-old woman with severe varicella pneumonia. Since then many case reviews have reported the beneficial effects of intravenous, or intravenous plus oral, acyclovir in treating cases of varicella pneumonitis[101,112–116]. A retrospective case-control study of intravenous acyclovir[117] (3–10 mg/kg every 8 h for five days) begun within 36 h of admission in 11 patients (followed by oral acyclovir in six) and compared with 27 patients who received no acyclovir, revealed significantly lower mean temperatures and respiratory rates and greater improvement in oxygenation evident within 5–6 days of hospitalization. There was also some evidence that early treatment with acyclovir resulted in a more rapid improvement in oxygenation[118]. Of the 22 mothers evaluated, three died of severe disease and no child had congenital or perinatal varicella. Another retrospective study using historical controls recommended that acyclovir might be of substantial benefit in reducing maternal mortality[102].

Thus, it seems reasonable to initiate intravenous acyclovir at the first evidence of respiratory involvement in pregnant patients with varicella infection. The dose should be adjusted for any fall in creatinine clearance. There are limitations and inherent biases associated with such studies together with the crucial contribution of improved intensive care over the years. Acyclovir treatment in varicella pneumonitis is appropriate, despite the lack of direct proof in prospective trials. The IV dose of aciclovir is 10 mg/kg three times daily for a minimum of five days[89,102,109,118,119]. An intravenous dose of 10 mg/kg acyclovir every eight hours yields mean steady-state plasma peak and trough concentrations of 92 and 10 μmol, respectively[120]. This is above the concentration of 1.4–6.4 μmol required for 50% inhibition of varicella-zoster virus *in vitro*[121]. However, impairment of renal function as a result of accumulation of acyclovir in the renal collecting system has been reported in patients who were inadequately hydrated[122]. Therefore, to maintain a good urine output acyclovir should be infused slowly with a litre of fluid for each gram of drug[123].

Oral therapy with acyclovir should not be the initial treatment for patients with varicella pneumonitis although some clinicians have reported success with substitution of oral acyclovir for intravenous therapy to enable completion of antiviral therapy on an outpatient basis[54]. Oral acyclovir is poorly, slowly and incompletely absorbed and concentrations of the drug sufficient to inhibit virus replication successfully, even with maximal dosing, may not be achieved to improve clinical outcome[124].

As with other causes of primary viral pneumonitis, secondary bacterial pneumonia is a potential complication of varicella pneumonitis, which has led many clinicians to prescribe antibiotic prophylaxis, particularly to smokers. Though there is no clear evidence that routine use of antibiotics is beneficial in viral pneumonitis[125], it is usual clinical practice to use these in pneumonitis complicating chickenpox. Concurrent bacterial sepsis during an episode of varicella pneumonitis is likely to be due to *Streptococcus pneumoniae*, *Staphylococcus aureus* and *Haemophilus influenzae*,[125] and suitable antibiotics include cefuroxime and co-amoxiclav.

Beneficial results have been reported from the use of hyperimmune globulin[126] or normal immune globulin in chickenpox pneumonia but these findings have not been confirmed in controlled studies. The role of corticosteroid treatment is uncertain and controversial as there have been no controlled studies to evaluate its effectiveness.

WHAT CONSTITUTES A SIGNIFICANT VARICELLA CONTACT FOR PREGNANT WOMEN?

The Pediatric Infectious Diseases Committee of the American Academy of Pediatrics[127] has arbitrarily defined a significant exposure as:

- household contact, i.e. living in the same household as a case of chickenpox or herpes-zoster;
- face-to-face contact or any close contact with a case of chickenpox for at least five minutes.
- contact indoors with a case of chickenpox or herpes-zoster for >1 h.

PREVENTION OF VARICELLA AND BENEFITS OF PROPHYLAXIS WITH ZOSTER IMMUNOGLOBULIN

There has been some question over the efficacy of varicella-zoster immune globulin (VZIG), but studies suggest that it may be used to modify or prevent disease in the mother[128,129,130]. It is recommended for susceptible pregnant mothers exposed to chickenpox[131,132]. In one study, 20 of 25 (80%) susceptible pregnant women did not develop clinical evidence of varicella infection when given 0.2 ml/kg VZIG within 24–96 h of exposure[133]. Clinical varicella infection developed in 16 of 18 (89%) susceptible women who did not receive VZIG. The potential severity of varicella infection in the pregnant adult justifies further studies of VZIG in susceptible pregnant women exposed to VZV[134].

For prophylaxis to be effective in chickenpox, immunoglobulin therapy should be instigated as early as possible following contact, although up to 20% of patients do not know the source of their infection. It is therefore crucial that adults, including pregnant women, seek medical attention immediately. Since the vast majority of pregnant women who have been exposed to varicella-zoster virus during pregnancy will have a history of chickenpox they can be reassured that they are immune and do not need immunoglobulin prophylaxis. If a pregnant woman is in contact with a case of chickenpox and knows she has no previous history of chickenpox or has a doubtful history, she should present for a VZV antibody immunity test. It appears that immunoglobulin is most efficacious if it is administered within 72 h of exposure but there is evidence to indicate benefit for up to 10 days following exposure. There is no benefit to the mother in the administration of immunoglobulin once she has developed chickenpox. There are, however, some data to support the use of VZIG to protect the fetus from the fetal varicella syndrome[129], though prospective studies are needed to clarify this point.

HERPES ZOSTER IN PREGNANCY

Shingles in pregnancy is an uncommon disease. The incidence in women of childbearing years is 2.58 (20–29 years), 2.29 (30–39 years) and 2.92 (40–49 years)/1000/year which is significantly lower than the incidence over 50 years of age (>5.09, increasing with age)[23]. The lower the age, the less likelihood there is to be significant acute-phase pain or extensive vesiculation. Similarly, neuralgic complications are rare as these are also age related. As VZV is not viraemic during herpes zoster in most immunocompetent patients, there is no risk of dissemination of the virus. Clearly, the fetus is not at risk of infection from the mother if there is no viraemic spread and the fetal varicella syndrome is not a feature of this disease. Occasional reports of an association between shingles and congenital abnormality have not been further substantiated and can be regarded as coincidental. There is no reason to believe that the natural immunosuppression of pregnancy increases the incidence of the shingles in the pregnant woman as men of the same age do not have a lower incidence of disease.

MANAGEMENT OF HERPES ZOSTER IN PREGNANCY

As shingles is often mild and pregnant patients are invariably under 50 years of age, antiviral therapy to control herpes zoster is usually an unnecessary and unjustifiable treatment. The management of the shingles rash should be conservative with topical lotions, e.g. calamine, and mild analgesics if acute pain is a problem. The vesicles contain infectious VZV and transmission to other susceptible patients is a possibility although less than that for varicella. Consequently, it is advisable for patients with shingles to cover the lesions, to wash their hands carefully after wound care and to avoid contact with other susceptible patients at risk of varicella. All patients with shingles should be carefully followed up for signs and symptoms of complications, although these are rarely seen. Ophthalmic complications are occasionally very serious and early referral to an ophthalmologist is advisable.

When appropriate, the use of topical acyclovir in the eye can be extremely beneficial and can prevent internal ophthalmic complications. The use of topical acyclovir in pregnancy is unlikely to result in significant systemic absorption of the drug and is justifiable when the eye is at risk of serious damage. After 20 weeks' gestation, oral acyclovir 800 mg five times daily for seven days can also be considered as an adjunct to topical ophthalmic therapy.

WHAT RISK DOES CHICKENPOX DURING PREGNANCY POSE FOR THE FETUS OR NEWBORN?

An infected mother may pass VZV to the fetus during transplacental viraemia and to the newborn by respiratory droplet/direct contact with infectious lesions after birth. The consequences depend on the timing of the infection and the gestational age. During the first 20 weeks of gestation there is a risk of the fetal varicella syndrome[135], intrauterine death[77,135,136,137], congenital varicella[138] (acquired around the time of delivery) and neonatal varicella which is postnatally acquired (Plate E).

THE FETAL VARICELLA SYNDROME

The fetal varicella syndrome (FVS) is characterized by a wide range of anomalies, including cicatricial lesions of the skin with hypoplasia of tissues in a dermatomal distribution, reduced birthweight, mental retardation, ophthalmological and central nervous system anomalies, neuropathic bladder and gastro-

intestinal anomalies. The syndrome occurring among the offspring of women with chickenpox in pregnancy, reported in retrospective studies, ranges from 0% to 9%[133,139–143] while a large prospective trial demonstrated an overall risk of ~1%[129]. Criteria for diagnosis of FVS have only relatively recently been documented[144].

PATHOGENESIS

The pattern of defects seen in FVS suggests that the condition results from intrauterine herpes zoster[145], the extremely short latent period between fetal infection and reactivation resulting from the lack of humoral or cell-mediated immunity in the first 20 weeks of gestation. The mechanism of injury lies in the known neurotropic nature of the virus and the main pathogenetic process leading to the array of anomalies is probably due to the effect of VZV on the fetal nervous system[146].

Whereas the latency established postnatally after primary varicella infection is held in check for several years or decades by effective T-cell immunity, the lack of immunological development in the fetus cannot prevent reactivation of fetal virus in neural tissue and can lead to fetal zoster at multiple sites[144,147]. In the fetus, the close relationship between innervation and tissue development at maturation may determine many of the described anomalies which result from uncontrolled and excessive viral replication in ganglia, neurones and innervated tissues. It has been suggested that the effects on the developing fetus may represent a spectrum of disease, ranging from segmental skin scarring to very severe malformations[145]. This depends on the stage of fetal development, the severity of herpes zoster and the specific neurones affected by herpes zoster *in utero*.

PREVALENCE

There are at least 71 cases of the FVS cited in the literature[128,129,133,140,148–183] resulting from intrauterine infections. However, congenital anomalies are rare when the many thousands of cases of varicella in pregnancy managed every year without serious disease are taken into account. The anomalies were first described in 1947[148] and the existence of FVS was initially postulated in 1974[153].

Evidence firmly suggests that the FVS is associated with maternal varicella infection within the first 20 weeks of pregnancy[129,133,139,144,180] although one recent report mentions congenital anomalies after maternal varicella at 25 weeks' gestation[183]. FVS is rare since most women of childbearing age have established immunity to the virus[133,139,184]. Although the incidence of FVS reported in retrospective studies was shown to range from 0% to 9% of at-risk pregnancies[133,139–143], this latter figure has proved to be excessively high, probably due to the low case numbers and possible selection bias. One prospective cohort study failed to confirm a statistically significant increase in congenital anomalies[139]. A further report[134] estimated the risk of fetal defects after first-trimester maternal varicella infection as 0.5% to 6.5% and 0% to 1.1% thereafter in the second and third trimesters of pregnancy.

A large prospective European trial has recently shown the overall risk of FVS to be ~1%[129]. The highest risk (2.0%) was seen between 13–20 weeks gestation, with a lower risk (0.4%) when maternal varicella occurred before 13 weeks[40]. Given that the incidence of varicella in pregnancy in the UK is three per 1000[130], the incidence of FVS is about 1.6 per 100 000 births[129]. The majority of women who contract varicella during pregnancy have children with no evidence of the FVS and who do not develop herpes zoster early in life.

Mothers who have herpes zoster during pregnancy pose little risk to the fetus[130, 142]. There are approximately 18 reported cases[145,158,185–189] among them one of skin scarring and limb hypoplasia in a baby born to a woman who developed disseminated cutaneous zoster at 12 weeks' gestation[145]. However, Eyal *et al.*[189], in reviewing the literature before 1983, were not convinced that these birth defects were attributable to localized maternal zoster. Herpes zoster in infancy without prior clinical varicella is thought to result from exposure to varicella-zoster virus *in utero*[190].

CLINICAL FEATURES

Low birthweight is an almost constant feature of FVS[139,140,149–151,153,154,158,160,167, 168,171,173,175–178,181]. The other features can be grouped as dermatological, neurological, ophthalmological, skeletal, gastrointestinal and genitourinary abnormalities.

Cicatricial skin lesions, in a dermatomal distribution suggestive of zoster infection with underlying hypoplasia of tissues, are well recognized[128,129,133,140,148–150,154, 158,165,168,171,173,176,180,181,183]. At birth, the skin lesions may look like areas of skin loss that become cicatricial after several weeks to months[148,149,151,154,167,171,180,183]. Skin lesions as the sole manifestation of FVS can occur[176] and among published reports, the skin lesions vary considerably[169], some being described as pale yellow lesions which may be 'pox-like'[149]. Connective tissue naevi in a child have been proposed as a further manifestation of intrauterine varicella infection[177]. Conversely, a majority of the features of FVS have been demonstrated in the absence of skin lesions[174].

Neurological abnormalities include mental retardation, seizures, and cortical atrophy[140, 148,149,151,153,154,165,171,181,183]. Spinal cord atrophy has also been described, in association with the other aspects of the syndrome[178,183]. Limb paresis, often with atrophy of the limbs, has been noted[1,2,4–6,19,26] and microcephaly may also be a feature[140,148,149,150–152,165], sometimes severe[179]. Other neurological anomalies reported include hypotonia, hyporeflexia, intermittent myoclonic seizures, encephalo-myelitis, dorsal radiculitis, Horner's syndrome and bulbar dysphagia, deafness, developmental delay and learning difficulties [149, 150,152,153,165,169,171,173,174,179,180,183]. Some authors [144,183] have noted that the level of neurological insult correlated with the level of skin dermatome involvement.

Ophthalmological abnormalities have been extensively reported and include choroido-retinitis, nystagmus, anisocoria, microphthalmia, enophthalmia, congenital cataract, corneal opacities, hypoplasia of the optic discs, optic atrophy and squint [128,130,139,149,151, 153,154,157,159,173,174,179–181].

Skeletal anomalies, such as limb hypoplasia associated with reduction deformities, have been well described [129,148–151,153,158,180, 181]. The hypoplasia may occasionally involve the mandible, clavicle, scapula, ribs, fingers and toes and can include equino-varus [148,174] and calcaneovalgus [175]. These anomalies arise either directly, due to cicatricial lesions causing reduction deformities, or secondary to denervation of limbs, which leads to diminished muscle mass and bone growth.

Gastrointestinal features include gastroeso-phageal reflux, duodenal stenosis, jejunal dilatation, microcolon and atresia of the sigmoid colon and anal sphincter malfunction [139,148,151,153,154,168,171,180,183]. These anomalies are probably a result of damage to the autonomic nervous system and the spinal cord.

Genitourinary abnormalities such as neurogenic bladder, sometimes associated with lax abdominal musculature, have been well described [148,151,153,154,168,180,183].

DIAGNOSIS

The criteria recommended for a diagnosis of fetal varicella syndrome have been described and include:

- maternal varicella infection during pregnancy;
- the presence of congenital skin lesions that correspond to a dermatomal distribution;
- immunological evidence of intrauterine varicella-zoster infection [144]. This should include either the demonstration of specific IgM antibodies to VZV after birth, or the persistence of IgG after six months of age [144,155,178].

During the pregnancy, cordocentesis could be performed to test for fetal varicella-specific IgM [175] but attempts to diagnosis fetal infection at an early stage are unreliable before 21 weeks, as IgM may not be detectable, even in infants who subsequently show typical features of the FVS [151]. The diagnosis of FVS by demonstrating persistent VZV IgG at one year of age is also unreliable as varicella-specific IgG may be undetectable, in spite of proven intrauterine infection [151].

Although herpesvirus particles have been demonstrated by electron microscopy in skin lesions at or near birth in a small number of cases [152,167], culture of varicella-zoster virus from infants with fetal malformations following maternal varicella infection during pregnancy yields poor results [191]. However, detection of the virus has been achieved in amniotic fluid and fetal blood using a DNA probe [192] and in two infants using dot-blot hybridization, where large volumes of post-mortem tissue were available for examination [175]. PCR testing of amniotic fluid and fetal blood is likely to replace the tests currently used to detect virions in fetal and placental tissue.

Major abnormalities including limb hypo-plasia and microcephaly can be diagnosed by ultrasound scan antenatally [141,175,193] but often these defects are not present until late in pregnancy. This can be due to virus not reactivating in the fetus until a few months after the primary infection or because the maternal varicella infection occurred late in the second trimester [145].

VARICELLA-ZOSTER IMMUNE GLOBULIN AND THE FETUS EXPOSED TO VZV

Some evidence now exists to show that VZIG may reduce the risk of FVS by preventing maternal viraemia[129] although long-term prospective studies are needed to clarify this point[194]. Anti-VZV IgM antibodies developed in only one of 89 infants (1.1%) born to mothers who had varicella during pregnancy, after postexposure prophylaxis with VZIG. Of 615 infants born to mothers with maternal varicella who were not given VZIG prophylaxis, 76 developed IgM antibodies (12.3%) (p=0.003)[129].

ACYCLOVIR THERAPY AND THE FETUS EXPOSED TO VZV

Acyclovir is currently not licensed for use in pregnancy and studies to evaluate any potential benefit with regard to FVS have not been undertaken. However, acyclovir is being used increasingly in pregnancy to prevent the complications of varicella and there is a tendency to be less, rather than more, concerned about the potential adverse effects that it may cause. The early concerns about the effects of acyclovir on the fetus have not been realized as associated fetal abnormalities were not seen in excess when acyclovir was used in early pregnancy[195–197]. Data collected from the GlaxoWellcome Acyclovir Pregnancy Registry in the nine years to June 1993 document the use of acyclovir in 811 pregnancies. Six hundred and one of these pregnancies have been followed to term and up to one year postnatally. No excess of birth defects was found in comparison to the background rate in the general US population[196,198]. However, the potential of treating maternal varicella to prevent the FVS should be balanced against the very small possible risk of adverse fetal effects of acyclovir[197]. Acyclovir crosses the placenta[198] and can be found in amniotic fluid, fetal tissues and cord blood[197]. It is

excreted by the fetal kidney and can be detected in infant urine[196,199].

PREVENTION

Due to the risk of FVS, varicella pneumonitis, premature labour and maternal mortality[198,200], women of childbearing age without a history of chickenpox should be screened for VZV antibody. Those without antibody to VZV and who are identified prior to becoming pregnant would be eligible for varicella vaccine in countries where this vaccine has become available[201,202]. Furthermore, pregnant women who are found to be susceptible to varicella infection when screened at booking or immediately following varicella contact should be told about the availability of VZIG and the need for early presentation to primary health-care physicians should clinical signs of varicella appear.

CONGENITAL VARICELLA

RISKS TO THE NEWBORN OF MATERNAL INFECTION IMMEDIATELY PRIOR TO DELIVERY

Chickenpox at 10 days of life or less is evidence of congenital varicella, i.e. definite intrauterine infection, as the incubation period is rarely <10 days and usually about 14 days. Congenital varicella should not be confused with the fetal varicella syndrome. Late-onset maternal varicella may:

● have no effect on the fetus (varicella in the newborn accounts for as little as 0.05% of reported cases)[203];
● cause typical varicella ~20% risk[139] (the first case was reported in 1978 with rash on day 1 and benign outcome[204]);
● cause fatal disseminated infection with widespread cutaneous and visceral lesions and death from respiratory distress within 4–6 days[205].

In 1944, Oppenheimer presented the first complete autopsy report of congenital varicella following maternal varicella five days before delivery. At seven days the baby developed a varicella rash and at 11 days died from respiratory distress. Autopsy showed macroscopic involvement of liver, spleen, kidneys and gastrointestinal tract. Microscopic examination revealed disseminated lesions almost everywhere in the body[206]. From a similar case in 1958, Ehrlich isolated VZV from lung extract and skin preparations[207]. In 1963, Pearson reported extensive focal invasion with destruction of epithelial and parenchymal cells in liver, kidney, adrenals, thymus, respiratory and gastrointestinal tracts[208]. Meyers estimates a case fatality ratio of 10%[139].

Records showing the time course of maternal vesicles document an interval between maternal and infant rash of 8–18 days[136,209], suggesting that the infection and incubation periods in mother and fetus are not simultaneous. Fetal infection is thought to occur at the end of the maternal incubation period, probably transplacentally during maternal viraemia[209]. Why only some infants are affected is not known, but the unpredictability of infection possibly reflects varying levels of maternal viraemia and differences in the protective efficacy of the placental barrier[208].

DOES THE TIMING OF THE MATERNAL OR NEONATAL RASH AFFECT THE PROGNOSIS IN UNTREATED CONGENITAL VARICELLA?

There is a predictable association between the timing of the maternal and the infant rash and infant prognosis[136,139,210–213]. Retrospective studies suggest that the infant born to a mother who develops varicella up to four days before to two days after delivery has a 20% risk of congenital chickenpox with a 20–30% risk of a fatal outcome[139,205], i.e. 5% of infants born to mothers with onset of varicella at four or less days from delivery, and untreated, may die of

disseminated infection[136]. These differences reflect the presence or absence of specific maternal anti-VZV antibodies in the infant circulation. A high maternal antibody titre is not realized until about the fifth day of her own exanthem. Maternal varicella 5–21 days predelivery usually results in benign neonatal chickenpox, the baby being protected by transplacentally acquired maternal antibody, detectable in the mother 4–5 days after the onset of her rash[214]. VZV IgG antibody readily crosses the placenta[215]. Gershon showed the protective effect of maternal antibodies, reporting two infants with mild varicella and cord IgG FAMA antibody titres of 1:64 and 1:32 following maternal varicella 2–3 weeks predelivery. Conversely, no antibody was found in an infant who died with congenital varicella following a maternal rash the day before delivery. Infection had disseminated to almost every organ, particularly lung, liver and brain, as one would expect in the immunocompromised[136].

A large prospective study of perinatal maternal VZV infection confirmed the increased risk of severe congenital varicella with the onset of the maternal rash between four days before and two days after delivery[213]. It suggested that the severity of neonatal varicella may be overestimated as only 21 deaths from this condition were reported in England and Wales from 1954 to 1973, before the availability of VZIG (the cited fatality rate of 30% is probably an overestimate caused by the selective reporting). The study also showed that infants born as late as seven days after the onset of maternal rash may be VZIG negative at birth. The clinical attack rate in 176 infants whose mothers' rash developed within seven days before to seven days after delivery was around 60%.

MANAGEMENT OF THE BABY AT RISK OF DEVELOPING CONGENITAL VARICELLA

Early administration of large doses of gammaglobulin to infants whose mothers had varicella within one week before delivery suggested that passive antibody may attenuate neonatal infection without preventing it[216,217]. The evidence shows that specific VZIG, if administered early enough, may even prevent infection[218] and, at least in the majority of cases, will modify the severity of any ensuing chickenpox[219,220], even in those at particular risk, i.e. neonates born to mothers with onset of varicella between four days before and two days after delivery[212].

The American CDC[211], the American Academy of Pediatrics and a consensus of American paediatricians[221] recommend VZIG for 'high-risk' infants (those born to mothers who develop chickenpox rash between five days before and 48 h after delivery), claiming that although the clinical attack rate may not be decreased, ensuing complications are less severe and deaths are rare. VZIG cannot, however, be relied upon in individual cases to prevent severe infection[222,223], even when administered on day one of life[212] or on the same day as the onset of the maternal rash[224,225]. Immature cell-mediated immunity is the likely deficiency allowing infection to break through[226,227].

Mothers with chickenpox near term have been given VZIG to try and give additional passive antibody to the baby. Recently prophylactic acyclovir has also been used in 'high-risk' neonates[228,229]. It is of the utmost importance to remember that the child may be clinically normal at birth. Close surveillance should continue for 14–16 days, i.e. safely to the end of any possible incubation period. Infants who develop neonatal varicella (whose mothers had chickenpox between five days before and 48 h after delivery) should receive intravenous acyclovir 10–15 mg/kg/dose eight hourly[211,223,225] to minimize the risk of severe infection, widespread vesiculation with haemorrhage and necrosis in multiple organs[139,230]. Intravenous acyclovir should be considered within 48 h of onset of the rash in other infants who have acquired varicella in the neonatal period.

CAN ACYCLOVIR GIVEN FOR VARICELLA IN LATE PREGNANCY PREVENT CONGENITAL VARICELLA?

There are insufficient data on acyclovir therapy in pregnancy to indicate efficacy in the prevention of congenital varicella. However, there is some evidence that it may inhibit intrauterine viral replication at the time of possible transplacental passage of VZV[231].

IS MATERNAL SHINGLES A RISK TO THE NEWBORN?

Maternal shingles at term does not constitute a risk to the newborn (or fetus) as the infection is not associated with a significant viraemia and the baby will be protected by adequate amounts of transplacentally transmitted maternal antibody.

POSTNATAL VARICELLA

Postnatal varicella in the newborn is rare. At least 85–90% of infant sera tested from cord blood are positive for VZV antibody, the titre usually being equal to maternal levels [232,233]. The majority of neonates, including low birthweight babies, are protected by passively acquired maternal antibody [234,235]. Even after nursery exposure, secondary cases are rare[208,234,236].

DOES PASSIVELY ACQUIRED MATERNAL ANTIBODY ALWAYS PROTECT THE NEWBORN?

Even when the mother is known to be immune, babies should be watched carefully when there has been intimate contact with chickenpox, as under these circumstances maternal antibody may not offer full protection. In an outbreak of varicella in a semi-closed domiciliary institution in Japan, all infants less than two months old were infected despite maternal antibody[237] and two cases of neonatal varicella caught from siblings with varicella have been described although both mothers were immune[238].

IS CHICKENPOX MORE SEVERE IN INFANTS?

The American IPAP[211] states that a normal infant who develops varicella after exposure is at no greater risk of complications than older children and the non-immune neonate who is exposed to varicella postnatally usually has normal childhood chickenpox. The more benign course than that seen in congenital varicella may be explained by the different route of infection and a lesser viral inoculum.

However, Preblud *et al.*[239] report a death: case ratio for children <1 year of age as fourfold that for 1–14-year-olds – 8/100000 compared to 2/100000. Rubin *et al.*[222] reported an apparently immunocompetent infant with severe cutaneous chickenpox, the rash first manifesting at 15 days, with visceral dissemination to the heart and lungs requiring intensive care and mechanical ventilation for respiratory distress and congestive cardiac failure. Four of 13 other cases of varicella at 11–28 days of age who had a severe illness were reviewed. Discrepancies between the epidemiological data and the finding that most clinical reports of postnatal varicella are generally mild may be partly explained by under-reporting of uncomplicated varicella in infants[237,239]. American data from 1972 (the first year that varicella became a nationally notifiable disease in the US) to 1978 showed that infants accounted for 1.4–3.3% of all reported cases but 6.0% of all varicella-associated deaths. The same figures from 1978 to 1982 were 1.5% and 7.6% respectively. The cause of death is usually pneumonitis at <6 months and encephalitis at >6 months.

SHOULD VZIG BE GIVEN TO ALL INFANTS FOLLOWING EXPOSURE TO VARICELLA?

The infant is at increased risk of severe infection compared to the older child but the risk of death is nonetheless low compared to other high-risk groups, i.e. 0.008% at <1 year, compared with 7% in the immunocompromised and 31% after intrauterine exposure. VZIG is not necessary for all infants exposed to varicella, but might be considered for selected neonates with significant exposure, e.g. premature and low birthweight babies whose mothers are immune, and to all babies born to mothers with a negative history of chickenpox[222,240]. The consensus advice of an expert group of American paediatricians is to err on the side of caution[221].

EXPOSURE TO VARICELLA PATIENTS IN THE NEONATAL INTENSIVE CARE UNIT

Horizontal transmission of varicella in maternity wards and nurseries is unusual[241]. Most neonates are protected by maternally derived antibody[242]. Infectious exposure times are usually brief but may be repeated, more prolonged and/or intimate where certain staff, e.g. the physiotherapist, are the source of infection[233,243]. Even premature and low birthweight infants usually have passively acquired VZV antibody[234,235, 243,244]. However, detectable VZV antibody may not confer protection after intimate contact[243] and neither birthweight nor gestational age can be relied upon as accurate indicators of likely neonatal serological status[234,235,244]. Prediction of serological status is made more difficult after neonatal transfusion with packed cells (reduction in antibody levels)[233] or whole blood and/or FFP (increase in antibody levels from VZV IgG present in the blood/blood product donation)[235].

Routine practice is to administer VZIG to all neonates following exposure[233,235,244]. If screening for VZV antibody can be done rapidly and reliably, unnecessary use of VZIG can be avoided and sensible isolation and cohorting of infants can be organized. Unless the FAMA or a sensitive ELISA test is locally available, some authorities recommend giving

VZIG to all exposed infants[244]. Others recommend, in the absence of effective screening, concentrating prophylaxis on those <30 weeks, <1 kg birthweight or where maternal history of varicella infection is negative or uncertain[212,235]. Application of these principles prevents outbreaks of varicella in neonatal intensive care units[233,235,244] but surveillance needs to be maintained and acyclovir should be given to any breakthrough cases.

ACKNOWLEDGEMENTS

The authors wish to acknowledge the contribution of the UK Advisory Group on Chickenpox and the Royal College of Obstetricians and Gynaecologists who have produced guidelines on the management of chickenpox. These guidelines have been published in the Varicella Supplement to the *Journal of Infection*[245] and as an RCOG Guideline[246].

Chickenpox in pregnancy

BACKGROUND

The individual recommendations in this guideline are based on the scheme endorsed by the NHS Executive.[1]

Varicella zoster (VZ) is a DNA virus of the herpes family that is highly contagious and transmitted by respiratory droplets and close personal contact. The primary infection is characterised by fever, malaise and a pruritic rash which develops into crops of maculopapules which become vesicular and crust over before healing. The incubation period is 10–20 days and **the disease is infectious 48 hours before the rash appears and lasts until the vesicles crust over.** Chickenpox (or primary VZ infection) is a common disease of childhood when it causes a mild infection, such that over 85% of the adult population is seropositive for VZ IgG antibody. Contact with chickenpox in pregnancy is common, but infection occurs in only one in 2000 pregnancies.[2,3] A higher proportion of adults from tropical and sub-tropical areas are susceptible to VZ infection.[4]

Following the primary infection, the virus remains dormant but can be re-activated to cause a vesicular erythematous skin rash in a dermatomal distribution known as Herpes Zoster (HZ). HZ in pregnancy does not usually result in intrauterine infection, although there is a case report of congenital Varicella Syndrome in an immunocompromised woman with disseminated HZ.[5]

Primary VZ infection in pregnancy can be associated with an adverse outcome in three possible ways:

1. **Maternal VZ infection**: Primary VZ infection can be more severe in adults and particularly in pregnancy. Pneumonia occurs in approximately 10% of cases. Mechanical ventilation may be required and mortality rates of up to 6% have been reported. Between 1985 and 1993, seven indirect maternal deaths and one late maternal death were reported in the UK in association with maternal Varicella pneumonia.[6]

2. **Congenital Varicella Syndrome** is secondary to primary VZ infection occurring before 20 weeks' gestation. The Syndrome includes one or more of the following:

> skin scarring in a dermatomal distribution;
> eye defects (microphthalmia, chorioretinitis, cataracts);
> hypoplasia of the limbs; and
> neurological abnormalities (microcephaly, cortical atrophy, mental retardation and dysfunction of bowel and bladder sphincters).

The risk is estimated to be approximately 2% and does not occur if the primary maternal infection occurs after 20 weeks' gestation.[7–9] The risk of spontaneous miscarriage after first trimester Varicella infection is not increased.[10] The prenatal diagnosis of congenital Varicella Syndrome is essentially by ultrasound. Poly-hydramnios, hyperechogenic foci in the liver and hydrops fetalis have been described.[11] Ultrasonography carried out five weeks after the primary infection may demonstrate structural changes. Cordocentesis and amniocentesis for VZ antibodies are of limited value.[12]

3. **Varicella infection of the newborn**: Transplacental passage of the virus appears to increase as gestation advances. Up to 50% of fetuses are infected when maternal infection occurs one to four weeks before delivery and one third of these babies develop clinical Varicella despite high titres of passively acquired maternal antibody.[13] This infection can be lethal in 20%–30% of infants if the maternal infection occurs four days before delivery and up to two days postpartum.[14] Babies with no clinical evidence of Varicella infection at birth can develop HZ in infancy, consistent with primary infection *in-utero*.

IMMUNISATION

Live attenuated Varicella vaccine has been shown to be safe and effective in preventing chickenpox in adults,[15] but it is not yet licensed for general use in the UK.[16] There may be a case for immunisation of all susceptible women prior to pregnancy[17] and also for immunising health care workers in contact with pregnant women. (This guideline will be reviewed when an appropriate vaccine becomes available.) Pending availability of live attenuated Varicella vaccine for primary prevention, passive immunisation is the only available strategy in cases of exposure in a susceptible pregnant woman. There is only limited evidence that passive immunisation with VZ IgG prevents or reduces the severity of maternal infection[13,18] or congenital Varicella Syndrome.[8] As the IgG is a blood product obtained from human volunteers with high titers its use is associated with the usual expense and risks. It must be given as soon as possible, preferably within 72 hours of contact with the infectious person, although there is some evidence of benefit up to 10 days after exposure.

RECOMMENDATIONS

All recommendations are **Grade C**.

1.   Management of a Woman with Suspected Varicella Contact in Pregnancy

1.1 It is very important to elucidate the contact history with particular respect to the certainty of the infection, the infectiousness (vesicular rash or development of rash within 48 hours of contact) and the degree of exposure (household face-to-face for five minutes or indoors contact for more than one hour).

1.2 If the pregnant woman has a previous history of Varicella it is reasonable to assume that she is immune to primary VZ infection. However, if there is any doubt then the VZ IgG titre should be checked.

1.3 If the pregnant woman has had a significant contact and no previous history of Varicella, then check for VZ IgG in the serum. At least 85% of women will be positive and can be reassured. The virology laboratory may be able to use serum stored from booking antenatal bloods thus saving time.

1.4 If the pregnant woman is not immune to VZ and the infection occurs before 20 weeks' gestation, then she should be given VZ IgG as soon as possible after contact.

1.5 Detection of IgM in maternal serum indicates primary VZ infection. If she develops primary VZ or shows serological evidence of sero-conversion in the first 20 weeks of pregnancy, then she has a 2% risk of congenital Varicella infection and will need to be informed of the implications.

1.6 Referral to a specialist centre for detailed ultrasound examination at 16–20 weeks' gestation or five weeks after infection, whichever is the sooner, should be considered.

1.7 Neonatal ophthalmic examination should be organised at birth.

1.8 If there is no previous history of Varicella and the contact occurs after 20 weeks, there is no risk of congenital Varicella infection, but the risk of maternal Varicella pneumonia remains. In these circumstances the administration of VZ IgG should be considered, although the evidence to support its use is not strong.

2.   Management of a Pregnant Woman who Presents with Chickenpox

2.1 The pregnant woman with Varicella should be isolated from all other pregnant women and neonates.

2.2 If the pregnant woman is in the second half of the pregnancy and is seen less than 24 hours after the development of the Varicella rash, then the administration of acyclovir may be expected to reduce the severity and duration of the illness (there are theoretical concerns about teratogenesis when acyclovir is used in the first trimester).

2.3 Where maternal infection occurs five days before or two days after delivery there is a 20%–30% risk of Varicella of the newborn. Thus where relevant and practical delivery should be delayed until 5–7 days after the onset of maternal illness to allow for passive transfer of antibodies.

2.4 If delivery occurs within five days of maternal infection, or if the mother develops primary Varicella infection within two days of giving birth, then the neonate should be given VZ IgG as soon as possible.

2.5 If neonatal infection occurs then this should be treated with acyclovir.

2.6 Hospitalisation and consultation with a specialist in infectious diseases is indicated if any respiratory symptoms occur in the infected woman, or if the lesions are dense and haemorrhagic, or if new lesions continue to develop six days after the onset.

2.7 Varicella pneumonia is an indication for treatment with intravenous acyclovir. In certain circumstances it may be necessary to consider mechanical ventilation. In the third trimester of pregnancy this may be facilitated by delivery, but elective delivery at this time will be associated with a high risk of neonatal Varicella.

3. Other Recommendations

3.1 On occasion a sibling has Varicella around the time mother and newborn baby are due for discharge from hospital. If the mother is immune to Varicella the risk to the newborn is minimal. However, if she is not immune both the newborn and the mother should be given VZ IgG.

3.2 All reasonable steps should be taken to isolate individuals, including health care professionals, with VZ infection, from pregnant women attending hospitals or general practitioner surgeries.

3.3 Staff who are thought (or known by previous testing) to be 'not immune' should avoid contact with varicella patients. However, those who are exposed, should be tested for varicella antibodies, and if found to be susceptible should be warned they may develop varicella. The incubation period is between two and three weeks.

REFERENCES

1. Mann T. Clinical Guidelines: Using clinical guidelines to improve patient care within the NHS, 1996. NHS Executive (Catalogue No 96CC0001).
2. Gershon, A A, Raker A, Steinburg S, Topf-Olstein B, Drusin L M. Antibody to varicella-zoster virus in parturient women and their offspring during the first year of the life. Pediatrics 1976, 58:692–6.
3. Sever J A, White L R. Intrauterine viral infections. Annu Rev Med 1969, 19:471–86.
4. Gershon A A. Chickenpox, measles and mumps. In: Infectious diseases of the fetus and newborn infant. Remington J S, Klein J O eds. 3rd Ed. Philadelphia W B Saunders, 1990:395–445.
5. Enders G, Miller E, Cradock-Watson J et al. Consequences of varicella and herpes zoster in pregnancy: prospective study of 1739 cases. Lancet 1994, 343:1548–51.
6. Reports on Confidential Enquiries into Maternal Deaths in the United Kingdom 1985–87, 1988–90 and 1991–93. London HMSO.

7. Preblud S R, Cochi S I, Orenstein W A. Varicella-zoster infection in pregnancy. N Engl J Med 1986, 315:1416–7.
8. Pastuszak A L, Levy M, Schick R N et al. Outcome after maternal varicella infection in the first 20 weeks of pregnancy. N Engl J Med 1994, 330:901–5.
9. Jones K L, Johnson K A, Chambers C D. Offspring of women infected with varicella during pregnancy: A prospective study. Teratology 1994, 49:29–32.
10. Siegel M, Fuerst H T, Peress N S. Comparative fetal mortality in maternal virus diseases. N Engl J Med 1966, 274:768–71.
11. Pretorius D H, Hayward I, Jones K L, Stamm E. Sonographic evaluation of pregnancies with maternal varicella infection. J Ultrasound Med 1992, 11:459–63.
12. Lecuru F, Taurelle R, Bernard J P et al. Varicella zoster virus infection during pregnancy: the limits of prenatal diagnosis. Euro J Obstet Gynecol Reprod Biol 1994, 56(1):67–8.
13. Miller E, Cradock-Watson J E, Ridehalgh M K S. Outcome in newborn babies given anti-varicella zoster immunoglobulin after perinatal maternal infection with varicella zoster virus. Lancet 1989, ii:371–3.
14. Zieger W, Friese K, Weigel M, Becker K P, Melchert F. Varicella infection at birth. Z Geburtshilfe Perinatol 1994 Aug 198:4,134–7 (in German).
15. Gershon A A, Steinberg S P. The National Institute of Allergy and Infectious Disease Varicella Vaccine Collaborative Study Group. Live attenuated varicella: protection in healthy adults compared with leukaemic children. J Infect Dis 1990, 158:661–6.
16. Immunisation against Infectious Disease 1996. HMSO.
17. Seidman D S, Stevenson D K, Arvin A M. Varicella vaccine in pregnancy. Br Med J 1996, 313:701–2.
18. Enders G. Management of varicella zoster contact and infection in pregnancy using a standardised varicella-zoster ELISA test. Postgrad Med J 1985, 61 (supp4):23–30.

Individual recommendations have been graded according to the level of evidence on which they are based using the scheme endorsed by the NHS Executive[1]:

Grade A: randomised trials

Grade B: other robust experimental or observational studies

Grade C: more limited evidence but the advice relies on expert opinion and has the endorsement of respected authorities

This guideline was produced under the direction of the Scientific Advisory Committee of the Royal College of Obstetricians and Gynaecologists as an educational aid to obstetricians and gynaecologists. This guideline does not define a standard of care, nor is it intended to dictate an exclusive course of management. It presents recognised methods and techniques of clinical practice for consideration by obstetricians/gynaecologists for incorporation into their practices. Variations of practice taking into account the needs of the individual patient, resources and limitations unique to the institution or type of practice may be appropriate.

Valid until June 2000
unless otherwise indicated

REFERENCES

1. Myers, M.G., Stanberry, L.R. and Edmond, B.J. (1985) Varicella-zoster virus infection of strain 2 guinea pigs. *J. Infect. Dis.*, **151**, 106–113.
2. Sadzot-Delvaux C., Merville-Louis, M.P., Delree, P. *et al.* (1990) An in vivo model of varicella-zoster virus latent infection of dorsal root ganglia. *J. Neurosci. Res.*, **26**, 83–89.
3. Davison, A.J. and Scott, J.E. (1986) The complete DNA sequence of varicella-zoster virus. *J. Gen. Virol.*, **67**, 1759–1816.
4. Cohen, J.L. and Seidel, K.E. (1993) Generation of varicella-zoster virus (VZV) and viral mutants from cosmid DNAs: VZV thymidylate synthetase is not essential for replication in vitro. *Proc. Natl Acad. Sci. USA*, **90**, 7376–7380.
5. Davison, A.J., Edson, C.M., Ellis, R.W. *et al.* (1986) A new common nomenclature for the glycoprotein genes of varicella-zoster virus and their glycosylated products. *J. Virol.*, **57**, 1195–1197.
6. Cohrs, R., Mahalingam, R., Dueland, A.N. *et al.* (1992) Restricted transcription of varicella-zoster virus in latently infected human trigeminal and thoracic ganglia. *J. Infect. Dis.*, **166**(suppl. 1), S24–S29.
7. Cohrs, R.J., Barbour, M.B., Mahalingam, R., Wellish, M. and Gilden, D.H. (1995) Varicella-zoster virus (VZV) transcription during latency in human ganglia; prevalence of VZV gene 21 transcripts in latently infected human ganglia. *J. Virol.*, **69**, 2674–2678.
8. Cohrs, R.J., Srock, K., Barbour M.B. *et al.* (1994) Varicella-zoster virus (VZV) transcription during latency in human ganglia: construction of a cDNA library from latently infected human trigeminal ganglia and detection of a VZV transcript. *J. Virol.*, **68**, 7900–7908.
9. Debrus, S., Sadzot-Delvaux, C., Nikkels, A.F., Piette, J. and Rentier, B. (1995) Varicella-zoster virus gene 63 encodes an immediate-early protein that is abundantly expressed during latency. *J. Virol.*, **69**, 3240–3245.
10. Takahashi, M. (1992) Current status and prospects of live varicella vaccine. *Vaccine*, **10**, 1007–1014.
11. Asano, Y., Suga, S., Yoshikawa, T. *et al.* (1994) Experience and reason: twenty-year follow-up of protective immunity of the Oka strain live varicella vaccine. *Pediatrics*, **94**, 524–526.
12. Gershon, A.A., LaRussa, P., Hardy, I., Steinberg, S. and Silverstein, S. (1991) Varicella vaccine: the American experience. *J. Infect. Dis.*, **166**(suppl. 1), S63–S68.
13. Johnson, C., Rome, L.P., Stancin, T. and Kamcar, M.L. (1989) Humoral immunity and clinical reinfections following varicella vaccine in healthy children. *Pediatrics*, **84**, 512–518.
14. Kuster, B.J., Weibel, R.E., Guess, H.A. *et al.* (1991) Oka/Merck varicella vaccine in healthy children: final report of a 2-year efficacy study and 7 year follow-up studies. *Vaccine*, **9**, 643–647.
15. Weibel, R.E., Neff, B.J., Kuter, B.J. *et al.* (1984) Live attenuated varicella virus vaccine: efficacy trial in healthy children. *N. Engl. J. Med.*, **310**, 1409–1415.
16. Arvin, A.M. (1995) Varicella-zoster virus. In *Virology*, 3rd edn, (Ed. B. Fields), Raven Press, New York.
17. Whitley, R.J. (1990) Varicella-zoster virus infections. In *Antiviral Agents and Viral Diseases of Man* (eds G.J. Galasso, R.J. Whitley and T.C. Merigan), Raven Press, New York.
18. Brunell, P.A. (1989) Transmission of chickenpox in a school setting prior to the observed exanthem. *Am. J. Dis. Child.*, **143**, 1451–1452.
19. Gustafson, T.L., Lavely, G.B., Brawner, E.R., Jr *et al.* (1982) An outbreak of airborne nosocomial varicella. *Pediatrics* **70**, 550–556.
20. Ross, A.H. (1962) Modification of chickenpox in family contacts by administration of gamma globulin. *N. Engl. J. Med.*, **267**, 369–376.
21. Ooi, P.L., Goh, K.T., Doraisingham S. and Ling, A.E. (1992) Prevalence of varicella-zoster virus infection in Singapore. *Southeast Asian J. Trop. Med. Public Health*, **23**, 22–25.
22. Gershon, A.A., Steinberg, S.P. and Gelb, L. (1984) Clinical reinfection with varicella-zoster virus. *J. Infect. Dis.*, **149**, 137–142.
23. Hope-Simpson, R.E. (1965) The nature of herpes zoster: a long-term study and a new hypothesis. *Proc. Roy. Soc. Med.*, **58**, 9–20.
24. Guess, H.A., Broughton, D.D., Melton, L.J. and Kurland, L.T. (1985) Epidemiology of herpes zoster in children and adolescents: a population-based study. *Pediatrics*, **76**, 512–518.
25. Koropchak, C.M., Solem, S.M., Diaz, P.S. and Arvin. A.M. (1989) Investigation of varicella-zoster virus infection of lymphocytes by in-situ hybridization. *J. Virol.*, **63**, 2392–2395.

26. Ozaki, T., Ichikawa, T., Matsui, Y. *et al.* (1986) Lymphocyte-associated viremia in varicella. *J. Med. Virol.*, **19**, 249–253.

27. Asano, Y., Itakura, N., Hiroishi Y. *et al.* (1985) Viremia is present in incubation period in non-immunocompromised children with varicella. *J. Infect. Dis.*, **106**, 69–71.

28. Asano, Y., Itakura, N., Hiroishi, Y. *et al.* (1985) Viral replication and immunologic responses in children naturally infected with varicella-zoster and in varicella vaccine recipients. *J. Infect. Dis.*, **152**, 863–868.

29. Gershon, A.A., Steinberg, S. and Silber, R. (1978) Varicella-zoster viremia. *J. Pediatr.*, **92**, 1033–1036.

30. Ozaki, T., Kajita, Y., Asano, Y., Aono, T. and Yamanishi, K. (1994) Detection of varicella-zoster virus DNA in blood of children with varicella. *J. Med. Virol.*, **19**, 249–253.

31. Ghatak, N.R. and Simmerman, H.M. (1973) Spinal ganglion in herpes zoster. *Arch. Pathol.*, **95**, 411–455.

32. Straus, S.E. and Meier, J.R. (1992) Comparative biology of latent varicella-zoster virus and herpes simplex virus infections. *J. Infect. Dis.*, **166**(suppl. 1), S13–S23.

33. Croen, K.D., Ostrove, J.M., Dragovic, L.J. and Straus, S.E. (1988) Patterns of gene expression and sites of latency in human nerve ganglia are different for varicella-zoster and herpes simplex viruses. *Proc. Natl Acad. Sci. USA*, **85**, 9773–9777.

34. Bullowa, J.G.M. and Wishik, S.M. (1935) Complications of varicella. I. Their occurrence among 2534 patients. *Am. J. Dis. Child.*, **49**, 923–926.

35. Guess, H.A., Broughton, D.D., Melton, L.J. and Kurland, L.T. (1987) Population-based studies of varicella complications. *Pediatrics*, **78**, 723–727.

36. Jackson, M.A., Burry, V.F. and Olson, L.C. (1992) Complications of varicella requiring hospitalization in previously healthy children. *Pediatrics*, **2**, 441–445.

37. Fleisher, G., Henry, W., Sorley, M., Arbeter, A. and Plotkin. S. (1981) Life-threatening complications of varicella. *Am. J. Dis. Child.*, **135**, 896–899.

38. Cowan, M.R., Primm, P.A., Scott, S.M., Abramo, T.J. and Wiebe. R.A. (1994) Serious group A beta-hemolytic streptococcal infections complicating varicella. *Ann. Emerg. Med.*, **23**, 818–822.

39. Ey, J.L. and Fulginiti, V.A. (1981) Varicella hepatitis without neurologic symptoms or findings. *Pediatrics*, **67**, 258–263.

40. Gogos, C.A., Bassaris, H.P. and Vagenakis, A.G. (1992) Varicella pneumonia in adults. A review of pulmonary manifestations, risk factors and treatment. *Respiration*, **59**, 339–343.

41. Krugman, S., Goodrich, C.H. and Ward, R. (1957) Primary varicella pneumonia. *N. Engl. J. Med.*, **257**, 843–847.

42. Lieu, T.A. and Urion, D.K. (1992) Pre-eruptive varicella encephalitis and cerebellar ataxia. *Pediatr. Neurol.*, **8**, 69–70.

43. Barnes, D.W. and Whitley, R.J. (1986) CNS diseases associated with varicella-zoster virus and herpes simplex virus infections: pathogenesis and current therapy. *Neurol. Clin.*, **4**, 265–283.

44. Johnson, R. and Milbourne, P.E. (1970) Central nervous system manifestations of chickenpox. *Can. Med. Assoc. J.*, **102**, 831–834.

45. Peters, A.C., Versteeg, J., Lindman, J. and Bots, G.T. (1978) Varicella and acute cerebellar ataxia. *Arch. Neurol.*, **35**, 769–771.

46. Wallace, M.R., Bowler, W.A., Murray, N.B., Brodine, S.K. and Oldfield, E.C. III. (1992) Treatment of adult varicella with oral acyclovir. A randomized placebo-controlled trial. *Ann. Intern. Med.*, **17**, 358–363.

47. Preblud, S.R., Orenstein, W.A. and Bart, K.J. (1984) Varicella: clinical manifestations, epidemiology and impact in children. *Pediatr. Infect. Dis. J.*, **3**, 505–509.

48. Preblud, S.R. (1981) Age specific risks of varicella complications. *Pediatrics*, **68**, 14–18.

49. Preblud, S.R. (1986). Varicella: complications and costs. *Pediatrics*, **78**, 728–735.

50. Feldman, S. (1986) Varicella zoster infections of the fetus, neonate and immunocompromised child. *Adv. Pediatr. Infect. Dis.*, **1**, 99–115.

51. Gilden, D.H., Dueland, A.N., Devlin, M.E., Mahalingam, R. and Cohrs, R. (1992) Varicella-zoster virus reactivation without rash. *J. Infect. Dis.*, **166**, (suppl. 1), S30–S34.

52. Gilden, D.H., Wright, R.R., Schneck, S.A., Gwaltney, J.M., Jr. and Mahalingam, R. (1994). Zoster sine herpete, a clinical variant. *Ann. Neurol.*, **35**, 530–533.

53. Bhala, B.B., Ramamoorhy C., Bowsher, D. and Yelnoorker, K.N. (1988) Shingles and postherpetic neuralgia. *Clin. J. Pain*, **4**, 169–174.

54. Karbassi, M., Raizman, M.B. and Schuman, J.S. (1992) Herpes zoster ophthalmicus. *Surv. Ophthalmol.*, **36**, 395–410.

55. Liesegang, T.J. (1991) Diagnosis and therapy of herpes zoster ophthalmicus. *Ophthalmology*, **98**, 1216–1229.

56. Englund, J.A., Suarez, C.S., Kelly, J., Tate, D.Y. and Balfour, H.H., Jr. (1989) Placebo-controlled trial of varicella vaccine given with or after measles-mumps, rubella vaccine. *J. Pediatr.*, **114**, 37–44.

57. Hellinger, W.C., Bolling, J.P., Smith, T.F. and Campbell, R.J. (1993) Varicella-zoster virus retinitis in a patient with AIDS related complex: case report and brief review of the acute retinal necrosis syndrome. *Clin. Infect. Dis.*, **16**, 208–212.

58. Wood, M.J. (1991) Herpes zoster and pain. *Scand. J. Infect. Dis.*, **78**(suppl), 53–61.

59. Jemsek, J.S., Greenberg, S.B. and Taber, L. (1983) Herpes zoster associated encephalitis: clinicopathologic report of 12 cases and review of the literature. *Medicine*, **62**, 81–88.

60. Reichman, R.C. (1978) Neurologic complications of varicella-zoster infections. *Ann. Intern. Med.*, **375**, 89–96.

61. Drew, W.L. and Mintz, L. (1980) Rapid diagnosis of varicella-zoster virus infection by direct immunofluorescence. *Am. J. Clin. Pathol.*, **73**, 699–701.

62. Gleaves, C.A., Lee, C.F., Bustamante, C.I. and Meyers, J.D. (1988). Use of murine monoclonal antibodies for laboratory diagnosis of varicella-zoster virus infection. *J. Clin. Microbiol.*, **26**, 1623–1625.

63. Perez, J.L., Garcia, A., Niubo, J. *et al.* (1994) Comparison of techniques and evaluation of three commercial monoclonal antibodies for laboratory diagnosis of varicella-zoster virus in muco-cutaneous specimens. *J. Clin. Microbiol.*, **32**, 1610–1613.

64. Rawlinson, W.D., Dwyer, D.E., Gibbons, V.L. and Cunningham, A.L. (1989) Rapid diagnosis of varicella-zoster virus infection with a monoclonal antibody based direct immunofluorescence technique. *J. Virol. Methods*, **23**, 13–18.

65. Schmidt, N.J., Gallo, D., Devlin, Y., Woodie, J.D. and Emmons., R.W. (1980). Direct immunofluorescence staining for detection of herpes simplex and varicella-zoster virus antigens in vesicular lesions and certain tissue specimens. *J. Clin. Microbiol.*, **12**, 651–655.

66. Nahass, G.T., Mandel, M.J., Cook, S., Fan, W. and Leonardi, C.L. (1995) Detection of herpes simplex and varicella-zoster infection from cutaneous lesions in different clinical stages with the polymerase chain reaction. *J. Am. Acad. Dermatol.*, **32**, 730–733.

67. Landry, M.L., Cohen, S.D., Mayo, D.R., Fong, C.K.Y. and Andiman., W.A. (1987) Comparison of fluorescent antibody-to-membrane-antigen test, indirect immunofluorescence assay, and a commercial enzyme-linked immunosorbent assay for determination of antibody to varicella-zoster virus. *J. Clin. Microbiol.*, **25**, 832–835.

68. Steinberg, S.P. and Gershon, A.A. (1991) Measurement of antibodies to varicella-zoster virus by using a latex agglutination test. *J. Clin. Microbiol.*, **29**, 1527–1529.

69. Miller, E., Vurdien, J. and Farrington, P. (1993) Shift in age in chickenpox. *Lancet*, **341**, 308–309.

70. Gray, G.C., Palinkas L.A. and Kelley P.W. (1990) Increasing incidence of varicella hospitalisations in the United States Army and Navy personnel: are today's teenagers becoming more susceptible? Should recruits be vaccinated? *Pediatrics*, **86**, 867–873.

71. Siegel, M., Fuerst, H.T. and Press, N.S. (1966) Comparative fetal mortality in maternal virus disease: a prospective study on rubella, measles, mumps, chickenpox and hepatitis. *N. Engl. J. Med.*, **274**, 768–774.

72. Enders, G. (1984) Varicella-zoster virus infection in pregnancy. *Prog. Med. Virol.*, **29**, 166–196.

73. Fox, G.N. and Strangarity, J.W. (1989) Varicella-zoster virus infection in pregnancy. *Am. Fam. Physician*, **39**, 89–99.

74. Stagno, S. and Whitley, R.J. (1985) Herpes virus infections of pregnancy. Part II: Herpes virus and varicella-zoster virus infections. *N. Engl. J. Med.*, **313**, 1327–1330.

75. Balducci, J., Rodis, J.E., Rosengren, S. *et al.* (1992) Pregnancy outcome following first trimester varicella infection. *Obstet. Gynecol.*, **79**, 5–6.

76. Preblud, S.R. (1986) Varicella complications and costs. *Pediatrics*, **78**, 728–735.

77. Siegel, M., Fuerst, H.T. and Peres, N.S. (1966) Comparative fetal mortality in maternal virus diseases. *N. Engl. J. Med.*, **274**, 768–771.

78. Paryani, S.G. and Arvin, A.M. (1986) Intrauterine infection with varicella-zoster virus

after maternal varicella. *N. Engl. J. Med.*, **314**, 1542–1546.

79. Dunkle, L.M., Arvin, A.M., Whitley R.J. *et al.* (1991) A controlled trial of acyclovir in otherwise normal children. *N. Engl. J. Med.*, **325**, 1539–1544.

80. Wallace, M.R., Bowler, W.A., Murray, N.B., Brodine, S.K. and Oldfield E.C. (1992) Treatment of adult varicella with oral acyclovir. *Ann. Intern. Med.*, **117**, 358–363.

81. Sterner, G, Granstrom G, Lidman K *et al.* (1988) Management of pregnant women with contagious infections at delivery. *Scand. J. Infect. Dis.*, **20**, 463–473.

82. Sterner, G., Forsgren, M., Enocksson, E., Grandien, M. and Granstrom, G. (1990) Varicella-zoster infections in late pregnancy. *Scand. J. Infect. Dis.*, **71**(suppl), 30–35.

83. Straus, S.E., Ostrove, J.M. and Inchauspe, G. (1988) NIH conference. Varicella-zoster virus infections: biology, natural history, treatment, and prevention. *Ann. Intern. Med.*, **108**(2), 221–237.

84. Triebwasser, J., Harris, R. and Bryant, L. (1982) Varicella pneumonia in adults. *Medicine*, 1982; **46**, 409–420.

85. Chodos, W.A.S. (1982) Varicella in pregnancy. Report of a case and review of the literature. *J. Am. Osteopath. Assoc.*, **81**, 644–666.

86. Harris, R.E. and Rhoades E.R. (1965) Varicella pneumonia complicating pregnancy: report of a case and review of the literature. *Obstet. Gynecol.*, **25**, 734–740.

87. Pickeard, R.E. (1968) Varicella pneumonia in pregnancy. *Am. J. Obstet. Gynecol.*, **101**, 504–506.

88. Mendelow, D.A. and Lewis, G.C. Jr. (1969) Varicella pneumonia during pregnancy. *Obstet. Gynecol.*, **33**, 98–100.

89. Clements, D.A. and Katz, S.L. (1993) Varicella in a susceptible pregnant woman. *Curr. Clin. Topics Infect. Dis.*, **13**, 123–130.

90. Paryani, S.G. and Arvin, A.M. (1984) Consequences of varicella or herpes zoster in pregnancy for mother and infant. Programs and Abstracts of the 24th ICAAC, Washington, October 8–10.

91. Siegel, M. (1973) Congenital malformations following chickenpox, measles, mumps and hepatitis. *JAMA*, **226**, 1521–1524.

92. Grayson, M.L. and Newton-John H. (1988) Smoking and varicella pneumonia. *J. Infect.*, **16**, 312.

93. Ellis, M.E., Neal, K.R. and Webb, A.K. (1987) Is smoking a risk factor for pneumonia in adults with chickenpox? *Br. Med. J.*, **294**, 1002.

94. Waring, J.J., Neuberger, K. and Geever, E.F. (1942) Severe forms of chickenpox in adults with autopsy observations in a case with associated pneumonia and encephalitis. *Arch. Intern. Med.*, **69**, 384–408.

95. Postal, M.J., Moreau, A. and Sors, C. (1987) Pulmonary manifestations of chickenpox. Report of a case. Reviews of the literature. *Ann. Med. Internae* (Paris), **138**(8), 670–672.

96. Dowell, S.F. and Bresse, J.S. (1993) Severe varicella associated with steroid use. *Paediatrics*, **92**, 223–228.

97. Reiches, N. and Jones, J.F. (1993) Steroids and varicella. *Paediatrics*, **92**, 288–289.

98. Editorial. (1994) Severe chickenpox associated with systemic corticosteroids. *Curr. Prob. Pharmacovigilance*, **20**, 1–2.

99. Stirrat, G.M. (1994) Pregnancy and immunity. *Br. Med. J.*, **308**, 1385–1386.

100. Hart, C.A. (1988) Pregnancy and host resistance. *Clin. Immunol. Allergy*, **2**, 735–757.

101. Broussard, R.C., Payne, D.K. and George, R.B. (1991) Treatment with acyclovir of varicella pneumonia in pregnancy. *Chest*, **99**, 1045–1047.

102. Smego, R.A. and Asperilla, M.O. (1991) Use of acyclovir for varicella pneumonia during pregnancy. *Obstet. Gynecol.*, **78**, 1112–1116.

103. Carstairs, L.S. and Emond, R.T.D. (1961) *Proc. Roy. Soc. Med.*, **55**, 456.

104. Bocles, J.S., Ehrenkranz, N.J. and Marks, A. (1964) Abnormalities of respiratory function in varicella pneumonia. *Ann. Intern. Med.*, **60**, 183–195.

105. Weinstein, L. and Meade, R. (1956) Respiratory manifestations of chickenpox. *Arch. Intern. Med.*, **98**, 91–99.

106. Knyvett, A.F. (1966) The pulmonary lesions of chickenpox. *Q. J. Med.*, **35**, 313–323.

107. Severinghaus, J.W., Naifeh, K.H. and Koh, S.O. (1989) Errors in 14 pulse oximeters during profound hypoxia. *J. Clin. Monit.*, **5**, 72.

108. Curley, F.J. and Smyrnios, N.A. (1991) Routine monitoring of critically ill patients. In: *Intensive Care Medicine*, 2nd edn, (eds J.M. Rippe, R.S. Irwin, J.S. Alpert and M.P. Fink), Little, Brown, Boston.

109. Brown, A.Z. and Baker, D.A. (1989) Acyclovir therapy during pregnancy. *Obstet. Gynecol.*, **73**(3), 526–531.

110. Watts, H.D. (1992) Antiviral agents. Antibiotic use in obstetrics and gynecology. *Obstet. Gynecol. Clin. North. Am.*, **19**(3), 563–585.

111. Andrews, E.B., Yankaskas, B.C. and Cordero, J.F. (1992) Acyclovir in pregnancy register. Six years experience. *Obstet. Gynecol.*, **79**, 7–13.

112. Van der Meer, J.W.M., Thompson, J., Tan, W.D. and Versteeg, J. (1980) Treatment of chickenpox pneumonia with acyclovir. *Lancet*, 473–474.

113. Roscan, M., Baumgarten, W. Jr. and Charles, B.H. (1953) Varicella pneumonia with shock and heart failure. *Ann. Intern. Med.*, **38**, 830–845.

114. Gogos, C.A., Bassaris, H.P. and Vagenakis, A.G. (1992) Varicella pneumonia in adults. A review of pulmonary manifestations, risk factors and treatment. *Respiration*, **59**, 339–343.

115. Boyd, K. and Walker, E. (1988) Use of acyclovir to treat chickenpox in pregnancy. *Br. Med. J.*, **296**, 393.

116. Lotshaw, R.R., Keegan, J.M. and Gordon, H.R. (1991) Parenteral and oral acyclovir for management of varicella pneumonia in pregnancy: a case report with review of the literature. *W. Virginia Med. J.*, **87**, 204–206.

117. Haake, D.A., Zakowski, P.C., Haake, D.L. and Bryson, Y.J. (1990) Early treatment with acyclovir for varicella pneumonia in otherwise healthy adults: retrospective controlled study and review. *Rev. Infect. Dis.*, **12**, 788–797.

118. Dorsky, D.I. and Crumpacker, C.S. (1987) Drugs five years later. Acyclovir. *Ann. Intern. Med.*, **107**, 859–874.

119. Peterslund, N.A. (1988) Management of varicella-zoster infections in immunocompetent hosts. *Am. J. Med.*, **85**(suppl 2A), 74–78.

120. Blum, M.R., Liao, S.H.T. and Miranda, P. (1982) Overview of acyclovir pharmacokinetic disposition in adults and children. *Am. J. Med.*, **73**(suppl), 186–192.

121. Biron, K.K. and Elion, G.B. (1980) In vitro susceptibility of varicella-zoster virus to acyclovir. *Antimicrob Agents Chemother*, **18**, 443–447.

122. Balfour, H.H. (1984) Intravenous acyclovir therapy for varicella in immunocompromised children. *J. Pediatr.*, **104**, 134.

123. Balfour, H.H. (1986) Acyclovir therapy for herpes zoster – advantages and adverse effects. *JAMA*, **255**, 387–388.

124. McKendrick, M., McGill, J.I. and Wood, M.J. (1986) Oral acyclovir in acute herpes zoster. *Br. Med. J.*, **293**, 1529–1532.

125. Ellenbogen, C., Graybill, J.R., Silva, J. Jr. and Homme, P.J. (1974) Bacterial pneumonia complicating adenoviral pneumonia: a comparison of respiratory tract bacterial culture sources and effectiveness of chemoprophylaxis against bacterial pneumonia. *Am. J. Med.*, **56**, 169–178.

126. Loebl, W.Y. and Taylor, C.E.D. (1966) Treatment of varicella. *Lancet*, **1**, 1037.

127. American Academy of Pediatrics. (1994) Varicella-zoster infection. In: *Report of the Committee on Infectious Diseases*, AAP, 23rd edn, 514.

128. Enders, G. (1985) Management of varicella-zoster contact and infection in pregnancy using a standardized varicella-zoster ELISA test. *Postgrad. Med. J.*, **61**, 23–30.

129. Enders, G., Miller, E., Cradock-Watson, J., Boley, I. and Ridelagh, M. (1994) Consequences of varicella and herpes zoster in pregnancy: prospective study of 1739 cases. *Lancet*, **343**, 1547–1550.

130. Miller, E., Marshall, R. and Vurdien, J. (1993) Epidemiology, outcome and control of varicella-zoster infection. *Rev. Med. Micro.*, **4**, 222–230.

131. Prober, C.G., Gershon, A.A., Grose, C., McCrachen, G.H. Jr. and Nelson, J.D. (1990) Consensus: varicella-zoster infections in pregnancy and the perinatal period. *Pediatr. Infect. Dis. J.*, **9**, 865–869.

132. Gilbert, G.L. (1993) Chickenpox during pregnancy. *Br. Med. J.*, **306**, 1079–1080.

133. Enders, G. (1984) Varicella-zoster virus infection in pregnancy. *Prog. Med. Virol.*, **29**, 166–196.

134. Greenspoon, J.S. and Masaki, D.I. (1988) Fetal varicella syndrome. *J. Pediatr.*, **112**, 505–506.

135. Enders, G., Miller, E., Cradock-Watson, J., Bolley, I. and Ridehalgh, M. (1994) Consequences of varicella and herpes zoster in pregnancy: prospective study of 1739 cases. *Lancet*, **343**, 1547–1550.

136. Gershon, A.A. (1975) Varicella in mother and infant: problems old and new. In: *Infections of the Fetus and Newborn. Progress in Clinical and Biological Research*, (eds S., Krugman and A.A. Gershan), Alan R. Liss, New York, pp. 79–95.

137. Michie, C.A., Acolet, D., Charlton, R. *et al.* (1992) Varicella zoster contracted in the second trimester of pregnancy. *Pediatr. Infect. Dis. J.*, **11**, 1050–1053.

138. Meyers, J.D. (1974) Congenital varicella in term infants: risk reconsidered. *J. Infect. Dis.*, **129**, 215–217.

139. Siegel, M. (1973) Congenital malformations following chickenpox, measles, mumps, and hepatitis: results of a cohort study. *JAMA*, **226**, 1521–1524.

140. Paryani, S.G. and Arvin, A.M. (1986) Intrauterine infection with varicella-zoster virus after maternal varicella. *N. Engl. J. Med.*, **314**, 1542–1546.

141. Balducci, J., Rodis, J.F., Rosengren, S. *et al.* (1992) Pregnancy outcome following first-trimester varicella infection. *Obstet. Gynecol.*, **79**, 5–6.

142. Preblud, S.R., Cochi, S.L. and Orenstein, W.A. (1986) Varicella-zoster infection in pregnancy. *N. Engl. J. Med.*, **315**, 1416–1417.

143. Hill, A.B., Doll, R., Galloway, T.McL. and Hughes, J.P.W. (1958) Virus diseases in pregnancy and congenital defects. *Br. J. Prev. Soc. Med.*, **12**, 1–7.

144. Alkalay, A.L., Pomerance, J.J. and Rimosin, D.L. (1987) Fetal varicella syndrome. *J. Pediatr.*, **111**, 320–323.

145. Higa, K., Dan, K. and Manabe, H. (1987) Varicella zoster virus infections during pregnancy: hypothesis concerning the mechanism of congenital malformations. *Obstet. Gynecol.*, **69**, 214–222.

146. Gershon, A.A. (1990) Chickenpox, measles and mumps. In: *Infectious Diseases of the Fetus and Newborn Infant*, 3rd edn, (eds J.S. Remington and J.O. Klein), W.B. Saunders, Philadelphia, pp. 395–445.

147. Brunell, P.A. (1966) Placental transfer of varicella-zoster antibody. *Pediatrics*, **38**, 1034–1036.

148. LaForet, E.G. and Lynch, C.L. Jr. (1947) Multiple congenital defects following maternal varicella. *N. Engl. J. Med.*, **236**, 534–537.

149. Rinvik, R. (1969) Congenital varicella encephalomyelitis in surviving newborn. *Am. J. Dis. Child.*, **117**, 231–235.

150. Savage, M.O., Moosa, A. and Gordon, R.R. (1973) Maternal varicella infection as a cause of fetal malformations. *Lancet*, **i**, 352.

151. McKendry, J.B.J. and Bailey, J.D. (1973) Congenital varicella associated with multiple defects. *Can. Med. Assoc. J.*, **108**, 66–68.

152. Dodion-Fransen, J., Dekegel, D. and Thiry, L. (1973) Congenital varicella-zoster infection related to maternal disease in early pregnancy. *Scand. J. Infect. Dis.*, **5**, 149–153.

153. Srabstein, J.C., Morris, N., Larke, R.B.P. *et al.* (1974) Is there a congenital varicella syndrome? *J. Pediatr.*, **84**, 239–243.

154. Brice, J.E.H. (1976) Congenital varicella resulting from infection during the second trimester of pregnancy. *Arch. Dis. Child.*, **51**, 474–476.

155. Frey, H.M., Bialkn, G. and Gershon, A.A. (1977) Congenital varicella: case report of a serologically proved long-term survivor. *Pediatrics*, **59**, 110–112.

156. Fucillo, D.A. (1977) Congenital varicella. *Teratology*, **15**, 329–330.

157. Charles, N.C., Benett, T.W. and Margolis, S. (1977) Ocular pathology of the congenital varicella syndrome. *Arch. Ophthalmol.*, **95**, 2034–2037.

158. Hanshaw, J.B. and Dudgeon, J.A. (1978) Varicella-zoster infections. In: *Major Problems in Clinical Paediatrics, Vol. XVII. Viral Diseases of the Fetus and Newborn*, (eds) W.B. Saunders, Philadelphia, pp. 192–208.

159. Cotlier, E. (1978) Congenital varicella cataract. *Am. J. Ophthalmol.*, **86**, 627–629.

160. Alexander, I. (1979) Congenital varicella. *Br. Med. J.*, **2**, 1074.

161. Asha Bai, P.V. and John, T.J. (1979) Congenital skin ulcers following varicella in late pregnancy. *J. Pediatr.*, **94**, 65–67.

162. Pettay, O. (1979) Intrauterine and perinatal infections. *Ann. Clin. Res.*, **11**, 258–266.

163. David, T.J. and Williams, M.L. (1979) Herpes zoster in infancy. *Scand. J. Infect. Dis.*, **11**, 185–186.

164. Taranger, J., Blomberg, J. and Strannegard, O. (1981) Intrauterine varicella: a report of two cases associated with hyper-A-immuno-globulinaemia. *Scand. J. Infect. Dis.*, **13**, 297–300.

165. Borzyskowski, M., Harris, R.F. and Jones, R.W.A. (1981) The congenital varicella syndrome. *Eur. J. Pediatr.*, **137**, 335–338.

166. Bailie, F.B. (1983) Aplasia cutis congenita of neck and shoulder requiring a skin graft: a case report. *Br. J. Plast. Surg.*, **36**, 72–74.

167. Enders, G. (1984) Varicella-zoster virus infection in pregnancy. *Prog. Med. Virol.*, **29**, 166–196.

168. Kotchman, G.S. Jr., Grose, C. and Brunell, P.A. (1984) Complete spectrum of the varicella congenital defects syndrome in a 5 year old child. *Pediatr. Infect. Dis. J.*, **3**, 142–145.

169. Alfonso, I., Palomino, J.A., De Quesada, G. and Munitz, I. (1984) Congenital varicella syndrome. *Am. J. Dis. Child.*, **138**, 603–604.

170. Hajdi, G., Mezner, Z., Nyerwes, W., Buky, B. and Simon, M. (1986) Congenital varicella syndrome. *Infection*, **14**, 177–180.

171. Alkalay, A.L., Pomerance, J.J., Yamamura, J.M., Sittler, S. and Baladi, K.S. (1987) Congenital anomalies associated with maternal varicella infections during early pregnancy. *J. Perinatol.*, **7**, 69–71.

172. Harding, B. and Baumer, J.A. (1988) Congenital varicella-zoster. A serologically proven case with necrotizing encephalitis and malformation. *Acta. Neuropathol. Berl.*, **76**, 311.

173. Lambert, S.R., Taylor, D., Kriss, A., Holzel, H. and Heard, S. (1989) Ocular manifestations of the congenital varicella syndrome. *Arch. Ophthalmol.*, **107**, 52–56.

174. Hammad, E., Helin, I. and Pacsa, A. (1989) Early pregnancy varicella and associated congenital anomalies. *Acta. Paediatr. Scand.*, **78**, 963–964.

175. Scharf, A., Scherr, O., Enders, G. and Helftenbein, E. (1990) Virus detection in the fetal tissue of a premature delivery with a congenital varicella syndrome. A case report. *J. Perinat. Med.*, **18**, 317–322.

176. Lloyd, K.M. and Dunne, J.L. (1990) Skin lesions as the sole manifestation of the fetal varicella syndrome. *Arch. Dermatol.*, **126**, 546–547.

177. White, M.I., Daly, B.M., Moffat, M.A.J. and Rankin, R. (1990) Connective tissue naevi in a child with intra-uterine varicella infection. *Clin. Exp. Dermatol.*, **15**, 149–151.

178. Da Silva, O., Hammerberg, O. and Chance, G.W. (1990) Fetal varicella syndrome. *Pediatr. Infect. Dis. J.*, **9**, 854–855.

179. Scheffer, I.E., Baraitser, M. and Brett, E.M. (1991) Severe microcephaly associated with congenital varicella infection. *Develop. Med. Child Neurol.*, **33**, 916–920.

180. Cradock-Watson, J. (1991) Varicella-zoster virus infection during pregnancy. In: *Current Topics in Clinical Virology*, (Ed. P. Morgan-Capner), Public Health Laboratory Service, London, pp. 1–27.

181. Mendivil, A., Mendivil, M.P. and Cuartero, V. (1992) Ocular manifestations of the congenital varicella-zoster syndrome. *Ophthalmologica*, **205**, 191–193.

182. Salzman, M.B. and Sood, S.K. (1992) Congenital anomalies resulting from maternal varicella at 25 and a half weeks of gestation. *Pediatr. Inf. Dis. J.*, **11**, 504–505.

183. Hitchcock, R., Birthistle, K., Carrington, D., Calvert, A. and Holmes, K. (1995) Colonic atresia and spinal cord atrophy associated with a case of fetal varicella syndrome. *J. Pediatr. Surg.*, **30**, 1344–1347.

184. Gershon, A.A., Raker, R., Steinberg, S., Topf-Olstein, B. and Drusin, L. (1976) Antibody to varicella-zoster virus in parturient women and their offspring during the first year of life. *Pediatrics*, **58**, 692–696.

185. Duehr, P. (1955) Herpes zoster as a cause of congenital cataract *Am. J. Ophthalmol.*, **39**, 157–161.

186. Michon, P.L., Aubertin, D. and Jager-Schmidt, G. (1959) Deux observations de malformations congenitales paraissant relever d'embryopathies zosteriennes. *Arch. Fr. Pediatr.*, **16**, 695–701.

187. Webster, M.H. and Smith, C.S. (1977) Congenital abnormalities and maternal herpes zoster. *Br. Med. J.*, **2**, 1193.

188. Brazin, S.A., Simkovich, J.W. and Johnson, W.T. (1979) Herpes zoster during pregnancy. *Obstet. Gynecol.*, **53**, 175–181.

189. Eyal, A., Friedman, M., Peretz, B.A. and Paldi, E. (1983) Pregnancy complicated by herpes zoster: a report of two cases and literature review. *J. Reprod. Med.*, **28**, 600–603.

190. Brunell, P.A. and Kotchmar, G.S. (1981) Zoster in infancy: failure to maintain virus latency following intrauterine latency. *J. Pediatr.*, **98**, 71–73.

191. Demetrick, D.J., Magliocci, A.M. and Hwang, W.S. (1993) Absence of varicella zoster DNA in varicella embryopathy tissue utilizing the polymerase chain reaction. *Pediatr. Pathol.*, **13**, 345–355.

192. Gottardi, H., Rebensteiner, A., Delucca, A. *et al.* (1991) Nachwies des Varicellenvirus mit der DNA-Sonde im fetalen Blut und im Fruchtwasser. *Geburtsh u Frauenheilk*, **51**, 63–64.

193. Pretorius, D.H., Hayward, I., Jones, K.L. and Stamm, E. (1992) Sonographic evaluation of pregnancies with maternal varicella infection. *J. Ultrasound Med.*, **11**, 459–463.

194. Brunell, P.A. (1992) Varicella in pregnancy, the fetus, and the newborn: problems in management. *J. Infect. Dis.*, **166**, (suppl 1): S42–47.

195. Boyd, K. and Walker, E. (1988) Use of acyclovir to treat chickenpox in pregnancy. *Br. Med. J.*, **296**, 393–394.

196. Brown, Z.A. and Baker, D.A. (1989) Acyclovir therapy during pregnancy. *Obstet. Gynecol.*, **73**, 526.

197. Andrews, E.B., Vankaskas, C.B., Cordero, J.F., Schoeffler, K. and Hampp, R.N. (1992)

Acyclovir in pregnancy registry: six years' experience. *Obstet. Gynecol.*, **79**, 7–13.

198. Eldridge, R., Andrews, E.B. and Tilson, H.H. (1994) Pregnancy outcome following systemic prenatal acyclovir exposure – June 1, 1984 to June 30, 1993. *Arch. Dermatol.*, **130**, 153–154.

199. Greffe, B.S., Dooley, S.L., Deddish, R.B. and Krasny, H.C. (1986) Transplacental passage of acyclovir. *J. Pediatr.*, **108**, 1020–1021.

200. Harris, R.E. and Rhoades, E.R. (1965) Varicella pneumonia complicating pregnancy: report of a case and review of the literature. *Obstet. Gynecol.*, **25**, 734–740.

201. Gershon, A.A., Steinberg, S.P., Gelb, L. *et al.* (1984) Live attenuated varicella vaccine: efficacy for children with leukaemia in remission. *JAMA*, **252**, 355–362.

202. Asano, Y., Albrecht, P., Vujcic, L.K. *et al.* (1983) Five-year follow-up study of recipients of live varicella vaccine using enhanced neutralization and fluorescent antibody membrane antigen assays. *Pediatrics*, **72**, 291–294.

203. Shuman, H.H. (1939) Varicella in the newborn. *Am. J. Dis. Child.*, **58**, 564–570.

204. Hubbard, T.W. (1978) Varicella occurring in an infant twenty-four hours after birth. *Br. Med. J.*, 822.

205. DeNicola, L.K. and Hanshaw, J.B. (1979) Congenital and neonatal varicella. *J. Pediatr.*, **94**, 175–176.

206. Oppenheimer, E.H. (1944) Congenital chickenpox with disseminated visceral lesions. *Bull. Johns Hopkins Hosp.*, **74**, 240–248.

207. Ehrlich, R.M., Turner, J.A.P. and Clarke, M. (1958) Neonatal varicella. A case report with isolation of the virus. *J. Pediatr.*, **53**, 139–147.

208. Pearson, H.E. (1964) Parturition varicella-zoster. *Obstet. Gynecol.*, **23**, 21–27.

209. Alber, C. (1964) Neonatal varicella. Occurrence in babies born of infected mothers. *Am. J. Dis. Child.*, **107**, 492–494.

210. Raine, D.N. (1966) Varicella infection contracted in utero: sex incidence and incubation period. *Am. J. Obstet. Gynecol.*, **94**, 1144–1145.

211. ACIP. (1984) Recommendations of the Immunization Practices Advisory Committee. Varicella-zoster immune globulin for the prevention of chickenpox. *MMWR*, **33**, 84–100.

212. Hanngren, K., Grandien, M. and Granstrom, G. (1985) Effect of zoster immunoglobulin for varicella prophylaxis in the newborn. *Scand. J. Infect. Dis.*, **17**, 343–347.

213. Miller, E., Cradock-Watson, J.E. and Ridehalgh, M. (1989) Outcome in newborn babies given anti-varicella-zoster immunoglobulin after perinatal maternal infection with varicella-zoster virus. *Lancet*, **ii**, 371–373.

214. Hermann, K.L. (1982) Congenital and perinatal varicella. *Clin. Obstet. Gynecol.*, **25**, 605–609.

215. Brunell, P.A. (1966) Placental transfer of varicella-zoster antibody. *Pediatrics*, **38**, 1034–1037.

216. Brunell, P.A. (1967) Varicella-zoster infections in pregnancy. *JAMA*, **199**, 315–317.

217. Ross, A.H. (1962) Modification of chickenpox in family contacts by administration of gamma globulin. *N. Engl. J. Med.*, **267**, 369–376.

218. Brunell, P.A., Ross, A., Miller, L.H. and Kuo, B. (1969) Prevention of varicella by zoster immune globulin. *N. Engl. J. Med.*, **280**, 1191–1194.

219. Gershon, A.A. (1984) Prevention and treatment of varicella-zoster virus infection. *Pediatr. Infect. Dis. J.*, **3** (Suppl), 34–36.

220. Bose, B., Kerr, M. and Brookes, E. (1986) Varicella zoster immunoglobulin to prevent neonatal chicken pox. *Lancet*, **1**, 449–450.

221. Prober, C.G., Gershon, A.A., Grose, C., McCracken, G.H. and Nelson, J.D. (1990) Consensus: varicella-zoster infections in pregnancy and the perinatal period. *Pediar. Infect. Dis. J.*, **9**, 865–869.

222. Rubin, L., Leggiadro, R., Elie, M.T. and Lipsitz, P. (1986) Disseminated varicella in a neonate: implications for immunoprophylaxis of neonates postnatally exposed to varicella. *Pediatr. Infect. Dis. J.*, **5**, 100–102.

223. Carter, P.E., Duffty, P. and Lloyd, D.J. (1986) Neonatal varicella infection. *Lancet*, **2**, 1459–1460.

224. Holland, P., Isaacs, D. and Moxon, E.R. (1986) Fatal neonatal varicella infection. *Lancet*, **2**, 1156.

225. King, S.M., Gorensek, M., Ford-Jones, E.L. and Read, S.E. (1986) Fatal varicella-zoster infection in a newborn treated with varicella-zoster immunoglobulin. *Pediatr. Infect. Dis. J.*, **5**, 588–589.

226. Hayward, A., Laszlo, M. and Vafai, A. (1989) Human newborn natural killer cell responses to activation by monoclonal antibodies. *J. Immunol.*, **142**, 1139–1143.

227. Grose, C. (1989) Congenital varicella-zoster virus infection and the failure to establish virus-specific cell-mediated immunity. *Mol. Biol. Med.*, **6**, 453–462.

228. Haddad, J., Simeoni, U., Messer, J. and Willard, D. (1986) Perinatal varicella. *Lancet*, **1**, 1494–1495.

229. Sills, J.A., Galloway, A., Amegavie, L. *et al.* (1987) Acyclovir in prophylaxis and perinatal varicella. *Lancet*, **1**, 161.

230. Gershon, A.A. (1975) Varicella in mother and infant, problems old and new. *Prog. Clin. Biol. Res.*, **3**, 79–95.

231. Haddad, J., Simeoni, U., Messer, J. and Willard, D. (1987) Transplacental passage of acyclovir. *J. Pediatr.*, **110**, 164.

232. Gershon, A.A., Raker, R., Steinberg, S., Topf-Olstein, B. and Drusin, L.M. (1976) Antibody to varicella-zoster virus in parturient women and their offspring during the first year of life. *Pediatrics*, **58**, 692–696.

233. Lipton, S.V. and Brunell, P.A. (1989) Management of varicella exposure in a neonatal intensive care unit. *JAMA*, **261**, 1782–1784.

234. Raker, R.K., Steinberg, S., Drusin, L.M. and Gershon, A. (1978) Antibody to varicella zoster virus in low-birth-weight newborn infants. *J. Pediatr.*, **93**, 505–506.

235. Wang, E.E.L., Prober, C.G. and Arvin, A.M. (1983) Varicella zoster virus antibody titres before and after administration of zoster immune globulin to neonates in an intensive care nursery. *J. Pediatr.*, **103**, 113–114.

236. Matseone, S.L. and Abler, C. (1965) Occurrence of neonatal varicella in a hospital nursery. *Am. J. Obstet. Gynecol.*, **92**, 575–576.

237. Baba, K., Yabuuchi, H., Takahashi, M. and Ogra, P.L. (1982) Immunologic and epidemiologic aspects of varicella infection acquired during infancy and early childhood. *J. Pediatr.*, **100**, 881–885.

238. Readett, M.D., Birm, M.B. and McGibbon, C. (1961) Neonatal varicella. *Lancet*, **1**, 644–645.

239. Preblud, S.R., Bregman, D.J. and Vernon, L.L. (1985) Deaths from varicella in infants. *Pediatr. Infect. Dis. J.*, **4**, 503–507.

240. Department of Health, Welsh Office, Scottish Office and Health Department, DHSS (Northern Ireland). (1992) *Immunisation against Infectious Disease*, HMSO London, p. 157.

241. Young, N.A. and Gershon, A.A. (1983) Chickenpox, measles and mumps. In: *Infectious Diseases of the Fetus and Newborn Infant*, (Eds J.S. Remington and J.O., Klein), WB Saunders, Philadelphia, pp. 375–427.

242. Gitlin, D. (1971) Development and metabolism of the immunoglobulin. In: *Immunologic Incompetence*, (Eds B.M. Kagan and E.R. Stiehm), Year Book Medical Publishers, Chicago, pp. 3–13.

243. Gustafson, T.L., Shehab, Z. and Brunell, P.A. (1984) Outbreak of varicella in a newborn intensive care nursery. *Am. J. Dis. Child.*, **138**, 548–550.

244. Gold, W.L., Boulton, J.E., Goldman, C. *et al.* (1993) Management of varicella exposures in the neonatal intensive care unit. *Pediatr. Infect. Dis. J.*, **12**, 954–955.

245. Carrington, D. and McKendrick, M.W. (1998) Varicella supplement. *J. Infect.*, **36**(suppl 1).

246. Royal College of Obstetricians and Gynaecologists (1997) *Guideline No. 13.*, RCOG, London.

C.E. Roth and D.W.G. Brown

INTRODUCTION

Measles is a highly infectious viral exanthem caused by a negative-sense RNA virus of the genus *Morbillivirus* in the family *Paramyxoviridae*. Measles virus (MV) is the only member of its genus which regularly causes human disease. It is an illness which yields significant morbidity and mortality and even today, in the postvaccine era, measles remains an important cause of death and disability in the developing world. Prior to the development of safe and effective vaccines, measles infection in pregnancy was a rare event[1], as almost all individuals became infected in childhood, conferring lifelong immunity to the disease. This situation altered with the implementation of vaccination programmes which left some of the population both unprotected and unexposed to natural infection, rendering them susceptible to disease when outbreaks later occurred. In both developing and developed countries there may be women of childbearing age at risk of measles infection and the obstetrician should be aware of the clinical features and complications of measles in pregnancy.

CHANGING EPIDEMIOLOGY DUE TO VACCINATION

It is thought that measles is a relatively recent human disease, probably deriving from rinderpest, an animal morbillivirus which it closely resembles[2,53]. MV is believed to have evolved when humans and cattle began to live in close proximity to one another. There is no animal reservoir for MV and mathematical modelling suggests that a population of between 250 000 and 500 000 is required to sustain continuity of transmission. It is thus very much a disease of civilization[3,4].

Measles is extremely contagious. A secondary attack rate in households of 76% of susceptibles has been reported, compared to 61% for chickenpox and 31% for mumps[5]. Prior to the availability of measles vaccines, infection was almost universal in childhood. Exceptions were to be found mainly in isolated population groups where there was no circulation of measles virus and the entire population was susceptible (so-called 'virgin soil' populations), experiencing explosive epidemics with a 100% attack rate when infection was introduced. This was observed on several occasions over the last two centuries in the Faroe Islands and more recently in Greenland[6,7]. Elsewhere, most children were infected by the age of 10 years. The average age of infection will depend on the interaction of several factors determining susceptibility and the frequency of contact with others. In the developing world, measles occurs at an earlier age than in developed countries due to earlier loss of maternal antibody, higher birth rates and crowded living conditions. For similar reasons, children in urban areas

Viral Infections in Obstetrics and Gynaecology. Edited by D.J. Jeffries and C.N. Hudson. Published in 1999 by Arnold, ISBN 0 340 74095 7.

contract measles at a younger age than those in rural areas[8]. The introduction of vaccination affects these patterns. As vaccine coverage increases, the average age of cases tends to rise, although total numbers are reduced. If high coverage is achieved, there follows a 'honeymoon period'[9] of low incidence of measles, and cohorts of unimmunized susceptible children age without exposure to infection. As the numbers of susceptibles accumulate, an 'epidemic threshold' is reached and 'post-honeymoon' outbreaks occur, affecting mainly older children and susceptible adults[8]. In the measles outbreaks which occurred during the resurgence of measles in the USA between 1988 and 1991, 40% of cases reported were in those of reproductive age[10] and many cases were documented in pregnant women.

PATHOGENESIS AND CLINICAL FEATURES

MV is spread by aerosols and enters primarily by the respiratory route[11]. The conjunctiva may also be a site of viral entry. The viral haemagglutinin binds to a cell surface receptor, the CD46 molecule, which is a complement regulatory protein[12] although evidence is accruing that other cell surface proteins may also be involved[13]. After binding, the viral fusion protein mediates fusion with the cell membrane and the virus enters the respiratory epithelial cell. MV replicates in the respiratory epithelium for 2–4 days and spreads to local lymphatic tissues. Amplification of replication takes place in local lymph nodes, resulting in a viraemia, with haematogenous dissemination of virus to numerous organs including skin, conjunctiva, kidney, lung, gastrointestinal tract, liver and respiratory tract mucosa. Replication of virus occurs at these sites in endothelial cells, epithelial cells, monocytes and macrophages. MV is released from these sites of replication and at this point, approximately four days before the onset of the rash, the virus may be cultured from the upper respiratory tract and conjunctiva and the

patient becomes infectious to non-immune contacts. Ten to 14 days after infection the prodromal phase of measles begins with fever (increasing to 39–40°C over three days), malaise, anorexia, cough, coryza and conjunctivitis. Koplik's spots, small white lesions with an erythematous margin, appear on the buccal mucosa. The prodrome persists for 2–3 days.

Viral replication also occurs in the endothelial cells of small vessels throughout the vasculature, resulting in vascular dilatation, increased vascular permeability, infiltration by mononuclear cells and spread of infection to adjacent tissues. Infection of the endothelial cells in the dermis leads to infection of the stratum granulosum of the epidermal epithelium. The subsequent mononuclear cell infiltrate, oedema and focal keratosis form the basis of the rash[11]. The prodrome ends with the onset of a maculopapular rash, which first appears behind the ears and on the forehead, then extends to the trunk and extremities. In uncomplicated cases, defervescence occurs over the next 2–3 days. The patient remains infectious until around three days after onset of the rash. The rash begins to fade after 3–4 days, taking up to 10 days to resolve, and may be followed by some fine desquamation. Cough may persist for several days after the acute illness[14].

Diagnosis of measles based on clinical features is not always straightforward; measles may easily be confused with a number of other viral exanthema[15,16,17] and the World Health Organization (WHO) has developed a case definition[18] for use when laboratory confirmation is not available.

COMPLICATIONS OF MEASLES

Measles can affect numerous organs and a broad spectrum of complications has been documented. Respiratory disease may be severe with laryngotracheobronchitis and pneumonia. In immunocompetent individuals, pneumonia is usually due to secondary bacterial or viral infection and may result in chronic pulmonary disease. Otitis media is also common. Immunocompromised patients are at risk of severe giant cell pneumonitis due to MV replication. Interstitial pneumonitis due to MV replication may be detected radiographically even in uncomplicated illness, but rarely has clinical consequence except in adult cases (including pregnant women), when it may be severe[11,19–22]. Gastrointestinal effects may present as vomiting and diarrhoea which may be prolonged in children in the developing world where they may be exacerbated by concurrent parasitic or bacterial infections[23]. Adults are more likely than children to experience clinical hepatitis[19,21,24,25].

Neurological complications include postinfectious encephalomyelitis (PIE), which manifests with fits, obtundation, focal neurological signs and fever within two weeks of the onset of clinically apparent measles. This demyelinating encephalitis is thought to be autoimmune in origin and is associated with a significant mortality and a high rate of severe neurological sequelae among survivors. The risk of PIE increases with increasing age at infection. Other important neurological syndromes associated with measles infection include measles inclusion body encephalitis (MIBE), a fatal complication affecting immunocompromised patients with an onset of 1–6 months following acute measles[26,11], and subacute sclerosing panencephalitis (SSPE), a rare, invariably fatal progressive neurodegenerative disease which presents an average of seven years after measles and is strongly associated with infection acquired in the first year of life[27,58]. Eye disease is common in measles in the developing world and is an important cause of blindness, the risk of which may be increased by nutritional deficiency of vitamin A[28]. Immune suppression as a direct consequence of measles infection contributes to the high rate of secondary infections complicating acute measles[29] and probably to the increased mortality observed

in the months following resolved measles infection in the developing world[30]. This immune suppression is characterized by a diminution of delayed-type hypersensitivity reactions to recall antigens and of both humoral and cellular responses to new antigens[31,32,33]. Monocyte dysfunction and altered production of some cytokines may contribute to these events[29].

The burden of measles illness is heavier in the developing world. Measles acute case fatality rates are 50 times higher in the developing world than in industrialized countries. The rates of serious complications and sequelae reported from developing nations are also much higher[30].

THE IMMUNOLOGICAL RESPONSE TO NATURAL INFECTION: DIAGNOSIS

MV-specific immune responses become detectable with the onset of clinical illness. T-cell activation, proliferation of PBMCs and polyclonal B-cell activation[34,29] may be found with the onset of the prodrome. Antimeasles antibody appears with the onset of the rash: IgM is detected first, followed by IgG1 and then IgG4[35]. IgA appears in secretions, as may IgG and IgM[16]. This marked MV-specific immune activation occurs against the background of immune suppression mentioned above.

Antibodies are raised against most viral proteins, but the N (nucleocapsid) protein elicits the greatest proportion of antibody. Reactivity to the N protein forms the basis of the complement fixation test, now superseded for measles diagnosis by more reliable and sensitive tests. Immunofluorescence assays and viral culture may be used for viral detection from nasopharyngeal secretions, urine or buffy coat specimens, but specimens must be correctly timed (from the prodrome to 1–3 days after onset of the rash), so they cannot be reliably used to exclude current or recent infection. The polymerase chain reaction (PCR) may be performed to amplify and detect the viral genome, but may only be positive during a limited period and is, in any case, not yet widely available. The mainstay of routine diagnosis of acute measles infection nowadays is the detection of MV-specific IgM by enzyme immunoassay (EIA) using sonicated virus or recombinant proteins, preferably in an antibody capture format. This has the advantage of requiring only a single serum specimen, although the detection of seroconversion to measles through a significant rise in IgG by EIA or CFT in early-acute and convalescent paired samples is an alternative[11]. Detection of IgM and IgG in salivary samples is also feasible; this is convenient because it is less invasive than obtaining a blood sample, but very sensitive methods such as radioimmunoassay (RIA) may be required[16].

The cell-mediated immune response to measles infection becomes detectable at around the same time as the humoral response. Evidence for activation of T-cells may be found in the prodromal phase with increased plasma levels of IFN-γ and soluble IL-2 receptor. After the onset of the rash, MV-specific CD8+ cytotoxic T-lymphocytes (CTLs) and proliferating CD8 T-cells are present in the blood. CD4+ T-cells are proliferating during the rash and soluble CD4 levels become elevated and remain so for several weeks[29].

The relative contributions of the humoral and cell-mediated immune responses in conferring protection from subsequent reinfection and disease have not yet been fully explored. Antibody can be observed to have protective activity through the effect of maternal antibody in infancy and immunoglobulin preparations in people with defective immunity. However, a humoral response is not necessarily required, as can be seen in the case of agammaglobulinaemic patients, who recover normally from natural measles infection and are apparently immune thereafter[36]. Patients with defects in cellular immunity or with combined cellular and humoral deficits develop progressive disease. Whatever the

respective roles of the humoral and cellular arms, immunity conferred by natural infection generally persists throughout life.

VACCINE-INDUCED IMMUNITY

The measles vaccines in current use are live, attenuated vaccines administered intramuscularly. They are highly immunogenic, but the presence of preformed, passively transmitted antibody (e.g. maternal or from immunoglobulin preparations) may interfere with seroconversion, so they must be given at appropriate ages and with attention to the clinical and epidemiological situation[30]. The antibody response is similar to that of natural infection, although levels may be somewhat lower and may decay more rapidly over time. The period of protection conferred by maternal antibody in the infant may be of shorter duration in mothers with vaccine-induced immunity compared to mothers who experienced natural infection[37] and this may affect the design of vaccination schedules. Antibody levels are still detectable in the majority of recipients many years after vaccination, but primary or secondary vaccine failure rates may warrant the inclusion of a booster dose in the immunization programme. The USA, the UK and a number of other European countries have now formally adopted a two-dose measles vaccination schedule. The possibility of primary or secondary vaccine failure means that there will be women of childbearing age who may contract measles during an epidemic despite a clear history of vaccination[19]. Seroconversion following vaccination may be confirmed by the same serological tests used after natural infection. The cell-mediated immune response to vaccine has been less extensively studied than the humoral response because the assays required are more complex, but there is some evidence that cellular responses were better sustained than antibody responses in a group of subjects who showed a limited humoral response[38].

MEASLES IN PREGNANCY

OVERVIEW

Before the middle of the last century, gestational measles, an unusual occurrence, was not considered a serious risk to mother or fetus. Panum's report of the 'virgin soil' epidemic in the Faroe Islands in 1846 did not record problems relating to pregnancy, although it is known that several women were pregnant when they contracted measles. A number of case reports, case series and literature reviews appeared after 1879 suggesting that fetal or maternal outcomes were adversely affected and by the early 1900s gestational measles was widely accepted to be a dangerous illness[19]. Two case series, from Oklahoma in 1940[39] and South Australia in 1950[40], concluded that effects on the fetus were less severe than had previously been believed and congenital malformation was not demonstrated to be a consequence of maternal infection. The 10 'virgin soil' measles epidemics in Greenland between 1951 and 1962 afforded the opportunity to examine the records of a large number of cases of gestational measles and to follow up a number of the children born from these pregnancies[41].

A prospective, case control study performed in New York from 1957 to 1964 addressed the issues of fetal mortality and congenital malformation in several maternal virus infections[42,43,44]. Apart from a few small or heavily selected series, there were no further important studies reported until the resurgence of measles in the Americas in the late 1980s led to outbreaks involving pregnant women[19,20].

SEVERITY OF MEASLES IN PREGNANT WOMEN

It is well known that measles occurring in adulthood has an increased risk of severe complications, but there is no definitive evidence that pregnancy further elevates that risk. There were no maternal deaths or severe complications reported in the 24 cases comprising the Oklahoma outbreak[39]. During the first Greenland epidemic in 1951[21], four of 83 pregnant women with measles died (4.9%) compared to 19 of 1099 non-pregnant women with measles (1.7%). Deaths and other complications in pregnant women in concurrently unaffected Greenland populations were not discussed. Heart failure was observed more frequently in pregnant (4/83) than non-pregnant women (6/1099), but pneumonia was not. A series of 12 pregnant women hospitalized for measles in Houston, Texas, during an epidemic in 1988–9 demonstrated a high rate of maternal complications[19], but this was clearly a highly selected series. Severe pneumonitis was observed in eight patients, leading to one death. A transient, biochemical hepatitis, not clinically significant, was noted in seven patients, one of whom was also hepatitis B surface antigen positive. This rate is similar to that reported for non-pregnant adults with measles[45].

A review of case records of 58 women identified as pregnant who received medical care for measles in Los Angeles, California, between 1988 and 1991[20] revealed that 35/58 (60.3%) were hospitalized, compared to 246/748 (32.9%) non-pregnant women with measles. Pneumonia was recorded in 15/58 (25.9%) pregnant and 73/748 (9.8%) non-pregnant women. Death occurred in two pregnant women (3.4%) and four non-pregnant women (0.5%). The clinical information for the two groups was derived from very different sources: the medical records of the pregnant cases were subjected to intensive review, whereas the non-pregnant comparator data were drawn from routine disease surveillance reports.

None of these studies were designed to establish conclusively the existence of an increased risk of measles complications in pregnant women compared with other adults, but they do confirm that whatever the comparative magnitude, the risks are substantial.

ADVERSE OUTCOME OF PREGNANCY – FETAL LOSS AND PREMATURITY

The only prospective, controlled study of the effect of gestational measles on fetal outcome[42,43,44], part of a broader study encompassing other maternal viral infections, only managed to recruit 66 pregnant women with measles over eight years. The small sample size renders some of the results inconclusive. When fetal death rates were analysed according to gestational age there was no significant difference between cases and pregnant controls without measles infection. There were five fetal deaths in the measles group, two of which occurred within two weeks of maternal infection, one of which occurred 2–4 weeks after onset of maternal measles and two 10 or more weeks after onset of maternal measles, demonstrating no strong temporal association between infection and fetal loss. The fetal tissues were not examined for evidence of measles. Although abortion was not associated with measles infection, there was a significant increase in premature infants born to cases (10/60) compared to controls (2/62) and the results were largely associated with premature onset of labour during maternal illness.

All the other modern studies of outbreaks or series (including those discussed above) report greater or smaller proportions of fetal loss and/or prematurity[46] but they are all uncontrolled and background rates are not provided. It is interesting to note that the related morbillivirus, rinderpest, which causes severe illness with a high mortality rate in cattle, has been reported to cause abortion in infected animals[47] (see Chapter 14).

TERATOGENICITY AND CONGENITAL MALFORMATIONS

Little, if any, evidence supports a role for measles as a teratogenic virus. A few isolated, older reports of unrelated fetal defects have been published[48,49,50] but again, no background data are considered and it is not clear that the diagnosis of measles would bear close scrutiny. Dyer reported no cases of fetal malformation in the mothers who contracted measles in the first trimester during the Oklahoma outbreak[39]. Following the epidemic of measles in South Australia, two congenital anomalies were identified from 18 cases of gestational measles: one case of Down's syndrome (measles in fifth week of gestation) and one child diagnosed with partial deafness at 10 months of age (measles in the eighth week of gestation). During the Greenland epidemics, five congenital malformations were noted from 58 pregnancies in which measles occurred in the first trimester. These comprised one case of cerebral leucodystrophy (measles in first month of gestation), one case of cyclopia with microcephaly and polydactyly (second month of gestation), one case with multiple cardiac defects (second month of gestation), one case of anal atresia (second month of gestation) and one with cleft lip and palate (third month of gestation). Of the two cases from the second trimester, one had spastic tetraplegia and one had pulmonary stenosis and there was one case from the third trimester with a patent ductus arteriosus[41].

The only other modern report of a congenital anomaly associated with measles came from the New York study of 1957–64[43]. The incidence of congenital defects was the same in the control group as in the study group (one each). The anomaly in the measles case was bilateral deafness and the control group infant suffered mental retardation.

No clear association of measles infection with teratogenicity or other cause of congenital malformation can be derived from these reports. A much larger and properly designed study would be required to confirm or refute the existence of a risk of a low rate of abnormality.

INTRAUTERINE AND CONGENITAL INFECTION

No cases of congenital measles were reported in the Houston or Los Angeles outbreaks. A smaller Israeli outbreak describing six cases of maternal measles acquired shortly before delivery also found no clinical congenital measles in the neonates, all of whom were premature[46]. This study and the Houston report are the only two recording the use of serology to confirm the diagnosis of measles in some mothers or infants; unfortunately this means that the question of intrauterine infection was not addressed for almost all of the cases and no serological follow-up appears to have been performed on the surviving infants to identify MV infection.

A 1957 case report describes a case of congenital measles in a premature (29 weeks) neonate born one day after the onset of maternal illness[50]. The mother was an adult who had always lived in an urban English environment. No clinical details were provided about the mother's illness, save that she had a rash which had disappeared by seven days. The infant developed a rash on day 2, had apnoeic episodes and suffered a respiratory arrest, from which it was resuscitated. Soon after the infant had a seizure and died. It was noted that the rash disappeared moments before death. The description of the maternal and neonatal illnesses leave one in doubt about the accuracy of a diagnosis of measles.

There were no cases of congenital measles identified in the Greenland epidemics from the 92 women who had measles in the third trimester[21,41]. Dyer describes three cases of congenital measles out of 24 infected women in the Oklahoma outbreak[39]. Prior to 1940, there are a number of case reports featuring congenital infection, going back to 1646 (reviewed by Atmar *et al.* in[19]). It is remarkable that this manifestation should be missing from all modern series and given the difficulty of distinguishing measles from several other viral exanthems[15,16,17], the absence of any

confirmatory tests or even strict case definitions, it is difficult to know whether congenital measles is a genuine clinical entity. There is one report of a fetal death at 25 weeks gestation following a maternal illness diagnosed as measles by CFT, in which evidence of measles infection was detected in placental syncytial trophoblastic cells and decidua using immunofluorescence and immunoperoxidase staining methods. Fetal tissues showed no evidence of MV infection[51]. Once again, it would be necessary to perform a well-controlled study using appropriate serological and molecular diagnostic methods to answer questions about whether wild-type measles virus crosses the placenta and causes intrauterine infection and to delineate the validity and severity of congenital measles.

Perinatal infection with measles was suggested as a risk factor for the subsequent development of Crohn's disease after a retrospective Swedish epidemiological study of 300 subjects with Crohn's disease found an excess (57) over the expected number (39) of subjects whose birthdates coincided with measles epidemics[54]. However, the epidemiological methods employed have been criticized[55,56] and a larger, case control study of 2522 Crohn's disease patients and 2379 controls in the UK did not demonstrate any such association[57].

MANAGEMENT

Although there are many qualitative and quantitative questions still to be answered regarding the impact of measles in pregnancy, there is no doubt that in pregnant women and young infants measles can be a dangerous illness. It is recommended that susceptible pregnant women, neonates and infants up to the age of their first measles vaccination who are in contact with a case of measles receive post-exposure prophylaxis with human normal immunoglobulin, at a dose of 0.25 ml/kg of bodyweight. This should preferably be administered within 72 h but may be given up to seven days after exposure[1]. Susceptibility may be determined by an absence of detectable measles IgG on serology using EIA. Live vaccine may be administered three months later when passively acquired antibody will have disappeared, if there are no contraindications to it. Pregnant women should not receive vaccine, though they may be safely vaccinated in the puerperium. There is a theoretical risk in giving measles vaccine to pregnant women, as it is a live vaccine; however, unlike rubella vaccine, there is no evidence that the vaccine strain crosses the placenta and infects the fetus[52].

Management of measles infection, once established, is largely supportive, with specific therapy directed to any secondary infections or other complications which may develop. Immunoglobulin is of no benefit in established disease in the immunocompetent patient. Ribavirin, an antiviral nucleoside analogue drug which has been demonstrated to have activity *in vitro* against a number of RNA and DNA viruses but which has never been proven to be effective *in vivo* against measles, was used by Atmar *et al.* in the Houston outbreak[19]. Use of ribavirin was restricted to women beyond 20 weeks gestation, as its teratogenic potential in humans is still uncertain. Neither benefit nor adverse events were apparent in mothers or infants in this outbreak.

Finally, attention should be given to reducing any risk of nosocomial transmission in the delivery unit or hospital ward. Pregnant women, or mother and neonate, should be isolated until no longer infectious or able to be discharged. Only immune staff and visitors should be permitted to enter the isolation cubicle. Many hospitals determine measles immunity in their staff at the pre-employment health check. Most staff and patients will be immune but a history of measles infection or vaccination should be sought from any who have been exposed to a case of measles. Serological evidence of immunity should be obtained if any doubt remains about immune

status. Those who lack evidence of immunity should be treated as contacts and offered appropriate prophylaxis. Non-immune staff or visitor contacts of a measles case should be excluded from the ward between five and 21 days from the date of exposure whether or not they have received post-exposure prophylaxis to cover the incubation and potential infectious period of natural measles and of modified measles, a milder form of the illness with a prolonged incubation phase which occasionally occurs after administration of immunoglobulin. Personnel who become ill should be excluded until seven days after the development of the rash[1].

REFERENCES

1. Centers for Disease Control (1989) Measles prevention: recommendations of the Immunization Practices Advisory Committee. *MMWR*, **38**, SUO9.
2. Norrby, E., Sheshberataran, H., McCullough, K.C., Carpenter, W.C. and Orvell, C. (1985) Is rinderpest virus the archevirus of the morbillivirus genus? *Intervirology*, **23**, 228–232.
3. McNeill, W.H. (1976) *Plagues and Peoples*. Anchor Press Doubleday, Garden City, New Jersey.
4. Black, F.L. (1966) Measles endemicity in insular populations: critical community size and its evolutionary implications. *J. Theoret. Biol.*, **11**, 207–211.
5. Hope-Simpson, R.E. (1952) Infectiousness of communicable diseases in the household (measles, chickenpox and mumps). *Lancet*, **2**, 549–554.
6. Panum, P.L. (1940) Observations made during the epidemic of measles on the Faroe Islands in the year 1846. Delta Omega Society, New York.
7. Christensen, P.E., Schmidt, H., Bang, H.O. *et al.* (1953) An epidemic of measles in Southern Greenland, 1951. Measles in virgin soil. I. *Acta Med. Scand.*, **144**, 313–322.
8. Clements, C.J. and Cutts, F.T. (1995) The epidemiology of measles: thirty years of vaccination. *Curr. Topics Microbiol. Immunol.*, **191**, 13–34.
9. McClean, A.R. and Anderson, R.M. (1988) Measles in developing countries. Part II. The predicted impact of mass immunisation. *Epidemiol. Infect.*, **100**, 419–442.

10. Centers for Disease Control (1991) Notifiable diseases: summary by age group. *MMWR*, **39** (53): 10.

11. Griffin, D.E. and Bellini, W.J. (1996) Measles virus. In: *Fields Virology*, (eds B.N. Fields, D.M. Knipe, D.M. Howley *et al.*), Lippincott-Raven, Philadelphia, pp. 1267–1312.

12. Naniche, D., Varior-Krishnan, G., Cervoni, F. *et al.* (1993) Human membrane cofactor protein (CD46) acts as a cellular receptor for measles virus. *J. Virol.*, **67**, 6025–6032.

13. Gerlier, D., Varior-Krishnan, G. and Devaux, P. (1995) CD-46 mediated measles virus entry: a first key to host specificity. *Trends. Microbiol.*, **3**, 338–345.

14. Katz, M. (1995) Clinical spectrum of measles and M.A. *Curr. Topics Microbiol. Immunol.*, **191**, 3–12.

15. Makhene, M.K. and Diaz, P.S. (1993) Clinical presentations and complications of suspected measles in hospitalized children. *Pediatr. Infect. Dis. J.*, **12**, 836–840.

16. Brown, D.W.G., Ramsey, M.E., Richards, A.F. and Miller, E. (1994) Salivary diagnosis of measles: a study of notified cases in the United Kingdom 1991–3. *Br. Med. J.*, **308**, 1015–1017.

17. Tait, D.R., Ward, K.N., Brown, D.W.G. and Miller, E. (1996) Exanthem subitum (roseola infantum) misdiagnosed in infants as measles and rubella. *Br. Med. J.*, **312**, 101–102.

18. World Health Organization (1983) *Expanded Program on Immunization. Provisional Guidelines for the Diagnosis and Classification of the EPI Target Diseases for Primary Health Care, Surveillance and Special Studies.* WHO, Geneva.

19. Atmar, R. (1992) Complications of measles during pregnancy. *Clin. Infect. Dis.*, **14**, 217–226.

20. Eberhart-Phillips, J.E., Frederick, P.D., Baron, R.C. and Mascola, L. (1993) Measles in pregnancy: a descriptive study of 58 cases. *Obstet. Gynecol.*, **82**, 797–801.

21. Christensen, P.E., Schmidt, H., Bang, H.O. *et al.* (1953) An epidemic of measles in Southern Greenland, 1951. Measles in virgin soil. II. The epidemic proper. *Acta. Med. Scand.*, **144**, 430–449.

22. Gremillion, D.H. and Crawford, G.E. (1981) Measles pneumonia in young adults. An analysis of 106 cases. *Am. J. Med.*, **71**, 539–542.

23. Monif, G.R. and Hood, C. (1970) Ileocolitis associated with measles (rubeola). *Am. J. Dis. Child.*, **102**, 245–247.

24. Gavish, D., Kleinman, Y., Morag, A. and Cha-jek-Shaul, T. (1983) Hepatitis and jaundice associated with measles in young adults: an analysis of 65 cases. *Arch. Intern. Med.*, **143**, 674–677.

25. Wong, R.D. and Goetz, M.B. (1993) Clinical and laboratory features of measles in hospitalized adults. *Am. J. Med.*, **95**, 377–383.

26. Aicardi, J., Goutieres, F., Arsenio-Nunes, M.-L. *et al.* (1977) Acute measles encephalitis in children with immunosuppression. *Pediatrics*, **59**, 232–239.

27. Detels, R., Brody, J.A., McNew, J. and Edgar, A.H. (1973) Further epidemiological studies of subacute sclerosing panencephalitis. *Lancet*, **2**, 11–14.

28. Sandford-Smith, J.H. and Whittle, H.C. (1979) Corneal ulceration following measles in Nigerian children. *Br. J. Ophthalmol.*, **63**, 720–724.

29. Griffin, D.E. (1995) Immune responses during measles virus infection. *Curr. Topics Microbiol. Immunol.*, **191**, 117–134.

30. Clements C.J., Strassburg, M., Cutts, F.T., Milstein, J. and Torel, C. (1993) Challenges for the global control of measles in the 1990's. In: *Measles and Poliomyelitis*, (ed. E. Kurstak), Vienna, pp. 13–24.

31. Tamashiro, V.G., Perez, H.H. and Griffin, D.E. (1987) Prospective study of the magnitude and duration of changes in tuberculin reactivity during complicated and uncomplicated measles. *Pediatr. Infect. Dis.*, **6**, 451–454.

32. Whittle, H.C., Dossetor, J., Oduloju, A., Bryce-son, A.D.M. and Greenwood, B.M. (1978) Cell-mediated immunity during natural measles infection. *J. Clin. Invest.*, **62**, 678–684.

33. Coovadia, H.M., Wesley, A. and Brain, P. (1978) Immunologic events in acute measles influencing outcome. *Arch. Dis. Child.*, **62**, 861–867.

34. Ward, B.J., Johnson, R.T., Vaisberg, A., Jauregui, E. and Griffin, D.E. (1990) Spontaneous proliferation of peripheral mononuclear cells in natural measles virus infection: identification of dividing cells and correlation with mitogen responsiveness. *Clin. Immunol. Immunopathol.*, **55**, 315–326.

35. Mathiesen, T., Hammarstrom, L., Fridell, T. *et al.* (1990) Aberrant IgG subclass distribution to measles in healthy seropositive individuals, in patients with SSPE and in immunoglobulin-deficient patients. *Clin. Exp. Immunol.*, **80**, 202–205.

36. Good, R.A. and Zak, S.J. (1956) Disturbances in gammaglobulin synthesis as 'experiments of nature'. *Pediatrics*, **18**, 109–149.

37. Maldonado, Y., Lawrence, E.C., DeHovitz, R., Hartzell, H. and Albrecht, P. (1995) Early loss of passive measles antibody in infants of mothers with vaccine-induced immunity. *Pediatrics*, **96**, 447–450.

38. Ward, B., Boulianne, N., Ratnam, S. *et al.* (1995) Cellular immunity in measles vaccine failure. *J. Infect. Dis.*, **172**, 1591–1595.

39. Dyer I. (1940) Measles complicating pregnancy. Report of twenty-four cases with three instances of congenital measles. *South. Med. J.*, **33**, 601–604.

40. Packer A.D. (1950) The influence of maternal measles (morbilli) on the unborn child. *Med. J. Aust.*, **1**, 835–838.

41. Jespersen, C.S., Lattauer, J. and Sagild, U. (1977) Measles as a cause of fetal defects: a retrospective study of ten measles epidemics in Greenland. *Acta. Pediatr. Scand.*, **66**, 367–372.

42. Siegel M., Fuerst H.T. and Peress N.S. (1966) Comparative fetal mortality in maternal virus diseases. A prospective study on rubella, measles, mumps, chickenpox and hepatitis. *N. Engl. J. Med.*, **274**, 768–771.

43. Siegel M. (1973) Congenital malformations following chickenpox, measles, mumps, and hepatitis. Results of a cohort study. *JAMA*, **226**, 1521–1524.

44. Siegel, M. and Fuerst, H.T. (1966) Low birth weight and maternal virus diseases. A prospective study of rubella measles, mumps, chickenpox, and hepatitis. *JAMA*, **197**, 680–684.

45. Mouallem, M., Friedman, E., Pauzner, R. and Farfel, Z. (1987) Measles epidemic in young adults: clinical manifestations and laboratory analysis in 40 patients. *Arch. Intern. Med.*, **147**, 111–113.

46. Gazala, E., Karplus, M., Liberman, J.R. and Sarov, I. (1985) The effect of maternal measles on the fetus. *Pediatr. Infect. Dis. J.*, **4**, 203–204.

47. Barrett, T. (1994) Rinderpest and distemper viruses. In: *Encyclopedia of Virology*, (eds R.G. Webster and A. Granoff), London, pp. 1260–1268.

48. Swan, C., Tostevin, A. and Black, G.H.B. (1946) Final observations on congenital defects in infants following infectious diseases during pregnancy, with special reference to rubella. *Med. J. Aust.*, **2**, 889.

49. Fox, M.J., Krumbiegel, E.R. and Teresi, J.L. (1948) Maternal measles, mumps, and chickenpox as a cause of congenital abnormalities, *Lancet*, **1**, 746–749.

50. Kugel, R.B. (1957) Measles in a newborn premature infant. *Am. J. Dis. Child.*, **93**, 306–307.

51. Moroi, K., Saito, S., Kurata, T. and Yanagida, M. (1991) Fetal death associated with measles virus infection of the placenta. *Am. J. Obstet. Gynecol.*, **164**, 1107–1108.

52. Markowitz, L. and Katz, S.L. (1994) Measles vaccine. In: *Vaccines*, (eds S.A. Plotkin and E.A. Mortimer), W.B. Saunders, Philadelphia, pp. 229–276.

53. Barrett, T., Visser, I, Mamaev, L. *et al.* (1993) Dolphin and porpoise morbilliviruses are genetically distinct from phocine distemper virus. *Virology*, **193**, 1010–1012.

54. Ekbom, A., Wakefield, A., Zack, M. and Adami, H. (1994) Perinatal measles infection and subsequent Crohn's disease. *Lancet*, **344**, 508–510.

55. Rothwell, P. (1994) Interpretation of temporal variation in patterns of birth. *Lancet*, **344**, 1161–1162.

56. Lione, A. and Scialli, A. (1997) Perinatal exposure to measles virus and the risk of inflammatory bowel disease. *Reprod. Toxicol.*, **11**, 647–652.

57. Thompson, N., Pounder, R. and Wakefield, A. (1995) Perinatal and childhood risk factors for inflammatory bowel disease: a case-control study. *Eur. J. Gastroenterol.*, **345**, 1071–1074.

58. Miller, C., Farrington, C.P. and Harbart, K. (1992) The epidemiology of subacute sclerosing panencephalitis in England and Wales 1970–1989. *Int. J. Epidemiol.*, **21**, 998–1006.

N.S. Brink and C.E. Jensen

INTRODUCTION

Parvovirus B19 was first described in the 1970s as a cause of false-positive reactivity in immunoelectrophoretic tests done for the detection of hepatitis B surface antigen[1]. The precipitin line that formed in the agarose gel was excised and electron microscopic examination showed parvovirus particles[2]. The sera used were derived from blood donors and the name B19 from the code (number 19, row B) given to one of the serum samples in which the virus was first identified[3]. Further characterization showed B19 to be a small, non-enveloped DNA virus.

The first disease linked to B19 infection was aplastic crisis in patients with sickle cell anaemia[4,5]. Since then an aetiological link between B19 infection and the common childhood disease erythema infectiosum, also known as fifth disease, has been established[6]. Other manifestations of B19 infection include non-immune hydrops fetalis[7], fetal death, polyarthropathy[8], chronic anaemia in immunocompromised patients[9] and thrombocytopenia[10,11]. Most recently, intrauterine infection has been linked with congenital anaemia[12].

THE VIRUS

The family Parvoviridae consists of small naked icosahedral viruses with a single-stranded DNA genome[3]. B19 has recently been reclassified within the Parvoviridae into a new genus called *Erythrovirus*[2]. Although only one stable antigenic type of B19 has been described, minor antigenic variation does occur. The latter is not thought to be of diagnostic or epidemiological significance and infection is usually followed by lifelong immunity[3]. The virus contains one non-structural protein (NS-1) and two structural proteins (VP-1 and VP-2) and replicates in human erythroid progenitor cells. Viral binding occurs to an antigen of the blood group P system, the P antigen or globoside[13]. The P antigen is found on mature erythrocytes, erythroid progenitors, megakaryocytes and endothelial cells as well as placenta and fetal liver and heart[2]; this tissue distribution of P antigen may have implications for the pathogenesis of B19-related disease. It has also been shown that people who do not have P antigen (p phenotype) are naturally resistant to infection with B19[14].

EPIDEMIOLOGY AND PATHOGENESIS

Parvovirus B19 is distributed worldwide and is a common infection in humans[2]. Although infection occurs throughout the year, outbreaks are more likely in the late winter, spring and early summer months in temperate climates[3]. Infection is usually acquired between the ages of four and 10 with

Viral Infections in Obstetrics and Gynaecology. Edited by D.J. Jeffries and C.N. Hudson. Published in 1999 by Arnold, ISBN 0 340 74095 7.

about 60% of the blood donor population having evidence of past infection with B19[15]. B19 may be spread via respiratory secretions, close contact and fomites, with spread from respiratory tract to respiratory tract being the most common route of transmission[3]. Infection via blood products, particularly pooled coagulation factor concentrates, has also been described[16].

The pathogenesis of B19-associated disease involves two distinct components: first, a lytic infection of susceptible dividing cells and second, an interaction with the host immune response[3]. This may result in a biphasic illness (Figure 6.1). The primary site for the replication of B19 is the erythroid progenitor cells. This lytic infection causes a transient failure in red blood cell maturation which results in a drop in the number of reticulocytes with a consequent decrease in haemoglobin. Although adults with normal haematopoiesis will tolerate this transient red cell aplasia, individuals with a rapid red blood cell turnover, for example patients with sickle cell anaemia and fetuses, may develop anaemia. Lymphopenia, neutropenia and thrombocytopenia may also occur[3]. This viraemic or first phase of the illness is associated with a non-specific febrile illness. Infection is usually terminated by the production of a neutralizing antibody response[2]; this immune response may be accompanied by the development of a rash and/or arthralgia. These effects, which are probably immune mediated, are clinical manifestations of the second phase of the illness[3].

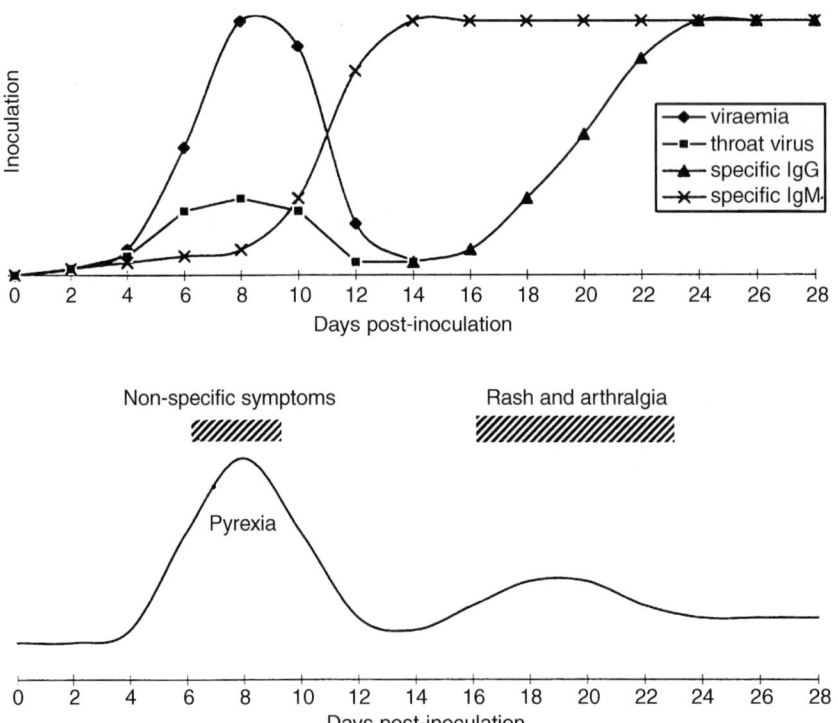

Figure 6.1 Schematic representation of the virological and clinical events during B19 virus infection. These findings resulted from experimental intranasal inoculation of susceptible volunteers, hence the use of the word 'inoculation' rather than 'infection' (modified from reference [3] with permission).

CLINICAL PRESENTATION

Infection with B19 may produce a spectrum of disease varying from asymptomatic infections to potentially fatal conditions. In individuals with an intact immune system infection may cause a non-specific febrile or 'flu-like' illness, a rash and/or arthralgia. Of note is that approximately 50% of infections are asymptomatic. In contrast to this, more severe disease, for example chronic anaemia, may occur in immunocompromised patients. Parvovirus infection in pregnancy will be discussed separately.

ERYTHEMA INFECTIOSUM

The most commonly recognized illness associated with B19 infection is the rash illness erythema infectiosum (EI)[16]. The association of this exanthem with B19 infection was first described by Anderson and colleagues during an outbreak in the United Kingdom[6]. Erythema infectiosum may be preceded by a non-specific febrile illness which usually occurs approximately seven days before the onset of the rash[3]. The exanthematous phase of the illness starts with a red rash on the cheeks (the so-called 'slapped-cheek' appearance) and is followed by the development of a rash on the trunk and extremities. The rash is initially erythematous and maculopapular but progresses into a lacy or reticular pattern (Plate F)[3]. In addition to the typical rash of EI, B19 infection may cause a variety of other exanthema varying from a faint fleeting rash to a rubella-like rash or a more florid exanthem.

ARTHROPATHY

Arthralgia and arthritis are the most common complications, usually occurring in adults and, in particular, females. In adult females joint complications are estimated to occur in about 80% of infections associated with a rash illness[3]. Of note is the fact that joint involvement may also occur in the absence of a rash. In adults the joint involvement is usually symmetrical, affecting the small joints of the hands, wrists and knees most commonly. In contrast to this, less symmetrical joint involvement has been reported in children[8]. In most cases the joint involvement will resolve within four weeks, but persistence for longer periods of time (months or even years) has been described[2].

APLASTIC CRISIS AND PERSISTENT INFECTION

Parvovirus B19 infection was first associated with aplastic crisis in patients with chronic haemolytic anaemia in the early 1980s[4,5]. These individuals usually present with lethargy and pallor and give a history of a recent viral-like illness. The minority of patients (less than 25%) have a rash. Laboratory examination shows anaemia, absence of reticulocytes in the peripheral blood and bone marrow erythroid hypoplasia[17]. B19 infection has also been associated with neutropenia and thrombocytopenia.

Infection in the immunocompromised individual, for example patients with congenital immunodeficiency, leukaemia and AIDS, may become chronic and result in persistent or relapsing anaemia. This may be severe, necessitating regular blood transfusions[2], and is due to a failure of virus-specific neutralizing antibody production[3,18]. As these individuals do not mount an adequate antibody response, they do not develop immune complex-mediated manifestations of disease, for example rash and/or arthropathy.

DIAGNOSIS

The diagnosis of B19 infection can be made by direct detection of virus or testing for a class-specific B19 antibody response. In addition, histological examination may show eosinophilic nuclear inclusions with peripheral condensation of chromatin in the erythroid precursors[16].

B19-specific antibody can be detected using serological assays, for example antibody capture radioimmunoassay or enzyme immunoassay. These are useful to diagnose the immune complex manifestations of disease[2]. Serological diagnosis of an acute or recent infection is usually dependent on the detection of a specific IgM response. Most laboratories report their serological results in arbitrary units (au). Levels of more than 10au of B19-specific IgM usually indicate a recent infection. Care must be taken, however, with the interpretation of a result of below 10au as sera containing a significant level of rubella-specific IgM may give a low level of reactivity when tested for B19-specific IgM[3,19]. In addition to this, B19-specific IgM may become undetectable 2–3 months after an acute infection[3]. This has important implications for the diagnosis of a fetal infection (see below). Under certain circumstances testing for B19-specific IgG may be of use in diagnosing a recent infection. If a serum sample predating the current illness is available (for example, a stored antenatal sample in a pregnant woman) the demonstration of a B19-specific IgG seroconversion may provide information on the timing of infection. An acute infection may also be diagnosed by the demonstration of a significant rise in IgG antibody titre between acute and convalescent serum samples.

There are a number of ways in which the virus can be detected. These include electron microscopy and immune electron microscopy which have been used on acute-phase sera taken from patients with an aplastic crisis[3]. In addition, the virus has been propagated *in vitro* in erythroid cells of human bone marrow and fetal liver. Virus culture remains a research technique, however, and is not used diagnostically. More recently, methods have been developed for the detection of B19-specific DNA using DNA hybridization or molecular amplification techniques[20].

Dot-blot hybridization will usually detect B19 DNA in sera from immunocompromised individuals with B19-related persistent or relapsing anaemia, in fetuses and in patients with a transient aplastic crisis. However, the more sensitive polymerase chain reaction is necessary to diagnose the persistent B19 infection in infants with congenital red cell aplasia; here B19 DNA may only be amplified from bone marrow[2].

MANAGEMENT

Management is supportive in the majority of cases with symptomatic relief for the arthritis/arthralgia and blood transfusion for an aplastic crisis[3]. Intravenous immunoglobulin has been used to treat persistent infection in immunocompromised patients; the rationale for this is that most commercial immunoglobulin preparations contain B19-specific neutralizing antibodies. The management of B19 infection in pregnancy is discussed below.

PARVOVIRUS INFECTION IN PREGNANCY

In 1984 B19 was reported as a cause of intrauterine death and hydrops fetalis[7]. This was followed shortly by the reassuring evidence that a normal pregnancy could follow despite a proven maternal and fetal infection[21]. However, because B19 infects rapidly dividing cells and, additionally, as some of the animal parvoviruses are known teratogens (see Chapter 14), infection in pregnancy has always been of considerable interest.

INCIDENCE AND CONSEQUENCES OF MATERNAL INFECTION

The incidence of acute infection in pregnant versus non-pregnant women appears to be similar. A study in Spain examined the incidence of acute B19 infection in a cohort of pregnant women; the measured incidence in this population was 3.7%[22] which is comparable to the reported incidence in a group of non-pregnant women[23]. Clearly this will vary between endemic and epidemic periods. It has also been shown that approximately 50% of pregnant women are immune to parvovirus B19[24]. Again, this is similar to the non-pregnant population.

Pregnant women do, however, have a higher incidence of asymptomatic acute infections when compared with the non-pregnant population. Only 30% of pregnant women in a large Spanish study had signs or symptoms suggestive of an acute infection (fever, rash or arthralgia)[22]. This contrasts with the lower incidence of asymptomatic infections reported in non-pregnant subjects[23]. This finding has been supported by a more recent study on a hospital outbreak of B19 infection where only three of 15 staff members infected were asymptomatic[25]. The higher incidence of subclinical infections in pregnancy is important as it means that many acute infections will go undiagnosed. It has also been suggested that there is a stronger association between subclinical maternal infection and the development of hydrops fetalis (plate G).

A recent study reported that six of 22 pregnant women with acute B19 infections were symptomatic. Seven cases of hydrops fetalis and one fetal death were associated with these maternal infections; all of the hydropic fetuses occurred in mothers with asymptomatic infections[26]. A possible explanation for this is that individuals with a symptomatic infection have a stronger immune response as the symptoms of rash and arthralgia are immune complex mediated. This is likely to result in a shorter period of viraemia with an associated decreased risk of fetal infection[27]. In addition to the lower incidence of subclinical infections in pregnancy, the clinical disease spectrum may vary with a pre-eclampsia-like syndrome with polyhydramnios and abdominal pain being described[28,29].

INCIDENCE AND CONSEQUENCES OF FETAL INFECTION

Whilst B19 infection in pregnancy is not uncommon and transplacental transmission of the virus occurs in a significant proportion of cases, most pregnancies have a satisfactory outcome. The possible consequences of fetal infection include a self-limiting infection, non-immune hydrops, fetal death or a persistent postnatal infection. The incidence of fetal infection has been estimated at between 25% and 33%[22,30]. The risk of fetal loss is, however, far lower. Initial small studies put the rate of fetal loss at between 26% and 38%[21,31,32]. More recent studies have, however, found a lower risk – 9% in a prospective study of B19 infection in pregnancy conducted by the Public Health Laboratory Service Working Party on Fifth Disease in the UK and 1.66% in a large study in Spain[22,30]. The results of the last two studies are not strictly comparable as the diagnosis of fetal loss due to B19 infection was made by DNA detection in fetal tissue in the PHLS study and by the observation of characteristic histological findings, together with the detection of B19 DNA, in the Spanish study. A further study showed a 2–3% increase in fetal deaths compared to a control group of patients[28,33].

Although the greatest risk of fetal loss is between weeks 10 and 20, B19 infection may cause early spontaneous abortion. Furthermore, fetal loss can also occur in the third trimester of pregnancy[28]. The interval between maternal illness and fetal death is usually between three and five weeks, but it may be as long as 11 weeks[30]. This suggests a specific incubation period rather than non-specific fetal loss resulting from a maternal febrile illness and has important implications for the diagnosis of B19-associated fetal loss (see below).

It has been suggested that the risk of fetal death in a pregnant woman with *unknown* immune status can be calculated as follows:

rate of susceptibility to infection × rate of maternal infection following exposure × risk of fetal death following confirmed maternal infection × 100[34]. The estimated susceptibility to B19 infection in pregnant women is approximately 50%. The rate of maternal infection depends, however, on the type of exposure. This has been estimated at approximately 50% for household contacts of patients with transient aplastic crisis or erythema infectiosum[35]. The attack rate among exposed non-immune school staff has been estimated at 20–30% and that of health-care workers at 35–47%[16,25,34]. The rate of fetal loss is usually estimated at between 1% and 9%. This enables the obstetrician caring for a pregnant woman with exposure to a B19 infection to provide some estimate of the risk of fetal loss. It is, however, preferable for a more precise diagnosis to be made. This includes the diagnosis of preexisting immunity in a pregnant woman with exposure to B19 and, if susceptible, laboratory follow-up for evidence of an acute infection (see below).

Hydrops fetalis is the commonest abnormality reported following B19 infection in pregnancy. A 10-year retrospective study conducted in Germany examined the prevalence of infection in 42 hydropic fetuses; B19 was identified in six (14.2%) cases[36]. This study included fetuses with rhesus incompatibility and congenital malformations. These results are broadly similar to those of Rogers and colleagues who reported a 16% incidence of fetal B19 infection in hydropic fetuses[37]. A further study selected for fetuses with anatomically normal non-immune hydrops. Here the incidence of B19-associated hydrops was, not surprisingly higher, accounting for 27% of the cases studied[38]. Of note is that differential infection with parvovirus B19 has also been described in a diamniotic dichorionic twin pregnancy with one twin developing hydrops fetalis whilst the second developed normally[39].

Because B19 infects rapidly dividing cells, concern has been expressed that infection during the critical embryonic stage may lead to congenital malformations. Furthermore, some of the animal parvoviruses are known to be teratogens[16]. However, no excess risk of birth defects was detected following clinically diagnosed outbreaks of erythema infectiosum[40]. In addition to this, congenital malformations have only rarely been associated with proven B19 infections. One fetus aborted in the first trimester had evidence of anomalies of the eye[41], and multiple structural defects including a cleft lip and palate; micrognathia and webbed joints were present in another fetus with a proven B19 infection[42]. However, there is no direct proof of a causal link between B19 infection and anatomical abnormalities; the frequency of congenital anatomical abnormalities in infants born to women with B19 infection in pregnancy is no higher than the background rates. Whilst this is reassuring it should be noted that in most of the studies the sample size is too small to detect a possible rare teratogenic effect[30].

POSTNATAL CONSEQUENCES OF CONGENITAL INFECTION

No neurodevelopmental abnormalities have been detected in infants surviving B19 infection *in utero*. In a large study, 60 pregnant women with acute infection during pregnancy were followed up, with the majority of infants (55) being assessed at one year of age. No congenital abnormalities or severe neurodevelopmental impairment were observed [22]. These results are similar to those of a study in the UK which followed up 114 infants whose mothers had serologically confirmed B19 infection in pregnancy. Again, no congenital anomalies or serious neurodevelopmental problems were noted[30]. Whilst this is reassuring to clinicians and parents alike, it is possible that congenitally infected babies may not have been followed up for long enough to detect more subtle neurodevelopmental or physical problems [30].

The question of viral persistence also needs further investigation. Persistent infection occurs in immunocompromised patients and may occur in fetuses due to their immunological immaturity. A recent report described persistent B19 infection in three infants with congenital red cell aplasia. All three fetuses developed hydrops fetalis and, after delivery, B19 DNA was detected in bone marrow. One of the children died and B19 DNA was also detected in various other tissues including liver, spleen, heart, thymus and brain. The other two patients remained persistently anaemic despite treatment with immunoglobulin. One had evidence of classical red cell aplasia and the second had marked dyserythropoiesis. Of note was the low level of B19 replication, with detectable virus in the bone marrow but not in the peripheral circulation. The authors concluded that persistent B19 infection should be considered in infants with congenital red cell aplasia [12]. It has also been suggested that B19 infection *in utero* may occasionally cause asymptomatic postnatal infection [43].

PATHOPHYSIOLOGY OF FETAL DISEASE

B19 infects mitotically active cells, in particular red blood cell progenitors. It is therefore logical that the greatest risk to the fetus is during the first 20 weeks of pregnancy (especially between weeks 10 and 20) as this coincides with the major development of the erythroid precursors. Fetal hydrops may result from a number of possible causes including high output cardiac failure secondary to fetal anaemia, myocarditis, anaemia with hypoxic cardiac and/or vascular damage and hepatic dysfunction with resultant hypoalbuminaemia and decreased oncotic pressure [44]. B19 infects the erythroid precursors which may result in erythroid hypoplasia and anaemia in the fetus [45] with haemoglobin levels as low as 1.7 g/dl having been reported [46]. This fetal anaemia causes tissue hypoxia which results in a compensatory increase in cardiac output,

leading to high output cardiac failure and fetal hydrops [34]. As B19 DNA has also been detected in cardiac tissue, a viral myocarditis with cardiac dysfunction has been suggested as a further possible cause of fetal hydrops [47].

The most striking postmortem findings include erythroid hypoplasia of the bone marrow with extramedullary haematopoiesis in organs such as the liver and spleen. The latter may result in marked hepatosplenomegaly [34]. Hepatic damage and giant cell hepatitis with cholestasis and haemosiderin deposition have also been described. It is not known whether these changes result primarily from the parvovirus B19 infection or occur because of excessive iron deposition [34]. The placenta is usually thick and oedematous with an excess of erythroblasts [7,34] and a vasculitis may be present in the placental villi [28,48]. Histologically, examination of tissue obtained from B19-infected fetuses shows the presence of typical intranuclear inclusions in the erythroid precursor cells. Inflammatory changes in the myocardium may also be evident. The histological features of B19 infection are similar across the range of gestational ages [48].

MANAGEMENT

Indications for investigation of a pregnant woman for suspected acute B19 infection include the following:

- a rash;
- unexplained polyarthralgia;
- maternal contact with a case of B19 infection;
- non-immune fetal hydrops;
- unexplained maternal polyhydramnios or elevation of maternal serum α-fetoprotein [44].

Elevation of maternal serum α-fetoprotein is sometimes used as an indication for B19-specific testing as several cases of documented fetal B19 infections have been associated with raised levels. These are likely to result from excessive leakage across a damaged placenta[28]. However, hydrops fetalis and fetal death secondary to B19 infection can also occur in the presence of unremarkable second-trimester maternal serum α-fetoprotein levels[49]. B19-specific testing is therefore the appropriate method of investigation.

Maternal serology may establish a recent infection by demonstrating the presence of a B19-specific IgM response, a rising IgG concentration or an IgG seroconversion. The latter is frequently possible as parallel testing of an acute-phase blood with a stored antenatal sample may be done. Care must be taken, however, when interpreting the IgM results. Fetal death can occur from one to 10 weeks after a clinical illness in the mother and maternal B19-specific IgM may become undetectable after 8–12 weeks. Fetal hydrops due to parvovirus B19 infection can therefore occur in the presence of a negative maternal IgM response[3]. In the case of maternal contact with a suspected acute infection, testing of stored antenatal blood may also be useful. The demonstration of B19-specific IgG in a blood sample that predates the contact indicates a past infection and presumed immunity to the virus. Those patients who are found to be B19 susceptible should be followed up serologically. B19-specific antibody testing should be done approximately four weeks after the contact or at the time of clinical symptoms if a rash or arthralgia occurs. Testing should be repeated if exposure continues[28]. Laboratory testing is important as the majority of patients with an acute infection in pregnancy will be asymptomatic[22]. Screening of pregnant women on the basis of clinical symptoms alone will therefore underestimate the incidence of acute infection.

If a symptomatic or asymptomatic parvovirus B19 infection is diagnosed during pregnancy the possible implications of infection should be discussed with the woman. Maternal infection is not considered to be an indication for termination of pregnancy.

However, careful follow-up of the fetus is indicated. This includes serial ultrasound examination every 1–2 weeks for a period of 12–14 weeks and, possibly, serum α-fetoprotein determinations (see above)[50]. Ascites, skin oedema, pleural or pericardial effusions, hepatomegaly, placentamegaly or an altered fetal biophysical profile (for example, decreased fetal movements) have been described as ultrasonographic indicators of fetal infection[51]. It has also been suggested that the biventricular outer dimension is the best predictor of perinatal outcome in cases of non-immune hydrops fetalis. A study by Carlson and colleagues showed that all 12 fetuses with non-immune hydrops and an enlarged biventricular outer dimension died, whereas the majority with a normal biventricular outer dimension lived[52]. Ultrasound examination may therefore provide valuable information on fetal well-being.

If fetal hydrops or maternal polyhydramnios is observed, a detailed ultrasound examination to exclude fetal anomalies should be done. In addition, fetal blood should be examined for the presence of B19 (see below) and to determine the haemoglobin concentration, karyotype and white blood cell and platelet counts. If the fetus is severely anaemic (for example, haemoglobin below 5 g/dl), fetal blood transfusion should be considered. If not, further follow-up, including weekly ultrasound examination, twice-weekly cardiotocographs and daily fetal movement recording, is indicated. If the fetus develops increasing hydrops, arrhythmia or an abnormal heart rate, further management depends on the gestational age. If this is more than 32 weeks, delivery with postnatal blood transfusion should be considered. In a fetus of less than 32 weeks gestation, diagnostic cordocentesis should be repeated and the haemoglobin re-estimated. If the fetus is severely anaemic fetal blood transfusion is indicated[53] (Figure 6.2); the degree of anaemia, rather than the presence or absence of hydrops, should be used to determine the need for fetal blood transfusion.

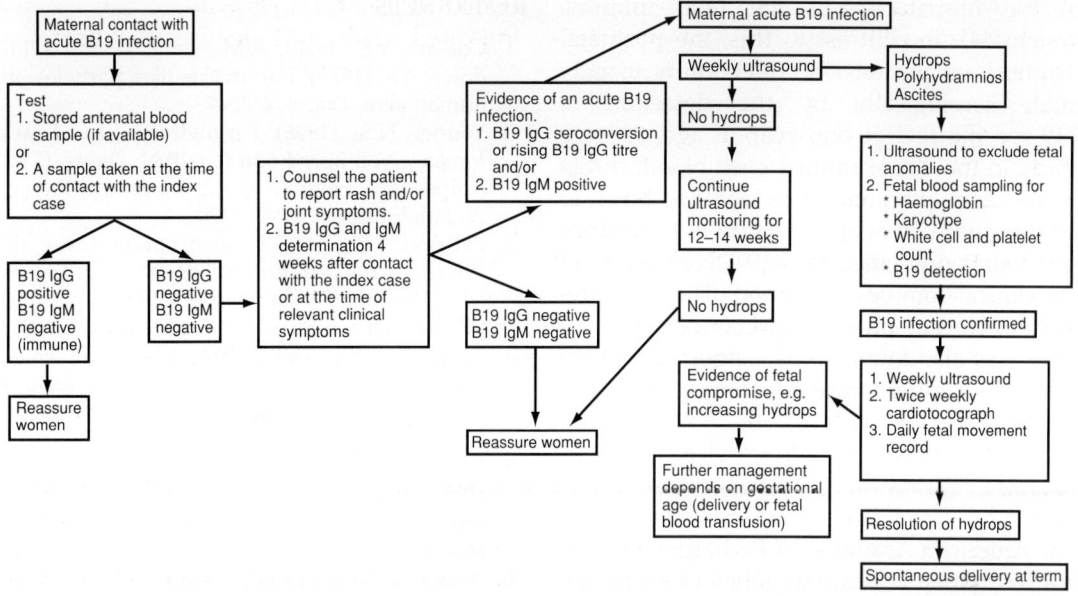

Figure 6.2 Schematic representation of the management of B19 infection in pregnancy (modified from reference [53] with permission).

The gestational age cut-off of 32 weeks may, of course, vary from unit to unit; this is not absolute and may need to be modified according to the clinical circumstances. For example, Donders and colleagues described the successful delivery of a 31-week hydropic fetus who was then transfused postnatally. Although persistent anaemia necessitated several blood transfusions up to the age of four months, the child was clinically and haematologically normal at two years of age[54]. If spontaneous resolution of hydrops occurs the woman should be allowed to continue to term and go into spontaneous labour[53].

Further specific intervention has also been described. As fetal hydrops may occur secondary to fetal myocarditis, direct fetal digitalization has been attempted. Although this led to a resolution of the fetal ascites within 72 h, fetal death occurred on day 5 of treatment[55]. In addition, high-dose intravenous immunoglobulin has also been used to treat severe pre-eclampsia with a compromised fetus in a pregnant women with a recent B19 infection. Selbing and colleagues described a 34-year-old woman admitted with severe pre-eclampsia and a proven maternal and fetal B19 infection. The administration of intravenous immunoglobulin resulted in a decrease in maternal proteinuria, normalization of blood pressure and a resolution of fetal ascites. Whilst it is difficult to draw firm conclusions from a single case report, the use of high-dose intravenous immunoglobulin is worth considering under the clinical circumstances described in this report[29].

DIAGNOSIS OF FETAL INFECTION

The diagnosis of fetal infection may be made by the observation of viral particles using electron microscopy or by direct detection of viral DNA in fetal blood samples. B19 DNA may also be detected in amniotic fluid or at autopsy[3,27]. Serological diagnosis of fetal infection is not reliable as most cases are negative for specific IgM, probably because of the immaturity of the fetal immune system[44]. In contrast to this, the postnatal diagnosis of intrauterine infection is usually made serologically by the detection of B19-specific IgG at one year of age. A large study in the UK examined cord blood, throat swabs and placenta from infants born to mothers with an acute infection in pregnancy and found no detectable B19 DNA in any of the clinical samples examined. The measurement of cord blood total IgM concentration at birth was also found to be a poor method of diagnosing intrauterine infections[30].

PREVENTION

The American Academy of Pediatricians does not recommend a routine policy of excluding pregnant workers or teachers from the workplace during an outbreak of EI. However, they do recommend that pregnant health-care workers should not care for patients with an aplastic crisis resulting from a B19 infection as such individuals may be highly contagious[56]. It is important to remember that once the rash of EI has developed the greatest risk of transmission has already occurred[17]. It is also likely that congenitally infected infants do not pose a significant risk of infection to their contacts as a large study failed to detect B19 DNA in any of the samples analysed from a cohort of infants infected *in utero*[30]. No vaccine is currently available. The role of prophylactic administration of human immunoglobulin to susceptible pregnant women after contact with a case of acute infection has yet to be determined.

ACKNOWLEDGEMENTS

The authors would like to thank Dr Wolfgang Preiser for his helpful comments and Ms Charlotte Aschen for preparing the diagrams.

REFERENCES

1. Cossart, Y.E., Field, A.M., Cant, B. and Widdows, D. (1975) Parvovirus-like particles in human sera. *Lancet*, **i**, 72–73.
2. Young, N.S. (1996) Parvoviruses. In: *Field's Virology*, Vol. 2, 3rd edn (eds B.N. Fields, D.M. Knipe, P.M. Howley *et al.*), Lippincott-Raven, Philadelphia, pp. 2199–2220.
3. Pattison, J.R. (1995) Human parvoviruses. In: *Principles and Practice of Clinical Virology*, 3rd edn, (eds A.J. Zuckerman, J.E. Banatvala and J.R. Pattison), John Wiley, Chichester.
4. Serjeant, G.R., Topley, J.M., Mason, K. *et al.* (1981) Outbreak of aplastic crises in sickle cell anaemia associated with parvovirus-like agent. *Lancet*, **ii**, 595–597.
5. Pattison, J.R., Jones, S.E., Hodgson, J. *et al.* (1981) Parvovirus infections and hypoplastic crisis in sickle-cell anaemia (letter). *Lancet*, **i**, 664–665.
6. Anderson, M.J., Lewis, E., Kidd, I.M., Hall, S.M. and Cohen, B.J. (1984) An outbreak of erythema infectiosum associated with human parvovirus infection. *J. Hygiene*, **93**, 85–93.
7. Brown, T., Anand, A., Ritchie, L.D., Clewley, J.P. and Reid, T.M. (1984) Intrauterine parvovirus infection associated with hydrops fetalis (letter). *Lancet*, **ii**, 1033–1034.
8. Reid, D.M., Reid, T.M., Brown, T., Rennie, J.A. and Eastmond, C.J. (1985) Human parvovirus-associated arthritis: a clinical and laboratory description. *Lancet*, **i**, 422–425.
9. Kurtzman, G.J., Ozawa, K., Cohen, B. *et al.* (1987) Chronic bone marrow failure due to persistent B19 parvovirus infection. *N. Engl. J. Med.*, **317**, 287–294.
10. Lefrere, J.J., Courouce, A.M. and Kaplan, C. (1989) Parvovirus and idiopathic thrombocytopenic purpura (letter). *Lancet*, **i**, 279.
11. Foreman, N.K., Oakhill, A. and Caul, E.O. (1988) Parvovirus associated thrombocytopenic purpura (letter). *Lancet*, **ii**, 1426–1427.
12. Brown, K.E., Green, S.W., de Mayolo, J.A. *et al.* (1994) Congenital anaemia after transplacental B19 parvovirus infection. *Lancet*, **343**, 895–896.
13. Brown, K.E., Anderson, S.M. and Young, N.S. (1993) Erythrocyte P antigen: cellular receptor for B19 parvovirus. *Science*, **262**, 114–117.
14. Brown, K.E., Hibbs, J.R., Gallinella, G. *et al.* (1994) Resistance to parvovirus B19 infection due to lack of virus receptor (erythrocyte P antigen). *N. Engl. J. Med.*, **330**, 1192–1196.

15. Cohen, B.J., Mortimer, P.P. and Pereira, M.S. (1983) Diagnostic assays with monoclonal antibodies for the human serum parvovirus-like virus (SPLV). *J. Hygiene*, **91**, 113–130.

16. Centers for Disease Control (1989) Risks associated with human parvovirus B19 infection. *MMWR*, **38**, 81–97.

17. Anderson, L.J. and Hurwitz, E.S. (1988) Human parvovirus B19 and pregnancy. *Clin. Perinatol.*, **15**, 273–286.

18. Frickhofen, N., Abkowitz, J.L., Safford, M. *et al.* (1990) Persistent parvovirus B19 infection in patients infected with human immunodeficiency virus type 1 (HIV-1): a treatable cause of anaemia in AIDS. *Ann. Intern. Med.*, **113**, 926–933.

19. Kurtz, J.B. and Anderson, M.J. (1985) Cross-reactions in rubella and parvovirus specific IgM tests (letter). *Lancet*, **ii**, 1356.

20. Tabrizi, S.N., Chen, S., Borg, A.J. and Garland, S.M. (1994) Use of polymerase chain reaction for detection of human parvovirus B19. *J. Infect. Dis.*, **170**, 1047–1048.

21. Mortimer, P.P., Cohen, B.J., Buckley, M.M. *et al.* (1985) Human parvovirus and the fetus (letter). *Lancet*, **ii**, 1012.

22. Gratacos, E., Torres, P-J., Vidal, J. *et al.* (1995) The incidence of human parvovirus B19 infection during pregnancy and its impact on perinatal outcome. *J. Infect. Dis.*, **171**, 1360–1363.

23. Adler, S.P., Manganello, A-M.A., Koch, W.C., Hempfling, S.H. and Best, A.M. (1993) Risk of human parvovirus B19 infections among school and hospital employees during endemic periods. *J. Infect. Dis.*, **168**, 361–368.

24. Cartter, M.L., Farley, T.A., Rosengre, S. *et al.* (1991) Occupational risk factors for infection with parvovirus B19 among pregnant women. *J. Infect. Dis.*, **163**, 282–285.

25. Seng, C., Watkins, P., Morse, D. *et al.* (1994) Parvovirus B19 outbreak on an adult ward. *Epidemiol. Infect.*, **113**, 345–353.

26. Smoleniec, J.S., Pillai, M., Caul, E.O. and Usher, J. (1994) Subclinical transplacental parvovirus B19 infection: an increased fetal risk? *Lancet*, **343**, 1100–1101.

27. Gay, N.J., Hesketh, L.M., Cohen, B.J. *et al.* (1994) Age specific antibody prevalence to parvovirus B19: how many women are infected in pregnancy? *Commun. Dis. Rep.*, **4**, R104–R107.

28. Hall, C.J. (1994) Parvovirus B19 infection in pregnancy. *Arch. Dis. Child.*, **71**, F4–F5.

29. Selbing, A., Josefsson, A., Dahle, L.O. and Lindgren, R. (1995) Parvovirus B19 infection during pregnancy treated with high dose intravenous gammaglobulin. *Lancet*, **345**, 660–661.

30. Public Health Laboratory Service Working Party on Fifth Disease (1990) Prospective study of human parvovirus (B19) infection in pregnancy. *Br. Med. J.*, **300**, 1166–1170.

31. Anand, A., Gray, E.S., Brown, T., Clewley, J.P. and Cohen, B.J. (1987). Human parvovirus infection in pregnancy and hydrops fetalis. *N. Engl. J. Med.*, **316**(4), 183–186.

32. Schwarz, T.F., Roggendorf, M., Hottemtrager, B. *et al.* (1988) Human parvovirus B19 infection in pregnancy (letter). *Lancet*, **ii**, 566–567.

33. Torok, T.J. (1990) Human parvovirus B19 infections in pregnancy. *Pediatr. Infect. Dis. J.*, **9**, 772–776.

34. Boley, T.J. and Popek, E.J. (1993) Parvovirus infection in pregnancy. *Semin. Perinatol.*, **17**, 410–419.

35. Chorba, T., Coccia, P., Holman, R.C. *et al.* (1986) The role of parvovirus B19 in aplastic crisis and erythema infectiosum (fifth disease). *J. Infect. Dis.*, **154**, 383–393.

36. Schwarz, T.F., Nerlich, A. and Hillemanns, P. (1993) Detection of parvovirus B19 in fetal autopsies. *Arch. Gynecol. Obstet.*, **253**, 207–213.

37. Rogers, B.B., Mark, Y. and Oyer, C.E. (1993) Diagnosis and incidence of fetal parvovirus infection in an autopsy series: I. Histology. *Pediatr. Pathol.*, **13**, 371–379.

38. Morey, A.L., Keeling, J.W., Porter, H.J. and Flemming, K.A. (1992) Clinical and histopathological features of parvovirus B19 infection in the human fetus. *Br. J. Obstet. Gynaecol.*, **99**, 566–574.

39. Pustilnik, T.B. and Cohen, A.W. (1994) Parvovirus B19 infection in a twin pregnancy. *Obstet. Gynecol.*, **83**, 834–836.

40. Ager, E.A., Chin, T.D. and Poland, J.D. (1966) Epidemic erythema infectiosum. *N. Engl. J. Med.*, **275**, 1326–1331.

41. Weiland, H.T., Vermey-Keers, C., Salimans, M.M. *et al.* (1987) Parvovirus B19 associated with fetal abnormality (letter). *Lancet*, **i**, 682–683.

42. Tiessen, R.G., van Elsacker-Niele, A.M.W., Vermeij-Keers, C.H.R. *et al.* (1994) A fetus with a parvovirus B19 infection and congenital anomalies. *Prenatal Diagn.*, **14**, 173–176.

43. Koch, W.C., Adler, S.P. and Harger, J. (1993) Intrauterine parvovirus B19 infection may

cause an asymptomatic or recurrent post-natal infection. *Pediatr. Infect. Dis. J.*, **12**, 747–750.

44. Sheikh, A.U. and Ernest, J.M. (1995) Clinical picture and consequences of fetal parvovirus B19 infection. *Ann. Intern. Med.*, **27**, 7–8.

45. Burton, P.A. and Caul, E.O. (1988) Fetal cell tropism of human parvovirus B19 (letter). *Lancet*, **i**, 767.

46. Anderson, M.J., Khousam, M.N., Maxwell, D.J. *et al.* (1988) Human parvovirus B19 and hydrops fetalis (letter). *Lancet*, **i**, 535.

47. Porter, H.J., Quantrill, A.M. and Flemming, K.A. (1988) B19 Parvovirus infection of myocardial cells (letter). *Lancet*, **i**, 535–536.

48. Morey, A.L., Porter, H.J., Keeling, J.W. and Flemming, K.A. (1992) Non-isotopic in situ hybridisation and immunophenotyping of infected cells in the investigation of human fetal parvovirus infection. *J. Clin. Pathol.*, **45**, 673–678.

49. Saller, D.N., Rogers, B.B. and Canick, J.A. (1993) Maternal serum biochemical markers in pregnancies with fetal parvovirus B19 infection. *Prenatal Diagn.*, **13**, 467–471.

50. Ghidini, A. and Lynch, L. (1994) Management strategies for congenital infections. *Mt. Sinai J. Med.*, **61**, 376–388.

51. Rodis, J.F., Quinn, D.L., Gary, G.W. *et al.* (1990) Management and outcomes of pregnancies complicated by human B19 parvovirus infection: a prospective study. *Am. J. Obstet. Gynecol.*, **163**, 1168–1171.

52. Carlson, D.E., Platt, L.D., Medearis, A.L. and Horenstein, J. (1990) Prognostic indicators of the resolution of nonimmune hydrops fetalis and survival of the fetus. *Am. J. Obstet. Gynecol.*, **163**, 1785–1787.

53. Sheikh, A.U., Ernest, J.M. and O'Shea, M. (1992) Long-term outcome in fetal hydrops from parvovirus B19 infection. *Am. J. Obstet. Gynecol.*, **167**, 337–341.

54. Donders, G.G.G., van Lierde, S., van Elsacker-Niele A-M.W. *et al.* (1994) Survival after intrauterine parvovirus B19 infection with persistence in early infancy: a two year follow-up. *Pediatr. Infect. Dis. J.*, **13**(3), 234–236.

55. Naides, S.J. and Weiner, C.P. (1989) Antenatal diagnosis and palliative treatment of nonimmune hydrops fetalis secondary to fetal parvovirus B19 infection. *Prenatal Diagn.*, **9**, 105–114.

56. American Academy of Pediatrics, Committee on Infectious Diseases (1990) Parvovirus, erythema infectiosum and pregnancy. *Pediatrics*, **85**, 131–133.

Herpes simplex virus infections in pregnancy

A. Mindel

THE VIRUS

There are two herpes simplex viruses designated herpes simplex type 1 (HSV1) and herpes simplex virus type 2 (HSV2)[1]. They are members of the alpha herpesvirinae sub-family of the Herpesviridae[2]. The only other human herpesvirus that is a member of this subfamily is varicella-zoster virus[2]. The classification into alpha herpesvirinae is based on a number of factors, the most important being the ability to establish latent infections mainly but not exclusively in neurological cells, in particular sensory ganglia[2]. In common with all members of the Herpesviridae family, these viruses consist of double-stranded DNA, an icosahedral capsid containing 162 capsomeres, amorphous material surrounding the capsid known as the tegument and an envelope containing viral protein spikes consisting of glycoproteins[3]. The two herpes simplex viruses have a considerable degree of genetic similarity with approximately 50% of the DNA sequences being highly conserved[3].

One major feature of herpes simplex virus infections is the ability to establish latency with subsequent reactivation. It is believed that once infected, latent virus remains with the individual for life and periodic reactivation, resulting either in asymptomatic viral excretion from skin or mucous membranes or clinical disease, occurs throughout the life of the individual[4].

EPIDEMIOLOGY

Herpes simplex virus (HSV) infections are among the commonest viral infections affecting humans[5]. HSV infections can occur around the mouth (cold sores), the genital area (genital herpes) and the eye (ophthalmic herpes) or disseminate to the brain (herpes simplex encephalitis), internal organs or the skin[5]. However, most individuals acquire the infection asymptomatically and probably remain asymptomatic for the rest of their lives. It is likely that most of these individuals will shed virus asymptomatically from time to time although some may have minor symptoms that they do not recognize as being due to herpes[6].

Until recently, serological tests were unable to differentiate accurately between HSV1 and HSV2 infection. However, type-specific serological tests, mainly using Western blot technology[7–9] have now been used in many epidemiological surveys. These studies suggest that infections with HSV1 and HSV2 are extremely common. HSV1 (buccal) infections are usually acquired in early childhood: by the age of five approximately 30% of North American children are infected with HSV1 and by the age of 15 approximately half will be infected[10]. Studies throughout the world have suggested that HSV1 seroprevalence in adults ranges between 40% and 95%[11].

In contrast, seroprevalence surveys have shown that HSV2 (genital) infection is

Viral Infections in Obstetrics and Gynaecology. Edited by D.J. Jeffries and C.N. Hudson. Published in 1999 by Arnold, ISBN 0 340 74095 7.

extremely rare in childhood but increases rapidly from the age of 15 to peak in the mid 30s[12–14]. These studies have shown that besides age, other important factors for acquisition of HSV2 include the number of sexual partners, acquisition of other STDs and gender (women are more likely to acquire the infection than men)[12,13]. Some studies have suggested that other factors may be important including race (in America, Afro-Americans have a higher seroprevalence than Caucasian Americans), social class (individuals coming from poor socioeconomic backgrounds are more likely to be seropositive than those coming from more wealthy backgrounds) and poor education levels[12].

Population-based surveys have shown that in the US between 1976 and 1980, the HSV2 seroprevalence in adults aged 15 years or over was 16.4%[12]. A subsequent survey conducted between 1988 and 1994 suggested that the seroprevalence had increased to 21.7%[15]. A study in Toronto between 1978 and 1980, using a non-type specific serological test which was thought to underestimate the seroprevalence of HSV2 by up to 30%, showed that HSV2 seroprevalence was 17.5%[16] and a study in San Francisco showed a seroprevalence of 33%[17]. Studies in selected population groups have shown extremely variable HSV2 seroprevalence. For example, among STD clinic attenders reported seroprevalence ranges from 8% to 83%[11,14, 18–20], among female prostitutes from 75% to 96%[11,20,21] and in blood donors from 5% to 18%[14–21].

EPIDEMIOLOGY OF HSV IN PREGNANCY

Most women who become pregnant have already been exposed to herpes simplex type 1 infection, with serological surveys in antenatal

Table 7.1 HSV 2 seroprevalence in antenatal clinic attenders

City	Number tested	Percentage positive	Test	Author and Reference
Toyko	90	6	gG2 Immunodot	Hashido[18]
Padua, Italy	NK	8.4	gG2 Immunodot	Nahmias[11]
Seville, Spain	NK	9.7	gG2 Immunodot	Nahmias[11]
Birmingham, Alabama (whites)	NK	11.4	gG2 Immunodot	Nahmias[11]
Taiwan	NK	13.5	gG2 Immunodot	Nahmias[11]
Sydney	229	14.5	gG2 ELISA	Cunningham[19]
Stockholm 1969	941	17	gG2 ELISA	Forsgren[22]
Lyon	NK	17.3	gG2 Immunodot	Nahmias[11]
Rejkjavik, Iceland	NK	18.8	gG2 Immunodot	Nahmias[11]
Stockholm 1983	1759	32	gG2 ELISA	Forsgren[22]
Stockholm 1989	1000	32	gG2 ELISA	Forsgren[22]
Stanford, USA 1991	277	32	gG2 ELISA	Kulhanjian[23]
Atlanta (whites)	NK	34.9	gG2 Immunodot	Nahmias[11]
Sao Paulo 1988–9 (low and middle class)	455	36	ELISA and Western blot	Weinberg[25]
Seattle, USA 1990	201	37.8	Western blot	Brown[24]
Sao Paulo 1988–9 (very low income)	200	42	ELISA and Western blot	Weinberg[25]
Atlanta (blacks)	NK	53.4	gG2 Immunodot	Nahmias[11]

NK, not known; ELISA, enzyme immunoassay; gG2, glycoprotein G2 clinics showing that 50–90% of women have previously been exposed to the virus[11]. The seroprevalence of HSV2 in antenatal clinic attenders is very variable (6–53%) and is summarized in Table 7.1[11,18,19,22–25]. The lowest seroprevalence (8%) noted was in Padua, Italy, and the highest (53%) in blacks in Atlanta, USA. However, the vast majority of women with HSV2 antibodies will not give a history of previous genital herpes. The incidence of clinically apparent recurrent genital herpes in pregnancy (see below) will be dependent upon the prevalence of this infection within the community.

The importance of antibody status in relation to pregnancy outcome in antenatal patients is discussed below.

DETECTED VERSUS UNRECOGNIZED HERPES

Several studies have tried to elucidate the relationship between the detection of HSV antibodies (mainly HSV2) and symptoms or signs suggesting herpetic infections[14,17,26–28]. One may divide these studies into two types: seroprevalence studies and prospective clinical studies. The seroprevalence studies (i.e. those where groups of individuals are screened for HSV antibodies and are asked about symptoms suggesting herpes) show that 70% of individuals with HSV antibodies are asymptomatic. However, studies where individuals with HSV antibodies are given information regarding the clinical manifestations of herpes and then prospectively followed suggest that 50% will be truly asymptomatic, 30% will have clinical disease and an additional 20% will have disease that would have been unrecognized had this procedure not been adopted[26,28].

The importance of these studies in relation to pregnancy is that many women will enter pregnancy with HSV2 infection and be unaware of their serostatus or that they may shed virus asymptomatically at term (see below).

CLINICAL MANIFESTATIONS OF GENITAL HERPES IN WOMEN

As mentioned above, genital herpes is often asymptomatic. However, following exposure, some individuals may develop severe primary episodes and many of these will go on to have clinical recurrences over many years[29]. Most genital infections are due to HSV2 although a considerable minority may be caused by HSV1[30,31]. The infection is transmitted via sexual intercourse, with genital HSV1 infections occurring as a consequence of orogenital sex. The clinical manifestations of the first episode caused by the two viruses are similar but genital infection with HSV2 recurs earlier and more frequently than genital infection with HSV1[32–34].

The severity of the first episode is affected by prior exposure to HSV infections, usually HSV-1 oral disease in childhood. Those who do not have antibodies tend to have more severe symptoms, particularly systemic symptoms, when compared with those who have antibodies[29].

The first symptoms usually occur anywhere between two and 14 days following exposure. The local symptoms consist of pain and dysuria and there may be a vaginal discharge noticed due to herpetic lesions occurring on the cervix (Plate I). The first sign of infection is erythema followed shortly by painful vesicles that rapidly burst to leave shallow painful ulcers. The vesicles and ulcers are often multiple and occur on the labia minora (Plate J), fourchette and cervix as well as other parts of the genitalia. The vesicles continue to occur in crops over two weeks and the entire illness lasts approximately three weeks from the first signs of the infection to the healing of the ulcers. Lesions occurring on dry skin will crust over, whereas those on the mucous membranes do not form crusts. The dysuria may be very severe, particularly if lesions are near the urethra. On occasion, the dysuria may be so severe that patients develop urinary retention[29]. The systemic symptoms consist of fever, malaise and myalgia which usually last up to five days[29].

Complications of first-episode genital herpes include self-limiting viral meningitis, dissemination to cutaneous sites distant from the genitalia, in particular thighs, buttocks and hands, secondary infection of lesions (this is uncommon) and a radiculomyelopathy involving the sacral nerves leading to difficulty with urination and defaecation and loss of sensation over the sacral dermatomes. This syndrome is more common in association with herpetic proctitis but can occasionally occur with vulval herpes[29].

Recurrences are usually less severe, lasting between five and seven days, and mostly consist of a single lesion or small crop of lesions on the external genitalia, thighs or buttocks. Some patients may develop prodromal or warning symptoms before the onset of lesions, usually consisting of a tingling sensation in the genitalia, thigh or buttock with general feelings of ill health occurring up to 24 h before the onset of lesions[29,35]. In addition, some patients develop a neuralgia-type pain in the dermatomal distribution of the lesions and for some individuals the prodromal symptoms and neuralgic pain may be more troublesome than the lesions themselves. The frequency of recurrences is extremely variable. Some individuals have either no recurrences or very occasional episodes whereas others have as many as 12 or 15 per year.

PRIMARY INFECTION DURING PREGNANCY

As mentioned above, the majority of infections acquired either before or during pregnancy are asymptomatic. In those situations where clinical disease does occur, the clinical features are usually very similar to those that occur in non-pregnant women[36]. However, occasionally severe disseminated HSV infections can occur. In the handful of cases that have been described, clinical features include cutaneous dissemination and spread to internal organs leading to necrotizing hepatitis which may be associated with thrombocytopenia, leucopenia, disseminated intravascular coagulation and encephalitis[37–41]. Without treatment, the mortality approaches 50%.

RECURRENT INFECTION IN PREGNANCY

The clinical features of recurrent genital herpes in pregnancy are similar to those occurring in non-pregnant women. However, some women find that recurrences are more frequent or more severe during pregnancy. Whether this is due to the effects of pregnancy or merely reflects the natural history of the infection remains to be determined.

EPIDEMIOLOGY OF NEONATAL HERPES

Neonatal herpes is a rare infection. In the USA the incidence per 100 000 live births is 20–50[42–44], in Australia 10[45], in Sweden six[46] and in the UK less than three[47]. The reasons for these differences probably relate to the prevalence of HSV1 in the community (HSV1 infections confer some protection against subsequent infection with HSV2)[48] and the incidence of HSV2, in particular the acquisition rates between the ages of 18 and 30[12]. One aspect that should be considered when interpreting these data is the fact that very few countries collect information prospectively regarding neonatal herpes and the reported incidence may be underestimated. For example, in Australia the rates are based on a single survey conducted at one hospital in Melbourne[45] and it is likely that the population attending that hospital was not representative of the country as a whole.

TRANSMISSION TO THE FETUS

There are several ways in which transmission to the fetus can occur, including *in utero*, at the time of delivery and postnatally. About 85% of the transmissions occur as a consequence of delivery through an infected birth canal, 5%

are acquired *in utero* and 10% are acquired postnatally [36].

Maternal infection occurring in early pregnancy (up to 20 weeks) can result in spontaneous abortion [49,50]. However, infection occurring later in pregnancy is not associated with spontaneous miscarriages but can result in intrauterine growth retardation [51]. The risk of spontaneous abortion associated with primary infection in pregnancy has been estimated to be up to 25% [52]. However, this information should be regarded with some caution as these studies have involved very small numbers of individuals.

Postnatal infection can occur via the mother, the father or another relative with herpes or from friends or associates or hospital personnel who come into contact with the baby [53–58]. It is presumed that most of these infections occur because of direct contact of the baby with infected secretions from a cold sore or herpetic lesion on the skin or as a result of breastfeeding from an infected nipple [58]. However, many individuals shed the virus asymptomatically from the mouth and presumably other skin sites and may constitute a risk to the baby. This risk has not yet been quantified in formal studies.

Transmission at the time of delivery is dependent upon a number of factors including the type of maternal infection (first episode compared with recurrences) [59], maternal HSV antibody status [60–62], time since rupture of the membranes [60], instrumentation (Plate H) [63,64], site of lesions and duration of the episode [29].

The type of maternal infection that occurs at or around the time of delivery is the most important determinant of the risk of acquisition of neonatal herpes, with first-episode genital herpes constituting a far greater risk than recurrent infection. The reasons for this difference are likely to be multiple and include the following:

- the first episode is usually more severe and longer lasting than recurrences;

- lesions often occur on the cervix with the first episode but this rarely occurs with recurrences;
- viral titres are much higher with the first episode compared with recurrences;
- duration of lesions and viral shedding are longer for the first episode compared with recurrences [29].

Overall, the risk of transmission following delivery through an infected birth canal with primary genital herpes is between 33% and 50% [51,65] compared with <5% if the woman has recurrent genital herpes at the time of delivery [59]. Some women acquire primary genital herpes during pregnancy without developing symptoms. However, the risk to the neonate, comparing symptomatic and asymptomatic primary infection, appears similar [59].

The observation that most women who acquire primary genital herpes during pregnancy are asymptomatic, and that asymptomatic viral shedding can occur with both primary and recurrent genital herpes, may help to explain why more than 70% of mothers of infants with neonatal herpes do not appear to have had any signs or symptoms suggesting herpes [66,67].

First-episode genital herpes can be divided into true primary or non-primary disease on the basis of prior HSV antibody status [29]. Individuals who have no prior HSV exposure and acquire genital herpes for the first time in late pregnancy (true primaries) have a high risk of transmission to the neonate [51]. However, the risk of transmission to the neonate associated with non-primary infection (previous exposure to HSV) appears to be negligible. A recent study from Seattle using type-specific serology on paired sera (using one sample from early in pregnancy and one at the time of delivery) has suggested that up to 2% of women in that city acquire HSV1 or HSV2 for the first time during pregnancy. However, only those women who acquire HSV very late in pregnancy, before seroconversion can be detected, appear to be at risk of transmitting HSV to their babies. The risk to the baby was independent of symptoms in the mother[67a]. The risks associated with asymptomatic viral shedding in conjunction with first episode and recurrent disease have recently been elucidated. Asymptomatic shedding in association with first-episode genital herpes was associated with neonatal herpes[59], low birthweight and preterm labour[68], whereas asymptomatic shedding in association with recurrent genital herpes was not associated with low birthweight or preterm labour[68] and only associated with neonatal herpes in one of 34 (3%) women[59].

The frequency of asymptomatic viral shedding in non-pregnant women is dependent on several factors including viral type, HSV antibody status and the time since acquisition of the infection[69]. There is no reason to believe that the situation in pregnant women is any different. Asymptomatic viral shedding occurs more frequently with HSV2 genital infection than HSV-1[69]. In addition, in the three months following the acquisition of primary HSV2 genital infection asymptomatic viral shedding occurs 2–3 times more frequently than later on[69]. This observation highlights the importance of inapparent primary HSV2 genital infection in late pregnancy. Women with existing HSV1 infections, who acquire genital HSV2, appear to be at a decreased risk of asymptomatic viral shedding from the vulva but not from the cervix[69].

There are numerous reports concerning the frequency of asymptomatic viral shedding at the time of delivery, which can occur in several different situations. Viral shedding without clinically obvious lesions occurs at the time of delivery in 1–2% of women with a history of recurrent genital herpes[70,71], in 0.2% of women with serological evidence of HSV2 infection[70] and in 23% of women with recent acquisition of HSV2[51] (see above).

Prior antibody status is also important. First, women with prior HSV1 infection are less likely to acquire HSV2 during pregnancy[26,27]. Second, babies born to mothers with prior HSV infection acquire antibody-dependent cell-mediated cytotoxic (ADCC) and neutralizing antibodies transplacentally[58]. Although the evidence concerning the benefit of transplacental antibodies is conflicting, both neutralizing and ADCC antibodies appear to offer at least some protection to the baby in terms of reduced acquisition of herpes and if the infection is acquired, it tends to be less severe[46,60–62,72–74]. The time since rupture of the membranes is also important and it has been suggested that if the membranes are ruptured for longer than eight hours, the risk of ascending infection increases and consequent benefits of caesarean section (see below) are reduced[73].

Finally, medical instrumentation may also be important, particularly the use of scalp electrodes which may offer a portal of entry for the virus (Plate H)[76,77].

CLINICAL MANIFESTATION OF NEONATAL HERPES

Neonatal herpes may be classified into infection acquired *in utero* and infection acquired via delivery through an infected birth canal[10]. As discussed above, infection acquired *in utero* is exceptionally rare but is the most severe form of neonatal herpetic infection. Infected babies may have involvement of the skin, the eyes and the brain. Skin manifestations include vesicles or scarring, eye involvement includes choroidoretinitis with or without keratoconjunctivitis. The brain involvement includes encephalitis usually in association with microcephaly or hydranencephaly[78].

Infection occurring from delivery through an infected birth canal can be further classified into localized infection, disseminated infection and encephalitis[74]. These three manifestations each appear to occur in approximately one-third of patients. However, there is some evidence to suggest that

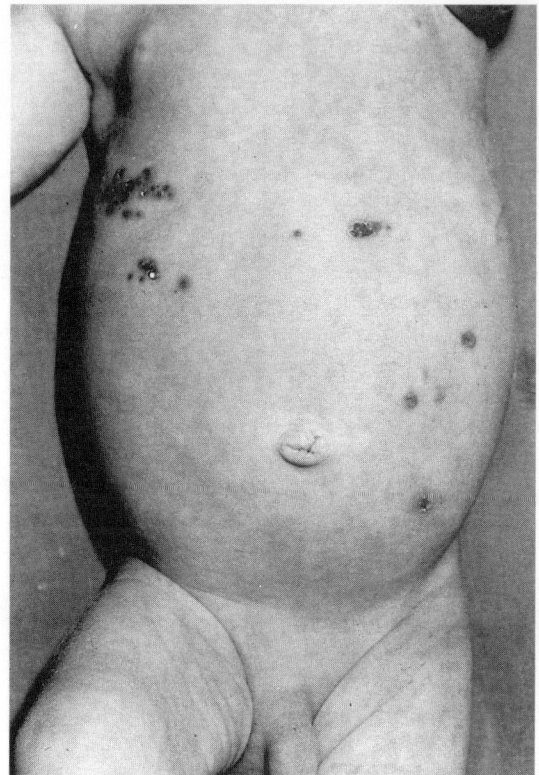

these proportions may have altered in recent years, with more babies presenting with skin, eye or mucous membrane infections and fewer presenting with disseminated infection than was the situation in the 1970s[74].

LOCALIZED INFECTION

Localized infection can occur on the skin or in the eye or mouth[60]. The skin manifestations include clusters of vesicles or crusts that may occur on any part of the body (Figures 7.1, 7.2, Plate H), although lesions on the presenting part are more common[60,75]. Occasionally the lesions are atypical, presenting as erythematous or purpuric maculae, erythema multiforme or zosteriform lesions[79].

Lesions can occur in the oral cavity, either alone or in conjunction with skin or eye disease, and ocular herpes also can occur alone or in conjunction with orolabial or cutaneous disease[80]. Any part of the eye can be infected but most commonly there is a blepharoconjunctivitis with vesicles on the eyelids and surrounding face[80,81]. Choroidoretinitis, conjunctivitis, keratitis, uveitis, retinal dysplasia, microphthalmia and cataracts can

Figure 7.1 Neonatal herpes. Crusted lesions on the abdomen of a 10-day-old neonate with herpes.

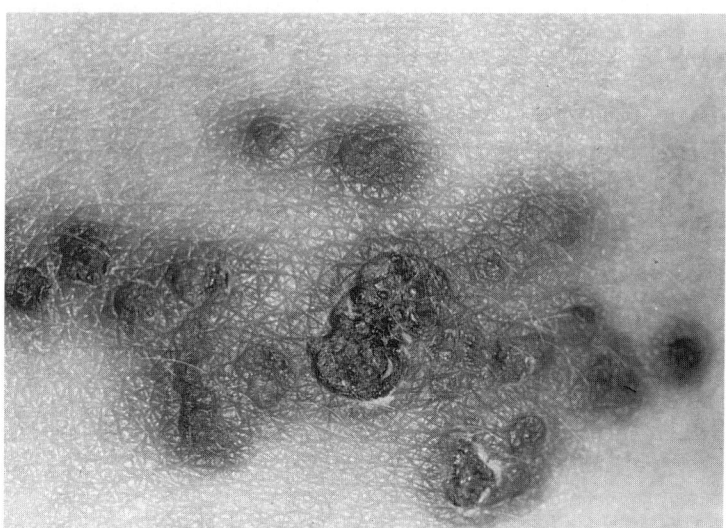

Figure 7.2 Neonatal herpes. Close-up view of crusted lesions on the abdomen.

occur [80–83]. Choroidoretinitis is almost invariably associated with encephalitis [84].

Localized disease is not associated with early mortality [74]. However, skin lesions may recur over many months resulting in scarring, particularly when secondary infection occurs, and eye disease may lead to visual loss or blindness [73]. Some of these babies also have evidence of neurological impairment that may not be apparent at birth and it may be 6–12 months after delivery that problems are detected. The important long-term neurological problems include microcephaly and spastic quadriplegia [73].

DISSEMINATED DISEASE

Infection can involve any internal organ, the commonest being the liver and the adrenals. Other organs that may be involved include the upper respiratory tract, the lungs, oesophagus, stomach, lower genital tract, spleen, kidneys, pancreas and even the heart [74]. The onset of the disease is usually insidious and non-specific and difficult to diagnose. Babies present with irritability, poor appetite and lethargy. Later on, fever, respiratory problems and seizures develop. On examination the babies may be noted to have hepatomegaly, jaundice or evidence of a bleeding diathesis [74]. Skin lesions may be present, which will aid in the diagnosis [75]. However, the majority of babies do not have skin lesions. Without therapy, mortality approaches 80%, with the babies dying of disseminated intravascular coagulation or pneumonia [10]. Up to three-quarters of all babies with disseminated herpes infection also have CNS involvement [74].

ENCEPHALITIS

One-third of babies with neonatal herpes have involvement of CNS alone. However, as mentioned above, the majority of those with disseminated infection also have CNS involvement [74]. Infection presents with lethargy, irritability, tremors and seizures. On examination, the temperature is usually raised, there is evidence of bulging fontanelles and pyramidal tract signs. Skin lesions may be present in about half of the babies [84,85].

The long-term prognosis is poor with 50% of the infants either dying or suffering severe neurological deficit including microcephaly, hydranencephaly, porencephalic cysts, spasticity, psychomotor disturbances and learning difficulties [74,75].

MANAGEMENT OF THE PREGNANT WOMAN WITH HERPES

FIRST EPISODE

Women who present with a first episode of genital herpes during pregnancy should be considered for antiviral therapy. Anecdotal evidence suggests that treatment with acyclovir may be very successful in reducing the severity of these infections and in decreasing mortality [86,87]. In the cases reported to date the dose of acyclovir was 7.5 mg/kg intravenously for 5–11 days. Intravenous acyclovir will reduce the duration and severity of the episode and is particularly helpful in those individuals who have a true primary infection (i.e., no previous HSV antibodies) [88]. However, the treatment should be used with caution in pregnancy, particularly in the first trimester, as the safety of acyclovir for the fetus has not been firmly established. Nonetheless, several anecdotal reports on the use of acyclovir for genital or orolabial herpes or varicella-zoster virus infection [86,87,89–93], together with cumulative data collected by the Acyclovir in Pregnancy Register [94], have to date not produced any adverse events attributable to the drug.

The Acyclovir in Pregnancy Register was set up to record all acyclovir use during pregnancy. Most of the reported acyclovir use was to treat preexisting herpes simplex infections. However, some physicians reported using the drug for severe or life-threatening infections. Between the beginning of June 1984 and the end of June 1993, 811 reports were received although adequate follow-up information was only available for 601 (74%). Acyclovir use occurred at different stages of pregnancy and comparisons with birth defects surveillance data maintained by the CDC suggested that there was no increase in birth defects in infants born to mothers who used the drug at any time during pregnancy[94]. These data are encouraging; however, the relatively small sample size, the loss to follow-up and under-reporting are of concern. Consequently, in the first trimester the potential benefits of acyclovir will need to be weighed against the possibility of any rare teratogenic effects.

Most women who have been treated in pregnancy have received standard doses of acyclovir, usually by mouth[94]. However, there is some evidence to suggest that the mean steady state of acyclovir may be lower in pregnant women probably due to an increase in body mass and higher basal metabolic rate[95,96], and higher doses may be appropriate. Further studies will be required to determine the optimum dose and duration of therapy in pregnancy.

The newer antiviral agents valaciclovir (a prodrug of acyclovir)[97] and famciclovir (a prodrug of penciclovir)[98] both have a similar mode of action to acyclovir by competing as a substrate for viral thymidine kinase. Both of these agents appear to have an advantage over acyclovir in terms of greater bioavailability and consequently less frequent daily dosing[97,98]. However, their long-term safety and efficacy are yet to be established and there is little evidence to suggest that their efficacy is better than that of acyclovir. Consequently, until further information is available, famciclovir and valaciclovir should be avoided in pregnancy.

RECURRENT GENITAL HERPES

In non-pregnant women, recurrent genital herpes can be managed either with intermittent antiviral therapy or with continuous suppression to prevent recurrences occurring[99–101]. The latter approach is particularly useful in women with frequent recurrences[101]. A similar approach can be used in pregnancy. However, as discussed above, although there is no evidence suggesting safety concerns with acyclovir in pregnancy, until further information is available it would seem prudent to avoid the drug in pregnancy, particularly during the first trimester.

The use of acyclovir suppression to reduce the likelihood of caesarean sections is discussed below.

TREATMENT OF THE INFECTED INFANT

Both acyclovir and vidarabine have considerable efficacy for the treatment of neonatal herpes. These two drugs were compared in a randomized, controlled, multicentre trial[75]. The dosage of vidarabine was 30 mg/kg/day administered by continuous intravenous infusion. The dose of acyclovir was 30 mg/kg/day intravenously in three divided doses. There were no statistically significant differences with respect to morbidity, mortality or toxicity between the two drugs. However, although both acyclovir and vidarabine reduced mortality, a considerable number of babies (in particular those who presented with CNS or disseminated infection) were left with serious long-term sequelae, mainly CNS damage. There are several possible reasons for this poor response including delay in diagnosis and initiation of therapy and extensive brain or other organ damage prior to the commencement of therapy.

Although there is no significant difference in efficacy between these two agents, the ease of administration of IV acyclovir and its better safety profile mean that most paediatricians now recommend this drug in preference to vidarabine. Trials evaluating valaciclovir and famciclovir are awaited with interest.

PREVENTION OF TRANSMISSION

PREVENTING INTRAPARTUM INFECTION

Although acyclovir has had a significant impact on reducing the mortality and morbidity of neonatal herpes, many infants are still left with serious morbidity, in particular neurological problems. Consequently, there has been considerable interest in the possibility of preventing transmission to the neonate. One of the major problems in formulating a management policy is that up to 70% of babies with neonatal herpes are born to mothers without any signs or symptoms suggestive of genital herpes[66,67]. Many prevention strategies have been used or suggested for use, although the majority of these have not been evaluated adequately. This has resulted in considerable confusion regarding the appropriate management of herpes simplex in pregnancy.

This matter was explored in a recent postal survey of obstetricians' attitudes to the management of genital herpes in the UK. One thousand two hundred and one obstetricians responded to the postal survey and of these, only 369 (31%) admitted to having a formal policy governing the management of herpes in pregnancy within their unit. In addition, 60% advocated regular screening and two-thirds of these performed regular antenatal swabs for viral culture. Indications for performing a caesarean section were equally diverse, with 92% offering caesarean section if an active lesion was seen at the time of labour, 50% offering it to those who had had a positive viral culture on the occasion prior to presentation in labour (even though 32% of these did not perform viral cultures!) and 36% thought it was appropriate to perform a caesarean section if the patient thought there was a recurrence even if no lesions were visible[102].

The current options available for prevention of neonatal herpes fall into three categories: detection and treatment of primary genital herpes, detection and treatment of recurrent genital herpes and the prevention of postnatal infection. However, despite the fact that the risks associated with recurrent genital herpes in pregnancy are small, efforts have been directed mainly at detecting the recurrent disease.

PREVENTING NEONATAL HERPES FROM PRIMARY MATERNAL GENITAL HERPES

In the first six months following primary herpes, there is a considerable risk of both clinical recurrences and asymptomatic viral shedding[69]. Consequently, these women are at particular risk of infecting the neonate at the time of delivery.

A recent study by Scott *et al.* has suggested that suppressive acyclovir used from 36 weeks gestation, in women who had had a first episode of genital herpes during that pregnancy, could significantly reduce the likelihood of having a caesarean section[103]. These authors conducted a randomized, double-blind, placebo-controlled trial in women with first-episode genital herpes. This study showed that none of the 21 acyclovir-treated patients and nine of the 25 (36%) placebo-treated patients had a caesarean section (odds ratio 0.04, 90% confidence interval 0.002–0.745, p=0.002). However, although the study clearly demonstrated a considerable advantage in terms of reducing the likelihood of caesarean section, there were no adverse fetal outcomes in either group and none of the patients had asymptomatic viral shedding at the time of delivery. On the basis of this study, it would seem reasonable to recommend suppressive acyclovir therapy for all women having a first episode of genital herpes from 36 weeks of pregnancy until the time of delivery. This approach would have a number of advantages, including a decrease in the proportion of women requiring caesarean sections and in the overall costs of these pregnancies. The optimum time to start therapy and the question of the appropriate dose are still to be addressed.

PREVENTING NEONATAL HERPES FROM RECURRENT MATERNAL GENITAL HERPES

Several strategies have been suggested, including:

- caesarean section to bypass the birth canal in women with recurrence of genital herpes at the time of delivery[104,105];
- suppressive antiviral therapy for the last few weeks of pregnancy in women with a history of recurrent genital herpes to reduce the risk of a clinical recurrence or asymptomatic viral shedding and the possible perceived need for caesarean section[106,107];
- antiviral therapy for newborns from all women with recurrent genital herpes to prevent infection in the newborn[108].

Caesarean section remains the main method for preventing neonatal herpes in women with recurrent genital herpes. However, there are no published studies to evaluate this intervention and considering the low risk of transmission (about 3%), the potential benefit needs to be weighed against the risks associated with caesarean section, including deep vein thrombosis and pulmonary embolism, operative blood loss and the need for transfusion, longer hospital stays, repeat caesarean section, uterine rupture and an increased risk of neonatal respiratory distress, damage to other organs, infection, pain and discomfort[109–111]. Although the mortality associated with caesarean section is low, it is at least twice that of vaginal delivery[109].

The decision to perform a caesarean section is usually based on one of several considerations including prodromal symptoms suggestive of an imminent genital recurrence, a clinically evident genital recurrence at the onset of labour, a positive viral culture during the time preceding labour and finally a maternal request for the procedure irrespective of clinical signs[102,104,105]. In recurrent genital herpes viral shedding only lasts a few days[29,35] and given that the results of viral culture are often not available for a week

or more, decisions based on viral culture may not reflect the situation at the time of delivery[112,113]. Current methods for the immediate detection of virus using cytology or direct immunofluorescence lack sensitivity[112,114].

The results of a study looking at the efficacy, risks and costs of caesarean section in women with a history of genital herpes were recently published[115]. Using evaluated information from published studies, the authors concluded that the practice of recommending caesarean section for women with a history of recurrent herpes who were having a recurrence at the time of delivery would result in more than 1580 excess caesarean deliveries for every case of neonatal herpes prevented. Consequently, some people have abandoned this approach, relying solely on the presence of a clinically apparent recurrence at the time of delivery. This approach will reduce the number of unnecessary caesarean sections, but will miss the occasional patient who will be shedding virus asymptomatically.

There has been considerable interest in the possibility of using suppressive acyclovir therapy during the last four weeks of pregnancy in an attempt to prevent viral reactivation, clinical recurrences and consequently the need for caesarean section. A study conducted in Norway attempted to address this issue[106]. Forty six women with recurrent genital herpes were treated with acyclovir 200 mg four times daily starting at least a week before expected term and a control group of 46 women did not receive any treatment. The authors failed to state how patients were allocated to each of the two arms. Acyclovir treatment was given for an average of 10 days (range 3–27 days). There were no recurrences in the 10 days prior to delivery or at the time of delivery in the acyclovir-treated group, compared with eight (17%) within 10 days before delivery in the untreated group and four recurrences at the time of delivery. The authors reported that these differences were statistically significant (p<0.001). In addition, there were no caesarean sections for maternal genital herpes in the acyclovir-treated group compared with nine (20%) in the group who did not receive acyclovir (p<0.001). Although this study suggests that oral acyclovir during the last few weeks of pregnancy may be useful in reducing the number of caesarean sections, the fact that the study was not randomized and placebo-controlled calls these results into question. More recently, a randomized placebo-controlled trial of suppressive acyclovir in late pregnancy in women with recurrent genital herpes infection has been published[107]. Unfortunately, poor recruitment resulted in early termination of the study. An additional problem was that the two study centres (London and Sheffield) had slightly different eligibility criteria prior to entry as well as differences in the mode of delivery. In London, women were eligible to enter the study if they had a history of recurrent genital herpes, whereas in Sheffield to be eligible for the trial all women needed to have experienced at least one symptomatic recurrence during the pregnancy before trial entry. In London, at the time of labour if there was evidence of recurrent herpes, a caesarean section was recommended. However, in Sheffield if the woman experienced a herpes recurrence at or after 38 weeks gestation then delivery by caesarean section was performed. An estimate of sample size in the study was based on the assumption that the frequency of caesarean section for genital herpes would be 25% in the placebo group and this would be reduced to 5% in the treatment group, giving a requirement of 120 patients i.e. 60 in each group. After four years, only 63 patients were recruited and the trial was terminated. Treatment was with acyclovir 200 mg four times day or matching placebo from 36 weeks of pregnancy until delivery. Thirty one patients received acyclovir and 32 received placebo. There were no significant differences between the two groups. Nine of the 31 (29%) acyclovir recipients had a recurrence after trial entry

compared with 11 of the 32 (34%) placebo recipients. In addition, there were four (13%) caesarean sections for herpes in the acyclovir group compared with eight (25%) in the placebo group. The odds ratio for delivery by caesarean section for women taking acyclovir compared with those taking placebo was 0.44 (95% CI 0.09–1.59).

This study provides useful information on the use of acyclovir in late pregnancy. First, the dosage used in the study may have been inadequate. Previous pharmacokinetic studies in women in late pregnancy have suggested that higher doses of acyclovir may be necessary to achieve therapeutic serum levels. In addition, the problems of compliance and the frequency of tablet taking need to be addressed[95,96]. In immunocompetent non-pregnant individuals, the frequency of tablet taking is more important than the total daily dose[116,117]. Compliance with therapy was not specifically addressed in the study and is obviously important. With a drug that has a relatively short half-life, compliance with therapy is essential.

What conclusions can be drawn from these studies? First, we urgently require further randomized placebo-controlled studies using appropriate doses of acyclovir in late pregnancy to determine whether this form of therapy can reduce the number of caesarean sections in this group of women. Second, women with recurrent herpes should be advised that there is no convincing evidence that acyclovir in standard therapeutic doses will reduce either the frequency of recurrences or the need for caesarean section in late pregnancy.

The possible use of acyclovir in infants born to mothers with a history of recurrent genital herpes, particularly those who have herpes at the time of delivery, has not been evaluated[108]. There are a number of possible drawbacks with this approach including treating a large number of newborns who would otherwise not require treatment, the appropriate dose to use and the duration of therapy.

Due to poor oral bioavailability, administration of acyclovir to neonates must be by the intravenous route. Until further information is available, this form of intervention should not be recommended.

On the basis of the evidence presented above, what is the appropriate management for women with a history of recurrent genital herpes? All women should be given the following information regarding herpes in pregnancy and the possible risks to the newborn. First, it should be stressed that risk of spread of infection to the newborn is small, even if a recurrence occurs at or around the time of delivery. Second, there is no convincing evidence that acyclovir at the usual doses used for suppression is of any proven benefit in the prevention of recurrences and the need for caesarean section in this circumstance. Third, women should be advised that due to the delay in obtaining the results of viral culture, regular swabbing for viral culture in late pregnancy is of limited value. Finally, although caesarean section is often recommend to bypass the birth canal, this procedure carries a significant morbidity and a mortality risk but nonetheless, in circumstances where a recurrence occurs at this time, it may still be recommended.

PREVENTING POSTNATAL INFECTION

Fortunately postnatal transmission is rare[53–58]. Health education for parents and risk reduction policies in neonatal units may help to reduce the risk still further. Nosocomial infections are of particular concern. A report using restriction endonuclease analysis has documented a hospital outbreak from a common source[56]. As a consequence, many neonatal units have instituted a policy of preventing health-care personnel with overt herpetic lesions from coming into contact with neonates[118]. However, this policy fails to recognize the relevance of asymptomatic viral shedding. Handwashing after contact with each patient, the use of gloves, and encouragement of staff to avoid kissing or cuddling neonates should help reduce this risk. In addition, relatives or friends with active cold sores should be discouraged from kissing the baby.

PREVENTION OF NEONATAL HERPES: FUTURE DEVELOPMENTS

To increase effectiveness in the prevention of neonatal herpes, more women at risk of transmitting the infection to their babies will need to be identified. Women may be classified into several groups according to risk, including those who acquire the infection for the first time in pregnancy, both symptomatically and asymptomatically, and those who have recurrent herpes and are shedding virus at the time of delivery, either symptomatically or asymptomatically. Women who acquire symptomatic genital herpes in pregnancy or who have a history of genital herpes can easily be detected. However, using type-specific HSV serology, it is now possible to detect women who have herpes but do not have symptoms[7–9]. An algorithm setting out this approach is shown in Figure 7.3. Women with a history of genital herpes should be advised about the risks, whereas those who do not have the infection, particularly if they have a partner who has HSV2 either symptomatically or asymptomatically, should be advised that they may be at risk of contracting the infection and that condoms may reduce this risk. A further development may be that couples thinking of having children will be advised to be screened before conceiving. Women who do not have antibodies to HSV2 could be vaccinated to prevent them acquiring the infection during pregnancy[119]. Further down the line would be the possibility of introducing vaccination for all girls before they become sexually active although the efficacy, safety, availability and cost effectiveness of such programmes will need to be carefully considered before implementation.

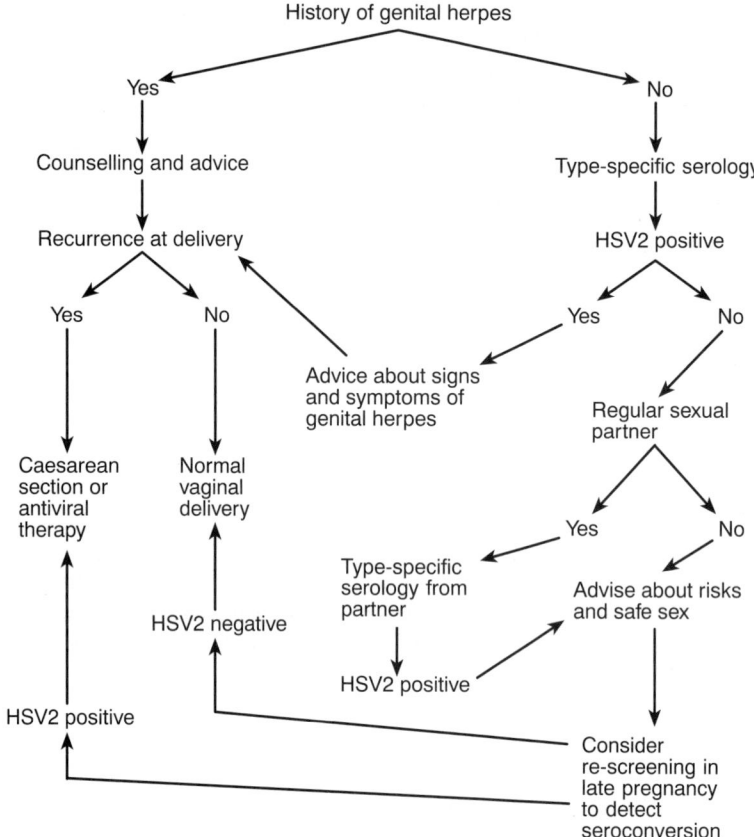

Figure 7.3 Algorithm for the management of herpes in pregnancy using clinical history and type-specific HSV serology in women and their partners.

REFERENCES

1. Schneweiss, K.E. (1962) Serologische untersuchungen zur typendifferen-zierung des herpesvirus hominis. *Z. Immuno-Forsch.*, **124**, 24–28.
2. Batterson, W. and Roizman, B. (1983) Characterization of the herpes simplex virion-associated factor responsible for the induction of α genes. *J. Virol.*, **46**, 371–377.
3. Roizman, B. (1993) The family Herpesviridae. A brief introduction. In *The Human Herpesviruses*, (eds B. Roizman, R.J. Whitley and C. Lopez), Raven Press, New York, pp. 1–9.
4. Roizman, B. and Sears, A.E. (1993) Herpes simplex viruses and their replication. In *The Human Herpesviruses*, (eds B. Roizman, R.J. Whitley and C. Lopez), Raven Press, New York, pp. 11–68.

5. Mindel. A. (1989) *Herpes Simplex Virus*, Springer Verlag, Berlin.
6. Mindel, A. (1994) Genital herpes – the forgotten epidemic. *Herpes*, **1**(2), 39–48.
7. Lee, F.K., Colernan, R.M., Pereira, L. *et al.* (1985) Detection of herpes simplex virus type 2 specific antibody with glycoprotein G. *J. Clin. Microbiol.*, **22**, 641–644.
8. Lee, F., Pereira, L., Griffin, C. *et al.* (1986) A novel glycoprotein for detection of herpes simplex virus type 1 specific antibodies. *J. Virol. Methods*, **14**, 111–118.
9. Ashley, R.L., Militoni, L., Lee, F. *et al.* (1988) Comparison of Western blot (immunoblot) and glycoprotein G specific immunodot enzyme assay for detecting antibodies to herpes simplex virus types 1 and 2 in human sera. *J. Clin. Microbiol.*, **26**, 662–667.

10. Whitley, R.L. and Gnann, J.W. Jr (1993) The epidemiology and clinical manifestations of herpes simplex virus infections. In *The Human Herpesviruses*, (eds B. Roizman, R.J. Whitley and C. Lopez), Raven Press, New York, pp. 69–105.

11. Nahmias, A.L., Lee, F.K. and Beckman-Nahmias, S. (1990) Sero-epidemiological and sociological patterns of herpes simplex virus infection in the world. *Scand. J. Infect. Dis.*, **69**, 19–36.

12. Johnson, R., Nahmias, A.I., Magder, L. *et al.* (1989) A seroepidemiological survey of the prevalence of herpes simplex virus type 2 in the United States. *N. Engl. J. Med.*, **321**, 7–12.

13. Christenson, B., Bottinger, M., Svensson, A. and Jeansson, S. (1992) A 15-year surveillance study of antibodies to herpes simplex virus types 1 and 2 in a cohort of young girls. *J. Infect. Dis.*, **25**, 147–154.

14. Cowan, E., Johnson, A.M., Ashley, R., Corey, L. and Mindel, A. (1994) Antibodies to herpes simplex virus type 2 as a serological marker of sexual lifestyle in populations. *Br. Med. J.*, **309**, 1325–1329.

15. Fleming D.T., McQuillan G.M., Johnson R.E. *et al.* (1997) Herpes simplex virus type 2 in the United States, 1976 to 1994. *N. Engl. J. Med.*, **337**, 1105–1111.

16. Stravraky, K.M., Rawls, W.E., Chiavetta, L. *et al.* (1983) Sexual and socioeconomic factors affecting the risk of past infections with herpes simplex virus type 2. *Am. J. Epidemiol.*, **118**, 109–121.

17. Siegel, D., Golden, E., Washington, E. *et al.* (1992) Prevalence and correlates of herpes simplex infections: a population-based AIDS in multi-ethnic neighbourhoods study. *JAMA*, **268**, 1702–1708.

18. Hashido, M., Kawana, T., Tsugemi, H. *et al.* (1990) The prevalence of type specific antibody to herpes simplex virus type 2 in Japan. *Igaku-no-ayumi*, **152**, 669–670.

19. Cunningham, A.L., Lee, F.K., Ho, D.W.T. *et al.* (1993) Herpes simplex virus type 2 antibody in patients attending antenatal or STD clinics. *Med. J. Aust.*, **158**, 525–528.

20. Corey, L. (1994) The current trend in genital herpes. Progress in prevention. *Sex. Trans. Dis.*, **21**(2), S38–S44.

21. Field, P.R., Ho, D.T.W. and Cunningham. A.L. (1993) Prevalence of herpes simplex virus type 2 (HSV-2) antibody in blood donors and children and patients attending antenatal and STD clinics in Sydney (abstract). *ASH Annual Scientific Meeting*, Perth.

22. Forsgren, M., Skoog, E., Jeansson, S. *et al.* (1994) Prevalence of antibodies to herpes simplex virus in pregnant women in Stockholm in 1969, 1983 and 1989: implications for STD epidemiology. *Int. J. STD AIDS*, **5**, 113–116.

23. Kulhanjian, J.A., Soroush, V., Au, D.S. *et al.* (1992) Identification of women at unsuspected risk of contracting primary herpes simplex virus type 2 infections during pregnancy. *N. Engl. J. Med.*, **326**(14), 916–920.

24. Brown, Z.A., Benedetti, K., Watts, H. *et al.* (1995) A comparison between detailed and simple histories in the diagnosis of genital herpes complicating pregnancy. *Am. J. Obstet. Gynecol.*, **172**, 1299–1303.

25. Weinberg, A., Canto, C.L.M., Pannuti, C.S. *et al.* (1993) Herpes simplex virus type 2 infection in pregnancy: asymptomatic viral excretion at delivery and seroepidemiologic survey of two socioeconomically distinct populations in Sao Paulo, Brazil. *Rev. Inst. Med. Trop. Sao Paulo*, **35**, 285–290.

26. Koutsky, L., Ashley, R., Holmes, K. *et al.* (1990) The frequency of unrecognised type 2 herpes simplex virus infection among women: implications for the control of genital herpes. *Sex. Trans. Dis.*, **17**, 90–94.

27. Breinig, M., Kingsley, L.A., Armstrong, J.A. *et al.* (1990) Epidemiology of genital herpes in Pittsburgh: serologic, sexual, and racial correlates of apparent and inapparent herpes simplex infections. *J. Infect. Dis.*, **162**, 306–312.

28. Langenberg, A., Benedetti, L., Jerkins, L. *et al.* (1989) Development of clinically recognisable genital lesions among women previously identified as having 'asymptomatic' herpes simplex virus type 2 infection. *Ann. Intern. Med.*, **110**, 882–887.

29. Corey, L., Adams, H.G., Brown, Z.A. and Holmes, K.K. (1983) Genital herpes simplex virus infections: clinical manifestations, course and complications. *Ann. Intern. Med.*, **98**, 958–972.

30. Barton, I.G., Kinghorn, G.R., Name, S. *et al.* (1982) Incidence of herpes simplex virus type 1 and 2 isolated in patients with herpes genitalis in Sheffield. *Br. J. Vener. Dis.*, **58**, 44–47.

31. Scoular, A., Leask, B. and Carrington, D. (1990) Changing trends in genital herpes due

to herpes simplex virus type 1 in Glasgow, 1985–88 (letter). *Genitourin. Med.*, **66**, 226.

32. Reeves, W.C., Corey, L., Adams, G.H. *et al.* (1981) Risk of recurrence after first episode of genital herpes. Relation to HSV type and antibody response. *N. Engl. J. Med.*, **305**, 315–319.

33. Mindel, A. and Sutherland, S. (1983) Genital herpes – the disease and its treatment including intravenous acyclovir. *J. Antimicrob. Chemother.*, **12**(B), 51–59.

34. Lafferty, W.E., Coombs, R.W., Benedetti, L. *et al.* (1987) Recurrences after oral and genital herpes simplex virus infection. Influence of site of infection and viral type. *N. Engl. J. Med.*, **316**, 1444–1449.

35. Mindel, A., Coker, D.M., Faherty, A. and Williams, P. (1988) Recurrent genital herpes: clinical and virological features in men and women. *Genitourin. Med.*, **64**, 103–106.

36. Whitley, R. (1994) Herpes simplex virus infections of women and their offspring: implications for a developed society. *Proc. Natl Acad. Sci. USA*, **91**, 2441–2447.

37. Anderson, J.M. and Nicholls, M.W.N. (1972) Herpes encephalitis in pregnancy. *Br. Med. J.*, **1**, 32.

38. Goyette, R.E., Donowho, E.M., Hieger, L.R. and Plunkett, G1. (1974) Fulminant herpesvirus hominis hepatitis during pregnancy. *Obstet. Gynecol.*, **43**, 91.

39. Young, E.L., Killam, A.R. and Greene, J.F. (1976) Disseminated herpes virus infection: associated with primary genital herpes in pregnancy. *JAMA*, **235**, 273.

40. Hensleigh, P.A., Glover, D.B. and Cannon, M. (1979) Systemic herpesvirus hominis in pregnancy. *J. Reprod. Med.*, **22**, 171.

41. Peacock, J.E. and Sarubbi, F.A. (1983) Disseminated herpes simplex virus infection during pregnancy. *Obstet. Gynecol.*, **61**, 13.

42. Prober, C. (1995) Herpes simplex infection in pregnancy: preventing neonatal herpes infection. In *Clinical Management of Herpes Viruses*, (eds S.L. Sacks, S.E. Straus, R.J. Whitley and P.D. Griffiths), 105 Press, Amsterdam, pp. 87–99.

43. Nahmias, A.L., Keyserling, H.L. and Lee, F.K. (1989) Herpes simplex viruses 1 and 2. In *Viral Infections of Humans. Epidemiology and Control*, 3rd edn, (ed. A.S. Evans), Plenum, New York, pp. 393–417.

44. Sullivan-Bolyai, L., Hull, H.F., Wilson, C. and Corey, L. (1983) Neonatal herpes simplex virus infection in King County, Washington: increasing incidence and epidemiologic correlates. *JAMA*, **250**, 3059.

45. Garland, S. (1992) Neonatal herpes simplex: Royal Women's Hospital 10 years experience with management guidelines for herpes in pregnancy. *Aust. NZ J. Obstet. Gynaecol.*, **32**, 331–334.

46. Malm, G., Berg, U. and Forsgren, M. (1995) Neonatal herpes simplex: clinical findings and outcome in relation to type of maternal infection. *Acta Paediatr.*, **84**, 256–260.

47. Hall, S.M. and Glickman. (1990) Report from the British Paediatric Surveillance Unit. *Arch. Dis. Child.*, **65**, 807–809.

48. Sturn, B. and Schneweiss, K.E. (1979) Protective effect of an oral infection with herpes simplex type 1 against subsequent genital infection with herpes simplex virus type 2. *Med. Microbiol. Immunol.*, **165**, 119–127.

49. Grossman, J.H. III., Wallen, W.C. and Sever, J.L. (1981) Management of genital herpes simplex virus infection during pregnancy. *Obstet. Gynecol.*, **58**, 1–4.

50. Harger, J.H., Pazin, G.L., Armstrong, J.A., Breinig, M.C. and Ho, M. (1983) Characteristics and management of pregnancy in women with genital herpes simplex virus infection. *Am. J. Obstet. Gynecol.*, **145**, 784–791.

51. Brown, Z.A., Vontver, L.A., Benedetti, L. *et al.* (1987) Effects on infants of a first episode of genital herpes during pregnancy. *N. Engl. J. Med.*, **317**, 1246–1251.

52. Nahmias, A.L., Josey, W.E., Naib, Z.M. *et al.* (1971) Perinatal risk associated with maternal genital herpes simplex virus infection. *Am. J. Obstet. Gynecol.*, **110**, 825–837.

53. Douglas, L., Schmidt, O. and Corey, L. (1983) Acquisition of neonatal HSV-1 infection from a paternal source contact. *J. Pediatr.*, **103**, 908.

54. Light, U. (1979) Postnatal acquisition of herpes simplex virus by the newborn infant: a review of the literature. *Pediatrics*, **63**, 480–482.

55. Francis, D.P., Hermann, K.L., MacMahon, J.R., Chivigny, K.H. and Sanderlin, K.C. (1975) Nosocomial and maternally acquired herpesvirus hominis infections, a report of four fatal cases in neonates. *Am. J. Dis. Child.*, **129**, 889.

56. Hammerberg, O., Wahs, L., Chernesky, M., Luchsinger, L. and Rawls, W. (1980) An outbreak of herpes simplex virus type 1 in an

intensive care nursery. *Pediatr. Infect. Dis.*, **2**, 290.

57. Linnemann, C.C., Jr, Buchman, T.G., Light, U.J., Ballard, J.L. and Roizman, B. (1978) Transmission of herpes simplex virus type 1 in a nursery for the newborn: identification of viral species isolated by DNA fingerprinting. *Lancet*, **1**, 964.

58. Sullivan-Bolyai, J.Z., Fife, K.H., Jacobs, R.F., Miller, Z. and Corey, L. (1983) Disseminated neonatal herpes simplex virus type 1 from a maternal lesion. *Pediatrics*, **71**, 455.

59. Brown, Z.A., Benedetti, L., Ashley, R. *et al.* (1991) Neonatal herpes simplex virus infection in relation to asymptomatic maternal infection at the time of labor. *N. Engl. J. Med.*, **324**, 1247–1252.

60. Whitley, R.J. (1990) Herpes simplex virus infections. In: *Infectious Diseases of the Fetus and Newborn Infant*, 3rd edn, (eds S. Remington and J.O. Klein), W.B. Saunders, Philadelphia, pp. 282–305.

61. Yeager, A.S., Arvin, A.M., Urbani, L.J. and Kemp, L.A. (1980) Relationship of antibody in outcome in neonatal herpes simplex virus infections. *Infect. Immun.*, **29**, 532–538.

62. Prober, C.G., Sullender, W.M., Yasukawa, L.L. *et al.* (1987) Low risk of herpes simplex virus infections in neonates exposed to the virus at the time of vaginal delivery to mothers with recurrent genital herpes simplex virus infections. *N. Engl. J. Med.*, **316**, 240–244.

63. Parvey, L.S. and Chien, L.T. (1980) Neonatal herpes simplex virus infection introduced by fetal monitor scalp electrode. *Pediatrics*, **65**, 1150–1153.

64. Kaye, E.M. and Dooling, E.C. (1981) Neonatal herpes simplex meningoencephalitis associated with fetal monitor scalp electrodes. *Neurology*, **3**(1), 1045–1055.

65. Nahmias, A.L., Josey, W.E., Naib, Z.M. *et al.* (1971) Perinatal risk associated with maternal genital herpes simplex virus infection. *Am. J. Obstet. Gynecol.*, **110**, 825–837.

66. Whitley, R.L., Nahmias, A.L., Visintine, A.M., Fleming, C.L. and Alford, C.A. (1980) The natural history of herpes simplex virus infection of mother and newborn. *Pediatrics*, **66**, 489–494.

67. Yeager, A.S. and Arvin, A.M. (1984) Reasons for the absence of a history of recurrent genital infections in mothers of neonates with herpes simplex virus. *Pediatrics*, **73**, 188–193.

67a. Brown, Z.A., Selke S., Zeh J. *et al.* (1997) The acquisition of herpes simplex virus during pregnancy. *N. Engl. J. Med.*, **337**, 509–515.

68. Brown, Z.A., Benedetti, L., Selke, S. *et al.* (1996) Asymptomatic maternal shedding of herpes simplex virus at the onset of labor: relationship to preterm labor. *Obstet. Gynecol.*, **87**(4), 483.

69. Koelle, D.M., Benedetti, L., Langenberg, A. and Corey, L. (1992) Asymptomatic reactivation of herpes simplex virus in women after the first episode of genital herpes. *Ann. Intern. Med.*, **116**(6), 433.

70. Arvin, A.M., Hensleigh, P.A., Prober, C.C. *et al.* (1986) Failure of antepartum maternal cultures to predict the infant's risk of exposure to herpes simplex virus at delivery. *N. Engl. J. Med.*, **315**, 796–800.

71. Prober, C.G., Hensleigh, P.A., Boucher, E.R. *et al.* (1988) Use of routine viral cultures at delivery to identify neonates exposed to herpes simplex virus. *N. Engl. J. Med.*, **318**, 887–889.

72. Kohl, S., West, M.S., Prober, C.G. *et al.* (1989) Neonatal antibody dependent cellular cytotoxic antibody levels are associated with the clinical presentation of neonatal herpes simplex virus infection. *J. Infect. Dis.*, **160**, 770–776.

73. Nahmias, A.L., Keyserling, H.L. and Kerrick, C.M. (1983) Herpes simplex. In: *Infectious Diseases of the Fetus and Newborn Infant*, 2nd edn, (eds S. Remington and J.O. Klein), W.B. Saunders, Philadelphia, p. 638.

74. Whitley, R.L., Corey, L., Arvin, A. *et al.* (1988) Changing presentation of neonatal herpes simplex virus infection. *J. Infect. Dis.*, **158**, 109–116.

75. Whitley, R.L., Arvin, A., Prober, C. *et al.* (1991) A controlled trial comparing vidarabine with acyclovir in neonatal herpes simplex virus infection. *N. Engl. J. Med.*, **324**, 444–449.

76. Parvey, L.S. and Chien, L.T. (1980) Neonatal herpes simplex virus infection introduced by fetal monitor scalp electrode. *Pediatrics*, **65**, 1150.

77. Kaye, E.M. and Dooling, E.C. (1981) Neonatal herpes simplex meningoencephalitis associated with fetal monitor scalp electrodes. *Neurology*, **3**(1), 1045.

78. Baldwin, S. and Whitley, R.J. (1989) Intrauterine HSV infection. *J. Teratol.*, **39**, 1–10.

79. Musci, S.E., Fine, E.M. and Togo, Y. (1971) Zoster-like disease in the newborn due to herpes simplex virus. *N. Engl. J. Med.*, **284**, 24.

80. Nahmias, A. and Hagler, W. (1972) Ocular manifestations of herpes simplex in the newborn. *Int. Ophthalmol. Clin.*, **12**, 191.

81. Nahmias, A., Visitine, A., Caldwell, A. and Wilson, C. (1976) Eye infections. *Surv. Ophthalmol.*, **21**, 100.

82. Cibis, A and Burde, R.M. (1971) Herpes simplex virus induced congenital cataracts. *Arch. Ophthalmol.*, **85**, 220–223.

83. Reersted, R. and Hansen, B. (1979) Chorioretinitis of the newborn with herpes simplex virus type 1: report of a case. *Acta. Ophthalmol.*, **57**, 1096–1100.

84. Arvin, A.M., Yeager, A.S., Bruhn, F.W. and Grossman, M. (1982) Neonatal herpes simplex infection in the absence of mucocutaneous lesions. *J. Pediatr.*, **100**, 7–15.

85. Sullivan-Boyle, L, Hull, H., Wilson, C. and Corey, L. Presentation of neonatal herpes simplex virus infections: implications for a change in therapeutic strategy. *Pediatr. Infect. Dis.*, **5**, 309.

86. Foidart, L.M. and Lambotte, R. (1988) Treatment of severe genital herpes simplex virus (HSV) infection during pregnancy with intravenous acyclovir (abstract 43–10). Second World Congress of Sexually Transmitted Diseases, Paris, June 25–28.

87. Spangler, L.G., Kirk, L.K. and Knudson, M.P. (1994) Uses and safety of acyclovir in pregnancy. *J. Fam. Pract.*, **38**, 186–191.

88. Mindel, A., Adler, M.W., Sutherland, S. and Fiddian, A.P. (1982) Intravenous acyclovir treatment for primary genital herpes. *Lancet*, **ii**, 697–700.

89. Cox, S.M., Cunningham, F.G. and Luby, J. (1995) Management of varicella pneumonia complicating pregnancy. *Am. J. Perinatol.*, **7**, 300–301.

90. Broussard, R.C., Payne, D.K. and George, R.B. (1991) Treatment with acyclovir of varicella pneumonia in pregnancy. *Chest*, **99**, 1045–1047.

91. Hankins, G.D.V., Gilstrap, L.C. and Patterson, A.R. (1987) Acyclovir treatment of varicella pneumonia in pregnancy (letter). *Crit. Care. Med.*, **15**, 336–337.

92. Landsberger E.J., Hager, D.W. and Grossman, J.H. (1986) Successful management of varicella pneumonia complicating pregnancy: a report of three cases. *J. Reprod. Med.*, **31**, 311–314.

93. Smego, R.A. and Asperilla, M.D. (1991) Use of acyclovir for varicella pneumonia during pregnancy. *J. Am. Coll. Obstet. Gynecol.*, **78**, 1112–1116.

94. CDC. (1993) Pregnancy outcomes following systemic prenatal acyclovir exposure: June 1, 1984 to June 30, 1993. *MMWR*, **42**(41), 806–889.

95. Frenkel, L., Brown, Z., Bryson, Y. *et al.* (1991) Pharmacokinetics of ACV in the term human pregnancy and neonate. *Am. J. Obstet. Gynecol.*, **164**, 569–576.

96. Haddad, L., Langer, B., Astruc, D., Messer, L. and Lokiec, F. (1993) Oral acyclovir and recurrent genital herpes during late pregnancy. *Obstet. Gynecol.*, **82**, 102–104.

97. Weller, S., Blum, M.R., Doucett, M. *et al.* (1993) Pharmacokinetics of the acyclovir prodrug, valacyclovir, after escalating single and multiple dose administration to normal volunteers. *Clin. Pharamcol. Ther.*, **54**, 595–605.

98. Boyd, M.R., Safrin, S. and Kern, E.R. (1993) Penciclovir: a review of spectrum of activity, selectivity, and cross-resistance pattern. *Antiviral Chem. Chemother.*, **4**(suppl), 3–11.

99. Guinan, M.E. (1986) Oral acyclovir for treatment and suppression of genital herpes simplex virus infection. *JAMA*, **255**, 1747–1749.

100. Mertz, G.J. (ed.) (1988) Long term acyclovir suppression of recurrent genital herpes. *STD Bull.*, **special issue**, 3–7.

101. Mindel, A. (1991) Antiviral chemotherapy for genital herpes. *Med. Virol.*, **1**, 111–118.

102. Brocklehurst, P., Carney, O., Ross. E. and Mindel, A. (1995) The management of recurrent genital herpes infection in pregnancy: a postal survey of obstetric practice. *Br. J. Obstet. Gynaecol.*, **102**, 791–797.

103. Scott, L.L., Sanchez, P.L., Jackson, G.L., Zeray, R. and Wendel, G.D. (1996) Acyclovir suppression to prevent cesarean delivery after first-episode genital herpes. *Obstet. Gynecol.*, **87**, 69–73.

104. Gibbs, R.S., Amstey, M.S., Sweet, R.L., Mead, P.B. and Sever, L.L. (1988) Management of genital herpes infection in pregnancy. *Obstet. Gynecol.*, **7**(1), 779–780.

105. American Academy of Pediatrics (1980) Perinatal herpes simplex virus infections. Committee on Fetus and Newborn and Infectious Diseases. *Pediatrics*, **66**, 147–148.

106. Stray-Pederson, B. (1990) Acyclovir in late pregnancy to prevent neonatal herpes simplex (letter). *Lancet*, **ii**, 756.

107. Brocklehurst, R., Kinghorn, G., Carney, O. *et al.* (1998) A randomised placebo controlled trial of suppressive acyclovir in late pregnancy in women with recurrent genital herpes infection. *Br. J. Obstet. Gynaecol.*, **105**, 275–280.

108. Lissauer, T. and Jeffries, D. (1989) Preventing neonatal herpes infection. *Br. J. Obstet. Gynaecol.*, **96**, 1015–1023.

109. Bashore, R.A., Phillips, W.H. and Brinkman, C.R. (1990) A comparison of the morbidity of midforceps and cesarean delivery. *Am. J. Obstet. Gynecol.*, **162**, 1428–1435.

110. Danforth, D.N. (1985) Cesarean section. *JAMA*, **253**, 811–818.

111. Alan Guttmacher Institute (1987) *Blessed Events and the Bottom Line: Financing Maternity Care in the United States*. Alan Guttmacher Institute, New York, p. 18.

112. Moseley, R.C., Corey, L., Benjamin, D., Winter, C. and Remington, M.L. (1981) Comparison of viral isolation, direct immunofluorescence, and indirect immuno-peroxidase techniques for detection of genital herpes simplex virus infection. *J. Clin. Microbiol.*, **13**, 913–918.

113. Mead, P.B. (1986) Proper methods of culturing herpes simplex virus. *J. Reprod. Med.*, **31**(5), 390–394.

114. Richman, D.D., Cleveland, P.H., Redfield, D.C., Oxman, M.N. and Wahl, G.M. (1984) Rapid viral diagnosis. *J. Infect. Dis.*, **149**, 298–310.

115. Randolph, A.G., Washington, A.E. and Prober, C.G. (1993) Cesarean delivery for women presenting with genital herpes lesions: efficacy, risks, and costs. *JAMA*, **270**, 77–82.

116. Mindel, A., Faherty, A., Carney, O. *et al.* (1988) Dosage and safety of long-term suppressive acyclovir therapy for recurrent genital herpes. *Lancet*, **i**, 926–928.

117. Kroon, S., Peterson, C.S., Andersen, L.P. *et al.* (1990) Long-term suppression of severe recurrent genital herpes simplex infections with oral acyclovir: a dose titration study. *Genitourin. Med.*, **66**, 101–104.

118. Whitley, R. (1995) Perinatal herpes simplex virus infections. In *Clinical Management of Herpes Viruses* (eds S.L. Sacks, S.E. Straus, R.J. Whitley and P.D. Griffiths), 105 Press, Amsterdam, pp. 101–116.

119. Mindel, A. (1995) Recent advances in genital herpes. *Ann. Acad. Med. Singapore*, **24**, 584–592.

M.-L. Newell and C. Peckham

INTRODUCTION

The human immunodeficiency virus (HIV) is a retrovirus, which causes immune suppression through destruction of CD4+ T-lymphocytes. This results in an increased susceptibility to common infections which in turn leads to acquired immune deficiency syndrome (AIDS). There are at least two types of HIV, of which HIV1 is the most prevalent and pathogenic. HIV2 is uncommon in Western countries and is less transmissible (see later). In this chapter we refer to HIV1.

HIV infection can be acquired through sexual contact, blood or blood products (which include injecting drug use with contaminated equipment) and vertically from mother to child. The World Health Organization estimates that there are currently more than 1 000 000 individuals with AIDS worldwide with, in most countries, similar numbers of men and women affected. In Europe, as elsewhere, the AIDS epidemic has emerged as a major health problem although its impact across regions and subpopulations within Europe is variable.

By October 1997, nearly 35 000 women had been reported with AIDS from 47 European countries[1]. The majority of these women reported a history of injecting drug use, but a substantial and increasing proportion had acquired their infection through heterosexual contact (Table 8.1). The proportion of female AIDS cases rose from 11% in 1986 to 20% in 1997[1]. In countries such as Italy and Spain, where the prevalence of HIV infection among intravenous drug users is high, the proportion of female AIDS cases is greater than in the Northern European countries, such as Sweden, Denmark and Germany, where there is a preponderance of AIDS cases among homosexual men.

Most of the women reported with AIDS are of childbearing age. This has implications for the number of children at risk of HIV infection, as vertical transmission is the main mode of acquisition of infection for children (Table 8.2). By October 1997, 7700 children had been diagnosed with AIDS in Europe, the majority from Romania (4400), France (680), Spain (830) and Italy (620)[1]. Most of the children with AIDS reported from Romania had acquired infection through the use of contaminated needles and syringes, which highlights the need for continued vigilance in the prevention of infection through this route. In the remaining countries, 84% of the 3200 children were infected as a result of mother-to-child transmission. About 40% of the mothers of the vertically infected children reported a history of intravenous drug use.

HIV INFECTION

Although AIDS surveillance is important, it is limited as an indicator of trends in HIV

Viral Infections in Obstetrics and Gynaecology. Edited by D.J. Jeffries and C.N. Hudson. Published in 1999 by Arnold, ISBN 0 340 74095 7.

Table 8.1 Adult AIDS cases by transmission group and sex, October 1997, WHO European region (adapted from reference[1])

Transmission group	Males	Females	Total
Homosexual male	67 546	–	67 546
Injecting drug user (IDU)	60 129	16 770	76 899
Homo/bisexual IDU	2 838	–	2 838
Blood/blood product	4 953	1 697	6 650
Heterosexual contact	16 022	12 784	28 806
Nosocomial infection	7	3	10
Other/undetermined	8 121	2 129	10 250
Total	159 616	33 383	192 999

Table 8.2 Paediatric AIDS, WHO European region, October 1997 (adapted from reference[1])

Transmission group	Males	Females	Total
Mother to child	1469	1402	2871 (38%)
Blood/blood product	793	468	1261 (17%)
Nosocomial infection	1181	843	2024 (27%)
Other/undetermined	779	577	1356 (18%)
Total	4222	3290	7512 (100%)

infection in adults because of the long latent period and under-reporting of AIDS[2]. In the future, comparisons of trends in adult AIDS will be increasingly difficult to interpret with the widening of the case definition of AIDS to include low CD4 cell counts in the USA[3] but not in Europe[4]. To predict the spread of the epidemic, monitoring of HIV prevalence is essential. Laboratory reports of first HIV-positive antibody tests are used in the UK to monitor the spread of HIV infection[5]. However, both laboratory and clinical reporting schemes are likely to underestimate the extent of the problem because of the bias inherent in any reporting system that relies on individuals presenting with symptoms or who come forward to be tested.

A more reliable approach for estimating the population prevalence of HIV infection is unlinked anonymous testing of blood taken for other purposes. Increasingly this approach is being used to monitor the epidemic, although it is important to appreciate that this is limited to people who have blood taken[6–9]. In parallel with AIDS reports, there are marked differences in the seroprevalence of HIV infection between European countries and between populations within one country[6,7,9]. However, the results of unlinked anonymous testing are limited in that they lack information on risk factors, such as injecting drug use or country of origin. Although they are restricted to sample populations in accessible groups, their strength is that they do not suffer from bias resulting from refusal to be tested or failure to identify people at risk. In relation to antenatal or neonatal seroprevalence, attempts have been made to overcome the problem of lack of identifiers by relating the results to population characteristics of women delivering in given areas[10].

In England, unlinked anonymous testing among pregnant women has been continuous in selected sites since the beginning of 1990[8]. Residual specimens from antenatal samples collected for rubella serology are tested for HIV antibody. HIV seroprevalence rates for women with live births are available for Italy, Southeast England and Scotland, based on unlinked anonymous testing of neonatal blood samples taken routinely from all newborns for metabolic screening[11,12]. Results from these screening programmes have been used to monitor the spread of infection in the community (Figure 8.1), to evaluate the success of antenatal screening programmes and to predict the future of the HIV epidemic[11,12].

Further information about characteristics of HIV-infected pregnant women is provided from the results of special studies, such as the European Collaborative Study, which started in 1986. In this study, which has enrolled infants born to HIV-infected women in 22 European centres in eight countries, the majority of women were white, primi-

gravidae, married or cohabiting and born in Europe[13,14]. About two-thirds had a history of injecting drug use and many had a partner with a history of injecting drug use. Although patterns of transmission varied across European centres, a relative increase in heterosexual transmission was observed after 1986. A similar study in France has enrolled a substantial number of women from sub-Saharan Africa, resident in France[15]. Information from American studies suggests that a disproportionate number of women from minority populations are HIV infected and that acquisition of infection is often associated with injecting drug use and multiple sexual partners[16].

OBSTETRIC AND PAEDIATRIC SURVEILLANCE

Confidential clinical reporting schemes in which HIV-seropositive pregnant women and/or HIV-seropositive children are notified centrally can provide useful surveillance information. However, these programmes are relatively costly and results are only of value if they include a substantial proportion of all infected women or children.

In the UK a national study of HIV in pregnancy was established in 1989, through the Royal College of Obstetricians and Gynaecologists, to establish a confidential register of known HIV-positive pregnancies[17]. The results of this surveillance programme have been used to assess current antenatal screening programmes by comparing cases reported to the register with results from the unlinked anonymous neonatal screening programme. This has provided an estimate of the extent to which HIV infection is not recognized in pregnant women[18].

In Italy the register of paediatric HIV infection and AIDS[19,20] has provided valuable information on children with infection, their presenting symptoms, the natural history of AIDS and survival. In the UK, a similar paediatric surveillance scheme exists,

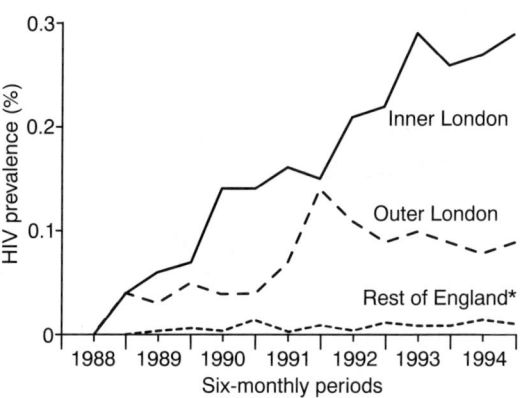

* Includes the Thames Regions outside London

Figure 8.1 Trends in prevalence of HIV 1 infection among pregnant women, by area of residence, 1988–94 (newborn infant dried blood spots taken for metabolic screening).

whereby paediatricians report on a monthly basis any child with HIV infection or born to an HIV-seropositive mother[21]. Nil returns are included and response rates are over 90%. This paediatric surveillance is linked to the obstetric surveillance scheme to give a comprehensive picture of vertically acquired infection in Britain[18]. In both the Italian and UK registers, follow-up information is also obtained on the children reported.

PREGNANCY IN HIV-INFECTED WOMEN

Results from a number of small studies suggest that pregnant women with HIV infection experience no increase in pregnancy-associated complications[22–24]. There is little information about labour and delivery complications, but the management of labour is becoming a focus of interest as several studies have shown that the risk of vertical transmission may be associated with events occurring at the time of delivery[25–27]. In a study in Edinburgh, Scotland, rates of induction of labour, use of epidural anaesthesia or oxytocin, assisted vaginal delivery, episiotomy and caesarean section were similar in HIV-infected and uninfected women[22]. In immunocompromised women, it is plausible that the risk of postoperative wound infection or postpartum endometritis may be greater[28]. The avoidance of fetal scalp sampling or application of scalp electrodes to avoid fetal exposure to contaminated maternal blood could possibly result in decisions to perform additional caesarean sections[29].

The obstetric management of HIV-infected pregnancies is similar to that of non-HIV-infected pregnancies[30]. Additional investigations focus on markers of progression of HIV disease. Although the risk of vertical transmission associated with the use of invasive procedures such as chorionic villus sampling and amniocentesis is unknown, these are best avoided because of the potential risk to the fetus[29].

HIV INFECTION AND PREGNANCY

Information on the natural history of the infection in pregnant women and its effect on pregnancy outcome is required, so that a woman identified as HIV infected before or during pregnancy can be adequately informed about the consequences for herself and her newborn infant. It has been suggested that pregnancy might enhance the immune suppression caused by HIV infection[31]. Early information based on case reports[32,33], series of women with symptomatic disease, or studies that lacked appropriate controls reported pregnancy-associated progression of disease. Subsequently, findings from prospective studies have suggested that pregnancy is unlikely to result in accelerated HIV disease progression in asymptomatic women[24,34–36]. This suggestion is supported by the absence of a gender effect in several natural history studies[37,38]. Comparisons have usually been based on differences in immunological changes (CD4+ cell, counts and CD4+/CD8+ cell ratios) in pregnancy between HIV-infected and HIV-uninfected women, rather than between pregnant and non-pregnant HIV-infected women with a similar duration of infection[36,39].

HIV INFECTION AND PREGNANCY OUTCOME

The question as to whether HIV infection adversely affects pregnancy outcome remains unresolved. A prospective study in the USA showed an increased rate of spontaneous fetal loss with detection of HIV in placental and fetal tissues in 50% of aborted fetuses. Mothers with AIDS were at especially high risk of miscarriage[40]. Studies reporting an increased risk of low birthweight associated with maternal HIV infection are mainly limited to symptomatic women and located in sub-Saharan African countries[41]. Conversely, studies of largely asymptomatic women, even in the African setting, have found no increased risk of prematurity or low birthweight and no increase in perinatal mortality rates[23,34,42]. The adverse outcome reported in studies in Africa and Haiti could reflect the social and health status of the mother, rather than the direct effect of HIV infection on the fetus or infant. Maternal weight gain, infant birthweight and placental weight have not been shown to be associated with maternal HIV infection status[34]. Based on a study in New York, Minkoff *et al.*[23] reported no association between maternal HIV infection and the incidence of chorioamnionitis or endometritis, mean birthweight, gestational age at delivery, head circumference and Apgar scores. No excess of congenital abnormalities or pattern of abnormalities has been reported in children born to women with HIV infection[42].

Although adverse pregnancy outcome may be associated with advanced maternal disease, comparisons of HIV-infected and uninfected infants born to HIV-infected mothers reveal no differences in birthweight, height, head circumference, gestational age or incidence of congenital malformations[42,43]. Birthweight is related to intravenous drug use during pregnancy and not to the infant's infection status; infants with drug-withdrawal symptoms are lighter than those whose mothers had not used intravenous drugs during pregnancy[42,44].

VERTICAL TRANSMISSION STUDIES IN EUROPE

Most children in Europe who acquire HIV infection do so through vertical transmission. The rate of vertical transmission in Europe before the introduction of zidovudine ranged between 15% and 20% and is currently 6–9% with more widespread use of antiretroviral therapy and in the absence of breastfeeding[15,27,45].

The risk of transmission of HIV2 infection is low. In the French collaborative study[46] based on 41 infants born to mothers who were HIV2 positive, the estimated risk of mother-to-child transmission of HIV2 was between 0% and 11%. Further evidence that the vertical transmission rate of HIV2 is likely to be low comes from the Ivory Coast, where the results of specific IgA and PCR tests at six months of age suggested that 28% (95% confidence interval 12–49%) of infants born to HIV1-infected mothers were infected compared with 3% (95% confidence interval 0–15%) of infants born to HIV2-infected mothers.

Vertical transmission of HIV infection may occur before, during or after delivery but the relative importance of each of these stages remains uncertain (Table 8.3). There is good evidence that intrauterine infection occurs, although its contribution to vertical transmission cannot be quantified. Studies based on placental and fetal tissues following termination of pregnancy in HIV-infected women give conflicting results. In an investigation of fetal thymuses, HIV was detected in only two of 100 tested and was not found in the

Table 8.3 Timing of vertical transmission

Intrauterine
- HIV detected in fetal material as early as 8 weeks
- Nearly half the infected infants show detectable virus in the first week of life
- Rapid disease progression in 15–25% of infected infants

Peripartum
- No excess of congenital abnormalities
- No association of birthweight with infection status
- Higher transmission risk for firstborn twin delivered vaginally
- Lack of detectable virus in a substantial number of infected infants in first few days of life
- Decreased transmission with caesarean section delivery

Postpartum
- Breastfeeding associated with increased transmission

92 fetuses that resulted from elective mid-trimester termination[47]. These results suggested a low frequency of early HIV infection *in utero* and have been supported by others[48]. In contrast, there have been reports of detection of virus in fetal tissue as early as 15 weeks gestation[49,50]. CD4+ cells have been identified in fetus-derived placental tissue and these could provide a mechanism for transplacental infection. However, placental infection does not necessarily imply fetal infection and the possibility of maternal contamination and false-positive results remains a problem.

There is increasing debate about the importance of intrapartum acquisition of infection. The exchange of blood between mother and child during labour and at the time of delivery, and the detection of virus in cervical secretions, make acquisition of infection at this stage plausible. Postnatal transmission of infection through breastfeeding can occur to infants born to women with established infection, as well as to infants born to mothers who become infected postnatally[51].

RISK FACTORS FOR VERTICAL TRANSMISSION

Transmission from mother to child has also been associated with certain maternal factors and/or events around the time of birth. The differences in vertical transmission rates between studies or populations are likely to reflect differences in the distribution of such factors[52].

Advanced maternal disease, as measured clinically by AIDS and immunologically by p24-antigenaemia, low CD4 count or low CD4: CD8 ratio and high plasma viral load, is associated with increased transmission risk[15,53–56]. Other maternal factors that may be associated with an increased likelihood of transmission include viral characteristics[57] and genetic factors which may be associated with immune responses[52].

Other sexually transmitted diseases which cause lesions in the cervix and/or chorio-amnionitis may result in an increase in HIV load in the genital tract and cause ascending infection or increased exposure to infection during delivery. As viral load varies with length of time since infection the risk of transmission is likely to be increased at times of high viral load, specifically in primary infection as well as in patients with advanced disease. The type of maternal immune response and its relation to risk of vertical transmission is still unresolved. Mother-to-child transmission may be influenced by both the viral phenotype and host-cell susceptibility to HIV infection[58]. It has also been suggested that certain HIV1 variants may be more transmissible than others[59].

Severe prematurity has been associated with increased risk of infection in the infant[55,60]. Infants born before the transfer of adequate levels of maternal antibodies, which occurs late in pregnancy, could be more susceptible to acquisition of infection during delivery.

There is increasing evidence to suggest that substantial transmission occurs around the time of delivery (Table 8.3). The findings of the international registry of HIV-exposed twins showed that the first twin was more likely to be infected than the second and the authors concluded that a significant proportion of HIV transmission occurs during passage through the birth canal[26]. The results from laboratory studies also lend support to the view that some infants acquire infection at birth[61] in that only about 40% of infants have evidence of infection shortly after birth (Figure 8.2). The time between rupture of membranes and delivery, as well as the duration of the second stage of labour, could influence the exposure of the infant to HIV-infected maternal fluids and may therefore affect the transmission risk. However, results from prospective studies are conflicting[25,27,62].

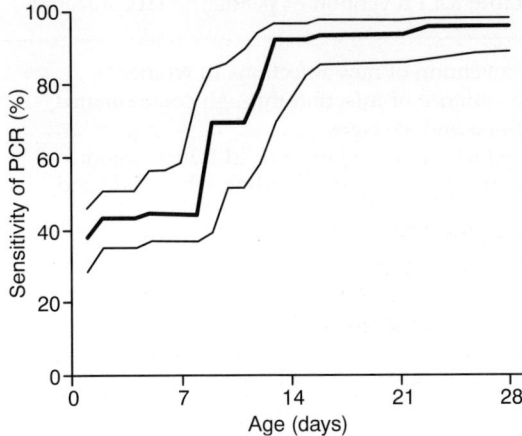

Figure 8.2 Estimates of PCR sensitivity by age, with 95% confidence intervals.

MODE OF DELIVERY

It has been proposed that elective caesarean delivery could reduce the rate of transmission by reducing exposure of the infant to contaminated blood or cervical secretions. In the European Collaborative Study, involving more than 1000 mother-child pairs, caesarean section delivery approximately halved the risk of transmission compared with vaginal delivery, even when allowing for factors known to be associated with vertical transmission (including maternal CD4 count)[27]. This translates as a reduction in vertical transmission rates from 18% to 9.7% and indicates that approximately 12 caesarean section operations would have to be performed to prevent one paediatric infection.

A subsequent meta-analysis of data from 11 prospective perinatal transmission studies, including 3202 mother-child pairs, showed a 20% reduction in risk of transmission following caesarean section delivery[63]. However, the two largest studies included in this analysis gave conflicting results: there was a 50% reduction associated with caesarean section deliveries in the European Collaborative Study, whereas in the French perinatal study there was little difference. This meta-analysis could not distinguish emergency from elective caesarean section nor could it allow for any other variables associated with vertical transmission. This meta-analysis is currently being updated with data from 15 prospective studies and nearly 9000 mother-child pairs. Preliminary information suggests that elective caesarean section delivery is associated with a significant reduction in the risk of vertical transmission

BREASTFEEDING

Transmission of HIV through breastfeeding has been described in situations where the mother acquired the infection shortly after birth (either through contaminated blood or through heterosexual contact)[64]. Seroconversion was reported in a breastfed child of 30 months shortly after his mother developed a serious breast abscess. The estimated risk of transmission of infection through breastfeeding in women infected postnatally is between 16% and 42%[51].

Infants of mothers with established infection at the time of delivery are likely to be at lower risk of infection from breastfeeding because they have maternal antibodies which may have a protective role and their mothers, unless symptomatic, are probably less infectious. Based on prospective studies on infants born to HIV-infected mothers, it has been estimated that in this group the additional risk of transmission through breastfeeding, over and above transmission *in utero* or during delivery, was between 7% and 22%[51]. In both the French perinatal study and the European Collaborative Study breastfeeding approximately doubled the risk of transmission[15,55].

In most Western countries and Thailand, HIV-infected women are advised not to breastfeed[64,65]. However, in many settings in the developing world the disadvantages of artificial feeding in terms of morbidity and mortality outweigh the reduction in the risk of HIV infection[66]. The World Health Organization continues to recommend breastfeeding in populations where malnutrition and infectious diseases are important causes of infant death[64].

To obtain a more precise estimate of the additional risk of transmission through breastfeeding, a randomized controlled trial of breastfeeding versus bottle feeding was set up in Nairobi, Kenya[67]. Concern has been expressed about the justification for such a trial. Much is already known about the risk of transmission through breastfeeding and it is unlikely that a more precise estimate of this risk will change current public health policies. However, harm could result from introducing the concept that bottle feeding may be the better method of feeding. It is known that in settings where infant mortality rates are high and often due to infectious diseases, bottle feeding carries significant additional risk. Although the trial makes special provisions to ensure that bottlefed infants are not disadvantaged, it remains dubious as to whether it will be possible to ensure this in a non-trial situation. Any estimates of the extent of morbidity and mortality associated with feeding method will only apply to the trial population[65].

INTERVENTIONS

Many of the current approaches to interventions to reduce vertical transmission of HIV are based on the premise that a substantial proportion of transmission from mother to child occurs in late pregnancy or at the time of delivery[48,55,68,69]. These include caesarean section delivery, vaginal lavage or cleansing of the birth canal, antiretroviral drugs, passive and active immunization and the administration of vitamin A to mother and child (Table 8.4).

MODE OF DELIVERY

Much attention has focused on caesarean section delivery as an approach to reducing mother-to-child transmission. However, avail-

Table 8.4 Prevention of paediatric HIV infection

Prevention of new infections in women
Avoidance of infection through contaminated blood and syringes
Reduction of mother-to-child transmission:
● avoidance of breastfeeding where safe and affordable
● therapeutic interventions:
　– antiretroviral therapy
　– vitamin A supplementation
　– immunotherapy
● modification of obstetric practices:
　– cleansing of the birth canal
　– caesarean section delivery
　– avoidance of scalp electrodes and fetal blood sampling

---

able evidence does not support the routine use of elective caesarean section for all HIV-infected women. Concern about maternal morbidity needs to be balanced against the potential benefit for the fetus[28]. A randomized, controlled trial has started in Europe to evaluate the effectiveness of elective caesarean section in preventing perinatal transmission.

VAGINAL LAVAGE

To avoid acquisition of infection during birth, cleansing of the birth canal with an antiseptic and/or virucidal agent has been proposed. Disinfectant can be administered to pregnant women during the last trimester of pregnancy and/or during labour and delivered by vaginal douching, local application or vaginal suppositories. The agent should inactivate HIV *in vitro*, have little or no local or systemic toxicity, be simple to apply and safe for the infant[70]. It is not clear what the most effective and safe agent is, nor whether a virucidal agent would be more beneficial than lavage.

Enrolment in a randomized controlled trial of chlorhexidine as cleansing agent has been completed in a study in Malawi[71]. Preliminary findings show a lack of effect overall, but a substantial reduction in vertical transmission rate in women in the treatment arm with duration of ruptured membranes longer than four hours. Further trials are planned in other sites in Africa.

Little information is available on HIV viral load in the vagina and cervix and its association with viraemia and advanced disease. Evidence from a small number of women studied suggests that viral load in the vagina/cervix is increased during pregnancy, although less than half of all pregnant women infected with HIV appear to harbour virus in the vagina/cervix. The expected effect of vaginal lavage on reduction of vertical transmission may therefore be limited. However, as an intervention it is relatively cheap, could be applied to all women irrespective of their HIV status and would avoid the necessity of antenatal testing as a prelude to planned intervention. It may also reduce the rate of neonatal complications resulting from other genital tract infections.

ANTIRETROVIRAL DRUGS

Antiretroviral drugs decrease maternal viral load and/or inhibit-4 viral replication in the infant, thereby decreasing the risk of transmission. Results from an American-French trial showed that antiretroviral therapy with zidovudine during pregnancy, labour and in the neonatal period significantly reduced the risk for the infant[72]. In the USA and elsewhere it is now recommended to offer zidovudine to all HIV positive pregnant women[73]. However, the optimum timing and method of therapeutic intervention is not known and information regarding the long-term effect of zidovudine treatment on the child, at least 80% of whom are uninfected anyway, is needed. Furthermore, it will be important to monitor the effect of temporary zidovudine treatment on the subsequent clinical management of the woman.

The findings reported from prospective studies suggest that the benefits of zidovudine in reducing vertical transmission may

extend to women with CD4 counts lower than those of the women included in the American-French trial and that treatment of the infant may not be necessary. These studies have revealed only mild reversible toxicity, such as anaemia, in the infant and have not shown teratogenicity or major maternal side effects[66,74].

Short-term zidovudine treatment in the asymptomatic stage of HIV infection may accelerate the selection of zidovudine-resistant strains. This would compromise the efficacy of zidovudine treatment and could result in the transmission of a primary zidovudine-resistant infection to the infant[75,76].

Other antiretroviral drugs, such as non-nucleoside reverse transcriptase, 3TC and protease inhibitors, particularly as combination therapy, are being or will be assessed. A trial has started in the USA in which nevirapine is being administered late in pregnancy to women receiving zidovudine therapy throughout pregnancy[66].

IMMUNIZATION

The maternal immune response, humoral and/or cellular, to HIV infection may play a role in preventing perinatal transmission. Antibodies might act to neutralize or otherwise destroy the virus either in the mother or the infant, while cell-mediated immunity might reduce the mother's viral load[65]. Protection could be achieved both by infusion of HIV-specific immunoglobulin and by monoclonal antibodies. The use of HIV immunoglobulin requires the selection of asymptomatic HIV-infected donors with high titres of neutralizing antibodies.

A randomized controlled trial of passive immunization has started in Uganda, using HIV-specific immunoglobulin. This trial involves women who have never received zidovudine and complements an American trial investigating the role of passive immunization in women already treated with zidovudine. Cell-mediated immune responses to highly conserved parts of the virus have been found both in HIV-infected individuals and in others who appear to have been exposed to the virus without becoming infected [77]. This would suggest that protective immunity could act through cell-related as well as antibody-mediated mechanisms. Active immunization is the most attractive approach because it can potentially induce long-lasting immunity in the mother and it may also induce fetal immunity. Several phase I trials in which pregnant HIV-infected women are immunized with recombinant envelope vaccines have been carried out in the USA. The optimal time for immunization is unknown and repeated doses may be required before significant neutralizing antibody titres are found. The risk of this therapeutic approach includes activation of the immune system that could increase maternal viral load. Additionally, two phase I/II trials of active immunization of infants and children against HIV have been carried out in the USA. One trial was aimed at prevention or postexposure prophylaxis of HIV infection acquired during the intrapartum period. The other was a therapeutic trial in which infants and children identified as HIV infected were immunized to delay progression of disease.

Evidence from anonymous unlinked antenatal and neonatal screening programmes has shown that many children at risk are not being identified. In view of the potential for reducing the risk of vertical transmission, increased efforts are now being made to identify HIV-infected women during pregnancy. The UK Department of Health encourages named voluntary HIV testing for all women antenatally in areas of high prevalence (as indicated by the results of anonymous antenatal or neonatal screening) and selective testing of women perceived to be at risk in lower prevalence areas. In the USA since the publication of the results of the zidovudine trial [72] the introduction of mandatory testing of all pregnant women has been proposed [78–81]. If voluntary antenatal testing is to be successful the provision of pre-test discussion and post-test counselling of women identified as HIV infected is an essential prerequisite. Satisfactory levels of uptake are a requirement of any antenatal testing programme. The benefits and risks to both mother and child, as well as the cost implications, must be carefully considered and the ethical issues surrounding testing addressed.

DIAGNOSIS OF INFECTION

As maternal HIV antibodies cross the placenta, serological diagnosis of infection in infants born to infected mothers is problematic in the first year of life. Passively acquired maternal antibodies may persist until 18 months of age, although the majority of uninfected children will have lost maternal antibodies before their first birthday [55]. An earlier diagnosis of infection can be made by virus culture, polymerase chain reaction, the detection of p24-antigen or HIV-specific IgA [82]. Culture of HIV is the definitive method of diagnosis but it is slow and expensive and its use is limited to specialized laboratories. The polymerase chain reaction, which detects and amplifies viral genetic material, is increasingly used to make an early diagnosis of infection in children born to HIV-infected mothers [61,82]. This method is less expensive and faster than viral culture. A child is considered not to be infected when he or she becomes seronegative in the absence of any clinical or virological evidence of infection. It is now possible to make a diagnosis of infection in most non-breastfed infants by three months of age.

NATURAL HISTORY

Prospective studies based on cohorts of children followed from birth are required to establish the natural history of vertically acquired HIV infection. Registers and surveillance provide information on the natural history of specific conditions, usually after the diagnosis of AIDS or HIV-related symptoms. The most common manifestation of HIV infection in early childhood is a combination of persistent generalized lymphadenopathy, hepatomegaly and splenomegaly. Persistent hypergammaglobulinaemia can occur early and may predate the onset of clinical symptoms or signs. About 25% of infected children develop AIDS within the first year of life and 14% die of an HIV-related disease[83,84].

It has been suggested that the early onset of severe disease may be associated with intra-uterine acquisition of infection or with advanced maternal disease. The most frequent AIDS-defining illness in the first year of life is *Pneumocystis carinii* pneumonia, whereas lymphoid interstitial pneumonitis is common at later ages. HIV-related encephalitis occurs in a proportion of infected children and is usually diagnosed in the second year of life. Recurrent and serious bacterial infections are AIDS-defining in vertically infected children. Although the majority of infected children show some manifestation of HIV infection before the age of 12 months, many improve over the second, third and subsequent years of life and are able to attend normal schools.

As the number of infected women and children increases, more attention is being given to issues relating to the care not only of the woman but also of her infected and uninfected children. Uninfected children born to infected mothers are also affected by their parents' disease. Many are born into socially disadvantaged families in which one or both parents may be an intravenous drug user. Prevention of infection in women of child-bearing age remains the first priority[85].

REFERENCES

1. WHO-EC Collaborating Centre on AIDS (1997) *AIDS Surveillance in Europe, Quarterly Report No. 55*. WHO, Paris.
2. McCormick, A. (1991) Unrecognised HIV related deaths. *Br. Med. J.*, **302**, 1365–1367.
3. Van Griensven, G.J.P., Boucher, E.C., Roos, M. and Coutinho, R.A. (1991) Expansion of AIDS case definition. *Lancet*, **338**, 1012–1013.
4. Ancelle-Park, R.A. (1992) European AIDS definition. *Lancet*, **339**, 671.
5. Waight, P.A., Rush, A.M. and Miller, E. (1992) Surveillance of HIV infection by voluntary testing in England. *CDR Rev.*, **2**, R85–R90.
6. Ades, A.E., Parker, S., Berry, T. *et al.* (1991) Prevalence of maternal HIV-1 infection in Thames regions: results from anonymous unlinked neonatal testing. *Lancet*, **337**, 1562–1564.
7. Ippolito, G., Costa, F., Stegagno, M. *et al.* (1991) Blind serosurvey of HIV antibodies in newborns in 92 Italian hospitals: a method for monitoring the infection rate in women at time of delivery. *J. Acq. Immune Defic. Syndr.*, **4**, 402–407.
8. Public Health Laboratory Service (1991) The unlinked anonymous HIV prevalence monitoring programme in England and Wales: preliminary results. *Commun. Dis. Rep.*, **1**(7), R69–75.
9. Tappin, D.M., Girdwood, R.W.A., Follett, E.A.C. *et al.* (1991) Prevalence of maternal HIV infection in Scotland based on unlinked anonymous testing of newborn babies. *Lancet*, **337**, 1565–1567.
10. Ades, A.E., Parker, S., Cubitt, D. *et al.* (1992) Two methods for assessing the risk factor composition of the HIV-1 epidemic in heterosexual women: South-East England, 1988–1991. *AIDS*, **6**, 1031–1036.
11. Unlinked Anonymous HIV Surveys Steering Group (1995) *Unlinked Anonymous HIV Prevalence Monitoring Programme: England and Wales*. HMSO, London, p. 33.
12. Holland, F.J., Ades, A.E., Davison, C.F. *et al.* (1994) Use of anonymous newborn serosurveys to evaluate antenatal HIV screening programmes. *J. Med. Screen.*, **1**, 176–179.
13. European Collaborative Study (1995) Clinical and immunological characteristics of HIV-1 infected pregnant women. *Br. J. Obstet. Gynaecol.*, **102**, 869–875.
14. European Collaborative Study (1995) Characteristics of pregnant HIV-1 infected women in Europe. *AIDS Care*, **8**, 33–42.
15. Mayaux, M-J., Blanche, S., Rouzioux, C. *et al.* (1995) Maternal factors associated with perinatal HIV-1 transmission: the French Cohort Study: 7 years of follow-up observation. *J. Acq. Immune Defic. Syndr.*, **8**, 188–194.

16. Edlin, B.R., Irwin, K.L., Faruque, S. *et al.* (1994) Intersecting epidemics – crack cocaine use and HIV infection among inner-city young adults. *N. Engl. J. Med.*, **331**, 1422–1427.
17. Davison, C.F., Ades, A.E., Hudson, C.N. and Peckham, C.S. (1989) Antenatal testing for human immunodeficiency virus. *Lancet*, **ii**, 1442–1444.
18. Davison, C.F., Holland, F.J., Newell, M-L., Hudson, C.N. and Peckham, C.S. (1992) Screening for HIV infection in pregnancy. *AIDS Care*, **5**, 135–140.
19. De Martino, M., Tovo, P., Galli, L. *et al.* (1991) Prognostic significance of immunologic changes in 675 infants perinatally exposed to human immunodeficiency virus. *J. Pediatr.*, **119**, 702–709.
20. Tovo, P.A., de Martino, M., Gabiano, C. *et al.* (1992) Prognostic factors and survival in children with perinatal HIV-1 infection. *Lancet*, **339**, 1249–1253.
21. Hall, S. and Glickman, M. (1988) The British Paediatric Surveillance Unit. *Arch. Dis. Child.*, **63**, 344–346.
22. Johnstone, F.D. (1993) Pregnancy outcome and pregnancy management in HIV-infected women. In: *HIV Infection in Women*, (eds M.A. Johnson and F.D. Johnstone), Churchill Livingstone, Edinburgh, pp. 187–198.
23. Minkoff, H.L., Henderson, C., Mendez, H. *et al.* (1990) Pregnancy outcomes among mothers infected with human immunodeficiency virus and uninfected control subjects. *Am. J. Obstet. Gynecol.*, **163**, 1598–1604.
24. Selwyn, P.A., Schoenbaum, E.E., Davenny, K. *et al.* (1989) Prospective study of human immunodeficiency virus infection and pregnancy outcomes in intravenous drug users. *JAMA*, **261**, 1289–1294.
25. Burns, D.N., Landesman, S., Muenz, L.R. *et al.* (1994) Cigarette smoking, premature rupture of membranes, and vertical transmission of HIV-1 among women with low CD4+ levels. *J. Acq. Immune. Defic. Syndr.*, **7**, 718–726.
26. Duliege, A-M., Amos, C.I., Felton, S. *et al.* (1995) Birth order, delivery route, and concordance in the transmission of human immunodeficiency virus type 1 from mothers to twins. *J. Pediatr.*, **126**, 625–632.
27. European Collaborative Study (1994) Caesarean section and risk of vertical transmission of HIV-1 infection. *Lancet*, **343**, 1464–1467.
28. Semprini, A.E., Castagna, C., Ravizza, M. *et al.* (1995) The incidence of complications after caesarean section in 156 HIV positive women. *AIDS*, **9**, 913–917.
29. Royal College of Obstetricians and Gynaecologists (1996) *Working Party Report on HIV Infection in Maternity Care and Gynaecology*. RCOG, London.
30. Scaravelli, G., Thorne, C. and Newell, M. (1995) The management of pregnancy and delivery in HIV infected women in Europe. *Eur. J. Obstet. Gynecol. Reprod. Biol.*, **62**, 7–13.
31. Mandelbrot, L. and Henrion, R. (1993) Does pregnancy accelerate disease progression in HIV-infected women? In: *HIV Infection in Women*, (eds M.A. Johnson and F.D. Johnstone), Churchill Livingstone, Edinburgh, pp. 157–171.
32. Minkoff, H.L. (1987) Care of pregnant women infected with human immunodeficiency virus. *JAMA*, **258**, 2714–2717.
33. Scott, G.B., Fischl, M.A., Klimas, N. *et al.* (1985) Mothers of infants with the acquired immunodeficiency syndrome: evidence for both symptomatic and asymptomatic carriers. *JAMA*, **253**, 363–366.
34. Alger, L.S., Farley, J.J., Robinson, B.A. *et al.* (1993) Interactions of human immunodeficiency virus infection and pregnancy. *Obstet. Gynecol.*, **82**, 787–796.
35. Mulcahy, F., Kelly, G and Tynan, M. (1994) The natural history of HIV infection in women attending a sexually transmitted disease clinic in Dublin. *Genitourin. Med.*, **70**, 81–83.
36. Temmerman, M., Nagelkerke, N., Bwayo, J. *et al.* (1995) HIV-1 and immunological changes during pregnancy: a comparison between HIV-1 seropositive and HIV-1 seronegative women in Nairobi, Kenya. *AIDS*, **9**, 1057–1060.
37. Lepri, A., Cozzi Pezzotti, P., Dorrucci, M., Phillips, A.N., Rezza, G. and the Italian Seroconversion Study (1994) HIV disease progression in 854 women and men infected through injecting drug use and heterosexual sex and followed for up to nine years from seroconversion. *Br. Med. J.*, **309**, 1537–1542.
38. Melnick, S.L., Sherer, R., Louis, T.A. *et al.* (1994) Survival and disease progression according to gender of patients with HIV infection. *JAMA*, **272**, 1915–1921.
39. Brettle, R.P., Raab, G.M., Ross, A. *et al.* (1995) HIV infection in women: immunological markers and the influence of pregnancy. *AIDS*, **9**, 1177–1184.

40. Langston, C., Lewis, D.E., Hamill, H.A. *et al.* (1995) Excess intrauterine fetal demise associated with maternal human immunodeficiency virus infection. *J. Infect. Dis.*, **172**, 1451–1460.

41. Temmerman, M., Chomba, E.N., Ndinya-Achola, J. *et al.* (1994) Maternal human immunodeficiency virus-1 infection and pregnancy outcome. *Obstet. Gynecol.*, **83**, 495–501.

42. European Collaborative Study (1994) Perinatal findings in children born to HIV-infected mothers. *Br. J. Obstet. Gynaecol.*, **101**, 136–141.

43. Mayaux, M., Burgard, M., Teglas, J. *et al.* (1996) Neonatal characteristics in rapidly progressive perinatally acquired HIV-1 disease. *JAMA*, **275**, 606–610.

44. Blanche, S., Rouzioux, C., Guihard Moscato, M.-L. *et al.* (1989) A prospective study of infants born to women seropositive for human immunodeficiency virus type 1. *N. Engl. J. Med.*, **320**, 1643–1648.

45. Kind, C., Brandle, B., Wyler, C-A. *et al.* (1992) Epidemiology of vertically transmitted HIV-1 infection in Switzerland: results of a nationwide prospective study. *Eur. J. Pediatr.*, **151**, 442–448.

46. HIV Infection In Newborns French Collaborative Study Group (1994) Comparison of vertical human immunodeficiency virus type 2 and human immunodeficiency virus type 1 transmission in the French prospective cohort. *Pediatr. Infect. Dis. J.*, **13**, 502–506.

47. Brossard, Y., Aubin, J.-T., Mandelbrot, L. *et al.* (1995) Frequency of early in utero HIV-1 infection: a blind DNA polymerase chain reaction study on 100 fetal thymuses. *AIDS*, **9**, 359–366.

48. Ehrnst, A., Lindgren, S., Dictor, M. *et al.* (1991) HIV in pregnant women and their offspring: evidence for late transmission. *Lancet*, **ii**, 203–207.

49. Lyman, W.D., Kress, Y., Kure, K. *et al.* (1990) Detection of HIV in fetal central nervous system tissue. *AIDS*, **4**, 917–920.

50. Sprecher, S., Soumerknoff, G., Puissant, F. and Degueldre, M. (1986) Vertical transmission of HIV in 15 week fetus. *Lancet*, **ii**, 288–289.

51. Dunn, D., Newell, M., Ades, A. and Peckham, C. (1992) Risk of human immunodeficiency virus type 1 transmission through breastfeeding. *Lancet*, **340**, 585–588.

52. Newell, M.L. and Peckham, C. (1993) Risk factors for vertical transmission of HIV-1 and early markers of HIV-1 infection in children. *AIDS*, **7**, S591–S597.

53. Borkowsky, W., Krasinski, K., Cao, Y. *et al.* (1994) Correlation of perinatal transmission of human immunodeficiency virus type 1 with maternal viremia and lymphocyte phenotypes. *J. Pediatr.*, **125**, 345–351.

54. Dickover, R.E., Garratty, E.M., Herman, S.A. *et al.* (1996) Identification of levels of maternal HIV-1 RNA associated with risk of perinatal transmission. *JAMA*, **275**, 599–605.

55. European Collaborative Study (1992) Risk factors for mother-to-child transmission of HIV-1. *Lancet*, **339**, 1007–1012.

56. Fang, G., Burger, H., Grimson, R. *et al.* (1995) Maternal plasma human immunodeficiency virus type 1 RNA level: a determinant and projected threshold for mother-to-child transmission. *Proc. Natl Acad. Sci. USA*, **92**, 12100–12104.

57. Ometto, L., Zanotto, C., Maccabruni, A. *et al.* (1995) Viral phenotype and host-cell susceptibility to HIV-1 infection as risk factors for mother-to-child HIV-1 transmission. *AIDS*, **9**, 427–434.

58. Tudor-Williams, G., St. Clair, M.H. and McKinney, R.E. (1992) HIV-1 sensitivity to zidovudine and clinical outcome in children. *Lancet*, **i**, 15–19.

59. Albert, J., Fiore, J., Fenyo, E.M. *et al.* (1995) Biological phenotype of HIV-1 and transmission. *AIDS*, **9**, 822–823.

60. Paik, M.C., Begg, M.D., El-Sadr, W., Gorman, J. and Stein, Z. (1995) Difference in clinical implications of CD4 counts among HIV-infected homosexual men and injection drug using men and women. *Stat. Med.*, **14**, 1889–1900.

61. Dunn, D.T., Brandt, C.D., Krivine, A. *et al.* (1995) The sensitivity of HIV-1 DNA polymerase chain reaction in the neonatal period and the relative contributions of intra-uterine and intra-partum transmission. *AIDS*, **9**, F7–7F11.

62. Imrie, J. and Coombes, Y. (1995) *No time to waste. The scale and dimensions of the problem of children affected by HIV/AIDS in the United Kingdom.* Barnardos, Ilford, Essex, p.80.

63. Dunn, D.T., Newell, M.L., Mayaux, M.J. *et al.* (1994) Mode of delivery and vertical transmission of HIV-1: a review of prospective studies. *J. Acq. Immune Defic. Syndr.*, **7**, 1064–1066.

64. World Health Organization (1992) Consensus statement from the WHO/UNICEF: consultation on HIV transmission and breast-feeding. *Wkly Epidemiol. Rec.*, **67**, 177–179.

65. Nicoll, A., Newell, M., van Praag, E., van de Perre, P. and Peckham, C. (1995) Infant feeding policy and practice in the presence of HIV-1 infection. *AIDS*, **9**, 107–119.

66. Fast, P., Newell, M-L., Mofenson, L., Ammann, A. and Rossi, P. (1995) Strategies for prevention of perinatal transmission of HIV infection. Report of a Consensus Workshop (II), Siena, Italy, June 3–6, 1993. *J. Acq. Immune Defic. Syndr.*, **8**, 161–175.

67. Nduati, R.W., John, G.C., Richardson, B.A. *et al.* (1995) Human immunodeficiency virus type 1-infected cells in breast milk: association with immunosuppression and vitamin A deficiency. *J. Infect. Dis.*, **172**, 1461–1468.

68. Goedert, J.J., Duliege, A-M., Amos, C.I., Felton, S., Biggar, R.J. and the International Registry of HIV-Exposed Twins (1991) High risk of infection with human immunodeficiency virus type I for first-born, vaginally delivered twins. *Lancet*, **338**, 1471–1475.

69. Krivine, A., Firtion, G., Cao, L. *et al.* (1992) HIV replication during the first few weeks of life. *Lancet*, **339**, 1187–1189.

70. Minkoff, H. and Mofenson, L.M. (1994) The role of obstetric interventions in the prevention of pediatric human immunodeficiency virus infection. *Am. J. Obstet. Gynecol.*, **171**, 1167–1175.

71. Dabis, F., Msellati, P., Newell, M-L. *et al.* (1995) Methodology of intervention trials to reduce mother to child transmission of HIV with special reference to developing countries. *AIDS*, **9**, S67–74.

72. Connor, E.M., Sperling, R.S., Gelber, R. *et al.* (1994) Reduction of maternal–infant transmission of human immunodeficiency virus type 1 with zidovudine treatment. *N. Engl. J. Med.*, **331**, 1173–1180.

73. Centers for Disease Control and Prevention (1994) Recommendations for the use of zidovudine to reduce perinatal transmission of human immunodeficiency virus. *MMWR*, **43 RR-11**, 1–20.

74. Newell, M. and Gibb, D. (1995) A risk-benefit assessment of zidovudine in the prevention of perinatal HIV transmission. *Drug Safety*, **12**, 274–282.

75. Loveday, C., Kaye, S., Tenant-Flowers, M. *et al.* (1995) HIV-1 RNA serum-load and resistant viral genotypes during early zidovudine therapy. *Lancet*, **345**, 820–824.

76. Siegrist, C., Yerly, S., Kaiser, L., Wyler, C. and Perrin, L. (1995) Mother to child transmission of zidovudine-resistant HIV-1. *Lancet*, **344**, 1771–1772.

77. Roques, P.A., Gras, G., Parnet-Mathieu, F. *et al.* (1995) Clearance of HIV infection in 12 perinatally infected children: clinical, virological and immunological data. *AIDS*, **9**, F19–26.

78. Bayer, R. (1995) Ethical issues in the use of zidovudine to reduce vertical transmission of HIV (letter). *N. Engl. J. Med.*, **332**, 892.

79. Bonkovsky, F.O. (1994) Ethical issues in perinatal HIV. *Clin. Perinatol.*, **21**, 15–28.

80. Hoffman, C.A. and Munson, R. (1995) Ethical issues in the use of zidovudine to reduce vertical transmission of HIV (letter). *N. Engl. J. Med.*, **332**, 891.

81. Wilfert, C.M. (1994) Mandatory screening of pregnant women for the human immunodeficiency virus. *Clin. Infect. Dis.*, **19**, 664–666.

82. Consensus Workshop on Early Diagnosis of HIV Infection (1992) Early diagnosis of HIV infection in infants: report of a consensus workshop held in Siena, Italy, January 1992. *J. Acq. Immune Defic. Syndr.*, **5**, 1169–1178.

83. Blanche, S., Newell, M.L., Mayeaux, M.J. *et al.* (1997) Morbidity and mortality in European children vertically infected by HIV-1. The French Pediatric HIV Infection Study Group and European Collaborative Study. *J. Acq. Immune Defic. Syndrome*, **14**, 442–450.

84. European Collaborative Study (1994) Natural history of vertically acquired human immunodeficiency virus-1 infection. *Pediatrics*, **94**, 815–819.

85. Royal College of Paediatrics and Child Health (1998) HIV infection: prevention of vertical transmission. Report of an intercollegiate working party.

J. McIntyre

HIV INFECTION IN AFRICAN WOMEN

Africa is the continent most affected by the HIV epidemic. In contrast to the industrialized world, the majority of infections are a result of heterosexual transmission and women are at the highest risk of infection[1,2]. Ninety percent of HIV-infected people by the year 2000 will be in the resource-deprived world, the majority in Africa, but a considerable number also in Asia[3]. UNAIDS estimated that there were 30.6 million people living with HIV/AIDS at the end of 1997, comprising 29.5 million adults and 1.1 million children[4]. Current estimates are that there are over 12 million HIV-infected persons in Africa and the epidemic has reached unprecedented levels in Africa south of the Sahara. Most of these infections occur in the reproductive age group with the peak prevalence in women being in the 20–25 age group. Close to 1.5 million HIV-positive African women become pregnant each year, 30% or more of whom will transmit the infection to their children. In many areas of Africa, HIV infection has become the most common medical complication of pregnancy and complications of HIV disease are starting to impact on maternal mortality rates. In Zimbabwe and Zambia, complications of HIV1 disease are already becoming more common causes of maternal mortality than eclampsia and haemorrhage.

AIDS has become the leading killer of young men and women in many parts of the world. In Africa south of the Sahara, HIV1-related disease is likely to account for over 75% of annual deaths in the 15–60 age group within the next 15–20 years. Life expectancy at age 15 in countries severely affected by the AIDS epidemic will drop from 50 to below 30 years[5].

The prevalence of HIV infection in Africa south of the Sahara has reached an average of 7.4% in the 15–49 age group, with an estimated 3.4 million new infections annually[4]. Southern Africa is the worst affected area. One adult in five in Zimbabwe was thought to be HIV infected in 1996[4]. There are few population-based studies of HIV1 seropositivity rates in Africa. A study in Rwanda in 1986 showed that 30% of adults in the 26–40 age group were infected[6]. In Tanzania a population-based study of over 4000 people showed a positive rate of 7.3%[7]. In Uganda, a 1990 population-based study showed that the ratio of HIV-infected women to HIV-infected men was 1.4 to 1[8]. In the KwaZulu-Natal province of South Africa, a rural area characterized by high levels of poverty and migrant labour, women had a 3.2-fold higher HIV prevalence than men[9]. Male-to-female ratios in urban African areas are likely to be closer to parity. Recently reported population-based seroprevalence figures were 20.9% for a rural Ugandan population, 9.9% in Cameroon and 2.2%

Viral Infections in Obstetrics and Gynaecology. Edited by D.J. Jeffries and C.N. Hudson. Published in 1999 by Arnold, ISBN 0 340 74095 7.

in Gabon [10,11,12]. In contrast to the rapidly increasing rates in southern Africa, recent reports from urban centres in Uganda have shown a drop of around 20% in prevalence rates, thought to be due to behaviour change [13].

Pregnant women provide an accessible group for HIV testing and the prevalence in these women is often taken as the best indicator of the level of HIV infection in the sexually active population. Despite this, sentinel surveillance at antenatal clinics may underestimate the population prevalence, as shown in a study in the Mwanza district of Tanzania, where the prevalence in antenatal attenders was below that of the general population by a factor of 0.75 [14].

Many studies have reported on HIV seroprevalence rates in pregnant women in Africa. Rates of HIV1 infection vary from below 1% to over 50% in some southern African clinics. Some recently reported infection rates from sentinel studies in pregnant women in Africa are shown in Table 9.1. In South Africa, national anonymous seroprevalence studies have demonstrated an increase in HIV infection rates from 0.76% in 1990 to 7.57% in 1994 and over 15% in 1996 [15,16,17]. There is a wide in-country geographical variation in prevalence in South Africa, highest in Kwa-Zulu-Natal at 25% and lowest in the Western Cape at 3%. In the absence of testing at antenatal clinics in most African countries, few HIV-infected women are aware of their infection and little can be done to identify them or implement strategies to reduce vertical transmission. Mother-to-child transmission is responsible for around 20% of all new infections in Africa and children of HIV-positive mothers, infected or not, face the prospect of losing their parents. It is estimated that there will be as many as 8.2 million AIDS orphans in the continent by the year 2000 and that the ability of the extended family system in Africa to care for these children may be severely strained [4,18].

HIV2

Infection with HIV2 is less common than HIV1. It is rare in east and southern Africa, except in Mozambique where it is endemic at a very low level. A recent study has also shown the presence of HIV2 infection in pregnant women in Zimbabwe, at a prevalence of 7.6% [19]. In central-west Africa the

Table 9.1 Reported rates of HIV1 seropositivity in women in Africa

Country	Group	Year reported	Percentage HIV1 seropositive	Reference
Burkina Faso	Pregnant women	1997	8.0%	[100]
Côte d'Ivoire	Pregnant women	1995	13.1%	[101]
Ethiopia	Pregnant women	1994	10.7%	[102]
Gabon	General population women	1998	2.0%	[103]
Ghana	Pregnant women	1995	1.6%–2.8%	[104]
Guinea Bissau	Pregnant women	1994	1.5%	[105]
Malawi	Pregnant women	1998	32.4%	[106]
South Africa	Pregnant women	1995	7.57%	[17]
Uganda	Pregnant women	1995	20%–21.2%	[107,108]
Zambia	Urban pregnant women	1992	33.6%	[109]
Zambia	Rural pregnant women	1992	13.1%	[109]
Zimbabwe	Pregnant women	1995	30.4%	[19]

prevalence is also low, although there is some infection present in northern Angola. The predominant area of HIV2 infection is in west Africa, where it was probably present for a long time before it was recognized [20,21]. The prevalence of HIV2 infection in affected areas has remained relatively stable over the past decade, while the prevalence of HIV1 infection has increased.

It appears that the clinical course of HIV2 infection is slower than that of HIV1, although HIV2 infection is associated with the development of AIDS. Dual infections are possible. It has been suggested that HIV2 infection may, in part, protect against the acquisition of HIV1 [22]. Transmission of HIV2 from mother to child has been demonstrated [23,24,25] but this occurs significantly less often than transmission of HIV1. Studies in Côte d'Ivoire and in France showed no transmission of HIV2 from mother to child [26,27] and a study in Senegal showed a transmission rate of 3.8% [28]. Both HIV1- and HIV2-infected women were more likely to have spontaneous abortions or stillbirths than uninfected women in Abidjan, although the mortality in children born to HIV2-positive women was not increased [26]. In view of the clinical and epidemiological differences between HIV1 and HIV2 infections, and the lesser effect of HIV2 infection on pregnancy, the discussion which follows will focus only on HIV1 infection.

WOMEN AT RISK FOR HIV

A number of factors, both sociological and biomedical, increase the risk of African women for HIV infection. While women are at the highest risk, societal pressures often prevent them from taking the necessary precautions to guard against infection, even when their male partners may have many other sexual partners. Women carry the dual burden of infection and of caring for infected family members and may also be incorrectly perceived as the source of HIV in the community [29]. Poverty, gender inequalities and lack of employment opportunities mean that many women are forced into commercial sex work in order to survive, which creates a high prevalence cohort of women in this situation [30].

VIROLOGICAL FACTORS

There is significant variation in viral subtypes of HIV1 around the world, as distinguished by DNA sequencing. Nine subtypes have been identified to date, with subtype B being the commonest in the United States, Europe and Australia. The widest variation of HIV1 subtype occurs in Africa. The predominant subtypes of HIV encountered in Africa are A and D in central Africa and A and C in east and southern Africa [31]. Subtypes E, G and H occur in central Africa [32,33]. Subtype B has a relatively low prevalence in Africa. Langerhans cells in the vagina and cervix provide a possible initial cell contact for HIV. Some HIV serotypes may have higher affinity for the Langerhans cells and are thus more efficient in heterosexual transmission. This has been demonstrated *in vitro* for subtype E and may be so for other non-B subtypes [34].

SEXUALLY TRANSMITTED DISEASES AND OTHER INFECTIONS

Sexually transmitted diseases (STDs) are very common in Africa: reported rates for gonorrhoea in pregnant women range from 5% to 15% and chlamydial infection is present in 6–20% [35,36,37]. Syphilis is diagnosed in around 10% of women in many African settings and rates of over 30% have been documented [38,39]. Genital ulcer disease has been implicated strongly as a co-factor in HIV transmission [40,41,42]. In a population-based study in Tanzania, 14.2% of men and 4.2% of women reported a history of genital ulceration [43]. The increased susceptibility to HIV infection caused by this high prevalence is enhanced by sexual practice: O'Farrell *et al.* [44] showed that both men and women with active genital ulceration continued with risky sexual behaviour. Genital warts, caused by human papillomaviruses, may also facilitate HIV transmission, particularly if secondarily infected[45].

While the strongest correlation between HIV acquisition and STDs exists with genital ulceration, the non-ulcerative infections have also been implicated as risk factors[46,47,48]. Pelvic inflammatory disease, in the absence of ulceration, has been implicated[48]. Women reporting a history of genital ulceration and pelvic inflammatory disease in Zimbabwe were 5.8 times more likely to be HIV positive[19]. Given the very large numbers of women with pelvic infection or non-ulcerating STDs, the lack of adequate or timely treatment in many African settings, the high rate of 'silent' or undiagnosed pelvic infections and the risk of reinfection, it is likely that the non-ulcerative STDs are more important in HIV transmission than was first realized. The control and treatment of STDs in Africa remains one of the most crucial HIV/AIDS prevention activities[49,50]. This is clearly demonstrated by the results of an intervention study providing improved STD services in the Mwanza region of Tanzania, where HIV incidence dropped by 40%[51].

Other, non-sexually transmitted infections and infestations may also place African women at risk. Schistosomiasis is common and may cause genital lesions or ulceration which could facilitate the spread of HIV[52]. It has been suggested that there is also an immunological basis for the increased susceptibility of Africans to HIV, related to the high prevalence of other infections, especially helminthic, in Africa. This may lead to an overactivation of the immune system making the hosts more open to HIV infection and less able to fight it[53].

CONTRACEPTIVE METHODS

There have been conflicting reports about the role of different contraceptive methods in women's susceptibility to HIV infection. The use of barrier methods, which provide some protection against HIV infection, is low in Africa. Oral contraceptives have been associated with HIV infection in research from Kenya[36]; this is possibly a result of the ectropion of the cervix related to oral contraceptive use, which may provide a vulnerable area for HIV transmission. However, other African studies have shown no association with oral contraceptive use or other hormonal contraceptive methods. Experimental animal evidence that progestogen contraceptives may thin the vaginal lining and make viral infection more likely has not been replicated in humans. There remains a concern about the effects of progestogen contraceptives in this regard, given the extremely high usage of injectable progestogen in Africa. The studies of contraceptive method use and HIV infection are largely cross-sectional and further prospective work is required before any definitive association can be proved or recommendation issued[54].

SOCIAL AND CULTURAL FACTORS

Many social and cultural factors and practices have been implicated in the vulnerability of African women to HIV infection. These and patterns of sexual networking differ from country to country, but there is a common thread of lack of gender equity and the resulting inability of African women to take control of their sexual behaviour. Some of these factors are shown in Table 9.2. So-called 'dry sex' practices, where women use objects, chemicals or herbal potions to tighten the vagina during sex, are common in southern and central Africa and have now been well documented[55,56,57]. The disruption of the vaginal mucosa and microlacerations which these practices can cause may increase the risk of infection. Hira[58] showed an increased rate of HIV infection in Zambian women who practised dry sex. An association has also been shown in Malawi[59] and in Zimbabwe,

Table 9.2 Sociocultural practices facilitating HIV1 infection of women in Africa

---

Polygamy
Multiple sexual partners
Early childbearing culture
Low educational level of women
Low employment level of women
Low condom use
The 'sugar-daddy' syndrome: men having sex
   with younger women to escape infection
Gifts: money or goods for sex
Fatalism
Lack of negotiation skills in sexual behaviour
Societal pressure and personal desire for children
Widow-cleansing practices
Belief in witchcraft as a cause of AIDS
Accepted practice of married men to have other
   sexual partners
Migrant labour
Male line inheritance traditions, forcing widows
   to exchange sex for financial support
Male circumcision traditions or lack thereof
Scarification by traditional healers
Dry sex practices
Herbal/traditional treatments for STDs
Non-consensual sex

---

where women who reported usage of intra-vaginal herbs were 1.4 times more likely to be HIV positive than non-users (95% CI 1.1–1.8)[19]. In north Africa, female genital mutilation remains a widespread practice, with a possible link to HIV susceptibility.

Traditional practices such as 'widow-cleansing', common in southern and central Africa, where a widow is expected to have sex with her late husband's brother as part of a 'cleansing' ritual, may be very dangerous in the age of AIDS[60]. Traditional cultural values promoting polygamy and early childbearing and the societal pressure on women to reproduce in order to prove their 'womanhood' lead to early sexual exposure and increased risks of infection. Migrant labour and rapid urbanization, common in many parts of Africa[61], disrupt families and promote the acquisition of new sexual partners, as well as placing a

financial imperative on the women left in the country to take new partners in exchange for gifts of money or goods[62].

In many parts of Africa, married men are very likely to have extramarital sexual partners. In a WHO-sponsored survey in six African countries, more than twice as many men as women reported sexual partners outside the marriage[63]. Condom usage is low in many African countries and there remains a lot of resistance to condoms from men. In Zambia, one of the countries hit hardest by the HIV/AIDS epidemic, condoms are used by only about 2% of the population[64]. Men also report significantly higher numbers of lifetime sexual partners. Even when a woman believes that she is in a monogamous relationship or reports only one lifetime sexual partner, she is at risk of HIV infection. Twenty one percent of HIV1-infected women in a Rwandan study reported only one sexual partner[65]. In many parts of Africa there are reports of men turning to younger women and girls for sex, as they are perceived to be 'less risky' in terms of HIV infection[61].

PREGNANCY AND HIV

ANTENATAL TESTING

There is a number of potential benefits to women of HIV testing prior to or during pregnancy. Where a woman is found to be infected, this knowledge can facilitate early treatment for her and appropriate treatment and follow-up of her child. It enables the woman to take decisions on continuation of the pregnancy and on future fertility, provides information to help her prevent transmission to sexual partners and allows an opportunity to attempt to prevent transmission to the child. If the test result is negative, women can be guided in appropriate HIV prevention measures and risk reduction behaviour.

Routine antenatal testing for HIV is not offered in many African settings, due to the cost involved. In many places, a diagnosis of HIV infection will thus only be made clinically. Reactions of women to antenatal HIV screening vary from country to country. In South Africa, where the epidemic is relatively young and most people have not seen people with AIDS-related diseases, testing is welcomed by women and there is an uptake in excess of 95%[66]. In other parts of Africa, where AIDS has become commonplace, women may be more reluctant to be tested, feeling that the test brings stigmatization and unhappiness, with no benefits[67]. In Kenya, only one-third of women who had given consent for testing for research projects returned to get their test result[68]. In addition, women may be at risk of domestic violence or loss of support if they inform partners of their HIV diagnosis[69,68].

As our knowledge of possible interventions to prevent perinatal transmission of HIV grows, so will the necessity to offer testing to all pregnant women, as most interventions will depend upon knowing the status of the mother. This will bring problems, not only in the attitudinal resistance of women to testing, but in the provision of a testing service for pregnant women which is accurate and affordable for resource-deprived countries.

EFFECT OF PREGNANCY ON HIV/AIDS

Although pregnancy itself is an immunomodulated state (see Chapter 1), it appears to have little or no effect on the progress of disease in asymptomatic HIV-positive women or in those with early infection. However, in women with late-stage HIV disease, there may be more rapid progression[70,71] and concern has been expressed that African women, with the additional factors of poor nutrition, multiple pregnancies and other infections, may have more rapid progression of HIV during their pregnancies than women in industrialized countries. This does not appear to be the case. CD4 and CD8 percentages were shown to be stable in HIV seropositive women in late

pregnancy and the postpartum period in a Malawian study, suggesting that pregnancy has little effect on immune status[37]. In a Kenyan study the changes during pregnancy in CD4 and CD8 cells and their ratio were not statistically significant[72]. These findings do not support the theory of a short-term synergistic effect of pregnancy and HIV1 infection on the immune system. As the epidemic progresses, HIV has become a more common cause of maternal mortality in some central African countries. This is thought to be due to women with advanced HIV disease becoming pregnant, rather than a pregnancy-induced acceleration of the HIV-related conditions.

PREGNANCY OUTCOME IN HIV-INFECTED WOMEN

It has been difficult to generalize research findings on pregnancy outcome from Europe and the United States to women in Africa. Unlike the industrialized world, where most HIV-infected women have additional risk factors in pregnancy related to drug use, infected women in Africa differ little from the general population. Adverse pregnancy outcomes have been reported in many African studies. These include complications of both early and late pregnancy, in addition to the transmission of HIV from mother to child. The general issues regarding transmission and pregnancy have been covered in Chapter 8 and this review will concentrate on findings in African studies.

Complications of pregnancy

Complications of early pregnancy have been reported in association with HIV1 infection in a number of African studies[37,70,73]. Both HIV1 and HIV2 infection in Africa have been associated with a higher rate of spontaneous abortion[23]. A Ugandan study showed that HIV-seropositive women were 1.47 times more likely to have had a previous spontaneous abortion and that this rose to 1.81 in

syphilis and HIV among sexually active subjects in Limbe district, South West Cameroon. *IXth International Conference on AIDS and STD in Africa*, Kampala, Uganda, December 10–14, abstract MoC014.

12. Peeters, M., Janssen, W., Dibanga, G. *et al.* (1995) Dynamic and molecular characteristics of HIV infection in Gabon (1985–1994). *IXth International Conference on AIDS and STD in Africa*, Kampala, Uganda, December 10–14, abstract TuA162.

13. Asiimwe-Okiror, G., Opio, A.A., Musinguzi, E. *et al.* (1997) Change in sexual behaviour and decline in HIV infection among young women in urban Uganda. *AIDS*, **11**, 1757–1763.

14. Borgdorff, M., Barongo, L., van Jaarsveld, E. *et al.* (1993) Sentinel surveillance for HIV-1 infection: how representative are blood donors, outpatients with fever, anaemia, or sexually transmitted diseases, and antenatal clinic attenders in Mwanza Region, Tanzania? *AIDS*, 7, 567–572.

15. Kustner, H.G.V., Swanevelder, J.P. and van Middelkoop, A. (1994) National HIV serosurveillance – South Africa, 1990–1992. *S. Afr. Med. J.*, **84**, 195–200.

16. Department of Health (1995) Fifth national HIV survey in women attending antenatal clinics of the public health services in South Africa, October/November 1994. *Epidemiol. Comments*, **22**(5): 90–100.

17. Department of Health (1996) *Summary of the Results of the Sixth National HIV Survey of Women Attending Antenatal Clinics of the Public Health Services in South Africa, October/November 1995*. Department of Health, Pretoria, South Africa.

18. Hunter, S. (1990) Orphans as a window on the AIDS epidemic in sub-Saharan Africa: initial results and implications of a study in Uganda. *Soc. Sci. Med.*, **31**, 681–690.

19. Mbizvo, M., Mashu, A., Chipato, T. *et al.* (1996) Trends in HIV-1 and HIV-2 prevalence and risk factors in pregnant women in Harare, Zimbabwe. *Cent. Afr. J. Med.*, **42**(1), 14–21.

20. Remy, G. (1993) L'espace epidemiologique de l'infection par le virus de l'immunodeficience humaine VIH2 en Afrique Sud Saharienne. *Med. Trop.*, **53**(4), 511–516.

21. Miyazaki, M. (1995) Epidemiological characteristics of human immunodeficiency virus type-2 infection in Africa. *Int. J. STD AIDS*, **6**(2): 75–80.

22. Kanki, P., Travers, K., Mboup, S. *et al.* (1995) HIV-2 provides natural protection against HIV-1 infection. *IXth International Conference on AIDS and STD in Africa*, Kampala, Uganda, December 10–14, abstract MoA026.

23. Gnaore, E., de Cock, K.M., Gayle, H. *et al.* (1989) Prevalence and mortality from HIV type 2 in Guinea Bissau, West Africa. *Lancet*, **334**, 513.

24. Matheron, S., Courpotin, C., Simon, F. *et al.* (1990) Vertical transmission of HIV-2. *Lancet*, **335**, 1103–1104.

25. Morgan, G., Wilkins, H.A., Pepin, J. *et al.* (1990) AIDS following mother to child transmission of HIV-2. *AIDS*, **4**, 879–882.

26. De Cock, K.M., Zadi, F., Adjorlolo G. *et al.* (1994) Retrospective study of maternal HIV-1 and HIV-2 infections and child survival in Abidjan, Côte d'Ivoire. *Br. Med. J.*, **308**, 441–443.

27. The HIV Infection in Newborns French Collaborative Group (1994) Comparison of vertical human immunodeficiency virus type 2 and human immunodeficiency virus type-1 transmission in the French prospective cohort. *Pediatr. Infect. Dis. J.*, **13**(6): 502–506.

28. Mbaye, N., Sarr, M., Fall, M. *et al.* (1995) Etude prospective de la transmission perinatale du VIH-2 a Dakar, Senegal. *IXth International Conference on AIDS and STD in Africa*, Kampala, Uganda, December 10–14, abstract ThC285.

29. UNAIDS (1997) *Reducing Women's Vulnerability to HIV Infection*. UNAIDS, Geneva, pp. 1–6.

30. Lamptey, P. and Potts, M. (1990) Targeting of prevention programs in Africa. in: *AIDS Prevention Handbook* (eds P. Lamptey and P. Piot), Family Health International, Durham, North Carolina.

31. Boswell, N.R., Carr, J.K., Salminen, M. *et al.* (1995) The distribution of HIV-1 serotypes in Africa. *IXth International Conference on AIDS and STD in Africa*, Kampala, Uganda, December 10–14, abstract MoA041.

32. Weniger, B.G., Takebe, Y., Ou, C-Y. and Yamazaki, S. (1994) Molecular epidemiology of HIV in Asia. *AIDS*, **8**(suppl 2), S13–S28.

33. Cunningham, A.L., Dwyer, D.E., Mills, J. and Montagnier, L. (1996) Managing HIV Part 3: Mechanisms of disease. *Med. J. Aust.*, **6**, 161–165.

34. Soto-Ramirez, L.E., Renjifo, B., McLane, M.F. *et al.* (1996) HIV-1 Langerhans' cell tropism

associated with heterosexual transmission of HIV. *Science*, **271**, 1291–1293.

35. Piot, P. and Tezzo, R. (1990) The epidemiology of HIV and other sexually transmitted infections in the developing world. *Scand. J. Infect. Dis.*, **69**(suppl), 89–97.

36. Plummer, F.A., Simonsen, J.N., Cameron, D.W. *et al.* (1991) Cofactors in male-female sexual transmission of human immunodeficiency virus type-1. *J. Infect. Dis.*, **163**, 233–239.

37. Miotti, P.G., Chiphangwi, J.D. and Dallabetta G. (1992) The situation in Africa. *Balliére's Clin. Obstet. Gynaecol.*, **6**(1), 165–185.

38. Mlisana, K.P., Monokoane, S., Hoosen, A.A. *et al.* (1992) Syphilis in the 'unbooked' pregnant woman. *S. Afr. Med. J.*, **82**, 18–20.

39. Qolohle, D.C., Hoosen, A.A., Moodley, J. *et al.* (1995) Serological screening for sexually transmitted infections in pregnancy: is there any value in re-screening for HIV and syphilis at the time of delivery? *Genitourin. Med.*, **71**, 65–67.

40. Latif, A.S., Katzenstein, D.A., Basset, M.T. *et al.* (1989) Genital ulcers and transmission of HIV among couples in Zimbabwe. *AIDS*, **3**, 519–523.

41. Johnson, A.M., Petherick, A., Davidson, S. *et al.* (1989) Transmission of HIV to sexual partners of infected men and women. *AIDS*, **3**, 367–372.

42. Plourde, P.J., Pepin, J., Agoki, E. *et al.* (1994) Human immunodeficiency virus type 1 seroconversion in women with genital ulcers. *J. Infect. Dis.*, **170**, 313–317.

43. Mosha, F., Nicoll, A., Barongo, L. *et al.* (1993) A population based study of syphilis and sexually transmitted diseases syndromes in north-western Tanzania. I. Prevalence and incidence. *Genitourin. Med.*, **69**, 415–420.

44. O'Farrell, N., Hoosen, A.A., Coetzee, K.D. and van den Ende, J. (1992) Sexual behaviour in Zulu men and women with genital ulcer disease. *Genitourin. Med.*, **68**(4), 245–248.

45. Miotti, P.G., Dallabetta, G.A., Daniel, R.W. *et al.* (1996) Cervical abnormalities, human papillomavirus and human immunodeficiency virus infections in women in Malawi. *J. Infect. Dis.*, **173**, 714–717.

46. Dallabetta, G. (1994) HIV and STDS: how are they linked? *Africa Health*, **November**, 19–20.

47. Hoegsberg, B., Abulafia, O., Sedlis, A. *et al.* (1990) Sexually transmitted diseases and human immunodeficiency virus infection among women with pelvic inflammatory disease. *Am. J. Obstet. Gynecol.*, **163**, 1135–1139.

48. Irwin, K. and Ellerbrock T. (1995) Does pelvic inflammatory disease increase the risk for acquisition of human immunodeficiency virus type 1? (letter). *J. Infect. Dis.*, **172**, 898–899.

49. Biggar, R.J. (1991) Preventing AIDS now. *Br. Med. J.*, **303**, 1150–1151.

50. Laga, M., Manoka, A., Kivuvu, M. *et al.* (1993) Non-ulcerative sexually transmitted diseases as risk factors for HIV-1 transmission in women: results from a cohort study. *AIDS*, **7**, 95–102.

51. Grosskurth, H., Mosha, F., Todd, J. *et al.* (1995) Impact of improved treatment of sexually transmitted diseases on HIV infection in northern Tanzania: randomised controlled trial. *Lancet*, **346**, 530–536.

52. Feldmeier, H., Krantz, I. and Poggensee, G. (1994) Female genital schistosomiasis as a risk factor for the transmission of HIV. *Int. J. STD AIDS*, **5**(5), 368–372.

53. Bentwich, Z., Kalinkovich, A. and Weisman Z. (1995) Immune activation is a dominant factor in the pathogenesis of African AIDS. *Immunol. Today*, **16**(4), 187–191.

54. Daly, C.C., Helling-Giese, G.E., Amti, J.K. and Hunter, D.J. (1994) Contraceptive methods and the transmission of HIV: implications for family planning. *Genitourin. Med.*, **70**(2), 110–117.

55. Runyanga, A., Pitts, M. and McMaster, J. (1992) The use of herbal and other agents to enhance sexual experience. *Soc. Sci. Med.*, **35**(8), 1037–1042.

56. Runyanga, A. and Kasule, J. (1995) The vaginal use of herbs/substances: an HIV-transmission facilitatory factor? *AIDS Care*, **7**(5), 639–645.

57. Civic, D. and Wilson, D. (1996) Dry sex in Zimbabwe and implications for condom use. *Soc. Sci. Med.*, **42**, 91–98.

58. Hira, S.K., Mangrola, U.G., Mwale, C. *et al.* (1990) Apparent vertical transmission of HIV-1 by breast feeding in Zambia. *J. Paediatr.*, **117**, 421–424.

59. Dallabetta, G., Miotti, P., Chiphangwi, J. *et al.* (1990) Vaginal agents as a risk factor for acquisition of HIV-1. *Fifth International Conference on AIDS in Africa*, Kinshasa, Abstract F0A2.

60. Campbell, T. and Kelly, M. (1995) Women and AIDS in Zambia: a review of the psychosocial

factors implicated in the transmission of HIV. *AIDS Care*, **7**, 365–373.

61. Decosas, J. and Pedneault, V. (1992) Women and AIDS in Africa: demographic implications for health promotion. *Health Policy and Planning*, **7**(3), 227–233.

62. Heise, L.L. and Elias, C. (1995) Transforming AIDS prevention to meet women's needs: a focus on developing countries. *Soc. Sci. Med.*, **40**(7), 931–943.

63. Carael, M., Cleland, J. and Adeokun, L. (1991) Overview and selected findings of sexual behavioural surveys. *AIDS*, **5**(suppl 1), S65–S74.

64. Gaisie, K., Cross, A.R. and Nsemukila, K. (1993) *Zambia Demographic and Health Survey 1992*. University of Zambia, Lusaka and Central Statistical Office and Macro International, Columbia, USA.

65. Allen, S., Lindan, C., Serufilira, A. *et al.* (1991) Human immunodeficiency virus infection in urban Rwanda: demographic and behavioural correlates in a representative sample of childbearing women. *JAMA*, **226**, 1657.

66. McIntyre, J.A. (1993) Pregnancy and HIV infection at Baragwanath Hospital, 1987–1993. *Eighth International Conference on AIDS and STD in Africa*, Marrakesh, Morocco, December 12–16, abstract ThOP 13.

67. Adu-Sarkodie, Y. (1996) Why Abena is not having an HIV test. *Br. Med. J.* (SA edition), **4**, 725.

68. Temmerman, M., Ndinya-Achola, J., Ambani, J. and Piot, P. (1995) The right not to know HIV test results. *Lancet*, **345**, 969–970.

69. Rothenberg, K.H. and Paskey, S.J. (1995) The risk of domestic violence and women with HIV infection: implications for partner notification, public policy and the law. *Am. J. Public Health*, **85**, 1569–1576.

70. Temmerman, M. (1994) Human immunodeficiency virus and women. *J. Obstet. Gynecol.*, **14**(suppl 2), S70–S75.

71. Ryder, R.W. and Temmerman, M. (1991) The effects of HIV-1 infection during pregnancy and the perinatal period on maternal and child health in Africa. *AIDS*, **5**(suppl 1), S75–S85.

72. Temmerman, M., Nagelkerke, N., Bwayo, J. *et al.* (1995) HIV-1 and immunological changes during pregnancy: a comparison between HIV-1-seropositive and HIV-1-seronegative women in Nairobi, Kenya. *AIDS*, **9**(9), 1057–1060.

73. Johnstone, F.D. (1993) Pregnancy outcome and pregnancy management in HIV-infected women. In: *HIV Infection in Women*, (eds M.A. Johnson and F.D. Johnstone), Churchill Livingstone, Edinburgh, pp. 187–198.

74. Byabamazina, C.R., Asiimwe, O.G., Malamba, S. *et al.* (1995) HIV/syphilis serology as an indicator of past pregnancy outcomes among antenatal attendees in Kampala. *IXth International Conference on AIDS and STD in Africa*, Kampala, Uganda, December 10–14, abstract TuC108.

75. Klugman, K.P., Patel, J., Sischy, A. and McIntyre, J.A. (1991) Serological markers of sexually transmitted diseases associated with HIV-1 infection in pregnant black women. *S. Afr. Med J.*, **80**, 243–244.

76. Leroy, V., de Clerq, A., Ladner, J., Bogaerts, J. *et al.* (1995) Should screening of genital infections be part of antenatal care in areas of high HIV prevalence? A prospective cohort study from Kigali, Rwanda. *Genitourin. Med.*, **71**(4), 207–211.

77. Minkoff, H.L., Willoughby, A., Mendez, H. *et al.* (1990) Serious infections during pregnancy among women with advanced human immunodeficiency virus infection. *Am. J. Obstet. Gynecol.*, **162**, 30–34.

78. Braddick, M.R., Kreiss, J.K., Embree, J.B. *et al.* (1990) Impact of maternal HIV infection on obstetrical and early pregnancy outcome. *AIDS*, **4**, 1001–1005.

79. Lallemant, M., Lallemant-Le, Coeur, S., Cheynier, D. *et al.* (1989) Mother to child transmission of HIV-1 and infant survival in Brazzaville, Congo. *AIDS*, **3**, 643–646.

80. Ryder, R.W., Nsa, W., Hassig, S.E. *et al.* (1989) Perinatal transmission of the human immunodeficiency virus type-1 to infants of seropositive women in Zaire. *N. Engl. J. Med.*, **320**, 1637–1642.

81. Temmerman, M., Plummer, F.A., Mirza, N.B. *et al.* (1990) Infection with HIV as a risk factor for adverse pregnancy outcome. *AIDS*, **4**, 139–144.

82. Lepage, P., Dabis, F., Htimana, D.G. *et al.* (1990) Perinatal transmission of HIV-1: lack of impact of maternal HIV infection on characteristics of livebirths and neonatal mortality in Kigali, Rwanda. *AIDS*, **5**, 295–300.

83. Gray, G., McIntyre, J.A. and Pettifor, J. (1995) Differences in growth and illness between

breastfed and formula fed infants born to HIV-positive women in Soweto. *IXth International Conference on AIDS and STD in Africa*, Kampala, Uganda, December 10–14, abstract ThB280.

84. The Working Group on Mother to Child Transmission of HIV (1995) Rates of mother to child transmission of HIV-1 in Africa, America and Europe. *J. Acq. Immune Defic. Syndr.*, **8**(5), 506–510.

85. Newell, M-L. and Peckham, C. (1993) Risk factors for vertical transmission of HIV-1 and early markers of HIV-1 infection in children. AIDS, 7(suppl 1), S91–S97.

86. Semba, R.D., Miotti, P.G., Chiphangwi, J.D. *et al.* (1994) Maternal Vitamin A deficiency and mother-to-child transmission of HIV-1. *Lancet*, **343**, 1593–1597.

87. Siena Consensus Workshop II (1995) Strategies for prevention of perinatal transmission of HIV infection. *J. Acq. Immune Defic. Syndr.*, **8**(2), 161–175.

88. Van de Perre, P., Simenon, A., Hitimana, D.-G. *et al.* (1993) Infective and anti-infective properties of breastmilk from HIV-1 infected women. *Lancet*, **341**, 914–918.

89. Van de Perre, P., Simenon, A., Msellati, P. *et al.* (1991) Postnatal transmission of human immunodeficiency virus type I from mother to infant. *N. Engl. J. Med.*, **325**, 593–598.

90. Ziegler, J.B. (1993) Breast feeding and HIV. *Lancet*, **342**, 1437–1438.

91. Kennedy, K.I., Fortney, J.A., Bonhomme, M.G. *et al.* (1990) Do the benefits of breastfeeding outweigh the risk of postnatal transmission of HIV via breastmilk? *Trop. Doct.*, **20**, 25–29.

92. UNAIDS (1996) *HIV and Infant Feeding*. UNAIDS, Geneva, pp. 1–2

93. Fowler, M.G. and Mofensan, H. (1997) Progress in the prevention of perinatal HIV-1. *Acta Pediatr.*, **421**, (suppl), 97–103.

94. McIntyre, J.A. (1996) Transmission of HIV from mother to child: strategies for prevention. *Maternal Child Health*, **21**(5), 116–118.

95. Connor, E.M., Sperling, R.S., Gelber, R. *et al.* (1994) Reduction of maternal-infant transmission of human immunodeficiency virus type 1 with zidovudine treatment. *N. Engl. J. Med.*, **331**(18), 1173–1180.

96. CDC (1998) Administration of zidovudine during late pregnancy and delivery to prevent perinatal HIV transmission. *MMWR*, **47**(8), 151–154.

97. Biggar, R.J., Miotti, P.G., Taha, T.E. *et al.* (1996) Perinatal intervention trial in Africa: effect of birth canal cleansing intervention to prevent HIV transmission. *Lancet*, **347**, 1647–1650.

98. Taha, T.E., Biggar, R.J., Broadhead R.L. *et al.* (1997) Effect of cleansing the birth canal with antiseptic solution on maternal and newborn morbidity and mortality in Malawi: clinical trial. *Br. Med. J.*, **315**(7102), 216–219.

99. Verkuyl, D.A. (1995) Practising obstetrics and gynaecology in areas with a high prevalence of HIV infection. *Lancet*, **346**, 293–296.

100. Sangare, L., Meda, N., Lankoande, S. *et al.* (1997) HIV infection among pregnant women in Burkina Faso: a nationwide serosurvey. *Int. J. STD AIDS*, **8**(10), 646–651.

101. Wiktor, S.Z., Ekpini, E., Dondero, T. *et al.* (1995) Feasibility of conducting a clinical trial to evaluate a short course of zidovudine to interrupt mother to child HIV-1 transmission in Abidjan, Cote d'Ivoire. *IXth International Conference on AIDS and STD in Africa*, Kampala, Uganda, December 10–14, abstract Tul26.

102. Kidan, K.G., Fantahun, M. and Azeze, B. (1995) Seroprevalence of human immunodeficiency virus infection and its association with syphilis seropositivity among antenatal clinic attenders at Debretabor Hospital, Ethiopia. *E. Afr. Med. J.*, **72**(9), 579–583.

103. Bertherat, E., Georges-Courbot, M.C., Nabias, R. *et al.* (1998) Seroprevalence of four sexually transmitted diseases in a semi-urban population of Gabon. *Int. J. STD AIDS*, **9**(1), 31–36.

104. Laarie, J. (1995) HIV sero-surveillance in Northern Ghana. *IXth International Conference on AIDS and STD in Africa*, Kampala, Uganda, December 10–14, abstract MoC015.

105. Nauclèr, A., Norrgren, H., Andersson, S. *et al.* (1995) Trends in HIV infection in Guinea Bissau. *IXth International Conference on AIDS and STD in Africa*, Kampala, Uganda, December, 10–14 abstract MoCO81.

106. Taha, T.E., Dallabetta, G.A., Hoover, D.R. *et al.* (1998) Trends of HIV-1 and sexually transmitted diseases among pregnant and postpartum women in urban Malawi. *AIDS*, **12**(2), 197–203.

107. Nabaitu, J., Ricard, D., Kengeya-Kayondo, J.F. and Nunn, A.J. (1995) HIV-1 seroprevalence and risk perception in a rural area of SW

Uganda. *IXth International Conference on AIDS and STD in Africa*, Kampala, Uganda, December 10–14, abstract MoC013.

108. Bagenda, D., Mmiro, F., Mirembe, F. *et al.* (1995) HIV-1 seroprevalence rates in women attending prenatal clinics in Kampala, Uganda. *IXth International Conference on AIDS and STD in Africa*, Kampala, Uganda, December 10–14, abstract MoCO16.

109. Msiska, R. (1992) *Overview of the HIV/AIDS Situation in Zambia*. Ministry of Health, Lusaka, Zambia.

110. Prazuck, T., Yameogo, J.M., Heylinck, B. *et al.* (1995) Mother-to-child transmission of human immunodeficiency virus type 1 and type 2 and due infection: a cohort study in Banfora, Burkina Faso. *Pediatr. Infect. Dis. `J.*, **14**, 940–947.

Viral hepatitis and pregnancy 10

D. Siebert, S. Locarnini and A. Cunningham

INTRODUCTION

In the decade since interferon was first subjected to clinical trial as a therapy for non-A non-B hepatitis there have been substantial gains in our understanding of the aetiology, pathogenesis, treatment and prevention of viral hepatitis. The significance of hepatitis B virus (HBV) alone is such that, even in countries with a low level of endemicity like the United States, it is a major cause of preventable chronic disease in young children. Only 2–10% of all HBV infections in the USA occur in the first year of life yet neonatal infection accounts for up to 30% of the chronic disease in adults[1,2,3]. While treatment with interferon and immunosuppressive drugs has met with limited success in established disease, early vaccination has been shown to have a profound effect on the incidence of chronic viral hepatitis B in children[4]. This single fact has raised the practice of modern obstetrics and neonatology to a leading role in the management and control of chronic viral hepatitis.

During this same 10-year period, three novel viruses have been characterized, quantitative virology has been developed as an investigational tool in clinical research and a number of new specific antiviral agents have been produced. The rapid acceleration in hepatitis research has been driven by the inexorable developments of molecular biology. Our text reviews the features of viral hepatitis in pregnant women, neonates and infants and summarizes the major advances in clinical management over the last 10 years.

CLINICAL FEATURES AND GENERAL MANAGEMENT OF HEPATITIS

The major types of viral hepatitis cannot be easily distinguished on clinical grounds. Each type of pathogenic agent, the host's age, immune status and the presence of coexisting liver disease influence the frequency of jaundice and other symptoms. However, a reliable diagnosis can usually be made with sensitive and specific laboratory tests for the known agents. Serology is the mainstay of diagnosis but virus detection assays, including nucleic acid techniques, may be required in the newborn.

ACUTE SYMPTOMATIC DISEASE IN ADULTS

In males, and females who are not pregnant, icteric attacks are usually associated with a prodrome, or pre-icteric illness, which is characterized by malaise, anorexia and nausea. Vomiting is a feature in some cases and fever is often present, especially with hepatitis A and E. Other symptoms include headaches and aversion to cigarettes and alcohol. In more indolent cases prodromal symptoms may persist for 2–3 weeks. Discomfort may

Viral Infections in Obstetrics and Gynaecology. Edited by D.J. Jeffries and C.N. Hudson. Published in 1999 by Arnold, ISBN 0 340 74095 7.

develop in the right upper abdominal quadrant and this may be exacerbated by sudden movements, manual pressure or tapping on the ribs.

When the urine darkens the colour of the faeces often pales, and the prodromal symptoms begin to abate as jaundice develops. Sometimes this is accompanied by transient pruritus. The liver is palpable in most patients and frequently tender. Splenomegaly occurs in 10–20% but signs of portal hypertension are absent in acute disease except during the late stages of very severe hepatitis. When hyperbilirubinaemia rises beyond 2.5–3.0 mg/dl, icterus becomes clinically apparent and, in a few cases, bradycardia can be detected when very high levels of bilirubin are present. In adults jaundice typically lasts 1–4 weeks, although it can remain for many weeks, while lassitude and fatigue can persist for several weeks further[5,6].

Acute viral hepatitis should be diagnosed with care. Virus incubation periods temporally overlap and some people experience only a brief flu-like illness or gastrointestinal upset without jaundice (Table 10.1). In addition, viral hepatitis might be omitted from the differential diagnosis in patients with minor symptoms when there is no history of exposure or of a recent event such as blood transfusion[6]. By contrast, ascending cholangitis and other forms of serious sepsis need to be excluded in a febrile, jaundiced patient.

Exclusion of non-viral disease should be based on history, physical findings and laboratory data. Both alanine aminotransferase (ALT) and aspartate aminotransferase (AST) are sensitive non-specific indicators of hepatocyte damage. In acute viral hepatitis they may exceed the normal range by 10-fold or more. The diagnosis should be confirmed by identification of the causal agent and, where appropriate, its source should be investigated. Atypical clinical or biochemical features such as evidence of cholestasis should also be investigated by early ultrasound imaging when appropriate[7].

Most patients can be managed at home with regular examination every few days until evidence of improvement occurs. Support in the form of good nutrition including frequent, small, high-carbohydrate, low-fat meals, adequate fluid intake and rest is necessary. Alcohol consumption should be avoided. Further treatment is necessary if there is evidence of hepatic decompensation. Reduction in liver size with deepening jaundice is serious and the transaminases, alkaline phosphatase, bilirubin concentration and prothrombin time should be rechecked. Patients with worsening disease and symptoms of volume depletion or those with no home support require hospital care.

Table 10.1 Classification and incubation periods of the major hepatotropic viruses

Virus	Family	Nucleic acid	Size	Incubation period (mean)	Incubation period (range)
HAV	*Picornaviridae*	SS (+) RNA	30 nm	21 days	15–45 days
HBV	*Hepadnaviridae*	DS DNA	42 nm	70 days	30–180 days
HCV	*Flaviviridae*	SS (+) RNA	60–80 nm	50 days	15–150 days
HDV	Virusoid	SS (–) RNA	37 nm	Unknown	21 days with HBV superinfection
HEV	*Caliciviridae*	SS (+) RNA	35 nm	40 days	15–60 days
HGV	*Flaviviridae*	SS (+) RNA	Unknown	Unknown	Unknown

DS, double stranded; SS, single stranded; (+), positive sense (mRNA like); (–), negative sense

ACUTE VIRAL HEPATITIS IN PREGNANCY

In industrialized countries the presentation of acute hepatitis in pregnant women does not differ significantly from the disease seen in other women or males[8]. Available data indicate that neither hepatitis A nor B is likely to be more severe during pregnancy than at other times. However, there are insufficient data to comment on this with respect to hepatitis C or the δ agent. Outside western countries the major cause of severe viral hepatitis in pregnancy is HEV[9].

Jaundice in pregnancy has a number of causes (Table 10.2), but in countries such as the United States and United Kingdom viral hepatitis is the most common[9]. Apart from infection with hepatitis A, B, C, D or E (and possibly HGV), primary infection with EBV, CMV or herpes simplex should also be considered along with more unusual agents such as enteroviruses[10]. The diagnostic algorithm includes conditions specific to pregnancy but high transaminase levels favour a diagnosis of viral hepatitis[11]. By contrast, the presence of low transaminase levels (AST <300 iu/l) does not exclude viral hepatitis. Hospital care should be considered for those with limited home support or progressive illness.

FULMINATING HEPATITIS IN PREGNANCY

With the exception of hepatitis E, fulminating viral hepatitis appears to be no more common during pregnancy than it is in women at other times or in men. This severe illness is characterized by the massive necrosis of hepatocytes. Typically the disease has a rapid onset and the patient develops deep jaundice followed by lethargy, vomiting, fetor hepaticus and then confusion as encephalopathy develops, often within a 10-day period. A minority of patients may present with an acute organic brain syndrome when the onset is so rapid that jaundice develops after the first stages of encephalopathy, but in general neurological symptoms follow within 4–8 weeks of the onset of jaundice. Asterixis is usually present during the second stage of encephalopathy but it may be only transient. The liver decreases in size and progressive dysfunction can be accompanied by fever and haemorrhage[6,12–14].

Fulminating disease is most often caused by hepatitis A or B in non-pregnant adults[7]. Not more than 0.35% of cases hospitalized for hepatitis die of fulminating hepatitis A in western countries[14]. Less than 1% of patients with HBV develop fulminating disease, but the mortality in such medically managed cases is of the order of 60%. For patients co-infected with HBV and HDV the occurrence of fulminating disease varies from 2% to 20% but it appears relatively more common in HDV superinfection of HBV (range 10–20% [15]). The frequency of fulminating disease after acute HCV appears to

Table 10.2 Causes of jaundice in pregnancy (adapted from references[7–11])

Intercurrent diseases during pregnancy (any trimester)	*Diseases of pregnancy (trimesters observed)*
Acute viral hepatitis	Hyperemesis gravidarum (1)
Cholelithiasis	Intrahepatic cholestasis of pregnancy (2/3)
Drug toxicity	Dubin–Johnson syndrome (2/3)
Underlying liver disease	Acute fatty liver of pregnancy (3)
Chronic viral hepatitis	Pre-eclampsia/eclampsia (2/3)
Autoimmune liver disease	HELLP syndrome (2/3)
Wilson's disease	
Primary biliary cirrhosis	

vary with geographical and socioeconomic factors. As few as 2% of patients with fulminating non-A non-B hepatitis have HCV in the majority of industrialized nations, but between 40% and 60% of selected patients in Japan, Taiwan and California have evidence of anti-HCV antibodies and/or HCV RNA in the serum[16,17]. The role of HGV in disease is controversial[18,19].

In resource-deprived nations HEV is a serious illness in pregnant women with a mortality rate of 17% in the third trimester[20]. The disease has not been reported amongst pregnant women in western countries but it should be considered in pregnant travellers returning from endemic areas with symptoms or signs of hepatitis. Liver biopsy of adult patients with acute HEV frequently reveals a characteristic histological pattern in which hepatocytes adopt an atypical pseudoglandular structure in affected areas. This can be associated with focal hepatic necrosis and intrahepatic cholestasis. An immune-mediated pathology is suspected because of the mixed cellularity of the inflammatory infiltrate and the associated disseminated intravascular coagulation that can accompany the hepatic necrosis[6,12,21].

There is no specific drug therapy for fulminating disease. At this late stage, viral replication has often ceased and antiviral medications themselves may further exacerbate hepatic damage. Emergency transplantation is highly successful but its role in pregnancy is completely unknown.

CHRONIC HEPATITIS IN PREGNANCY

Three agents are known to produce chronic hepatitis. HBV is the most frequent cause of the condition with almost 350 million cases of chronic HBV worldwide[22]. Twenty five percent of those infected as children are likely to die of HBV-induced liver disease[7,23]. Patients with chronic HBV may also have HDV co-infection or superinfection but the incidence of dual infection

varies widely with geographic location. In addition, more than 50% of patients with HCV are likely to develop persistent disease[24].

Due to the high rate of chronic hepatitis among certain ethnic groups and amongst risk groups, such as injecting drug users (IDUs) in western countries, the majority of neonatal hepatitis cases originate from women who are chronically infected with one or more of the persistent agents. Maternal co-infection with HIV increases the risk of disease progression in the hepatitis carrier and also increases the risk of viral transmission to the newborn[25,26]. In addition, it would appear that women infected with mutant strains of HBV (usually precore mutants) may also have a greater potential to transmit HBV to their offspring, who may then face an increased risk of fulminating infection with the mutant strain[27,28,29]. However, the relative risks of adverse outcomes are yet to be firmly established in these groups of patients.

The use of interferon to treat chronic hepatitis is contraindicated in pregnant women. The major therapeutic intervention associated with pregnancy is vaccination of the newborn in order to avoid perinatal transmission of HBV. There is also an evolving role for antiviral drugs. At present, the transmission of HIV from infected pregnant women to the fetus and neonate can be reduced using zidovudine but the role of drugs during pregnancy may evolve further[30,31], particularly as some nucleoside analogues developed for HIV treatment are also active against HBV (see later).

RELAPSING AND REACTIVATING HEPATITIS

A relapsing or polyphasic course of hepatitis has been reported in some patients with acute HAV, HDV and HCV. The relapses which occur more than eight weeks after the primary illness are almost certainly due to recurrent viral replication during convalescence[7]. Recurrence of HAV has been associated with alcohol consumption in a number of cases[6].

Reactivation of viral replication is also a well-recognized complication in patients with chronic infection, especially following cyto-toxic or immunosuppressive therapy. Pregnancy itself does not appear to have a major effect on the progression of chronic HBV or HCV[32]. However, clinical flares of chronic HBV have been reported to occur with increased frequency in some pregnant women[33]. Viral replication increases during such flares and is characterized by rising transaminase levels and increased conjugated hyperbilirubinaemia[7]. Flares of hepatitis do not usually require hospital care unless progressive liver dysfunction occurs.

EXTRAHEPATIC SYMPTOMS

Between 5% and 15% of adults with acute hepatitis can develop a triad of symptoms that includes fever, urticarial rash and arthritis (or arthralgia)[34]. This condition is analogous to serum sickness and is due to the deposition of virus–antibody immune complexes. It is most commonly observed in people with acute HBV but has been reported in some cases of HAV. The syndrome occurs during the pre-icteric phase of hepatitis and almost always improves with the onset of jaundice[6]. Poly-arteritis nodosa has been observed in some cases of acute and chronic HBV infection and both glomerulonephritis and mixed cryoglo-bulinaemia can be associated with either HBV or HCV infection[35,36,37]. HCV infection has recently been linked with an acquired form of porphyria cutanea tarda[38,39]. Neurological complications including Guillain–Barré syndrome have been associated with all forms of viral hepatitis and, on occasion, Raynaud's phenomenon and erythema nodosum have been reported in patients with acute infections[6]. The frequency of these complications in pregnant women is unknown but no reports of increased risk have been published.

HEPATOCELLULAR CARCINOMA IN PREGNANCY

Primary hepatocellular carcinoma HCC has a strong epidemiological link to both HBV and HCV infection[40–43]. The condition occurs in 25–40% of chronic HBV carriers infected as young children in highly endemic countries but less than 1% of those infected as adolescents or adults in most industrialized countries[44,45]. However, even in highly endemic areas where the prevalence of HBV serological markers closely matches the incidence of HCC (e.g. sub-Saharan Africa, China, Taiwan, Oceania, Italy and Greece), HCC is a rare disease in pregnant women[40,46]. Less than 30 case reports of HCC in pregnancy were published prior to 1996[47].

This tumour occurs predominantly in males and between 60% and 90% of affected patients have pre-existing cirrhosis. Reduced fertility in women with cirrhosis and a relatively late age of onset of HCC compared with men may explain why HBV-associated disease is not seen more often in pregnant women[47]. α-Fetoprotein in maternal serum can be significantly raised above normal in pregnant women with HCC but some authors have indicated that the level is normal in amniotic fluid[48–50]. Termination of pregnancy with subsequent chemotherapy for HCC has been attempted[51].

HCC associated with HCV has not been reported in pregnancy. Perinatal infection or acquisition of HCV in early life is relatively rare compared with HBV infection. In women who acquire HCV in adult life the risk of progression to hepatoma may be less likely to overlap with the reproductive years.

ACUTE VIRAL HEPATITIS IN THE NEWBORN

Viral hepatitis is usually an asymptomatic infection in newborns and infants. The vast majority of neonatal infections with hepatotropic agents (A, B, C, D and E) occur perinatally so that the rise in serum bilirubin or the presence of symptoms such as jaundice will coincide with the incubation period of the virus, calculated either from the time of birth or another potential exposure such as a blood product transfusion (see Table 10.1). HBV is the agent of greatest significance because 80–95% of neonates infected with HBV develop persistent infection[52]. Prenatal infections *in utero* are more likely with agents such as cytomegalovirus (CMV) or rubella and children born with established infection and signs of liver disease will generally be symptomatic within a few days of delivery when infected with either of these agents. Postnatal and perinatal infections with rubella or CMV are less likely to produce the severe hepatitis that may be part of the congenital syndromes[53].

In western countries acute HAV is rare in newborns. Asymptomatic infection occurs in 84% of children infected between the ages of one and two years[54]. However, in one series of 281 symptomatic children between three months and 12 years of age the spectrum of illness included jaundice (99%), dark urine (85%), anorexia (83%), lethargy (81%), vomiting (72%), abdominal pain (64%) and fever (57%)[55]. More than 99.9% of children with HAV recover[56].

Like HAV, HEV is transmitted by the faecal-oral route but acute disease is rarely reported in children. In resource-deprived countries the prevalence of anti-HEV antibodies was first reported to be as low as 1.4% in those under the age of 14 years[57]. However, neonatal deaths have recently been reported in India amongst offspring of women with fulminating HEV in late pregnancy[58].

The bloodborne hepatitis agents (HBV, HCV, HDV and HGV) are also rare causes of icteric disease in neonates and infants. Acute HBV has been well described but the major feature of this infection in neonates is the high frequency of chronic disease in children born to mothers positive for both HBsAg and HBeAg[52]. Disease progression in infants with symptomatic HBV is slower and more indolent than that of HAV but more than 90% of children with acute symptoms recover and the majority have parameters of liver function which return to normal within a year, despite the high risk of chronic infection[56].

Although δ hepatitis can occur as either superinfection or co-infection with HBV in young children, acquisition at birth is infrequent and acute severe disease in very early life has not been reported. Even in areas such as the Amazon basin where 40% of HBV-positive adults have HDV, the seroprevalence is less than 5% in children under 10 years of age[59].

Seroconversion to HCV is an uncommon event in newborns and evidence of symptomatic acute perinatal hepatitis C has not been published. Prior to the advent of screening tests in donors, blood product transfusion was the single most important cause of HCV in children[60]. There are insufficient data to comment on HGV symptoms in children.

With symptomatic illness, investigations to distinguish hepatocellular disease and biliary obstruction in newborns and infants should include serology for the major causes of viral hepatitis. Liver biopsy may ultimately be necessary to identify idiopathic neonatal hepatitis as this condition may account for up to 75% of cases of the neonatal hepatitis syndrome. Other causes of conjugated hyperbilirubinaemia include metabolic liver disease, biliary atresia and, in the first or second week, erythroblastosis with cholestasis[53].

FULMINATING HEPATITIS IN THE NEWBORN

Despite being a relatively benign illness in early childhood, perinatally acquired HBV has been found to trigger fulminant disease in some infants. This generally occurs between two and six months of age. The mother is frequently positive for anti-HBeAg antibody[61]. High serum viral titres in the mother have been implicated as the major risk factor for fatal hepatitis in two cases of HBV in neonates born in sequence to the same parent[62]. Precore mutant forms of HBV can circulate at high titre in anti-HBeAg-positive carriers and such mutants have been implicated in some cases of fulminating hepatitis in infancy[29,63]. Congenital α1-antitrypsin deficiency has also been linked to fatal cases of HBV in children in the UK[64]. Fulminating hepatitis does occur in older children due to HBV alone but it is more likely during co-infection or superinfection of HBV with HDV[65]. Currently, there are no detailed descriptions of fulminating HCV or HGV in the newborn.

The most likely infectious causes of fulminating hepatitis in the neonate are herpesviruses, enteroviruses, adenoviruses and HBV. The success of orthotopic liver transplantation in children with viral hepatitis, under two years of age, is lower than that achieved in children with metabolic liver disease and biliary atresia[66].

CHRONIC HEPATITIS IN CHILDREN

Children infected with HBV at birth or in early life face the greatest risk of adverse outcomes due to chronic hepatitis. In the USA between 1% and 10% of all HBV infections occur in neonates but these children account for 20–30% of the cases of chronic HBV[1,2,3]. Less than 1% of chronically infected children clear HBsAg annually but seroconversion from HBeAg to anti-HBe-Ag is usually accompanied by histological remission[67]. Longitudinal studies of HBV in children have shown that male sex is a risk factor for aggressive HBV disease and progression to cirrhosis[68]. Among Italian children 57% of the patients in one study had chronic active disease and 3% had cirrhosis, but no children with chronic active disease developed cirrhosis during the follow-up period[69]. Similarly there was no symptomatic disease noted in a four year study of 51 children in China who were asymptomatic carriers at diagnosis[70]. The incidence of cirrhosis during the childhood years is therefore difficult to establish.

In Italian children, chronic HCV most often occurred after transfusion during treatment for congenital or neoplastic haematological disease[60]. While birth to an HCV-seropositive mother was reported as the second most important risk factor in this study, long-term follow-up studies of children infected perinatally with HCV are yet to be published. The rate of chronic active disease in this group of children is unknown. However, cirrhosis due to HCV has been recorded in up to 11% of children with transfusion-associated hepatitis[71,72]. The role of hepatitis G in paediatric hepatitis is yet to be defined.

Interferon therapy of children with chronic hepatitis B and C has met with some qualified success (see later).

RELAPSING AND REACTIVATING HEPATITIS IN CHILDREN

Relapse of HAV has been reported in 23 children who experienced icteric disease but it has not been reported in neonatal cases[73]. The rare reactivation of HBV in children is frequently associated with the selection of precore mutant strains[74]. While acute HCV appears to run a fairly benign course in the young, the natural history of infection in children needs more detailed study.

EXTRAHEPATIC SYMPTOMS IN CHILDREN

While cholestatic disease has been noted in a number of paediatric HAV cases, extrahepatic manifestations include rash and arthritis in 5–7% of symptomatic children[55]. Young infants are reported to have evidence of failure to thrive, poor feeding and persistently loose, pale stools. Abdominal distension, vomiting, mild respiratory symptoms and fever may also be present[75].

Arthritis and skin eruptions have been associated with HBV infection in 10–14% of symptomatic children. Some of these cases exhibit a papular acrodermatitis with fever, adenopathy and liver enlargement (Gianotti–Crosti syndrome)[76,77].

HEPATOCELLULAR CARCINOMA IN CHILDREN

Paediatric HCC associated with HBV is rare[78]. It usually presents after the age of five and appears to be more common in males[53]. While HCC in adults can be resected when detected early, it frequently presents at a late stage[79,80].

HCC has also been associated with HCV in adults but if this carcinoma occurs in children with HCV, it is extremely rare.

ENTERICALLY TRANSMITTED HEPATITIS AGENTS

HEPATITIS A

Epidemiology

Hepatitis A is transmitted by the faecal–oral route. In resource-deprived nations it is usually an anicteric infection of young children but in highly industrialized countries it is seen most commonly in young adults in whom it produces jaundice in 80% of cases[81]. In areas of low endemicity, such as western countries, epidemic HAV is relatively infrequent and although it can result from common source outbreaks, spread by person-to-person contact is more common, exhibits a sporadic pattern, and is responsible for most cases of the disease[82]. At-risk individuals are the close contacts of those acutely infected with HAV, including people housed in group settings (families, children in day care, military personnel, students at boarding schools, the mentally handicapped and prison inmates), the sexual partners of infected homosexual men and IDUs[83–87]. Post-transfusion HAV has been reported but it is an uncommon event[88,89].

Hepatitis A in pregnancy

In the last 20 years several investigators have been unable to detect evidence of transmission from mother to baby at any stage of pregnancy[90–92]. However, a study in 1993 demonstrated perinatal transmission of HAV from an acutely infected mother to her premature infant either during birth or by close contact during breastfeeding. There was subsequent horizontal spread to four infants and 10 neonatal intensive care staff[93].

A recent report noted jaundice in a mother immediately after giving birth at 33 weeks of gestation. She was HAV-specific IgM positive. Her male partner and two older children later developed hepatitis. The premature infant was isolated and treated with immune serum globulin (100 mg/kg) five days after birth. HAV-specific IgM was not detected in cord blood or later samples. However, HAV RNA sequences were detected in the infant's sera and faeces on day 17 and day 32 using RT-PCR with HAV-specific primers[94]. This evidence supports intrapartum exposure of the infant to HAV.

Two observations can be made with respect to HAV transmission in newborns. First, HAV infection is an infrequent clinical entity near the time of birth. Nosocomial transmission in the postnatal period is a hazard in neonatology units where the morbidity and cost of outbreaks are significant. However, exposure to bloodborne HAV by transfusion is relatively unlikely, due to the short period of viraemia expected in a blood donor acutely infected with HAV. Close contact and faecal cross-contamination between patients and care-givers is the most likely source of transmission in hospital.

Second, prematurity is a factor in reported cases. One study has demonstrated prolonged excretion of HAV in the faeces of secondarily infected premature infants. It was concluded that the prolonged shedding was due to the immaturity of the immune system in these children[95]. The age of the host is a significant factor in the pathogenesis of HAV.

Molecular virology

HAV is a non-enveloped virus which is ether-resistant, stable at pH 3.0 and relatively resistant to heat. It is inactivated by ultraviolet irradiation, formaldehyde and chlorine [96,97]. The mature virion measures 27–32 nm in diameter. It is classified as the type species of the genus Hepatovirus, within the family Picornaviridae[98].

The virion contains a linear genome of single-stranded positive-sense RNA approximately 7500 nucleotides in length. A single open reading frame (ORF) extends from nucleotide 735 at the 5′ terminal end to about 60 nucleotides in advance of the 3′ terminal poly(A) tract. This sequence encodes a protein with a molecular weight of about 250 000 daltons (2200 amino acids). The genome organization of HAV is similar to that of other picornaviruses. A short viral protein (VPg) is covalently attached to the 5′ end of virion RNA, whilst the 3′ end terminates in a poly(A) tail[98]. The 5′ region of the genome codes for the four viral capsid proteins (VP1–4), with polymerase, helicase and proteinase motifs at the 3′ end[99]. The precise cleavage junctions of most HAV proteins are presently being characterized.

Replication strategy and pathogenesis

The acid resistance of HAV allows it to survive the gastric environment and pass, by an unknown mechanism, across the mucosa of the gastrointestinal tract. HAV enters hepatocytes via a calcium-dependent process[100,101]. The virus primarily replicated in the hepatocytes of experimentally infected marmosets but also in the intestinal mucosa[102].

Once inside the hepatocyte, the HAV RNA genome is uncoated and serves as a template for translation of viral proteins as well as for transcription of negative RNA strand replicative intermediates in the cytoplasm. These intermediates subsequently serve as templates for the synthesis of the virion and genomic (+) RNA[103,104]. The translation product from the polycistronic viral mRNA is a polyprotein which is cleaved into structural proteins and

enzymes, including helicases and polymerases. Three major structural proteins (VP0, VP1 and VP3) assemble in the cytoplasm to form subviral particles, first as pentamers and then procapsids, which interact with newly synthesized viral genomic (+) RNA to form nucleocapsid particles[105]. Finally, cleavage of the VP0 precursor into VP2 and VP4 produces the mature virion. Virus is then secreted in vesicles into bile as mature infectious virions[98]. In infected liver, most of the replication of HAV and associated changes in the hepatic parenchyma are periportal. Viral antigen is localized in the cytoplasm of hepatocytes and Kupffer cells and can be readily demonstrated by immunofluorescence[97].

The cell-mediated immune response may be primarily responsible for the clearance of HAV and the cytopathology in liver tissue. Natural killer cells and HAV-specific CD8+ cytotoxic T-cells from infected patients have been shown to lyse HAV-infected cells *in vitro*[106,107]. It is not known whether the appearance of anti-HAV antibody is a significant contributor to hepatocyte damage but complement-dependent cytotoxic antibodies have not been detected[108,109]. Host-generated interferon may also play a role in reducing HAV replication at the onset of clinical symptoms[110,111,112].

Laboratory diagnosis

There is a variety of tests for the diagnosis of HAV. The most frequently used tests today are variants of enzyme immunoassays (EIA), such as the microparticle enzyme immunoassay (MEIA), that detect anti-HAV specific IgM. This antibody appears in serum at the onset of disease and can usually be detected by the time the patient seeks medical attention. Normally HAV-specific IgG rises along with anti-HAV IgM but it climbs at a slower rate and peaks between six and 12 months after infection (Figure 10.1).

A single anti-HAV IgG titre is of little diagnostic value in acute disease. Rising titres

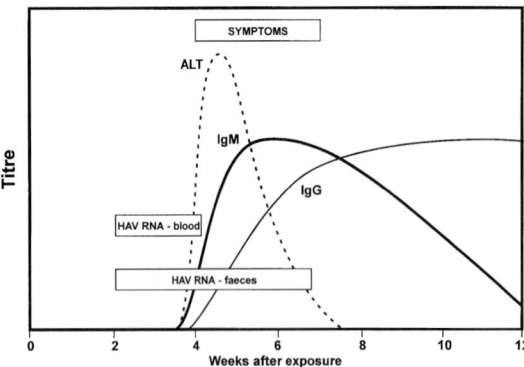

Figure 10.1 Virological and serological events in hepatitis A infection. ALT, alanine aminotransferase; Ig, immunoglobulin; titre refers to analyte titre.

of IgG can only be detected using both early acute and late convalescent sera. Older techniques for diagnosis included complement-fixation tests, immune-adherence haemagglutination, immune-electron microscopy, immunofluorescence and radioimmunoassay (RIA). A fourfold rise in total anti-HAV titre can be demonstrated with older 'paired-serum' techniques provided the first blood sample was taken sufficiently early. Patients who sought attention after their urine became dark would have close to peak total antibody titres, making it difficult to detect significant changes in the titre of total antibody[113].

The newer commercial IgM assays are the most reliable and are highly specific, most being capture assays targeting the μ chain of the pentameric immunoglobulin. Jaundice is often absent in neonates and children infected with HAV and the diagnosis will often rely on laboratory confirmation after a non-specific illness with a biochemical abnormality has been noted in the newborn or the disease has become clinically apparent in the mother or close contacts.

Direct detection of HAV particles or components was originally achieved using immune-electron microscopy (IEM) to detect the virus in the faeces of symptomatic patients and experimental primates. The limit of sensitivity

for IEM was from 1×10^5 to 1×10^6 particles per ml and although recently developed assays are a little more sensitive, it remains an experimental tool[114]. IEM has little if any place in routine diagnosis. In addition, while HAV antigen has been detected in faeces and in cell cultures using RIA and EIA, its use is limited to research and vaccine development[115]. HAV is a fastidious agent so that while some strains can be adapted to cell culture over many weeks, routine culture for HAV has no role in laboratory diagnosis.

Detection of HAV RNA has been achieved by using molecular hybridization assays and PCR. Both techniques have a role in basic research, public health and food laboratories and PCR is an evolving investigational tool in clinical research.

Prevention and treatment

Pregnancy does not influence the outcome of HAV infection in the mother as the morbidity and mortality do not differ significantly from those in other members of the population. In addition, there is no excess fetal loss associated with maternal infection[92].

The treatment of acute HAV usually involves supporting an ambulant patient with adequate hydration and nutrition, especially where vomiting is an early feature. Alcohol intake can make symptoms worse and traditionally abstinence is recommended to avoid a relapse of jaundice[67]. The very rare fulminating cases require hospital care and symptomatic treatment. Up to 80% of selected patients treated by orthotopic liver transplantation survive but there are no data on its use in pregnant women or the newborn with fulminating HAV[14].

Infected patients should not prepare or handle food for others until fully recovered. Advice regarding handwashing and personal hygiene within the family should be offered, along with immune serum globulin (ISG) for susceptible household contacts including the newborn. Postexposure prophylaxis is highly effective and will reduce the incidence of new cases by up to 90%. The neonate should be given ISG if the mother is icteric or thought to have been incubating HAV near the time of birth. The conventional dose is a single intramuscular injection of 0.02–0.06 ml/kg of bodyweight. This will provide 2–6 months of protection depending on the size of the dose and the titre of anti-HAV antibody in the ISG. ISG is given intramuscularly at all times and should never be given intravenously[116].

The immunoglobulin is safe to use in pregnant women newly exposed to HAV and is recommended for post-exposure prophylaxis by the American College of Obstetricians and Gynecologists[117]. There should be a clear indication for passive immunization of pregnant women which includes prolonged or household contact with an acutely infected person or occupational exposure during events such as outbreaks in schools or daycare centres.

There is no known risk of parenteral virus transmission associated with ISG given intramuscularly. However, transmission of HCV has been reported with the use of intravenous immunoglobulins and anti-RhD immunoglobulin. The risk of virus transmission in these products has been related to the method used for the plasma extraction of the immunoglobulin fraction[118,119].

The role of ISG in pre-exposure prophylaxis has been largely superseded by the advent of inactivated HAV vaccines. There are limited data on the safety of the currently available inactivated whole-virus vaccines in pregnancy. All have an excellent safety record but active vaccination in pregnancy should be considered only when there is a clear risk of HAV infection. This would include travel to areas of high endemicity from industrialized countries[120]. Screening to check for immune status will avoid unnecessary vaccination in pregnant women but ISG should be considered in those who are travelling urgently to high-risk destinations with insufficient time to develop active immunity by vaccination.

HEPATITIS E

Epidemiology

Hepatitis E is transmitted by the faecal–oral route and is the major cause of epidemic and sporadic hepatitis in many resource-deprived countries[121,122]. Most epidemics of HEV are associated with ingestion of virus-contaminated water, unlike epidemic HAV which is more commonly foodborne and is particularly associated with shellfish consumption[123]. Outbreaks of HEV in resource-deprived countries generally occur in the wake of flooding, where there has been extensive faecal contamination of local water supplies[121,124]. Epidemic HEV has been recorded in northern and north-eastern Africa, India, Nepal, Pakistan, Burma, the Kirzig Republic (former USSR), China, Borneo and Mexico[121–126].

High anti-HEV seroprevalence rates have been recorded in Egypt (24%) and India (49%)[121,127]. Intermediate levels of anti-HEV seroprevalence (near 10%) have been detected in Saudi Arabia, Nepal and Taiwan[121,127,128]. Industrialized nations have a low seroprevalence of anti-HEV: 0.5% in Australia, 1% in the USA, 1.7% in the UK and 2% in Germany[121,129,130]. However, the present status of serological tests is such that it is possible to underestimate the seroprevalence of anti-HEV depending on the origin of the test antigens[131].

In India and China, where sporadic infection is common, clinical disease associated with HEV is an illness of young adults and is more prevalent than HAV, which tends to cause asymptomatic infection in more juvenile age cohorts[121,125,132,133]. However, the seroprevalence of anti-HEV is reported to be between 1.4% and 10% among children under 10 years of age living in endemic areas[57,133]. In western nations the disease is most often reported in adults returning after travel to endemic areas.

Only 5% of anti-HEV antibody-positive individuals report a history of jaundice compared with 10–80% of anti-HAV-positive subjects[134]. Icterus was absent in the 67% of western aid workers who seroconverted to HEV while working in Somalia in 1993–4[135]. Symptomatic people develop an abrupt, often febrile (50%) illness with a pre-icteric phase lasting 1–10 days. This can be accompanied by abdominal pain, nausea and vomiting. The viraemia occurs during this pre-icteric phase and peaks with the rise in ALT. Most, if not all, symptomatic patients develop jaundice. This lasts 10–15 days and is accompanied by dark urine and hepatomegaly in up to 80% of cases. The majority of patients recover within one month[122–128,136].

Hepatitis E in pregnancy

During outbreaks of hepatitis E in endemic countries the mortality amongst women in the third trimester of pregnancy has usually ranged from 10% to 17%[21,121,124,136]. A mortality of 39% was recorded in one Indian outbreak in 1979[21]. Among Chinese women, maternal mortality was 1% in the first trimester, 8.5% in the second and 21% in the third[125]. In adult males and women who are not pregnant, the illness is usually self-limited, although it may cause fulminating hepatitis in 1–5% of icteric cases[122,124,136]. No carrier state has been identified.

There has been a single report of late antenatal mother-to-baby transmission of HEV in eight pregnant Indian women. Two children were born unaffected but maternal and cord blood was HEV RNA positive by PCR in five of the eight subjects and their respective neonates. Six children had anti-HEV IgG titres which persisted beyond six months of age, including all five who were positive for HEV RNA. One of these six children was icteric at birth; two other children died within 24 h of birth to mothers with fulminating hepatic failure. While one of the deceased was born at 34 weeks' gestation, the rest were born at term. Prenatal transmission of HEV appears to be possible in the third

trimester. The risks in the first and second trimester are ill-defined but abortion and intrauterine death appear to be more common in pregnant women with hepatitis E[58].

In one experiment, in which rhesus monkeys were employed as an animal model, investigators did not detect mother-to-infant transmission in six pregnant animals infected with human HEV and did not demonstrate the severe form of illness seen in pregnant humans. The pathogenesis of this disease is still poorly understood[137].

MOLECULAR VIROLOGY AND REPLICATION STRATEGY

HEV appears to be extremely labile. It does not tolerate high concentrations of salt including caesium chloride. It is difficult to recover from faecal specimens. The majority of viral particles are 32–34 nm in diameter but the size ranges from 27 nm to 38 nm. Virions are spherical and non-enveloped, exhibiting spikes and indentations on the surface[138].

The HEV genome is a single positive-sense RNA molecule of 7194 nucleotides with a 5′ methylguanosine cap and a 3′ polyadenylated tail. Three open reading frames have been identified (ORFs 1,2 and 3). The first encodes non-structural proteins including methyltransferase, helicase and RNA polymerase domains[139]. It is approximately 5000 nucleotides long and is found at the 5′ end of the genome. ORF2 occurs at the 3′ end and its almost 2000 nucleotides encode the sequence for the viral capsid protein VP1. Finally, ORF3, which is only 369 nucleotides long, partially overlaps the other two reading frames and is believed to encode a nucleoprotein[140].

Two strains of HEV, originating from Mexico and Burma, show distinct amino acid and nucleotide sequence divergence[141]. Most other characterized variants share homology with the Burmese strain[142]. HEV has been provisionally classified in the family

Caliciviridae based on its morphology, genetic structure and expression of subviral mRNA transcripts [7,139]. However the methyltransferase responsible for the 5′ capping of genomic HEV resembles that of the alphavirus, Sindbis. The domain for such a protein is not found in caliciviruses and HEV may require a new taxonomic niche [140].

Pathogenesis

Little is known about the attachment, entry, uncoating or replication of HEV virions. Partial characterization of capsid antigen formation has been described in mammalian cells transfected with a SV40 vector and capable of expressing the ORF2 product VP1 [140]. The release of virions from hepatocytes into biliary canaliculi is yet to be described in detail [121].

In acute infection, the histology of the hepatic lobules is disarrayed and the portal tracts enlarged. Kupffer cell proliferation, focal hepatic necrosis and bridging necrosis are seen. Ballooning and acidophilic degeneration of hepatocytes are accompanied by a mononuclear cell infiltrate [12,125]. In fulminating disease massive hepatocyte necrosis leads to collapse of the liver lobules. Swollen and foamy hepatocytes can develop an acinar arrangement. Phlebitis of the portal tract is associated with lymphocytic and polymorphonuclear neutrophil infiltration. Cholestasis is a feature of both acute and fulminating disease [12,21,125]. It has been proposed that the lymphocytic responses in severe disease may be triggered by the release of cytokines and vasoactive substances from damaged Kupffer cells [143,144].

Laboratory diagnosis

HEV-specific IgG can be demonstrated in the acute stage of HEV infection using enzyme immunoassays and immunoblots based on recombinant antigens [145,146]. HEV-specific IgM also appears during the acute illness but

reliable tests are yet to be developed for commercial use and the pathogenesis of HEV remains to be fully explored. Using currently available antigens, the titre of HEV-specific IgG appears to decline rapidly with a half-life of approximately six months [147]. Total antibody has, however, been recorded to persist for up to 12 years (Figure 10.2) [148]. An EIA based on recombinant VP1, expressed in a baculovirus vector, has recently been found to be sensitive and specific for anti-HEV antibody up to 24 months after infection [133,149]. The humoral immune response can also be measured by older, less sensitive methods including IEM and immunofluorescence [7].

Virus particles can be detected in serum and faeces up to 20 days prior to the onset of symptoms using RT-PCR [136,150]. Viraemia and especially faecal shedding rapidly decline after the onset of jaundice, although viraemia has been shown to persist in some patients [151]. Direct detection of the virus in faeces by IEM remains a research protocol as it is a relatively insensitive technique in the diagnostic laboratory [7].

Although HEV has recently been grown in fibroblasts, A549 cells and primary macaque hepatocytes, the virus is fastidious and routine culture for diagnosis is impracticable [152,153].

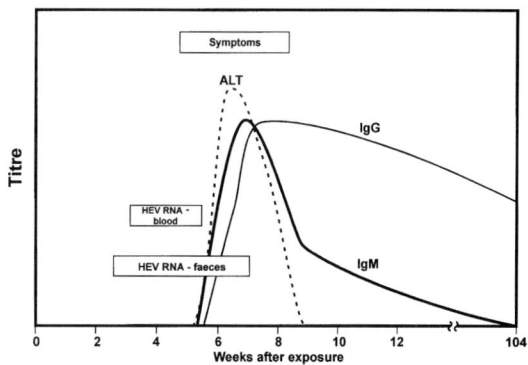

Figure 10.2 Virological and serological events in hepatitis E infection. ALT, alanine aminotransferase; Ig, immunoglobulin; titre refers to analyte titre.

Prevention and treatment

There is no therapy specific for HEV infection. While the condition is seen mostly in resource-deprived countries, poor nutrition and socio-economic circumstances do not contribute to the adverse outcome observed in pregnant women[154]. A detailed understanding of its pathogenesis during pregnancy will be required if rational principles are to be applied to the management of fulminating HEV hepatitis in this group. *In vitro*, HEV appears to respond to α-interferon and ribavirin in primary hepatocyte cultures but there are currently no suitable animal models of the disease in which to trial specific therapies[144]. Neither of these therapeutic agents is suitable for use in pregnancy.

Prevention relies mainly on the availability of clean water supplies. Person-to-person spread accounts for only 2.4–7% of cases but good personal hygiene, including handwashing, should still be advocated for households where cases of HEV have occurred[12,122]. HEV has recently been found in domestic pigs in Nepal but their potential to act as a source of human infection is unknown[155].

Passive immunization against HEV has been demonstrated in non-human primates but it requires large volumes of high-titre antiserum[156]. There have been no controlled human trials of anti-HEV-specific antisera nor attempts to establish a standardized titre. Existing stocks of ISG in western countries are unlikely to contain significant amounts of anti-HEV and safely obtaining large amounts of convalescent serum will be difficult[122].

Prevention of HEV awaits the development of an active vaccine[156].

BLOODBORNE AGENTS OF HEPATITIS

These agents include hepatitis B (HBV), hepatitis D (HDV), hepatitis C (HCV) and hepatitis G (HGV). Except for HDV which requires the presence of HBV to establish infection, all of these agents can infect the host as a single entity. However, co-infection or superinfection with more than one agent is common, especially amongst high-risk groups such as IDUs and people who have received multiple transfusions with blood or blood products. In addition, the presence of HIV infection in a person co-infected with a viral hepatitis agent (or agents) alters the pathogenesis of the liver disease and the risk of transmission to the newborn.

HEPATITIS B

Epidemiology

Hepatitis B may occur as either an acute or chronic infection. The presence of HBsAg in the patient's blood is the definitive marker of HBV infection in both situations[7]. The virus is transmitted by blood and body fluids, but while HBsAg is found in most body secretions, definitive transmission has been established only for blood and its derivatives, saliva and genital secretions[9]. The epidemiology of hepatitis B has been extensively reviewed and most cases in the newborn occur at, or soon after, birth to mothers who are chronic carriers of HBV[157,159].

Hepatitis B in pregnancy

The vast majority of mother-to-infant HBV infections are transmitted perinatally rather than *in utero*. Intrapartum or puerperal exposure to maternal blood is the major risk to the neonate. The point of entry is likely to be via minor abrasions to the skin acquired during birth, or across mucous membranes[9]. There is some evidence that HBsAg can be found in the gastric contents of infants born by normal vaginal delivery to carrier mothers. It appears that vaginal contents can be infectious to the infant via the oral route but this requires up to 50 times the parenteral inoculum[160]. Another possible oral route may be by exposure to colostrum containing potentially infectious virions[161,162]. The risk of transmission via oral ingestion is relatively small and can be regarded as low when compared with parenteral exposure.

Prenatal transmission of HBV does occur but is relatively rare. One Japanese study of five HBeAg-positive women demonstrated that *in utero* transmission is closely linked to 'placental leakage'. In this situation the maternal blood is thought to infect the fetus by passing across the placenta during threatened abortion or during premature labour as a result of partial breakdown of the villi. Such events are not apparent in all cases of suspected intrauterine transmission and subclinical placental leakage was proposed in two out of five pregnancies in HBeAg-positive mothers[163].

Postnatally, children who are born to chronic HBV carrier mothers are at greater risk of acquiring the infection than those in families where there is a chronic carrier other than the mother. This increased risk extends well into adult life and appears to be greater in children of mothers who are HBeAg positive. However, prior to mass vaccination for HBV in Taiwan, up to 50% of carriers were infected in childhood from sources other than their mothers[52,164]. Horizontal transmission in childhood is common in highly endemic countries[165]. In low prevalence countries such as the USA, familial clustering also occurs but close and long-term contact with household members other than the mother, especially siblings, represents the greatest risk[166].

In chronic HBV infection the presence of HBeAg or high levels of HBV DNA are consistently associated with viral burdens of up to 1×10^8 HBV particles/ml of serum[7, 167]. Generally, the risk of HBV transmission is dependent upon the burden of disease in the community and the viral load in the mother at the time of birth.

During the mid 1970s, the prevalence of chronic HBV in the people of Taiwan was between 5% and 20% and the rate of mother-to-infant transmission exceeded 40%[168].

At about the same time, the population prevalence in Pakistan was 1.5% and the transmission rate was < 4% while in the USA mother-to-infant transmission occurred at a rate of between 4.8% and 8.3% where the population prevalence was less than 1%[169,170,171]. Therefore, in high prevalence countries the risk of HBV transmission was significantly greater than in those countries where the disease was less of a burden.

Among Japanese women the presence of HBeAg in asymptomatic HBV carriers was a positive indicator of potential transmission and the presence of anti-HBe antibody was a negative indicator for transmission of HBV[172]. The prevalence of HBeAg carriage varies geographically, being high, prior to mass vaccination, in countries such as Japan and Taiwan[52]. Maternal viral load is high in HBeAg-positive carriers and infants born to mothers positive for HBeAg have a 70–80% risk of HBV infection, but mothers who are anti-HBe antibody positive pose a less than 10% risk to their newborns[173,174]. Even amongst women who are HBeAg positive, the risk of transmission is less than 10% when the viral load is no greater than 10 pg/ml. However, when the load exceeds this concentration, the transmission rate rises to about 80%[174].

The presence of a high community burden of mothers with a high viral load appears to ensure a perpetual cycle of reinfection with HBV in early life. This cycle is maintained because unlike adults, who develop chronic HBV in less than 10% of cases after acute infection, young children have an 80–90% chance of developing chronic HBV after infection in early life[52]. There is evidence that HBeAg crosses the placenta and can induce a state of tolerance in the fetus and neonate[175,176]. In transgenic mice, T-cell tolerance of HBeAg is epitope-specific and this appears to include amino acid residues 129 to 140. HBeAg-specific Th2 lymphocytes may influence the initiation or maintenance of the HBV carrier state[177].

Acute HBV infection in pregnancy is less common than chronic HBV but poses an increased risk for transmission to the newborn[178]. Schweitzer *et al.* showed that acute maternal HBV in the third trimester or early postpartum period resulted in a mother-to-infant transmission rate of 76% but that this rate was only 10% if acute disease occurred in the first or second trimester[179]. Other authors have confirmed these findings and have concluded that HBV is transmitted either at the time of delivery or soon after[180,181]. Transmission of HBV acquired in early pregnancy will not occur unless the chronic carrier state ensues. HBsAg does not appear to cross the placenta as readily as maternal anti-HBsAg antibody. Presumably the viral titre in acute infection is much higher at, or near the time of, birth when acute infection develops in late pregnancy, but may be low or absent if the infection occurs in the earlier stages of gestation. This has yet to be demonstrated, as has the exact point at which a newborn first acquires HBV[178].

Molecular virology

Human HBV is a compact 42 nm particle sensitive to acids and non-polar solvents (Figure 10.3). It is a DNA virus with an outer envelope composed of protein, lipid and carbohydrate. The major surface glycoproteins are a mosaic of antigens collectively referred to as hepatitis B surface antigen (HBsAg). A secondary internal structure is the 27 nm icosahedral nucleocapsid, or core, constructed from 180 core antigen (HBcAg) subunits. The core encloses both the viral genome, which is a circular, partially incomplete double helix, and a tightly-associated DNA polymerase[7,182].

One full-length DNA strand, the L or minus strand, is 3200 nucleotides long and codes for all the viral proteins (Figure 10.4). The complementary plus (or S) strand is shorter and therefore incomplete. The 5' end of the minus strand has a nick (partial discontinuity) at

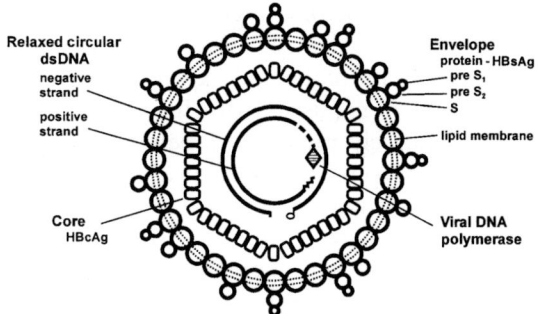

Figure 10.3 The structure of the hepatitis B (HBV) virion. Note the partially complete double-stranded DNA. HBsAg, hepatitis B surface antigen; HBcAg, hepatitis B core antigen.

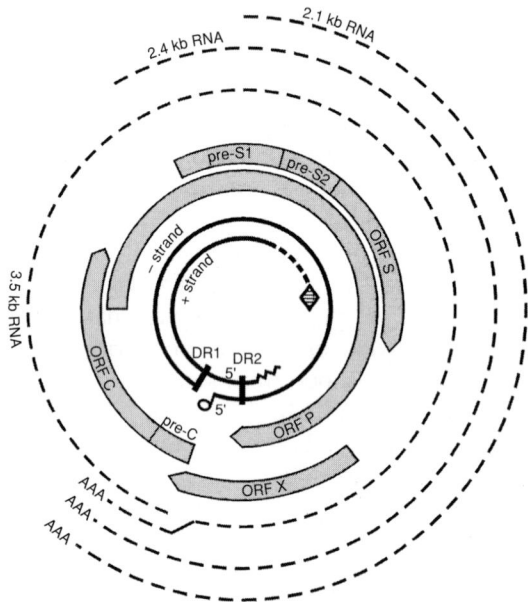

Figure 10.4 A physical and genetic map of the partially double-stranded HBV genome, its RNA transcripts and corresponding reading frames (ORFs). The 2.4 kb RNA transcript codes for all three surface antigen components while the 2.1 kb transcript codes only for S and pre-S2 components. Pre-genomic RNA is a 3.4 kb transcript which codes for the core protein and viral DNA polymerase. Some pre-genomic transcripts are packaged into new viral capsids along with new copies of the polymerase enzyme. This permits the synthesis of viral DNA to be completed within new virions. DR_1 and DR_2, direct repeat sequences; shaded boxes, ORF frames; heavy dashed lines, RNA transcripts.

nucleotide 1230 and a viral protein covalently bound to its terminus. Short direct repeat sequences, DR_1 and DR_2, are found on both DNA strands at the respective 5' ends. These two regions straddle the nick in the minus strand in order to hold the relaxed circular structure together by complementary base-pairing between opposing strands[183,184].

Four open reading frames are found on the HBV minus strand. These gene-like regions are the pre-S_1/preS_2/S ORF, the pre-C/C ORF, the P (or POL) ORF and the X region[184,185]. The long polymerase or P coding region overlaps all the other regions. It codes for the terminal protein and a DNA polymerase which has three distinct catalytic functions[186,187,188]. The envelope protein is generated from two mRNA species which code for the small, medium and large iso-forms of HBsAg[189]. A domain within the pre-S_1 region codes for the hepatocyte recep-tor-binding site on the larger of the three surface proteins[7,190].

The core gene possesses two initiation sites, nominally the pre-C and C start codons, which initiate production of the HBeAg and the shorter HBcAg respectively[191]. Finally, the X gene encodes a transactivating protein which upregulates transcription from a num-ber of viral and cellular promoters[192,193].

Viral replication

Replication of HBV follows attachment, pene-tration and uncoating of the virus in hep-atocytes. The virus attaches to permissive cells using at least one protein including the pre-S protein of the viral envelope. Penetration is thought to occur via receptor-mediated endo-cytosis, although a receptor is yet to be characterized[194–197]. After uncoating in the cytoplasm, the viral genome is translocated to the nucleus. Here the plus strand of HBV DNA is extended to its full length and the entire genome is enzymatically converted to covalently-closed circular (CCC) DNA, the vast majority of which exists in supercoiled

form[198,199]. Supercoiled DNA functions as a template for viral mRNA synthesis using host cell RNA polymerase II[200,201]. Three viral mRNA species are transcribed from the coding strand including a full-length 3.4 kb pre-genomic mRNA. Both pre-genomic mRNA and the viral polymerase are packaged into immature nucleocapsids whose units are first synthesized from the pre-genomic nucleic acid strand[202,203].

Viral DNA polymerase reverse-transcribes the long mRNA into a new minus strand of viral DNA, degrading the pre-genome as it proceeds along the messenger strand. A new plus strand is partially synthesized as the core of the virion is completed[204,205]. New cores interact with envelope proteins, synthesized in the endoplasmic reticulum from the two smaller mRNA species to form mature virions which are then released from the cell[206]. Some new cores can be recycled into the nucleus to amplify the further production of HBV[207].

Pathogenesis

Hepatitis B is an immunologically mediated disease and under normal circumstances, viral replication itself does not appear to be directly cytocidal to hepatocytes[7]. In both acute and chronic disease, hepatocyte damage follows the peak of viral DNA synthesis, correspond-ing to a period of immune lysis of infected cells[7,208]. However, accumulation of HBcAg or pre-S protein may be cytotoxic in certain situations[209]. Cell lysis could be triggered at high rates of replication, partic-ularly when immune responses are pro-foundly suppressed[210,211].

Recovery from HBV is largely due to the cellular immune response, particularly CD8+ T-cell responses, to the major epitopes of HBcAg and HBeAg[176]. In acute HBV infection, non-specific natural killer cells and cytotoxic CD8+ T-cells respond to viral anti-gens on the cell surface. Neutralizing anti-body to HBsAg prevents the spread of HBV to uninfected cells and is responsible for immunity to reinfection[212].

In chronic HBV the expression of HLA class I antigens is less than that observed during acute disease. Lymphocyte activity and hepatocellular necrosis are concomitantly reduced and this may be partially responsible for the persistence of viral infection[213]. In addition, HBeAg appears to be capable of interfering with MHC class II T-helper cells responsible for enhancing activity against the core antigen. In children, this may be responsible for the development of the carrier state[176]. Production of endogenous interferons is reduced in chronic carriers and this too is likely to contribute to viral persistence[214]. Abortive immunological responses to HBV may result in the selection of HBV mutants that prove even more difficult to clear[215]. HBV DNA traces may persist at very low levels even after successful cytotoxic T-lymphocyte (CTL) responses to acute infection. In some patients a persistent CTL response may be necessary to keep the virus in check for life[216].

Laboratory diagnosis

Acute and chronic HBV are best considered separately although they are overlapping stages within the natural history of HBV infection. The tests applied to distinguish these clinical stages are not mutually exclusive but are applied in order to define the pathological markers which characterize each stage. Surface antigen (HBsAg) is nearly always present in the serum of patients with active HBV and is the primary marker of both acute and chronic infection. While 'HBsAg-negative HBV' has been described, it is uncommon. Diagnosis of this condition usually relies on the detection of antibodies to the core antigen and of viral DNA[217].

Acute hepatitis B

During acute hepatitis B, HBsAg first appears in the early replicative phase of the infection.

This antigen is followed by the appearance of HBeAg, HBV DNA and the viral DNA polymerase which peak in the serum just before or at the time of the initial rise in alanine aminotransferase (ALT) (Figure 10.5). By the time most patients have symptoms, all of these markers of replication have declined in titre and will disappear within 1–8 weeks, leaving only surface antigen. The non-replicative phase of acute HBV is marked by the continued presence of surface antigen which, in most cases, remains detectable until early convalescence. Ultimately, in those who clear surface antigen, clinical recovery is complete with no evidence of residual liver damage[7]. If the antigenaemia persists beyond 13 weeks then chronic infection is the usual outcome[218]. In adults, more than 90% of patients recover from acute infection but among children under three years of age less than 10% will clear HBsAg and the infection will persist[9].

Antibodies to HBV markers start to appear during the first few days of symptomatic infection. The first humoral marker to appear is anti-HBc antibody[219]. The stimulus for its production is core antigen, a product of the core gene, which is present in hepatocytes and

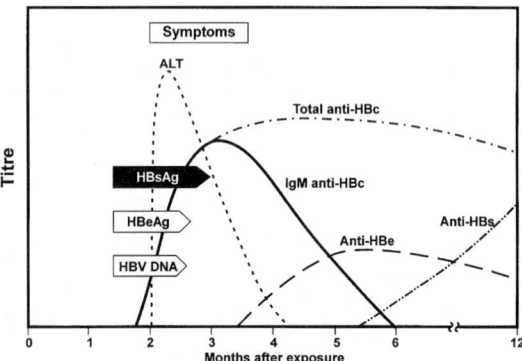

Figure 10.5 The major serological events in acute hepatitis B. Viral markers; hepatitis B surface antigen (HBsAg) and hepatitis B core-specific IgM are bold. Total anti-HBc = anti-HBc IgM and IgG. Hepatitis B e antigen (HBeAg) and anti-HBe are also indicated.

is not secreted into the blood in free form. In conjunction with the presence of surface antigen, the appearance of anti-HBc IgM is the definitive marker of acute HBV. At first, this antibody predominates and peaks in early convalescence, declining over 3–12 months to be gradually replaced by anti-core IgG. The second product of the HBV core gene is HBeAg. Production of anti-HBeAg antibody occurs early in acute infection and coincides with a rapid decline in serum HBeAg and HBV DNA levels[7].

Finally the appearance of antibody to HBsAg is the marker of recovery from acute infection. There may be a 'window' period between the loss of surface antigen and the appearance of anti-HBs but anti-HBc IgM remains positive at this time and the window is less apparent using more sensitive tests. Some patients who clear HBsAg develop only low levels of anti-HBsAg antibody and up to 15% may never produce any such antibody despite successfully clearing the infection[7].

Chronic hepatitis B

An individual who fails to eliminate HBV and remains HBsAg positive for a period of six months or more, has chronic infection and is referred to as a carrier of HBV (Figure 10.6). The initial pathogenesis is identical to that of acute infection but as transaminase levels decline HBsAg persists. Unlike acute disease, the HBV DNA, HBeAg and viral DNA

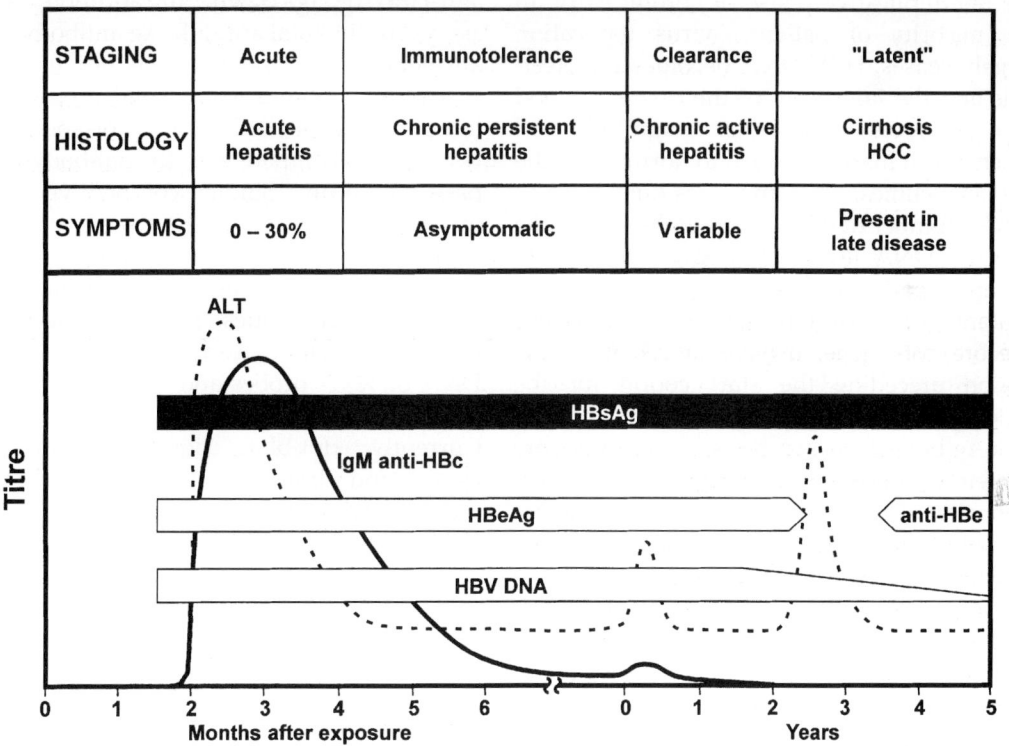

Figure 10.6 The clinical, histological and serological events of chronic hepatitis B. The infection is subclinical in the great majority of infected neonates born to HBsAg-positive mothers. ALT, alanine aminotransferase; HBsAg, hepatitis B surface antigen; HBeAg, hepatitis B e antigen; IgM anti-HBc, anti-hepatitis B core-specific IgM.

polymerase are not eliminated and all persist as markers of chronic infection[220].

The antibody response in chronic HBV is at first restricted to anti-core (anti-HBcAg antibody), which persists at high titre from the time of the first rise in ALT. All other antibody tests remain negative in chronic HBV, while the virus continues to replicate. Anti-HBsAg antibody can coexist with HBs antigenaemia but only at low titre until antigen is eventually cleared.

In chronic infection, seroconversion to anti-HBeAg occurs at the rate of 5–25% per annum. This usually coincides with a fall in the level of circulating viral DNA and DNA polymerase[221]. It is sometimes accompanied by a 'flare' in disease activity known as the seroconversion illness. This event marks the conversion from the replicative phase to the non-replicative phase of chronic HBV. In the majority of patients, virus replication largely ceases, HBV DNA becomes undetectable and the infectivity of the carrier's blood falls by several orders of magnitude. All biochemical markers return to normal and the patient's clinical state improves quickly[222].

In a number of cases, despite the loss of the HBeAg, DNA levels can remain high. This group of patients most often carry a 'precore mutant' strain of HBV. A mutation in the precore/core gene, usually at $\Delta 1896$ in the region preceding the start codon for the HBeAg mRNA, stops production of the HBeAg but allows synthesis of a shorter core protein to proceed from a downstream initiation site of translation. These mutants are thought to arise from a process of immune selection in the host and appear to lead to higher levels of viraemia, progressive disease and a more rapid evolution to endstage liver failure. The significance of neonatal infection with such mutants is yet to be established[223]. There is a marked geographical variation in the prevalence of infections with such mutants. Increased frequency of the mutant virus in adult populations correlates with an early age of acquisition[157].

Detection of hepatitis B markers

To confirm infection with HBV the presence of HBsAg can be established by antigen detection techniques. The assays most frequently used today are enzyme immunoassays (EIA) and radioimmunoassays (RIA)[224]. Although older EIAs lost some specificity in comparison with RIA tests, the newer enzyme-based immunoassays are more sensitive and equally specific (based on manufacturers' data) and do not require the use of radioisotopes. HBeAg is detected using the same technology.

To detect anti-HBsAg antibody, which is produced in both convalescent and vaccinated people, most currently available assays use an EIA format. Immunoglobulin class-capture EIAs are also widely used for the detection of anti-HBc-Ag IgM[225]. In addition, some assays for the total anti-HBcAg antibody were developed as competitive tests in which core antigen was bound to the solid phase and a test antibody labelled with ^{125}I or an enzyme was used to compete with the antibody in the patient's serum. Similar competitive assays for anti-HBeAg and HBeAg have also been developed.

HBV DNA can be detected in serum using a number of techniques. These include molecular hybridization assays which use either DNA or RNA probes and a variety of radioactive and non-radioactive detection methods. Currently dot-blot, liquid hybridization assays and 'branched-chain DNA' (bDNA) methods are in use. Gene amplification techniques including PCR have entered wider commercial production.

Quantification of viral load is now possible with some techniques, more recently with bDNA and QC-PCR (quantitative competitive PCR). Assays of this type have applications in monitoring the therapy of chronic HBV but prospective clinical studies will be required to determine if virus quantification has value in predicting the risk of HBV transmission to the newborn, and whether it is cost-effective to provide such information. One major advantage of such assays is their ability to detect virus in the HBeAg-negative patient, especially in those infected with precore mutant viruses. A major drawback, however, is the degree of variation in quantitative measurements between the various techniques and the lack of an international standard for HBV DNA quantification[226].

Treatment and prevention of hepatitis B

Immunoprophylaxis

Prospective studies have established that neonatal HBV can be prevented in up to 94% of children, born to carrier mothers, by using a combination of HBsAg-based vaccine and high-titre HBIG (hepatitis B immune globulin), commencing at the time of birth[227]. It is recommended that all expectant mothers be screened for HBsAg carriage prenatally even in low prevalence areas[228]. Administration of HBIG alone, close to the time of delivery, has been shown to reduce the infection rate by 70–80% in infants born to HBeAg-positive mothers[229,230]. Little protection was afforded to children who were given low doses of HBIG or received the first dose more than 48 h after birth[231]. In addition, passive immunization alone results in a significant risk of delayed HBV infection, unless it is accompanied by full vaccination[232].

The response to HBsAg-based vaccines is age-dependent and while the seroconversion rate in neonates is at least 95%, this still leaves a small percentage unprotected. Vaccine alone gives protection at rates similar to those for HBIG (70–80%) while using the two in combination is the most efficacious regimen with protection rates of up to 96%[227]. In neonates the vaccine is most effective when injected into the lateral aspect of the thigh and not the buttock, which has led to seroconversion rates as low as 60%[233]. The recommended dosage schedule is 0.5 ml of HBIG (100 iu) IM at delivery along with 0.5 ml of vaccine

($10 \, \mu g/ml$) at the same time or within the first week of life. A further 0.5 ml dose of vaccine should be administered at one month and then at six months of age. The greatest risk of transmission occurs with HBeAg-positive mothers but it is recommended that the infants of anti-HBeAg antibody-positive mothers be managed with the same regimen[234]. Multivalent paediatric vaccines which combine DTP and HBV antigens for use at 0, two and six months are currently being assessed in clinical trials.

Modern recombinant vaccines are composed of highly purified HBsAg particles expressed in yeast (*Saccharomyces cerevisiae*) and have vaccine efficacy and immunogenicity equivalent to that of the older serum derived forms which are still used in some countries (e.g. China)[235]. The reported side effects include local redness and soreness in 12% of individuals and some mild constitutional symptoms, including fever, which occur in up to 3% of recipients[236]. There are very few reports of severe reactions attributed directly to recombinant HBsAg vaccines. Some authors counsel against the use of vaccine in individuals with a history of yeast allergy but the significance of maternal yeast allergy in neonatal vaccination is unknown. Neurological complaints including Guillain–Barré syndrome have been reported in some vaccinees but at present the incidence of these disorders is no more frequent than in the background population. Rare cases of erythema nodosum and polyarthralgia have been reported after repeated doses of HBsAg vaccine[6]. 'Antigenaemia' due to the vaccine itself has been reported in newborns and infants[237].

Additional precautions to minimize the risk of the vertical transmission of HBV include:

- urgent screening of women who make their first presentation in late pregnancy or labour and give a history of IDU or other risk factors and early vaccination of at-risk infants[9];

- minimization of intrapartum procedures and instrumentation that involve or risk skin puncture of the child (e.g. scalp electrodes);
- gentle resuscitation, avoiding trauma to the pharynx and airway that may breach the mucosa and introduce HBV.

Some authors recommend that consideration be given to elective caesarean section and avoidance of breastfeeding in HBeAg and HBV DNA-positive mothers and that gastric aspiration be used to remove blood and vaginal fluids swallowed during birth[178]. There is some evidence that caesarean section is effective in reducing viral transmission of HIV and HCV from infected women but conflicting evidence with respect to women who are HBV carriers[9,25,238]. Breastfeeding by HBV carrier mothers will be safe in adequately vaccinated children although opinion has been divided on the relative risk to the neonates of HBeAg-positive carriers in low-prevalence countries[9,239]. The value of gastric aspiration has not been established and passing a gastric tube would seem to contradict the aim of minimal instrumentation.

In the long term, control of HBV depends largely on public health initiatives. Until recently, one of two strategies had been adopted: either population-based mass-vaccination programmes or risk group-targeted strategies. In Taiwan, the newborns of HBsAg-positive mothers were first targeted in 1984 but by 1987 all newborns and preschool children were routinely vaccinated against HBV. Between 1984 and 1989 the prevalence of HBsAg in children 0–12 years of age fell from 9.8% to 4.8%. In children under five years it fell from 9.3% to almost 2% over the same period. The decline in the number of pre-school children with detectable HBsAg was greater than expected and has been attributed to a reduction in childhood horizontal transmission as well as neonatal transmission in the hyperendemic population[240]. This phenomenon has also been noted in Indonesia although reversion to a risk group-targeted strategy has recently been advocated in Taiwan[241,242].

In low-prevalence countries such as the United States or Australia the prevailing vaccination strategies have been targeted at high-risk groups and this has included the newborns of high-risk parents or carrier mothers. Apart from children born to HBV carriers, the children at risk have included neonates in families that have migrated from highly endemic countries in Asia, Oceania and Africa, those born in high-risk indigenous groups and the children of parenteral drug users. In practice, this strategy has been ineffective due to factors such as poor follow-up by treatment centres, low compliance in some risk groups, such as injecting drug users, and an inability to track those who need to complete treatment regimes. One study has shown that only 65% of at-risk individuals received HBIG and HBV within seven days of delivery[243]. In another, only 59% of at-risk individuals received the full course of HBIG and three doses of HBV vaccine[244]. A revision of immunization strategy by the Immunization Practices Committee of the CDC led to recommendations for the prenatal screening for HBsAg in all pregnant women in 1988, and in 1991 a strategy for universal childhood vaccination[228]. A recent analysis has shown that infant vaccination is cost effective in low-prevalence countries such as the United States and, indeed, adolescent vaccination also compares favourably with other vaccines when cost per life-year saved is calculated[3]. In addition, an enhanced case management system has been shown to improve compliance with the full treatment regimen from 67% to 91%[245].

Seventy five countries with moderate to high levels of endemic HBV have commenced vaccination of infants[246]. It is yet to be determined if booster dosing will be required in adolescents vaccinated as young children. Several studies have shown that young adults are still protected after early childhood vaccination[3]. Countries with a low level of HBV endemicity should have instituted their own vaccination programmes by the end of 1997. Ten western nations have already introduced early childhood HBV vaccination or have adopted preadolescent vaccination programmes prior to the incorporation of recombinant HBsAg vaccines into existing multivalent paediatric vaccines[247].

Active treatment of hepatitis B

Up to 6% of vaccinated neonates are not protected by combined passive and active vaccination. The reasons for vaccine failure are poorly understood but overwhelming exposure to high titres of HBV, infection with a surface antigen escape mutant and infection *in utero* account for a number of cases[163,248]. Most children who acquire HBV perinatally become chronic carriers. As adults, 30–45% of HBeAg and HBV DNA positive carriers eliminate HBeAg and seroconvert to anti-HBeAg antibody after treatment with recombinant or lymphoblastoid α-interferon (IFN-α; 2.5–18 mU administered three times per week). Relapse, with the return of viraemia, occurs in up to 50% of patients[249]. Between 5% and 15% of untreated controls remit spontaneously each year, but less than 20% of treated individuals will lose their HBsAg-positive status after interferon-α 2a therapy. Interferon therapy is, however, contraindicated in pregnant women[250].

Most trials of interferons in children have been conducted on groups of 10–35 patients with chronic HBV, using recombinant α-interferon-2a. The best results were reported in a Spanish study of 12 children with active HBV disease. High-dose, $10 \, mU/m^2$ IFN-α was given three times a week for six months and 50% of treated patients cleared HBeAg compared with 17% of controls[251]. The majority of other trials have been disappointing although more recent studies show that the rate of HBeAg clearance is increased by IFN-α 2a, and the factors which predict response are comparable to those in adults[252,253]. In general, adult responders are HBeAg positive, have biopsy-proven evidence of active hepatitis and raised ALT levels, but have low serum HBV DNA concentration[254–257]. This phase in the natural history of the disease is known as the interferon window[257].

Low-dose therapy of less than 24 weeks' duration in children appears to be associated with less successful outcomes[258]. Combination therapy with steroids (prednisolone priming) may have additional benefit in children, although this is not the case in adults[7,259].

Children with high serum HBV DNA levels are less likely to have a persistent response to IFN-α once therapy has ceased and are more likely to develop progressive liver disease[259]. Patients with HBeAg-negative disease are often infected with precore mutant strains of HBV and usually have high levels of HBV in the circulation. However, seroconversion to anti-HBeAg antibody in children appears to be independent of viraemia due to either a wild-type virus population or a mixed population consisting of HBeAg-negative and wild-type virus[260].

Newer antiviral agents such as the nucleoside analogue lamivudine (3TC) have been shown to reduce HBV viral load to undetectable levels in chronically infected adults[261]. This drug appears to be more effective than IFN-α alone and far less toxic than older antiviral agents such as ara AMP. Other agents such as famciclovir and PMEA are under trial. Large antiviral drug trials are yet to be conducted in children with chronic HBV but with the trend toward multidrug therapy in chronic infections such as HIV, it may be that new multidrug or drug-cytokine combinations will be of greater benefit to younger patients with HBV.

Orthotopic liver transplantation is the only direct intervention available in fulminating hepatic failure or endstage chronic liver disease. In adults, those treated for acute fulminating HBV generally have a better prognosis and better long-term outcome than people who receive a transplanted organ for chronic HBV. Viral load prior to transplantation is the major predictor of post-transplant reinfection[7]. Graft reinfection with HBeAg-negative strains has a poor prognosis in adults but there are no data for children[262]. In children with fulminating hepatitis an INR ≥4 is a poor prognostic indicator. The allograft survival rate is below the rate for children who receive transplants for metabolic liver disease (74%) and biliary atresia (68%) and overall substantially lower (22%) in children under two years[66].

There are only limited data on drug therapy of fulminating hepatitis. Foscarnet has been shown to work in a small, selected group of adults who were HBV DNA positive when therapy commenced, although most patients with fulminating HBV do not appear to show evidence of active high-level viral replication by the time encephalopathy develops [263,264].

A further role for drug therapy might evolve in patients who have HBV co-infection with HIV. Azidothymidine (AZT, zidovudine) has been shown to reduce HIV transmission from mother to infant[30,265,266]. In addition, hepatitis B vaccine is effective in preventing HBV in the neonates of mothers infected with both HIV and HBV but is less successful than it is for neonates of chronic HBV carriers not infected with HIV[267]. It is tempting to speculate that an antiviral drug combination could be devised not only to reduce the risk of HIV transmission but also to help prevent the perinatal transmission of HBV. Potentially, neonatal vaccination could be used in conjunction with near-term antiviral therapy for HBV in HBeAg-positive or HBV DNA-positive mothers who have exceptionally high levels of HBV viraemia associated with HIV infection. Extending the use of antiviral drugs to women not co-infected with HIV would require more careful consideration of the risks and benefits associated with the prevention of HBV infection in 'high-risk' neonates (those born to mothers with high HBV DNA levels or women infected with escape mutants of HBV). A case for active intervention in this situation would have to account for the high level of protection now available with passive and active vaccines, comparing it with the cost and relatively low success rate of delayed treatment in children chronically infected with HBV. However, new vaccines may further reduce the risk of neonatal transmission[22].

HEPATITIS D (delta agent)

Epidemiology and perinatal transmission

The delta hepatitis agent (HDV) is transmitted only in the presence of HBV, either as a superinfection in a chronic HBV carrier or as a co-infection in a new host. The prevalence of HDV shows marked geographical variation with up to 23% of HBV carriers in southern Italy and 47% in Senegal being anti-HDV antibody positive[268,269]. However, in most western countries the rate is less than 10% and the disease occurs as localized epidemics in high-risk groups[270]. The common routes of transmission are close familial contact, sexual intercourse and parenteral exposure through injecting drug use, transfusion and nosocomial infection[270]. Little is known about the risk of HDV transmission from women to the newborn although one study has reported transmission of HDV from an HBeAg-positive mother, but no evidence of transmission from six anti-HBe antibody-positive mothers infected with both HBV and HDV[271].

Molecular virology

The HDV particle is an oval structure between 35 nm and 40 nm in diameter[270] (Figure 10.7). Unique among the intracellular parasites of mammals, it is really a subviral agent and depends on HBV to build infectious particles[272]. The outer coat of HDV is an aegis composed of HBsAg units which directs

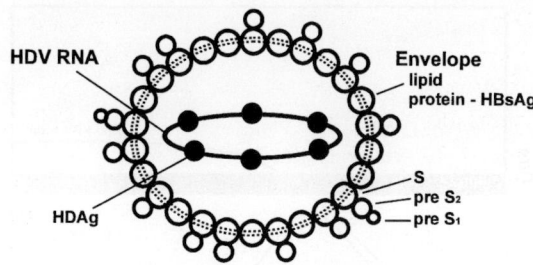

Figure 10.7 Structure of the δ hepatitis particle, HDV. HBsAg, hepatitis B surface antigen; HDAg, hepatitis δ antigen.

the genomic RNA of HDV to infect hepatocytes. However, like some plant viroids, free negative-sense HDV RNA is able to undergo both self-cleavage (ribozyme-like activity) and ligation in artificial cellular and cell-free systems[270]. The genome is a covalently-closed single strand of RNA which forms a circle. By base-pairing across its own sequences, it forms a folded rod in the shape of a safety pin[273]. This structure has no homology to cellular or hepadnaviral DNA and is subclassified into three genotypes[270,272].

Hepatocytes infected with HDV produce both genomic (minus sense) and antigenomic (plus sense) RNAs, each 1.7 kilobases (kb) in length[7,272]. The only known gene product, hepatitis δ antigen (HDAg), is translated from a single antigenomic open reading frame and has three established functions. δ antigen binds genomic RNA and acts as an amorphous nucleocapsid beneath the HBsAg cloak[274,275]. In addition, a leucine zipper motif appears to promote HDAg protein-to-protein interactions during HDV assembly[276–278]. Finally, the antigen contains a nuclear localization signal which is thought to direct newly synthesized HDAg to the viral replication site[279]. During the later stages of HDV replication the viral RNA undergoes a self-editing function resulting in the production of a second isoform of HDAg. The two HDAg species, S-HDAg (p24) and L-HDAg (p27), have opposing biological properties.

S-HDAg is required for HDV replication while the L-HDAg helps shut down replication and promotes virus assembly[280–283].

Replication

HDV RNA replication takes place in the nucleus of the hepatocyte. The processes of attachment, entry and uncoating are ill defined but HDAg is thought to be necessary for HDV RNA to enter the nucleus[272]. Within the nucleus the host cell RNA polymerase II then transcribes two complementary RNA forms from the minus sense HDV RNA template[272,283,284]. The first is a 0.8 kb plus-sense RNA with a polyadenylated tail. This product enters the cytoplasm and acts as mRNA for further HDAg synthesis.

The second transcript is a plus-sense antigenomic copy of HDV. By a process known as double rolling circle replication, the genomic template rolls as multimeric copies of the antigenome are synthesized[285,286]. As new HDAg migrates into the nucleus it accumulates and prevents further polyadenylation of the smaller nascent plus-sense RNA transcript. Synthesis of the antigenome is then enhanced. The natural ribozyme-like activity of the antigenome cleaves the multimeric RNA into monomeric units as soon as each new plus strand incorporates the ribozyme domain[272,285]. Linear antigenomes are then ligated to form closed circular plus-sense RNA[287]. A mirror image of the preceding events then generates new copies of the negative-sense RNA genome from the antigenomic templates[272].

Interaction with hepatitis B

Superinfection of HBV carriers with HDV not only results in HDV replication and expression, but also a significant reduction in HBV replication[288]. This could in theory be due to competition between viral templates for host cell RNA polymerase II, nucleotides and other enzymes in the hepatocyte nucleus[7].

The pathogenesis of the infection may be due in part to a cytotoxic effect of HDAg, immunological responses and/or interactions between HBV and HDV[272]. HDV genotype III appears to be responsible for a more severe form of HDV seen in South America but the responsible genetic sequences are unknown[272,289].

Laboratory diagnosis

The natural history of acute co-infection of HBV with HDV is more severe than for acute HBV alone although 90–95% of these patients recover. By contrast, 70–90% of patients with acute superinfection develop chronic hepatitis[269].

During acute co-infection the appearance of surface antigen is followed by HDV RNA and HDV antigen. Serum ALT then rises, often exhibiting a biphasic elevation which later falls to normal as the major viral markers and nucleic acids are cleared. Anti-HDV antibody, including HDV-specific IgM, rises soon after the onset of symptoms. The period of HDV antigenaemia is brief. Patients with acute HBV should be routinely tested for anti-HDV antibody along with HBV core-specific IgM. Repeated sampling may be required to exclude HDV[7].

The outcome of HDV superinfection is most frequently a progressive chronic hepatitis that leads to cirrhosis in over 70% of cases[290]. Acute superinfection occurs in the presence of established HBV and therefore HBV core-specific IgM is usually absent (Figure 10.8). HDV-specific IgM is present in most new cases alongside a rising titre of total anti-HDV antibody. In established infection, while the total anti-HDV antibody titre remains high, detection of HDV-specific RNA in plasma is the most reliable marker of chronic infection. Quantification of RNA markers is useful as a marker of recovery and therapeutic response[7].

The most readily available assays for anti-HDV antibodies are solid-phase immunoas-

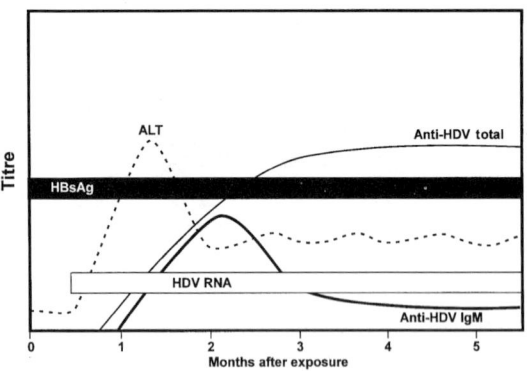

Figure 10.8 Serological events associated with HDV superinfection of a patient with chronic HBV. HBsAg, hepatitis B surface antigen; anti-HDV IgM, specific acute-phase immunoglobulin.

says including RIA and EIA. Over 90% of patients with acute HDV become HDV-specific IgM antibody positive. By contrast, immunoassays for HDV antigen can be quite insensitive. This may be related to the timing of blood sampling as HDV antigenaemia lasts only 1–2 weeks. Western blotting for the p24 and p26 antigens of HDV are most sensitive but are currently technically difficult and require the use of radiolabelled markers. Very few specialist centres make this available and it should not be considered in routine testing[291].

The 'gold standard' for the diagnosis of HDV is the detection of HDV antigen in hepatocytes using immunofluorescence- or immunoperoxidase-staining of liver biopsy material. However, with disease of more than 10 years duration only 50% of biopsy specimens stain positive for HDAg[292]. HDV RNA can also be detected in the cytoplasm of antigen-positive cells using hybridization assays[293]. Detection of the RNA in plasma, for HDV diagnosis and monitoring, is also possible with hybridization assays and, more recently, PCR, but there is no agreed standard and commercial systems are yet to be marketed[294]. The role of nucleic acid assays is expanding and major reference laboratories should have the capacity to perform at least one form of plasma assay on request[291].

Prevention and treatment

Perinatal HDV appears to be a very rare event, even in highly endemic areas, where horizontal transmission in later years is more common[271]. It is tempting to speculate whether the down-regulation of HBV viraemia by HDV in chronic carriers reduces the HBV viral load and therefore the infectivity of HBV/HDV-co-infected mothers to their neonates. This might account for the apparently relatively low incidence of dual infection in the newborn. There are as yet no studies which have examined the risk of HDV infection in neonates born to mothers who are immunocompromised and carry both HBV and HDV. Those on immunosuppressive therapy after organ transplantation or women with HIV might be expected to have a higher risk of HDV transmission. The measures used to control HBV transmission should also apply to children exposed to HDV.

There is no specific treatment for chronic HDV infection. IFN-α has been studied in small-scale trials for periods of up to 12 months. Despite an initial response, the histological improvement is lost and the markers of replication and disease activity reappear. Antiviral drugs such as ribavirin and levamisole provide no lasting benefit and immunosuppressive agents such as prednisolone and azathioprine are ineffective. Survival after orthotopic liver transplantation is as high as 70% in patients treated for fulminating HDV[7,269,270]. There is no specific drug therapy for acute HDV in pregnancy.

HEPATITIS C

Epidemiology

The most efficient routes of transmission of HCV are parenteral. Transfusion with infected blood or blood products, organ transplantation from HCV-positive donors, the sharing of contaminated needles by injecting drug users and occupational exposure to contaminated needles and medical equipment, all pose significant risk[295–299]. However, the risk to users of blood products has declined with the advent of donor blood screening and it is apparent that 20–50% of affected people do not have a defined history of parenteral exposure[300,301]. Case reports and small studies have shown that household, sexual and perinatal transmission of HCV are uncommon, but do occur[302,303].

Hepatitis C in pregnancy

Early studies of mother-to-infant transmission failed to show a significant rate of neonatal infection. Some of these studies relied on less sensitive first-generation serological assays for anti-HCV antibody, contained small numbers of mother–infant pairs, or had relatively short periods of follow-up to determine the risk of transmission.

Recently PCR-based assays have been used to detect HCV viraemia and to provide evidence to confirm a low rate of mother-to-infant transmission of between 1.8% and 6.1% in anti-HCV-positive mothers. Using genotyping and sequence analysis to establish homology between mother and infant plasma HCV, in conjunction with quantitative PCR and serological tests, one Japanese study has demonstrated a correlation between the titre of HCV in maternal blood and the risk of perinatal transmission. Twenty two of 53 antibody-positive mothers had no detectable HCV RNA in their plasma and did not transmit the virus to their infants. However, among HCV RNA-positive mothers (31/53), those whose titre of virus exceeded 1×10^6 virus copies per millilitre (3/31) transmitted the virus to their newborns[304]. Similar findings have been made in two smaller studies[305,306].

Some groups have detected higher rates of mother-to-infant HCV transmission in mothers co-infected with HCV and HIV, but other studies have concluded that the rates are no greater than those in women infected only with HCV[307,308]. Among women with

HCV viraemia the transmission rate has been reported to be between 0% and 25% but if co-infected with HIV, this increases to between 25% and 44% [304–310]. In adults, the severity of hepatitis and the titre of HCV RNA are higher as a result of increased HCV replication during HIV-induced immunosuppression. It is assumed that the higher transmission rate of HCV to neonates whose mothers have HIV is due to a high HCV viral load, but larger, more detailed studies will be required to verify these conclusions [32,311].

Hepatitis C genotype and vaginal delivery may influence the risk of transmission to the neonate but sufficient data are yet to be gathered [25,312]. However, the level of maternal HCV viraemia is the most consistent feature associated with persistent HCV viraemia in infants. The effect of high virus titre on the risk of HCV transmission is analogous to that which occurs with HBV, where those who are HBeAg positive or have high HBV DNA levels are more likely to transmit the virus to the newborn. This risk is maximal at the time of birth, presumably because that is when exposure to maternal blood and body fluids reaches its zenith.

Prenatal transmission of HCV may occur but it is yet to be clearly demonstrated. Transmission by postnatal exposure to breast milk is yet to be reported and none of the small investigations completed have yielded positive results [307,313,314]. Most of the studies of mother-to-infant transmission of HCV are composed of small patient cohorts. There is a need for large, prospective studies of sufficient duration to examine the effects of the severity of maternal disease, viral load, genotype and method of delivery as well as other factors which may influence the risk of transmission to the newborn.

Molecular virology

Hepatitis C has the physicochemical properties of an enveloped virus and is sensitive to chloroform and heat [315–317]. Infectious virions are less than 80 nm in diameter and are strongly associated with the lipoprotein fraction of human serum [318,319].

Complete HCV virions enclose a positive-sense 9.5 kb single-stranded RNA genome. One long open reading frame encodes a polyprotein of 3010 to 3033 amino acids flanked at each terminus by a 5′ untranslated region (UTR) and 3′ UTR respectively (Figure 10.9). The 5′ UTR is thought to function as an internal ribosome entry site for the translation of RNA while the recently sequenced 3′ UTR appears to be a determinant of infectivity with a role in initiating RNA replication [320–323].

The first 25% of the HCV ORF codes for three structural genes: core (C) and the envelope proteins E1 and E2-p7. These viral proteins appear to be cleaved from the initial polyprotein transcript by host cell signalases [320,324,325]. Sequences distal to the E2-p7 code for the non-structural proteins NS2 to NS5B.

NS2 protein incorporates a zinc-dependent metalloproteinase, responsible for the cleavage of the NS2/3 junction when associated with the aminoterminus of NS-3. The other functions of NS2 are unknown [320,326]. By contrast, the complete NS3 protein has a serine proteinase domain responsible for sequential cleavage of the viral polyprotein between NS3 and NS5B [320]. In addition, a helicase motif of NS3 may promote unwinding of newly synthesized RNA [327]. The NS4A product acts as a co-factor to NS3 in most of the later cleavage events [328]. Finally NS5 has the predicted structure of an RNA-dependent RNA polymerase involved in viral RNA replication [327].

Characterization of these features has shown HCV to be similar but distinct from both the Pestivirus and Flavivirus genera of the Flaviviridae [320]. A minimum of six genotypes of HCV can be distinguished based on the sequence heterogeneity within non-coding and coding regions of the genome. However, phylogenetic relationships do not

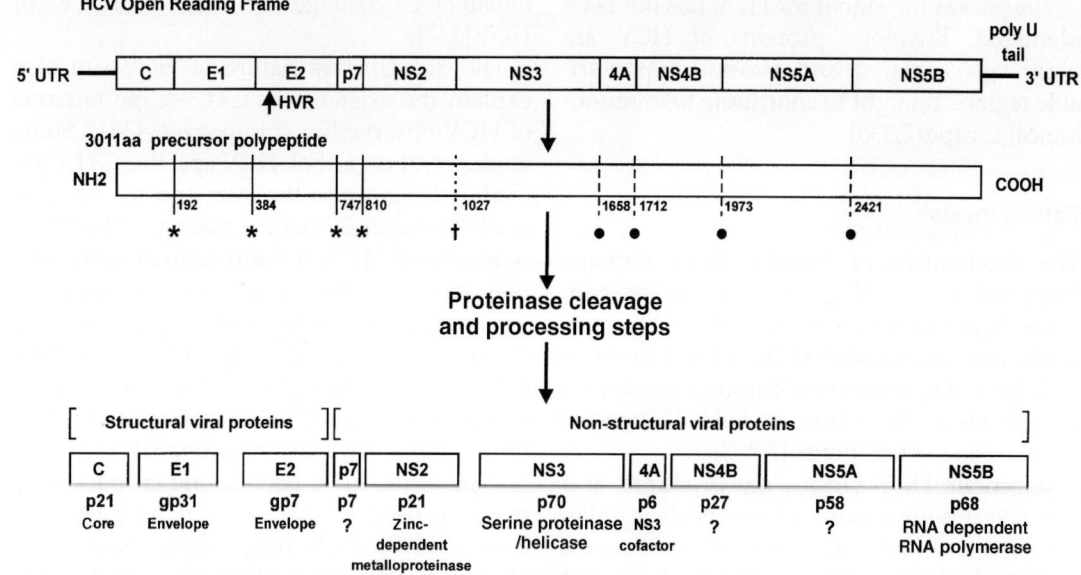

Figure 10.9 The physical and genetic map of HCV RNA. Cleavage of the viral polyprotein is carried out at the designated sites by host cell signalases (asterisks and lines) in the ER, the NS2–3 zinc-dependent proteinase (black crucifix and dashed line) and NS3-NS4A serine proteinase (black circles and dashed lines). Envelope glycoproteins are designated gp. The known functions of the viral proteins are included.

always hold true for the more conserved 5′ UTR and the hypervariable regions (e.g. E2-HVR) when compared with those obtained for individual genes such as core, E1, NS5B and the entire genomic sequence. Therefore, a consensus on genotyping is yet to be established[330,331,332].

Viral replication

Little is known about the attachment, entry and uncoating of HCV. Some recent evidence supports a model of HCV replication analogous to the known *in vitro* systems used to study flaviviruses and pestiviruses[7,329, 333,334].

HCV viral RNA replication most likely occurs in the smooth ER membranes which proliferate as replication continues[317,335]. Following the early synthesis of replicative proteins from the infecting genomic (+) RNA, a complex of these early products, including NS-3, NS-4 and NS-5 components, is likely to mediate the production of RNA replicative intermediates[7,329,334]. In flavivirus models, genomic length (GL) RNA is converted first to a double-stranded replicative form (RF). Through a partially single-stranded replicative intermediate (RI) there is preferential synthesis of new positive-sense genomic RNA from the RF dimer[333]. Dimeric hairpin-like HCV RNAs have been generated *in vitro*. This supports the concept that HCV polymerization is primed from a GL template. However, the identity of dimeric HCV RNA needs further definition[329].

It is presumed that unwinding of the dimeric RF by HCV NS-3 helicase would allow the synthesis of new plus-sense RNA from the negative strand[7]. *In vitro* polymerase assays have also demonstrated that a single-stranded RI-like molecule appears to be present during HCV RNA synthesis[334]. Much of this work requires confirmation.

The packaging signal for HCV has not been identified. Envelope proteins of HCV are highly glycosylated and possess hypervariable regions thought to contribute to immunological escape[7,336].

Pathogenesis

The mechanism of hepatocellular damage triggered by HCV is poorly understood. Direct hepatocyte damage due to viral components and cell-mediated immune responses may both play a role. Few chronically infected people clear the virus and HCV persists despite the host response[7,337].

Infectious HCV virions are produced at a low rate and the genome cannot be detected in the serum without the use of nucleic acid tests[338]. Native HCV antigens have not been detected at the hepatocyte surface and so attenuation of both replication and antigen production may contribute to the host's inability to clear the virus[337,338,339].

Production of RNA intermediates during viral replication can be cytotoxic. Double-stranded viral RNA triggers host cell defences including RNase L, which degrades RNA, and a protein kinase which stops the initiation of RNA translation. Interferon switches on the pathways that induce these two enzymes and could exert its major antiviral effect on HCV in this way[7].

HCV exists as a quasispecies, a population composed of a dominant master sequence and many variants exhibiting <1–2% sequence diversity from the master strain[338]. Because neutralizing antibodies are strain-specific, the quasispecies nature of the virus allows new strains to emerge when antibodies capable of clearing the dominant strain are produced[337, 340]. Envelope gene sequences code for hypervariable regions and glycosylation sites on the E1 and E2 proteins, increasing the frequency with which escape mutants can be produced[7,336]. Antibody-mediated pathways are unlikely to be responsible for either hepatocyte damage or the clearance of HCV[337].

The quasispecies nature of HCV can also explain the existence of CTL escape mutants of HCV observed in chimpanzees[341]. Some evidence shows that HCV-specific CTLs are confined mainly to the liver and the number of HCV-specific CTLs circulating in the blood is quite low[342,343]. Short-term immunosuppression has a beneficial effect on liver cell injury and in addition, some patients with demonstrable HCV-specific CTL activity have higher serum ALT levels and more active histological disease[7,344]. Increased numbers of inflammatory cells, including CD8+ mononuclear cells, have been found in periportal tissue, especially that affected by piecemeal necrosis[345]. CD4+ lymphocyte responses to HCV core and NS4 proteins have been found in some patients, but their pathogenic significance is unknown[346].

Finally, HCV is both hepatotropic and lymphotropic. Lymphocytes may act as a persistent extrahepatic reservoir for HCV[337,347].

Laboratory diagnosis

With currently available second- and third-generation screening assays, seroconversion to HCV generally occurs 6–8 weeks after primary infection (sensitivity of >99.7% for genotype 1 strains)[348]. More than half of all patients develop persistent disease and in both viraemic and convalescent patients the screening tests remain positive. In countries where genotype 1 is the predominant strain, less than 1% of screening tests performed using second-generation and third-generation assays are false positives[7,348].

The diagnosis of hepatitis C is complicated by the fact that viral antigens cannot be detected in the blood using existing technology, and serodiagnosis alone does not distinguish acute infection from chronic infection and convalescence. Until recently, PCR was the only available nucleic acid assay that could readily detect HCV viraemia[349]. A bDNA assay is now available and quantitative tests using either format have been marketed[350,351].

Typically, HCV RNA can be present in the blood as early as 14 days after acute infection[352]. Anti-HCV antibodies usually appear after the first rise in hepatic transaminases (Figure 10.10). Antibody to the C100–3 recombinant peptide, corresponding to part of the NS-4 viral protein, appears 8–12 weeks after acute infection but does occasionally rise even later. More recently developed assays contain recombinant core protein fragments and additional non-structural viral antigens[7,348].

Anti-HCV core IgG can be detected as early as six weeks after infection. However, there are no commercial assays available for HCV-specific IgM because it is difficult to detect reliably. In the research setting, the IgM can persist in patients with chronic HCV and most often disappears in those with self-limited disease or persons on interferon therapy[348,353].

In 50–80% of HCV-infected adults the viraemia persists for more than six months and is consistent with chronic infection. The genome can usually be detected by PCR whether the transaminases are normal or raised. Typically, aminotransferase levels fluctuate for several years during chronic infection, returning to normal in at least half of all cases[8]. The disappearance of HCV RNA is generally associated with biochemical and histological improvement in the patient[354].

The anti-HCV antibody detected in neonates is often due to passive transfer of maternal IgG. When the child is not infected

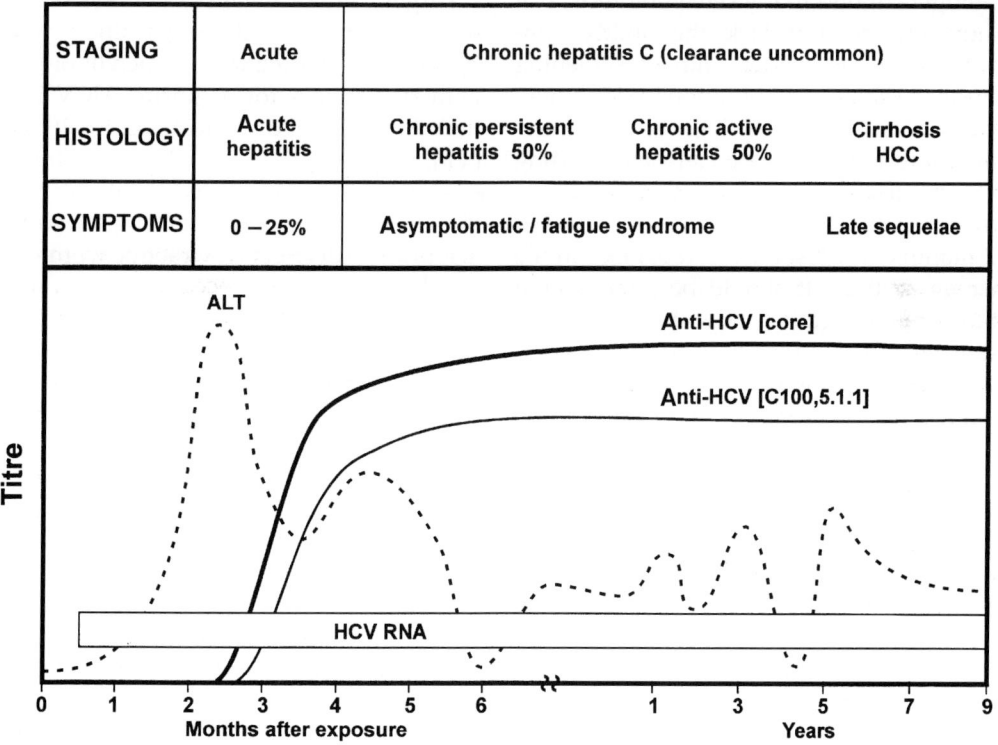

Figure 10.10 Clinical, histological and serological events of acute HCV followed by chronic infection. The timing of seroconversion varies with the type and specificity of the antigens used in tests for anti-HCV antibodies. The viraemia is not always continuous and may be intermittent.

this should begin to decline after six months of age[310]. In the first year of life the diagnosis of HCV will usually rely on biochemical evidence of hepatitis and the detection of HCV RNA. The rate of acute infection and the fraction of neonates who develop persistent disease after perinatal exposure to HCV need further definition.

One notable problem with HCV diagnosis has been the lack of confirmatory serological tests. In some laboratories a positive screening test for HCV is followed by a repeat test using an HCV assay containing a different set of antigens (or the same antigens produced using a different recombinant vector). If both tests are positive the result is said to be confirmed but if the second test is negative the result is reported as indeterminant.

Recombinant immunoblot assays (RIBA) and related tests, which separate the respective antigens found in the screening tests, can predict viraemia but lack the ability consistently to resolve indeterminant screening assays, especially in populations with a low prevalence of HCV[348,355]. Where indeterminant results cannot be clarified by using additional tests such as PCR, a series of follow-up serological assays over a period of 6–12 months may resolve discrepancies in the screening method. It should be remembered that a single negative PCR test does not exclude infection with HCV nor do persistently indeterminant serological results confirm infection.

Prevention

At present there are few effective countermeasures proven to prevent mother-to-infant transmission of hepatitis C. One small study has shown a reduction in vertical transmission from 32% to 6% among the newborns delivered by caesarean section to women infected with HCV and HIV[25]. Small-scale trials of ISG have shown that it does not appear to offer any significant protection against the neonatal acquisition of HCV.

Indeed, patients who are already seropositive for HCV can be reinfected with new strains of the virus. Unfortunately, the short-term prospects for an active vaccine are also limited[356].

Assuming that immunoprophylaxis or even drug therapy to reduce HCV viraemia and transmission can be developed, a number of issues will have to be addressed before a cost-effective prophylactic strategy can be designed. HCV is prevalent in 0.5–2.5% of adults in western countries but in some high-risk groups such as blood product recipients and IV drug users, up to 80% are seropositive[295,296]. Despite this, transmission to the neonate remains unusual except in mothers with HCV viraemia that exceeds 1×10^6/ml[304]. This also includes a group of women who are both HIV positive and HCV positive[25].

Larger, more detailed surveys of HCV seroprevalence will determine whether screening of all pregnant women or only those with risk factors for acquiring HCV is justified. As the level of viraemia ($\geq 1 \times 10^6$ copies per ml) appears to predict the risk of transmission, it will be necessary to investigate the therapeutic value of quantifying the viral load just prior to delivery in viraemic women[304]. In addition, if vaginal delivery is a consistent risk factor for the transmission of HCV from viraemic women, it will be important to determine if caesarean section will reduce the transmission rate sufficiently to eliminate the adverse long-term outcomes of HCV infection and whether operative intervention is justified. At present caesarean section to prevent HCV transmission is not recommended.

Among prospective mothers who have both HCV and HIV infections it would be useful to know if the reduction in HIV viral load achieved with zidovudine (or multidrug therapy) will not only reduce the risk of HIV transmission but also indirectly alter the concentration of HCV in the maternal blood and thereby reduce the risk of HCV transmission.

Treatment

Acute hepatitis C infection in pregnancy is a rare event. Although there are case reports of seroconversion to anti-HCV antibody during pregnancy, the rate of serious acute disease in the mother and subsequent transmission to the newborn is unknown[357]. Active treatment is necessary only in cases of fulminating hepatitis.

α-Interferon 2a is the most successful treatment for chronic hepatitis C and remains so after the first trial in patients with non A-non B hepatitis in 1986[358]. Several large trials have now been published and it is apparent that biochemical remission occurs in 50–75% of adult patients undergoing therapy for chronic active hepatitis, but ultimately biochemical improvement, loss of HCV viraemia and histological remission are achieved in only 15–30% of patients once interferon is ceased[7,250]. The majority of studies were initially carried out in patients with both biochemical and histological evidence of active hepatitis C. A significant fraction of patients with ALT levels that are normal or less than twice the normal range also have histological evidence of ongoing hepatic inflammation. One study has shown that treatment of such patients with IFN-α 2b can produce a 65% overall response rate with remission in 24 out of 37 patients, when viraemia was detected by PCR[359]. In general the factors that predict a permanent response to interferons in adults infected with HCV are the mode of acquisition, the severity of liver disease, the viral load and the genotype of HCV. Injecting drug users, those with chronic active hepatitis, a low viral load and those infected with genotypes other than type 1 are more likely to respond[360–362].

Small trials of interferons in children using lymphoblastoid IFN, recombinant IFN-α 2a and IFN-β have been encouraging[363,364]. An uncontrolled trial in 12 Spanish children showed reduction in ALT in 91% (11 of 12) children at 15 months and 45% at 24 months using low-dose IFN-α therapy[364]. More recent Italian and Japanese studies have shown 43% (six of 14 children) and 56% (10 of 18 children) biochemical remission rates associated with the loss of serum HCV RNA after 12 months of recombinant IFN-α in the first study and six months of lymphoblastoid IFN in the second[365,366]. Both studies followed patients for at least two years after ceasing therapy but only the second showed that low pretreatment HCV titre ($<10^7$ copies HCV/ml) was a predictor of therapeutic response. In both studies the majority of children had acquired HCV by parenteral routes. HCV acquired perinatally may be less likely to respond to interferons. These medications are relatively well tolerated in children but larger studies will be necessary to confirm the benefits of IFN-α therapy. Ribavirin and ribavirin-interferon combination trials are currently under way[367]. In the future, drugs which inhibit the NS-3/NS-4a proteinase complex may be one of the alternative strategies to reach the stage of clinical trial[368].

Orthotopic liver transplantation (OLT) for chronic HCV is successful in adults. Graft reinfection does occur but it does not usually lead to major graft dysfunction. HCV seropositive status is not therefore regarded as a contraindication to OLT for chronic hepatitis[7]. Between 60% and 68% of children undergoing OLT for fulminating hepatic failure survive, but outcome is worse in children under two years and the role of HCV in this group has not been defined[66,369,370]. Chronic HCV in children is most often an asymptomatic or relatively mild illness and early transplantation is usually unnecessary[60].

Co-infection of HCV with HBV is well known in adults but publications on the subject are few. In a Japanese study of 82 HBV-infected patients, 18 were co-infected with HCV and nine of these were HCV RNA positive by PCR. Fifteen of the 18 co-infected patients were seronegative for HBeAg and the replication of HBV in this group was reduced.

It was concluded that HCV was primarily responsible for the active hepatitis in the co-infected group[371]. However, HBV can coexist with hepatitis C[372]. Few if any studies on the therapy of this condition have been published and its significance in children is unknown[373].

HEPATITIS G

Epidemiology

Currently there is only limited information about the epidemiology, pathogenesis and outcome of HGV infection. Debate exists about whether it is a true hepatotropic agent and, indeed, its capacity to produce both acute and chronic clinical liver disease is yet to be defined.

The virus is able to establish chronic infection in humans but it appears that between 50% and 75% of infected persons eliminate HGV and develop a subsequent antibody response[374,375]. The prevalence of anti-HGV antibody-positive individuals is believed to be 2–3 times the prevalence of HGV RNA-positive individuals and the two groups are almost mutually exclusive[376,377]. However, specific serological assays for anti-HGV antibody have proved difficult to construct so that most of the information about the prevalence and transmission of HGV is based on virus detection using PCR.

The established data show that the virus is endemic worldwide. Parenteral transmission is common with a prevalence of 20–50% in IDUs, people with haemophilia and those receiving multiple transfusions. Approximately 20% of anti-HCV-positive individuals in Australia are HGV RNA positive and in industrialized countries between 1.5% and 4.2% of unpaid, highly screened blood donors are HGV RNA positive[18,147].

One west African population has an HGV carriage rate of 15%, with an overall prevalence ranging from 8% to 20% across all ages but no difference in prevalence between the sexes. Individuals in this population remained persistently HGV RNA positive, suggesting acquisition at an early age and a high chronic carriage rate analogous to that for HBV. This may reflect either a perinatal or early horizontal transmission pattern in resource-deprived countries[375,378].

Hepatitis G in pregnancy

Two case reports of mother-to-infant transmission have been made. Feucht *et al.* reported that three out of nine babies born to mothers who were HGV positive by PCR subsequently developed HGV infection. In these cases two of the mothers were co-infected with HIV and another with HCV[379]. A second report of HGV infection in a newborn demonstrated viraemia in a pregnant health-care worker and later in the newborn at four and six weeks post partum, after an initial cord blood specimen was negative for HGV sequences[378].

Molecular virology and pathogenesis

Hepatitis G is a member of the Flaviviridae with a genomic organization similar to HCV (Figure 10.11). The original cDNA clone of HGV identified a plus-strand RNA virus of 9392 nucleotides with a single ORF encoding a polyprotein of 2873 amino acids[18]. The physical properties of the virus are yet to be described but full-length clones have revealed 5' and 3' UTRs, core and envelope domains and putative non structural genes for a metalloproteinase, a serine proteinase, a helicase and a RNA-dependent RNA polymerase[380,381]. The replication strategy of HGV is likely to parallel that of other Flaviviridae but the pathogenesis of this infection is unclear[382].

Laboratory diagnosis

At present, there are no reliable serological assays for the diagnosis of HGV. In western countries the condition is usually considered when a patient presents with clinical or

HGV Open Reading Frame

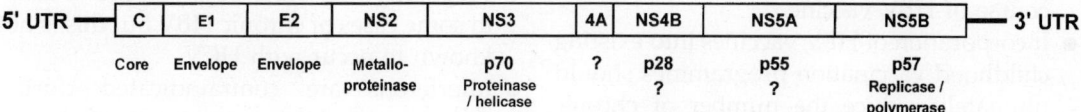

Figure 10.11 Physical and genetic map of the HGV open reading frame. The size and putative function(s) of the respective protein translation products are indicated.

biochemical evidence of hepatitis and tests for the other major causes of viral hepatitis are negative. In patients such as IDUs co-infection with HCV is common so that HGV infection should also be considered in people with active HCV disease[18]. Currently the only available test for HGV is a PCR assay. Research laboratories now have access to up to six different PCR primers and probes[378]. These are used to target either the 5′ UTR or genes for the putative NS3 or NS5 non-structural regions of the genome. The natural history of HGV infection and a complete diagnostic algorithm are yet to be established. Quantitative PCR or bDNA assays should soon become available in order to permit the assessment of viral load and its relevance to the risk of transmission.

Prevention and treatment

There have been some preliminary studies on the treatment of hepatitis G. It would appear logical to establish the role of inter-ferons in the treatment of patients who have HCV and HGV co-infections[380]. It is yet to be established whether there are sufficient adverse outcomes of HGV infection alone to justify specific drug therapy. At present, there are no data on treatment with other antiviral drugs.

Prevention of mother-to-infant transmission would need to follow the principles that apply to the management of women infected with HCV or both HIV and HCV. However, there are currently no data to support active inter-vention to prevent HGV transmission.

SUMMARY OF PRACTICAL MANAGEMENT ISSUES

MANAGEMENT OF VIRAL HEPATITIS IN PREGNANT WOMEN

Prevention and pregnancy

Screening

- All prospective mothers should be screened for HBsAg (and/or anti-HBc). The prevention of HBV in the neonates of carrier mothers will be a major part of any strategy to eradicate chronic HBV in children.
- The decision to screen for anti-HCV in pregnant women should be based on local epidemiological data and patient history. It may not be cost-effective to screen some low prevalence groups. Women with a history of recreational or frequent IDU, STD, blood product exposure and organ transplantation should be screened for anti-HCV. (Up to 50% of transplant recipients with HCV viraemia do not have antibodies to the virus.)

Vaccination

- Immune serum globulin (ISG) is indicated for pregnant women at risk of HAV after household or localized outbreaks. (ISG is not indicated for the prevention of HCV or HEV.)
- Pregnant women travelling to areas of high HAV endemicity from areas of low endemicity should be offered killed HAV vaccine.

- Non-immune pregnant women exposed to HBV should receive HBIG and the full course of HBV vaccine.
- Incorporation of HBV vaccines into existing childhood vaccination programmes should ultimately reduce the number of chronic carrier mothers who will in turn pose a risk to their own children.

Acute viral hepatitis

- Suspected viral hepatitis in pregnant women should always be confirmed by laboratory diagnosis.
- With regular review the majority of pregnant women who have acute viral hepatitis can be managed as ambulant patients. Symptomatic relief, avoidance of alcohol and maintenance of adequate nutrition and hydration are necessary but not always sufficient for the patient to cope outside hospital.
- Progressive jaundice, change in liver span (especially shrinkage), increasing transaminase levels and prothrombin times are evidence of decompensation. When hospital management is necessary, a hepatologist should be consulted.
- Acute HBV in late pregnancy increases the risk of mother-to-infant transmission compared with that due to chronic maternal infection.

Fulminating disease

- Fulminating hepatitis is a significant cause of maternal mortality in late pregnancy during outbreaks of HEV in developing countries.
- Hepatitis A and hepatitis B are rare but significant causes of fulminating hepatitis in adults worldwide.
- Acyclovir has been used successfully in known cases of severe HSV hepatitis in pregnancy.
- The role of therapeutic abortion and orthotopic liver transplantation in the pregnant woman has not been defined.

Chronic hepatitis in pregnancy

- Pregnancy may occasionally trigger a 'flare' in some cases of chronic HBV but this is not known to occur with HCV.
- Interferons are contraindicated during pregnancy and active treatment of chronic hepatitis is not required unless rapidly progressive disease occurs.
- The major risk of HBV and HCV transmission occurs at the time of delivery. This risk is increased (in part) by high viral loads especially in patients co-infected with HIV.
- Use of caesarean section to prevent transmission of HBV or HCV is not justified based on current data.

MANAGEMENT OF VIRAL HEPATITIS IN THE NEWBORN

Prevention of neonatal hepatitis

Screening

- Donor blood for premature and term newborn transfusions should come from donors screened for HBsAg as well as CMV, HCV and HIV antibodies. Anti-HAV-positive blood products should be used where possible.

Vaccination

- All children born to HBsAg carriers and women with acute HBV in the third trimester of pregnancy (including HIV carriers) should commence HBIG and HBV vaccine prophylaxis within 48 h of birth. HBV vaccine should not be delayed more than seven days.
- All children born to HBV screen-negative women should receive HBV vaccine according to the local standard vaccination schedule.
- Children born to households where HAV cases have been identified should receive

ISG prophylaxis as per the standard schedule.

- There is no indication for ISG prophylaxis in cases of maternal HCV or HEV.

Prophylaxis

- Where possible, mothers with acute HAV and HEV should not prepare food until they recover and should be counselled about the prevention of faecal–oral transmission by appropriate handwashing.
- Breastfeeding is not contraindicated in children vaccinated for HBV who are born to HBV carriers (or HCV carriers), unless the mother is co-infected with HIV.

Acute neonatal hepatitis

- All newborns with clinical or biochemical evidence of hepatitis or obstructive jaundice should have viral hepatitis excluded by laboratory tests. HEV causes significant mortality in newborns in endemic areas.
- In neonates, laboratory diagnosis of hepatitis should include culture for herpesviruses, adenoviruses and enteroviruses, serology for IgM to herpes viruses and nucleic acid assays where available. Hepatitis B is the most common hepatotropic agent causing infection in newborns.
- Most newborns require no hospital care unless clinical and biochemical evidence of progressive disease ensues.

Fulminating neonatal hepatitis

- A viral diagnosis should be attempted in all cases of fulminating neonatal hepatitis.
- An international normalized ratio (INR) ≥4 is indicative of poor prognosis.
- Orthotopic liver transplantation is indicated in children with severe progressive disease. However, children under two years of age have less successful outcomes than older children.

INFECTION CONTROL AND OCCUPATIONAL HEALTH

Screening

- All pregnant women should be screened for HBsAg (and/or anti-HBc). Women with a risk factor for HCV should be screened for anti-HCV.
- All patients with a risk factor for HIV or evidence of HBV or HCV infection should be asked to consent to HIV antibody screening (because of the risks associated with vertical transmission).
- All health-care workers, paramedical staff and carers of infants in day care and people in residential facilities should know their anti-HBs status. Anti-HBs-negative staff should know their HBsAg status.

Vaccination

- All health-care workers, paramedical staff and carers of infants in day care and residential facilities should be vaccinated against HBV. Seroconversion to vaccine should be verified by a test for anti-HBs. Revaccination policy will depend on consultation with a local authority until an international standard is developed.
- HBV vaccine non-responders should be offered HBIG and revaccination within 72 h of significant blood exposure.
- HAV vaccination should be considered for health-care providers working in communities with a high prevalence of HAV (e.g. indigenous populations in western countries).
- HAV and HBV vaccination with passive and active vaccines should be provided to exposed health-care workers not previously vaccinated against either agent.

FUTURE TRENDS IN OBSTETRIC VIROLOGY

A number of significant issues face practitioners of antenatal and obstetric care in the near future. Firstly, successful control of HAV outbreaks has recently been demonstrated using killed HAV vaccine instead of ISG[383]. Vaccine could be an effective substitute for ISG in pregnant women exposed to HAV. More aggressive vaccination programmes aimed at eradicating HAV in the wider community are technically possible[384]. In addition, it may be useful to consider routine HAV vaccination of neonatal intensive care staff working in high-prevalence areas, to assist in reducing the secondary cases of HAV after primary infection in a newborn.

Drugs which simultaneously reduce both HIV and HBV viraemia (e.g. lamivudine and adefovir dipivoxil) may prove useful in preventing the simultaneous transmission of both agents.

The potential for cervical shedding of agents such as HBV, HCV and HGV should be investigated. Newer, more sensitive molecular techniques could be used to assess both the risk of transmission and effects of intervention.

Wider study of the transmission of HCV and the risk of breastfeeding is a relatively high priority, as is the development of HCV-specific antiviral agents and a vaccine. In addition, the significance of HGV as a human pathogen needs further clarification. If maternal and mother-to-infant infection are significant, prevention strategies should be considered and developed.

Finally, in global terms two interventions have the greatest potential to reduce the burden of disease created by hepatotropic viruses. Coordinated vaccination programmes to prevent HBV in both the newborns of carrier mothers and other infants are the first priority. Recent evidence from Taiwan shows that the incidence of paediatric HCC has been significantly reduced by early vaccination against HBV[385]. In addition, further characterization of HEV pathogenesis in pregnant women and the newborn should help identify targets for both vaccine research and direct intervention in fulminating HEV.

REFERENCES

1. McMahon, B.J., Alward, W.L.M., Hall, D.B. *et al.* (1985) Acute hepatitis B infection: relation of age to the clinical expression of disease and subsequent development of the carrier state. *J. Infect. Dis.*, **151**, 599–603.
2. Margolis, H.S., Alter, M.J. and Hadler, S.C. (1991) Hepatitis B: evolving epidemiology and implications for control. *Semin. Liver Dis.*, **11**, 84–92.
3. Margolis, H.S., Coleman, P.J., Brown, R.E. *et al.* (1995) Prevention of hepatitis B virus transmission by immunization: an economic analysis of current recommendations. *JAMA*, **274**, 1201–1208.
4. Tsen, Y.J., Chang, M.H., Hsu, H.Y. *et al.* (1991) Seroprevalence of hepatitis B infection in children in Taipei, 1989: five years after a mass hepatitis B vaccination programme. *J. Med. Virol.*, **34**, 96–99.
5. Sherlock, S. (1993) Clinical features of hepatitis. In: *Viral Hepatitis: Scientific Basies and Clinical Management*, (eds A.J. Zuckerman and H.C. Thomas), Churchill Livingstone, Edinburgh, pp. 1–20.
6. Hsu, H.H., Feinstone, S.M. and Hoofnagle, J.H. (1995) Acute viral hepatitis. In: *Mandell, Douglas and Bennett's Principles and Practice of Infectious Diseases*, (eds G.L. Mandell, J.E. Bennett and R. Dolin), Churchill Livingstone, New York, pp. 1136–1153.
7. Locarnini, S.A. and Cunningham, A.L. (1995) Clinical treatment of viral hepatitis. In: *Antiviral Chemotherapy*, (eds D.J. Jeffries and E. De Clerq), John Wiley, Chichester, pp. 441–530.
8. Dinsmoor, M.J. (1997) Hepatitis in the obstetric patient. *Infect. Dis. Clin. North Am.*, **11**, 77–91.
9. Mishra, L. and Seef, L.B. (1993) Viral hepatitis A through E complicating pregnancy. *Gastroenterol. Clin. North Am.*, **21**(4) 873–887.
10. Klein, N.A., Mabie, W.C., Shaver, D.C. *et al.* (1991) Herpes simplex virus hepatitis in pregnancy: two patients successfully treated with acyclovir. *Gastroenterology*, **100**, 239–244.
11. Knox, T.A. and Olans, L.B. (1996) Liver disease in pregnancy. *N. Engl. J. Med.*, **335**(8), 569–576.
12. Krawczynski, K. (1993) Hepatitis E. *Hepatology*, **17**, 932–941.
13. Bernuau, J., Rueff, B. and Benhamou, J.P. (1986) Fulminant and subfulminant liver failure. *Semin. Liver Dis.*, **6**, 97–106.

14. O'Grady, J. (1992) Management of acute and fulminant hepatitis A. *Vaccine*, **10**(1), 521–523.

15. Conjeevaran, H.S. and di Bisceglie, A.M. (1993) Natural history (hepatitis D). In: *Viral Hepatitis: Scientific Basis and Clinical Management*, (eds A.J. Zuckerman and H.C. Thomas), Churchill Livingstone, Edinburgh, pp. 341–349.

16. Villamil, F.G., Ha, K.Q., Ya, C.H. *et al.* (1995) Detection of hepatitis C virus with RNA polymerase chain reaction in fulminant hepatic failure. *Hepatology*, **22**, 1379–1386.

17. Farci, P., Alter, H.J., Shimoda, A. *et al.* (1996) Hepatitis C virus-associated fulminant hepatic failure. *N. Engl. J. Med.*, **335**(9), 631–634.

18. Linnen, J., Wages, J., Zhen-Yong, Z.K. *et al.* (1996) Molecular cloning and disease association of hepatitis G virus: a transfusion-transmissible agent. *Science*, **271**, 505–508.

19. Heringlake, S., Ostercamp, S., Trautwein, C. *et al.* (1996) Association between fulminant hepatic failure and a strain of GBV virus C. *Lancet*, **348**, 1626–1629.

20. Khuroo, M.S., Teli, M.R., Skidmore, S. *et al.* (1981) Incidence and severity of viral hepatitis in pregnancy. *Am. J. Med.*, **70**, 252–255.

21. Hamid, S., Wasim Jafri, S., Khan, H. *et al.* (1996) Fulminant hepatic failure in pregnant women: acute fatty liver or acute viral hepatitis? *J. Hepatol.*, **25**, 20–27.

22. Zuckerman, J.N., Sabin, C. Craig, F.M. *et al.* (1997) Immune response to a new hepatitis B vaccine in healthcare workers who had not responded to standard vaccine: randomized double blind dose response study. *Br. Med. J.*, **314**, 329–333.

23. Gust, I.D. (1992) Control of hepatitis B in Australia: the case for alternative strategies. *Med. J. Aust.*, **156**, 819–821.

24. Di Bisceglie, A.M., Goodman, D., Ishak, K.G. *et al.* (1991) Long-term clinical and histopathological follow up of chronic post-transfusion hepatitis. *Hepatology*, **14**, 969–974.

25. Paccagnini, S., Principi, N., Massironi, E. *et al.* (1995) Perinatal transmission and manifestation of hepatitis C virus infection in a high risk population. *Paediatr. Infect. Dis. J.*, **14**, 195–199.

26. Zanetti, A.R., Tanzi, E., Paccagnini, S. *et al.* (1995) Mother to infant transmission of hepatitis C virus. *Lancet*, **345**, 289–291.

27. Brown, J.L., Carman, W.F. and Thomas, H.C. (1992) The clinical significance of molecular variation within the hepatitis B genome. *Hepatology*, **15**, 144.

28. Beath, S.V., Boxall, E.H., Watson, R.M. *et al.* (1992) Fulminant hepatitis B in infants born to anti-HBe hepatitis B carrier mothers. *Br. Med. J.*, **304**, 1169–1170.

29. Weizsacher, F., Pult, I., Geiss, K., Wirth, S. and Blum, H.E. (1995) Selective transmission of variant genomes from mother to infant in neonatal hepatitis B. *Hepatology*, **21**, 8–13.

30. Cooper, E.R., Nugent, R.P., Diaz, C. *et al.* (1996) After AIDS Clinical Trial 076: the changing pattern of zidovudine use during pregnancy, and the subsequent reduction in the vertical transmission of human immunodeficiency virus in a cohort of infected women and their infants. *J. Infect. Dis.*, **174**, 1207–1211.

31. Mayaux, M.J., Dussaix, E., Isopet, J. *et al.* (1997) Maternal virus load during pregnancy and mother to child transmission of human immunodeficiency virus type 1: the French perinatal cohort studies. *J. Infect. Dis.*, **175**, 172–175.

32. Floreani, A., Paternoster, D., Zappala, F. *et al.* (1996) Hepatitis C infection in pregnancy. *Br. J. Obstet. Gynaecol.*, **103**, 325–329.

33. Dr Peter Angus, personal communication.

34. Alpert, E., Isselbacher, K.J. and Schur, P.H. (1971) The pathogenesis of arthritis associated with viral hepatitis. *N. Engl. J. Med.*, **285**, 185.

35. Lisker-Melman, M., Webb, D., di Bisceglie, A.M. *et al.* (1989) Glomerulonephritis caused by chronic hepatitis B infection: treatment with recombinant human alpha interferon. *Ann. Intern. Med.*, **111**, 479–483.

36. Levo, Y., Gorevic, P.D., Kassah, H.J. *et al.* (1977) Association between hepatitis B and essential mixed cryoglobulinaemia. *N. Engl. J. Med.*, **296**, 1501–1504.

37. Wong, V.S., Egner, W., Brown, D. and Alexander, G.J. (1996) Incidence character and clinical relevance of mixed cryoglobulinaemia in patients with chronic hepatitis C virus infection. *Clin. Exper. Immunol.*, **104**(1), 25–31.

38. Fargion, S., Piperno, A., Cappellini, M.D. *et al.* (1992) Hepatitis C and porphyria cutanea tarda: evidence of a strong association. *Hepatology*, **16**(6), 1322–1326.

39. Cribier, B., Petrau, P., Keller, F. *et al.* (1995) Porphyria cutanea tarda and hepatitis C viral

infection: a clinical and virological study. *Arch. Dermatol.*, **131**(7), 801–804.

40. Szmuness, W. (1978) Hepatocellular carcinoma and the hepatitis B virus: evidence for a causal association. *Prog. Med. Virol.*, **24**, 40.

41. Beasley, R.P., Lin, C.C., Huang, L.Y. *et al.* (1981) Hepatocellular carcinoma and hepatitis B virus. A prospective study of 22,707 men in Taiwan. *Lancet*, **2**, 1129–1133.

42. Saito, I., Miyamura, T., Ohibayashki, A. *et al.* (1991) Hepatitis C infection is associated with the development of hepatocellular carcinoma. *Proc. Natl Acad. Sci. USA*, **87**, 6547–6549.

43. Shimotohuo, K. (1993) Hepatocellular carcinoma in Japan and its linkage to infection with hepatitis C virus. *Semin. Virol.*, **4**, 305–312.

44. Beasley, R.P. (1988) Hepatitis B virus – the major etiology of hepatocellular carcinoma. *Cancer*, **61**, 1942–1956.

45. Popper, H., Sharifritz, D.A. and Hoofnagle, J.H. (1987) Relation of hepatitis B carrier state to hepatocellular carcinoma. *Hepatology*, **7**, 764–772.

46. Ozoh, J.O., Onuigbo, M.A., Umeral, B.C. and Mgbor, S.P. (1992) Hepatoma in pregnancy. *Trop. Geogr. Med.*, **44**, 72–74.

47. Lau, W.Y., Leung, W.T., Ho, S. *et al.* (1995) Hepatocellular carcinoma during pregnancy. *Cancer*, **75**(11), 2669–2676.

48. Jeng, L.B., Lee, W.C., Wang, C.C. *et al.* (1995) Hepatocellular carcinoma in a pregnant woman detected by routine screening of maternal alpha-fetoprotein. *Am. J. Obstet. Gynecol.*, **172**, 219–220.

49. To, W.K. and Ghosl, A. (1993) Primary liver carcinoma complicating pregnancy. *Aust. NZ J. Obstet. Gynaecol.*, **33**, 325–326.

50. Wang, L.R., Jeng, C.J. and Chu, J.S. (1993) Pregnancy associated with primary hepatocellular carcinoma. *Obstet. Gynaecol.*, **81**, 811–813.

51. Goldberg, I., Hod, M., Katz, I. *et al.* (1991) A case of hepatocellular carcinoma in pregnancy detected by routine screening of maternal alpha-fetoprotein. *Acta Obstet. Gynecolog. Scand.*, **70**, 241–242.

52. Stevens, C.E., Neurath, R.E., Beasley, R.S. and Szmuness, W. (1979) HBeAg and anti-HBc detection by radioimmunoassay: correlation of vertical transmission in Taiwan. *J. Med. Virol.*, **3**, 237–241.

53. Sherlock, S. and Dooley, J. (1993) *Diseases of the Liver and Biliary System. Blackwell Scientific*, London, pp. 434–451.

54. Hadler, S.C., Webster, H.M., Erben, J.J. *et al.* (1980) Hepatitis A in day care centres: a community wide assessment. *N. Engl. J. Med.*, **302**, 1222–1227.

55. Chow, C.B., Lau, T.T.Y., Leung, N.K. and Chang, W.K. (1989) Acute viral hepatitis aetiology and evolution. *Arch. Dis. Child.*, **64**, 211–213.

56. Gregiorio, G.V., Miele-Vergani, G. and Mowat, A.P. (1993) Neonatal and paediatric infection. In: *Viral Hepatitis: Scientific Basis and Clinical Management*, (eds A.J. Zuckerman and H. Thomas), Churchill Livingstone, Edinburgh, pp. 541–563.

57. Bradley, D.W. (1990) Enterically transmitted non-A non-B hepatitis. *Br. Med. Bull.*, **46**, 442–461.

58. Khuroo, M.S., Kamili, S. and Jameel, S. (1995) Vertical transmission of hepatitis E. *Lancet*, **345**, 1025–1026.

59. Bensabath, G., Hadler, SC., Soares, M.C. *et al.* (1987) Hepatitis delta virus infection and Labraea hepatitis. Prevalence and role in fulminant hepatitis in the Amazon basin. *JAMA*, **258**, 479–483.

60. Bortolotti, F., Jara, P., Diaz, C. *et al.* (1994) Postransfusion and community acquired hepatitis C in childhood. *J. Paediatr. Gastroenterol. Nutrition*, **18**, 279–283.

61. Chang, M.H., Lee, C.Y., Chen, D.S. *et al.* (1987) Fulminant hepatitis in children in Taiwan: the important role of hepatitis B virus. *J. Paediatrics*, **111**, 34–39.

62. Fawaz, K.A., Gray, G.F., Kaplan, M.M. *et al.* (1975) Repetitive maternal-fetal transmission of hepatitis B. *N. Engl. J. Med.*, **293**, 1357–1359.

63. Omata, M., Ehata, T., Yokosuka, O. *et al.* (1991) Mutations in the pre-core region of hepatitis B DNA in patients with fulminant and severe hepatitis. *N. Engl. J. Med.*, **324**, 1699–1704.

64. Porter, C.A., Mowat, A.P., Cook, P.J.L. *et al.* (1972) Alpha-1 antitrypsin deficiency and neonatal hepatitis. *Br. Med. J.*, **3**, 435.

65. Farci, T., Barbera, C., Lavone, C. *et al.* (1985) Infection with delta agent in children. *Gut*, **26**, 4–7.

66. Bhaduri, B.R. and Meli-Vergani, G. (1996) Fulminant hepatic failure: paediatric aspects. *Semin. Liver Dis.*, **16**, 349–355.

67. Maggiore, G. (1995) Chronic hepatitis in children. *Curr. Opin. Paediatr.*, **7**, 539–546.

68. Hsu, H.C., Lin, Y.H., Chang, M.H. *et al.* (1988) Pathology of chronic hepatitis B infection in children with special reference to the intrahepatic expression of hepatitis virus antigens. *Hepatology*, **8**, 378–382.

69. Bortolotti, F., Calazia, R., Cadrobbi, P. *et al.* (1986) Liver cirrhosis associated with chronic hepatitis B infection in childhood. *J. Paediatrics*, **198**, 224–227.

70. Lok, A.S.F. and Lai, C.L. (1988) A longitudinal follow up of asymptomatic hepatitis B surface antigen positive Chinese children. *Hepatology*, **8**, 1130–1133.

71. Lai, M.E., de Virgilis, S., Argioulu, F. *et al.* (1993) Evaluation of antibodies to hepatitis C virus on a long term prospective study of post-transfusion hepatitis among thalassaemic children: comparison between first and second generation assay. *J. Paediatr. Gastroenterol. Nutrition*, **16**, 458–464.

72. Matmoka, S., Tatara, K., Hayabuchi, Y. *et al.* (1994) Serologic, virologic and histologic characteristics of chronic phase hepatitis C virus in children infected by transfusion. *Paediatrics*, **94**, 919–922.

73. Chiriaco, P., Guadalupi, C., Armigliato, M. *et al.* (1986) Polyphasic course of hepatitis A in children. *J. Infect. Dis.*, **153**, 378–379.

74. Bortolotti, F., Crivellareo, C., Brunetto, M.R. *et al.* (1993) Selection of a pre-core mutant of hepatitis B virus and reactivation of chronic hepatitis B acquired in childhood. *J. Paediatrics*, **123**, 583–585.

75. Capp, R.B., Bennett, A.M., Mills, E.H. *et al.* (1955) Infectious hepatitis in infants and small children. The clinical and laboratory picture with special reference to the non-icteric form. *Am. J. Dis. Child.*, **89**, 701.

76. Schmacher, H.R. and Ball, E.P. (1974) Arthritis in acute and chronic hepatitis. *Am. J. Med.*, **57**, 655.

77. Draelos, Z.K., Hansen, R.C., James, W.D. *et al.* (1986) Gianotti–Crosti syndrome associated with infections other than hepatitis B. *JAMA*, **256**, 2386–2388.

78. Chang, M.H., Hsu, H.Y., Hsu, H.C. *et al.* (1995) The significance of spontaneous hepatitis B e antigen seroconversion in childhood: with special emphasis on the clearance of hepatitis B e antigen before 3 years of age. *Hepatology*, **22**, 1387–1392.

79. Esquivel, C.O., Gutierrez, C., Cox, K.L. *et al.* (1994) Hepatocellular carcinoma and liver cell dysplasia in children with chronic liver disease. *J. Paediatr. Surg.*, **29**, 1465–1469.

80. Mazzaferro, V., Regalia, E., Doci, R. *et al.* (1996) Liver transplantation for the treatment of small hepatocellular carcinomas in patients with cirrhosis. *N. Engl. J. Med.*, **334**, 728–729.

81. Krugman, S., Ward, R. and Giles, J.P. (1962) The natural history of infectious hepatitis. *Am. J. Med.*, **32**, 717–728.

82. Gust, I.D. (1992) Epidemiological pattern of hepatitis A in different parts of the world. *Vaccine*, **10**(1), 56–58.

83. Hadler, S.C., Webster, H.M., Erben, J.J. *et al.* (1982) Hepatitis A in day care centres: a community wide assessment. *N. Engl. J. Med.*, **302**, 12–22.

84. Lendar, W.M., Lemon, S.M., Kirkpatrick, J.W. *et al.* (1985) Frequency of illness associated with hepatitis A virus infection in adults. *Am. J. Epidemiol.*, **122**, 226–233.

85. Hadler, S.C. and McFarland, L. (1986) Hepatitis A in day care centers: epidemiology and prevention. *Rev. Infect. Dis.*, **8**, 548–557.

86. Centers for Disease Control (1992) Hepatitis A in homosexual men. *MMWR*, **41**, 155–164.

87. Koff, R.S. (1995) Seroepidemiology of hepatitis A in the United States. *J. Infect. Dis.*, **171**, (suppl 1), S19–23.

88. Azimi, P.H., Roberts, R.R., Guralnik, J. *et al.* (1986) Transfusion acquired hepatitis A in a premature infant with secondary spread in an intensive care nursery. *Am. J. Dis. Child.*, **140**, 23–27.

89. Nobel, R.C., Kane, M.A., Reeves, S.A. and Roechel, I. (1989) Post-transfusion hepatitis A in a neonatal intensive care unit. *JAMA*, **252**, 2711–2715.

90. Schwer, M. and Moosa, A. (1978) Effects of hepatitis A and B in pregnancy on the mother and fetus. *S. Afr. Med. J.*, **54**, 1092–1095.

91. Tong, M.J., Thursby, M., Rakela, J. *et al.* (1981) Studies on the maternal infant transmission of the viruses which cause acute hepatitis. *Gastroenterology*, **80**, 999–1004.

92. Zhang, R.L., Zeng, J.S. and Zhang, H.Z. (1990) Survey of 34 pregnant women with hepatitis A and their neonates. *Chinese Med. J.* (English), **103**, 552–555.

93. Watson, J.C., Hemming, D.W., Borella, A.J. *et al.* (1993) Vertical transmission of hepatitis A resulting in an outbreak in a neonatal intensive care unit. *J. Infect. Dis.*, **167**, 567–571.

94. Tanaka, I., Shima, M., Kubota, Y. *et al.* (1995) Vertical transmission of hepatitis A. *Lancet,* **345,** 397.

95. Rosenblum, L.S., Villarino, M.E., Nainam, O.V. *et al.* (1991) Hepatitis A outbreak in a neonatal intensive care unit: risk factors for transmission and evidence of prolonged viral excretion among preterm infants. *J. Infect. Dis.,* **164,** 476–482.

96. Coulepis, A.G., Locarnini, S.A., Westaway, E.G. *et al.* (1982) Biophysical and biochemical characterization of hepatitis A virus. *Intervirology,* **18,** 107–127.

97. Gust, I.D., Coulepis, A.G., Feinstone, S.M. *et al.* (1983) Taxonomic classification of hepatitis A virus. *Intervirology,* **20,** 1–7.

98. Lemon, S.M. (1992) Hepatitis A virus: current concepts of the molecular virology, immunobiology and approaches to vaccine development. *Rev. Med. Virol.,* **2,** 73–87.

99. Cohen, J.I., Ticehurst, J.R., Purcell, R.H. *et al.* (1987) Complete nucleotide sequence of wild-type hepatitis A virus: comparison with different strains of hepatitis A virus and other picornaviruses. *J. Virol.,* **61,** 50–59.

100. Stapleton, J.T., Frederick, J. and Meyer, B. (1991) Hepatitis A virus attachment to cultured cell lines. *J. Infect. Dis.,* **164,** 1098–1103.

101. Zajac, A.J., Amphlitt, E.M., Rowlands, D.J. and Sangar, D.V. (1991) Parameters influencing the attachment of hepatitis A to a variety of continuous cell lines. *J. General Virol.,* **72,** 1667–1675.

102. Karayiannis, P., Jowett, T., Enticott, M. *et al.* (1986) Hepatitis A virus replication in tamarins and host immune response in relation to pathogenesis of liver damage. *J. Med. Virol.,* **18,** 261–276.

103. Locarnini, S.A., Coulepis, A.G., Westaway, E.G. and Gust, I.D. (1981) Restricted replication of human hepatitis A virus in cell culture: an intracellular biochemical study. *J. Virol.,* **37,** 216–225.

104. Anderson, D.A., Ross, B.C. and Locarnini S.A. (1988) Restricted replication of hepatitis A virus in cell culture: encapsidation of viral RNA depletes the pool of RNA available for replication. *J. Virol.,* **62,** 4201–4206.

105. Anderson, D.A. and Ross, B.C. (1990) Morphogenesis of hepatitis A virus: isolation and characterization of subviral particles. *J. Virol.,* **64,** 5284–5289.

106. Kurane, I., Binn, L.N., Bancroft, W.H. and Ennis, F.A. (1985) Human lymphocyte responses to hepatitis A virus infected cells: interferon production and lysis of infected cells. *J. Immunol.,* **135,** 2140–2144.

107. Vallbracht, A., Maier, K., Stierhof, Y.D. *et al.* (1989) Liver derived cytotoxic T cells in hepatitis A infection. *J. Infect. Dis.,* **160,** 209–217.

108. Gabriel, P., Vallbracht, A. and Flehmig, B. (1986) Lack of complement dependent cytotoxic antibodies in hepatitis A infection. *J. Med. Virol.,* **20,** 23–31.

109. Slusarczyk, J., Hansson, B.G., Nordenfeldt, E. *et al.* (1984) Etiopathogenic aspects of hepatitis A II. Specific and non-specific humoral immune response during the course of infection. *J. Med. Virol.,* **14,** 269–276.

110. Davis, G.L., Hoofnagle, J.H. and Waggoner, J.F. (1984) Acute type A hepatitis during chronic hepatitis B infection: association of depressed hepatitis B virus replication with appearance of endogenous alpha interferon. *J. Med. Virol.,* **14,** 141–147.

111. Levin, S. and Hahn, T. 1982. Interferon system in acute viral hepatitis. *Lancet,* **1,** 592–594.

112. Zachoval, R., Abb, J., Zachoval, V. and Deinhardt, F. (1986) Circulating interferon in patients with acute hepatitis A. *J. Infect. Dis.,* **153,** 1174–1175.

113. Gust, I. and Feinstone, S.M. (1988) *Hepatitis A,* CRC Press, Boca Raton, pp. 153–54.

114. Humphrey, C.D., Cook, E.H. Jr. and Bradley, D.W. (1990) Identification of enterically transmitted hepatitis virus particles by solid phase immune electron microscopy. *J. Virolog. Methods,* **29,** 177–188.

115. Locarnini, S.A., Garland, S.M., Lehmann, N.I., Pringle, R.C. and Gust, I.D. (1978) Solid-phase enzyme immunoassay for detection of hepatitis A virus. *J. Clin. Microsc.,* **9,** 459–465.

116. Winokar, P.L. and Stapleton, J.T. (1992) Immunoglobulin prophylaxis for hepatitis A. *Clin. Infect. Dis.,* **14,** 580–586.

117. American College of Obstetricians and Gynecologists (1991) *Immunization during pregnancy. Technical Bulletin,* No. 160. ACOG.

118. Power, J.P., Lawlor, E., Davidson, F. *et al.* (1995) Molecular epidemiology of an outbreak of infection with hepatitis C in recipients of anti-D immunoglobulin. *Lancet,* **345,** 1211–1213.

119. Yap, P.L., McOmish, F., Webster, A.D.B. *et al.* (1994) Hepatitis C virus transmission by intravenous immunoglobulin. *J. Hepatol.,* **21,** 455–466.

120. Theilmann, L., Kallinowski, B., Ganelin, K. *et al.* (1992) Reactogenicity and immunogenicity of three different lots of hepatitis A vaccine. *Vaccine*, **10**, (suppl 1), 131–134.

121. Bradley, D.W., Krawcznski, K. and Purdy, M.A. (1993) Hepatitis E: epidemiology, natural history and experimental models. In: *Viral Hepatitis: Scientific Basis and Clinical Management*, (eds A.J. Zuckerman and H.C. Thomas), Churchill Livingstone, Edinburgh, pp. 379–383.

122. Purcell, R.H. (1996) Hepatitis E virus. In: *Fields' Virology*, (eds B.N. Fields, D.M. Knipe and P.M. Howley), Lippincott-Raven, Philadelphia, pp. 2831–2843.

123. Xu, Zhi-Yi., Li, Zi-Hua., Wang, Jian-Xieng. *et al.* (1992) Ecology and prevention of a shellfish-associated hepatitis A epidemic in Shanghai, China. *Vaccine*, **10**(suppl 1), 67–68.

124. Bile, K., Isse, O., Mohamud, P. *et al.* (1994) Contrasting roles of rivers and wells as sources of drinking water on attack and fatality rates in a hepatitis E epidemic in Somalia. *Am. J. Trop. Med. Hygiene*, **51**(4), 466–474.

125. Zhuang, H. (1992) *Hepatitis E and Strategies for Its Control. Monographs in Virology* **19**. Karger, Basel, pp. 126–139.

126. Tavera, C., Velasquez, O., Avila, C. *et al.* (1987) Enterically transmitted nonA-nonB hepatitis in Mexico. *MMWR*, **36**, 597.

127. Arankalle, V.A., Chanda, M., Tsarev, S. *et al.* (1994) Seroepidemiology of waterborne hepatitis in India and evidence for a third enterically transmitted hepatitis agent. *Proc. Natl Acad. Sci. USA*, **91**, 3428–3432.

128. Lee, S.D., Wang, Y.J., Lu, R.H. *et al.* (1994) Seroprevalence of antibody to hepatitis E virus among Chinese subjects in Taiwan. *Hepatology*, **19**, 866–870.

129. Moaven, L.M., van Asten, M., Crofts, N. and Locarnini, S. (1995) Seroepidemiology of hepatitis E in selected Australian populations. *J. Med. Virol.*, **45**, 326–330.

130. Skidmore, S. and Sherrat, L. (1996) Hepatitis E in the UK. *J. Viral Hepatitis*, **3**, 103–105.

131. Mast, E., Alter, M., Holland, P. and Purcell, R. (1996) Evaluation of assays for antibody to hepatitis E by a serum panel. *IIX Triennial International Symposium on Viral Hepatitis and Liver Disease*, Rome, Italy.

132. Wong, D.C., Purcell, R.H., Greenivasan, M.A. *et al.* (1980) Epidemic and endemic hepatitis in India: evidence for nonA-nonB hepatitis virus aetiology. *Lancet*, **2**, 876–878.

133. Arankalle, V.A., Tsarev, S., Chadha, M. *et al.* (1995) Age specific prevalence of antibodies to hepatitis A and E in Pune, India, 1982 and 1992. *J. Infect. Dis.*, **171**, 447–450.

134. Dawson, G. (1992) Advances in diagnosing hepatitis E virus infection. *Today's Life Sci.*, October, 38–43.

135. Burans, J., Sharp, T. and Wallace, M. (1994) Threat of hepatitis E infection in Somalia during Operation Restore Hope. *Clin. Infect. Dis.*, **18**, 100–102.

136. Clayson, E., Myint, R., Smitbhan, D. *et al.* (1995) Viraemia, faecal shedding and IgM and IgG responses in patients with hepatitis E. *J. Infect. Dis.*, **172**, 927–933.

137. Tsarev, S.A., Tsareva, T.S., Emerson, S.U. *et al.* (1995) Experimental hepatitis E in pregnant Rhesus monkeys: failure to transmit hepatitis E virus (HEV) to offspring and evidence of naturally acquired antibodies to HEV. *J. Infect. Dis.*, **172**, 31–37.

138. Bradley, D.W. (1992) Hepatitis E: epidemiology, aetiology and molecular biology. *Rev. Med. Virol.*, **2**, 19–28.

139. Purdy, M., Tam, A., Huang, P. *et al.* (1993) Hepatitis E virus: a non-enveloped member of the 'alpha-like' RNA superfamily? *Semin. Virol.*, **41**, 90–94.

140. Jameel, S., Zafrullah, M., Ozdener, M. and Panda, S. (1996) Expression in animal cells and characterization of the hepatitis E structural proteins. *J. Virol.*, **70**, 207–216.

141. Huang, R., Nakazono, K., Ishii, K. *et al.* (1995) Existing variations on the genome of hepatitis E virus strains from some regions of China. *J. Med. Virol.*, **47**, 303–308.

142. Yin, S., Tsarev, S., Purcell, R. and Emmerson, S. (1995) Partial sequence comparison of eight new Chinese strains of hepatitis E suggest the genome sequence is relatively stable. *J. Med. Virol.*, **41**, 230–241.

143. Brown, E.A., Ticehurst, J. and Lemon, S.M. (1994) Immunopathology of hepatitis A and hepatitis E infections. In: *Immunology of Liver Diseases*, (eds H.C. Thomas and J. Waters), Kluwer Academic Publishers, Dordrecht, pp. 11–37.

144. Lemon, S.M. (1995) Hepatitis E virus. In: *Mandell, Douglas and Bennett's Principles and Practice of Infectious Diseases*, (eds G.L. Mandell, J.E. Bennett and R. Dolin), Churchill Livingstone, New York, pp. 1663–1665.

145. Dawson, G.J., Chau, K.H., Cabal, P.O. *et al.* (1992) Solid-phase enzyme linked immunosorbant assay for hepatitis E virus IgG and IgM antibodies using recombinant antigens and synthetic peptides. *J. Virolog. Methods*, **38**, 175–186.

146. Favorov, M.O., Fields, H.A., Purdy, T.L. *et al.* (1992) Serological identification of hepatitis E virus infections in epidemic and endemic settings. *J. Med. Virol.*, **36**, 246–250.

147. Bryan, J.P., Tsarev, S.A., Igbal, M. *et al.* (1994) Epidemic hepatitis E in Pakistan: patterns of serological response and evidence that antibody against hepatitis E protects against disease. *J. Infect. Dis.*, **170**, 517–521.

148. Khuroo, M.S., Kamili, S., Dar, M.Y. *et al.* (1993) Hepatitis E and long term antibody status. *Lancet*, **341**, 1335.

149. Tsarev, S., Tsareva, S., Emerson, A. *et al.* (1993) ELISA for antibody to hepatitis E virus (HEV) based on complete open-reading frame-2 protein expressed in insect cells: identification of HEV infection in primates. *J. Infect. Dis.*, **168**, 364–378.

150. Chauhan, A., Jamcel, S., Dilawari, J.B. *et al.* (1993) Hepatitis E virus transmission to a volunteer. *Lancet*, **341**, 149–150.

151. Nanda, S.K., Ansari, T.H., Acharya, S.K. *et al.* (1995) Protracted viraemia during sporadic hepatitis E infection. *Gastroenterology*, **108**, 225–230.

152. Huang, R., Nakazono, K., Ishii, O. *et al.* (1995) Hepatitis E virus (87A strain) propagated in A549 cells. *J. Med. Virol.*, **47**, 299–302.

153. Tam, A., White, R., Reed, E. *et al.* (1996) *In vitro* propagation of hepatitis E virus from *in vivo* infected primary macaque cells. *Virology*, **215**, 1–9.

154. Tsega, E., Hanson, B., Krawczynski, K. and Nordenfeldt, E. (1992) Acute sporadic viral hepatitis in Ethiopia: causes, risk factors and effects on pregnancy. *J. Infect. Dis.*, **14**, 961–965.

155. Clayson, E., Innis, B., Myint, K. *et al.* (1995) Detection of hepatitis E infections among domestic swine in the Kathmandu Valley of Nepal. *Am. J. Trop. Med. Hygiene*, **53**, 228–232.

156. Tsarev, S., Tsareva, T., Emmerson, S. *et al.* (1994) Successful passive and active immunization of cynomolgus monkeys against hepatitis E. *Proc. Natl Acad. Sci. USA*, **91**, 10198–10202.

157. Hadziyannis, S. (1995) Hepatitis B e antigen negative chronic hepatitis B: from clinical recognition to pathogenesis and treatment. *Viral Hepatitis Rev.*, **1**, 7–36.

158. Lok, A.S.F. and Lai, C-L. (1990) Acute exacerbations in Chinese patients with chronic hepatitis B (HBV) infection. Incidence predisposing factors and etiology. *J. Hepatol.*, **10**, 29–34.

159. Bortolotti, F. (1994) Chronic hepatitis B in childhood: unanswered questions and evolving issues. *J. Hepatol.*, **21**, 904–909.

160. Derso, A., Boxall, E.H., Tarlow, M.J. *et al.* (1978) Transmission of surface antigen from mother to infant in 4 ethnic groups. *Br. Med. J.*, **1**, 949–952.

161. Boxall, E.H., Flewett, T.H., Dane, D.S. *et al.* (1974) Hepatitis B surface antigen in breast milk. *Lancet*, **2**, 1007–1008.

162. Lin, Ho-Hsiung, Hsu, Hong-Yian, Chang, Mei-Hwei. *et al.* (1993) Hepatitis B virus in the colostra of HBe-positive carrier mothers. *J. Paediatr. Gastroenterol. Nutrition*, **17**, 207–210.

163. Ohto, H., Lin, H., Kawana, T. *et al.* (1987) Intrauterine transmission of hepatitis B virus is closely related to placental leakage. *J. Med. Virol.*, **21**, 1–6.

164. Beasley, R.P., Hwang, L.Y., Lin, C.C. *et al.* (1982) Incidence of hepatitis B virus infections in pre-school children in Taiwan. *J. Infect. Dis.*, **146**, 198–204.

165. Both, J.F., Ritchie, M.J.J., Duskeiko, G.M. *et al.* (1984) Hepatitis B virus carrier state in Ovamboland: role of perinatal and horizontal infection. *Lancet*, **1**, 1984.

166. Szmuness, W., Prince, A.M., Hirsch, R.L. *et al.* (1973) Familial clustering of hepatitis B infection. *N. Engl. J. Med.*, **289**, 1162–1166.

167. Gerlich, W. (1993) Structure and molecular virology (hepatitis B). In: *Viral Hepatitis: Scientific Basis and Clinical Management*, (eds A.J. Zuckerman and H.C. Thomas), Churchill Livingstone, Edinburgh, pp. 82–113.

168. Stevens, C.E., Beasley, R.P., Tsiu, J. *et al.* (1975) Vertical transmission of hepatitis B in Taiwan. *N. Engl. J. Med.*, **292**, 771–774.

169. Aziz, M.A., Khan, G., Khanum, T. *et al.* (1973) Transplacental and post-natal transmission of the hepatitis associated antigen. *J. Infect. Dis.*, **127**, 110–112.

170. Schweitzer, I.L., Moseley, J.W., Ashcavai, M. *et al.* (1973) Factors influencing neonatal infection by hepatitis B virus. *Gastroenterology*, **65**, 227–283.

171. Schweitzer, I.L. (1975) Vertical transmission of the hepatitis B surface antigen. *Am. J. Med. Sci.*, **270**, 287–291.

172. Okada, K., Kamigama, I., Inomata, M. *et al.* (1976) e antigen and anti-e in the serum of asymptomatic carrier mothers as indicators of positive and negative transmission of hepatitis B virus to their infants. *N. Engl. J. Med.*, **294**, 746–749.

173. Beasley, R.P., Trepo, C., Stevens, C.E. and Szmuness, W. (1977) e antigen and vertical transmission of hepatitis B. *Am. J. Epidemiol.*, **105**, 94–98.

174. Lelic, P.N., Ip, H.M.H., Reesink, H.W. *et al.* (1991) Prevention of the hepatitis B carrier state in infants of mothers with high and low levels of HBV-DNA. In: *Viral Hepatitis and Liver Disease*, (eds F.B. Hollinger, S.M. Lemon and H.S. Margolis), Williams and Wilkins, Baltimore, pp. 753–756.

175. Thomas, H.C., Jacyna, M., Waters, H. and Main, H. (1988) Virus-host interaction in chronic hepatitis B infection. *Semin. Liver Dis.*, **8**, 342–349.

176. Milich, D.R., Jones, J.E., Hughes, J.L. *et al.* (1990) Is a function of HBeAg to induce immunologic tolerance in utero? *Proc. Natl Acad. Sci. USA*, **87**, 6599–6603.

177. Milich, D.R., Schodel, F., Peterson, D.L. *et al.* (1995) Characterization of self reactive T cells that evade tolerance in hepatitis e antigen transgenic mice. *Eur. J. Immunol.*, **25**, 1663–1673.

178. Zeldis, J.B. and Crumpacker, C.S. (1995) Hepatitis. In: *Infectious Diseases of the Fetus and Newborn Infant*, 4th edn, (eds J.S. Remington and J.O. Klein), W.B. Saunders, Philadelphia, pp. 805–834.

179. Schweitzer, I.L., Dunn, A.E., Peters, R.L. *et al.* (1973) Viral hepatitis B in neonates and infants. *Am. J. Med.*, **55**, 762–771.

180. Cossart, Y.E. (1974) Acquisition of hepatitis B antigen in the newborn period. *Postgrad. Med. J.*, **50**, 334–337.

181. Merrill, D.A., DuBois, R.S. and Kohler, P.F. (1972) Neonatal onset of the hepatitis-associated antigen carrier state. *N. Engl. J. Med.*, **287**, 1280–1282.

182. Locarnini, S.A. and Gust, I.D. (1988) Hepadnaviridae: hepatitis B virus and the delta virus. In: *Laboratory Diagnosis of Infectious Diseases: Principles and Practice*, (eds E.H. Lenette, P. Halonen and F.A. Murphy), Springer-Verlag, New York, pp. 750–796.

183. Robinson, W.S. (1977) The genome of hepatitis B virus. *Annu. Rev. Microbiol.*, **31**, 357–377.

184. Tiollais, P., Pourcel, C. and Degean, A. (1985) The hepatitis B virus. *Nature*, **317**, 489–495.

185. Seeger, C., Summers, J. and Mason, W.S. (1991) Viral DNA synthesis. *Curr. Topics Microbiol. Immunol.*, **168**, 41–60.

186. Toh, H., Hayashida, H. and Miyata, T. (1983) Sequence homology between retroviral reverse transcriptase and putative polymerase of hepatitis B virus and cauliflower mosaic virus. *Nature*, **305**, 827–828.

187. Radziwill, G., Tucker, W. and Schaller, H. (1990) Mutational analysis of the hepatitis B P gene product domain structures and RNAase H activity. *J. Virol.*, **64**, 613–620.

188. Bartenschlarger, R. and Schaller, H. (1988) The amino-terminal domain of the hepadnaviral P gene encodes the terminal protein (genome linked protein) believed to prime reverse transcription. *EMBO J.*, **7**, 4185–4192.

189. Ueda, K., Tsurimoto, T. and Matsubara, K. (1991) Three envelope proteins of hepatitis B virus: large S, middle S and major S proteins needed for the formation of Dane particles. *J. Virol.*, **65**, 3521–3529.

190. Philipson, L. (1981) Virus receptors. In: *Receptors and Recognition*, B Series (eds K. Longberg-Holm and L. Philipson), Chapman and Hall, New York, pp. 11–36.

191. Weimer, T., Salfeld, J. and Will, H. (1987) Expression of the hepatitis B core gene. *In vitro* and *in vivo*. *J. Virol.*, **61**, 3109–3113.

192. Siddiqui, A., Jamcel, S. and Mapoles, J. (1986) Transcriptional control elements of hepatitis B surface antigen gene. *Proc. Natl Acad. Sci. USA*, **83**, 566–570.

193. Lau, J.Y.N. and Wright, T.L. (1993) Molecular virology and pathogenesis of hepatitis B. *Lancet*, **342**, 1335–1340.

194. Luscombe, C.A., Pederson, J., Bowden, S. *et al.* (1994) Alterations in intrahepatic expression of duck hepatitis B viral markers with ganciclovir chemotherapy. *Liver*, **14**, 182–192.

195. Blum, H.E., Stowring, L., Figus, A. *et al.* (1983) Detection of hepatitis virus DNA in hepatocytes, bile duct epithelium, and vascular elements by *in situ* hybridization. *Proc. Natl Acad. Sci. USA*, **80**, 6685–6688.

196. Delladetsima, J.K., Vafiadis, I., Tassopolous, N.C. *et al.* (1994) HBcAg and HBsAg expression in ductular cells in chronic hepatitis B. *Liver*, **14**, 71–75.

197. Jilbert, A.R., Freiman, J.S., Gowans, E.J. *et al.* (1992) Duck hepatitis B virus in liver, spleen and pancreas: analysis by *in situ* and Southern blot hybridization. *Virology,* **158**, 330–338.

198. Hruska, J.F., Clayton, D.A., Rubenstein, L.J.R. and Robinson, W.S. (1977) Structure of hepatitis B Dane particle DNA before and after the Dane particle DNA polymerase secretion. *J. Virol.,* **21**, 666–672.

199. Koch, J. and Schlict, H-J. (1993) Analysis of the earliest steps of hepadnaviral replication: genome repair after infectious entry into hepatocytes does not depend on viral polymerase activity. *J. Virol.,* **67**, 4874–4876.

200. Fowler, M.J.F., Monjardino, J., Tsiquaye, K.N. *et al.* (1984) The mechanism of replication of hepatitis B virus: evidence of asymmetric replication of the two DNA strands. *J. Med. Virol.,* **13**, 83–91.

201. Seeger, C., Ganem, D. and Varmus, H.E. (1986) Biochemical and genetic evidence for the hepatitis B virus replication strategy. *Science,* **232**, 477–484.

202. Buescher, M., Reiser, W., Will, H. and Schaller, H. (1985) Characterization of transcripts and the potential RNA pre-genome of duck hepatitis B virus: implication for replication by reverse transcription. *Cell,* **40**, 717–724.

203. Robinson, W.S., Miller, R.H. and Marion, P.L. (1987) Hepadnaviruses and retroviruses share genome homology and features of replication. *Hepatology,* **7**, 64s–73s.

204. Wang, G.H. and Seeger, C. (1993) Novel mechanism for reverse transcription in hepatitis B viruses. *J. Virol.,* **67**, 6507–6512.

205. Tavis, J.E., Perri, S. and Ganem, D. (1994) Hepadnavirus reverse transcription initiates the stem loop of the RNA packaging signal and employs a novel strand transfer. *J. Virol.,* **68**, 3536–3543.

206. Gudat, R. and Bianchi, L. (1977) Evidence for phasic sequences in HBcAg formation and cell membrane-directed flow of core particles in chronic hepatitis B. *Gastroenterology,* **73**, 1194–1197.

207. Tuttleman, J.S., Pourcel, C. and Summers, J. (1986) Formation of a pool of covalently closed circular viral DNA in hepadnavirus infected cells. *Cell,* **47**, 451–460.

208. Weissberg, J.I., Andres, L.L., Smith, C.L. *et al.* (1984) Survival in chronic hepatitis G: an analysis of 397 patients. *Ann. Intern. Med.,* **101**, 613–616.

209. Lau, J.Y.N., Bain, V.G., Davies, S.E. *et al.* (1992) High level of expression of hepatitis B viral antigens in fibrosing cholestatic hepatitis. *Gastroenterology,* **102**, 956–962.

210. Demetris, A.J. (1992) Hepatitis B after liver transplantation: new names for unusual presentations. *Gastroenterology,* **103**, 1355–1356.

211. Lau, J.Y.N., Bain, V.G., Davies, S.E. *et al.* (1991) Export of intracellular HBsAg in chronic hepatitis B virus infection is related to viral replication. *Hepatology,* **14**, 416–421.

212. Eddleston, A. (1987) Immunological aspects of hepatitis B infection. In: *Viral Hepatitis and Liver Disease,* (ed A. Zuckerman), Alan R. Liss, New York, pp. 603–605.

213. Peters, M., Vierling, J., Gershwin, M.E. *et al.* (1991) Immunology and the liver. *Hepatology,* **13**, 977–994.

214. Onji, M., Lever, A.M.L., Saito, I. and Thomas, H.C. (1989) Defective response to interferons in cells transfected with the hepatitis B virus genome. *Hepatology,* **9**, 92–96.

215. Chisari, F. and Ferrari, C. (1995) Hepatitis B virus immunopathogenesis. *Annu. Rev. Immunol.,* **13**, 29–60.

216. Rehermann, B., Ferrari, C., Pasquinelli, C. and Chisari, F.V. (1996) The hepatitis B virus persists for decades after patients recover from acute viral hepatitis despite active maintenance of a cytotoxic T-lymphocyte response. *Nature Med.,* **2**, 1104–1108.

217. Thiers, V., Nakajima, E. and Kremsdorf, D. (1988) Transmission of hepatitis B from hepatitis B seronegative subjects. *Lancet,* **2**, 1273–1276.

218. Nielsen, J.D., Dietrichson, O. and Elling, P. (1981) Incidence and meaning of persistence of Australia antigen in patients with acute viral hepatitis: development of chronic hepatitis. *N. Engl. J. Med.,* **285**, 1157–1160.

219. Hoofnagle, J.H. and Schafer, D.F. (1986) Serological markers of hepatitis B virus infection. *Semin. Liver Dis.,* **6**, 1–10.

220. Locarnini, S.A. and Gust, I. (1988) Hepadnaviridae: hepatitis B virus and the delta virus. In: *Laboratory Diagnosis of Infectious Diseases. Principles and Practice, Volume II, Viral, Rickettsial and Chlamydial Diseases,* (eds E.H. Lennette, P. Halonen and F.A. Murphy), Springer-Verlag, New York, pp. 750–796.

221. Sjogren, M. and Hoofnagle, J.H. (1985) Immunoglobulin M antibody to hepatitis B core

antigen in patients with chronic type B hepatitis. *Gastroenterology*, **89**, 252–258.

222. Hoofnagle, J.H. and Alter, H.J. (1984) Chronic viral hepatitis. In: *Viral Hepatitis and Liver Disease*, (eds G.N. Vyas, J.L. Dienstag and J.H. Hoofnagle), Grune and Stratton, New York, pp. 97–113.

223. Hsu, H-Y., Chang, M-H., Lee, C-Y. *et al.* (1995) Precore mutant hepatitis B virus in childhood hepatitis B: an infrequent association. *J. Infect. Dis.*, **171**, 776–781.

224. Decker, R.H. (1991) New diagnostic technologies: automation of immunoassays for hepatitis markers and solution hybridization for HBV DNA. In: *Viral Hepatitis and Liver Disease*, (eds F.B. Hollinger, S.M. Lemon and H. Margolis), Williams and Wilkins, Baltimore, pp. 795–798.

225. Gerlich, W.H., Luer, W. and Thomssen, R. (1980) Diagnosis of acute and inapparent hepatitis B infection by measurement of IgM antibody to hepatitis B core antigen. *J. Infect. Dis.*, **142**, 95–101.

226. Gerlich, W.H., Heermann, K.H., Thomssen, R. and the Eurohep Group (1995) Quantitative assays for hepatitis B virus DNA: standardization and quality control. *Viral Hepatitis Rev.*, **1**, 53–58.

227. Beasley, R.P., Hwang, L.Y., Lee, G.C. *et al.* (1983) Prevention of perinatally transmitted hepatitis B virus infections with hepatitis B immunoglobulin and hepatitis B vaccine. *Lancet*, **2**, 1099–1102.

228. Centers for Disease Control (1990) Hepatitis B virus. A comprehensive strategy for eliminating transmission in the United States through universal childhood vaccination. *MMWR*, **40**, 1–25.

229. Reesink, H.W., Reesink-Brongers, E.E., Lafher-Schut, B.J.T. *et al.* (1979) Prevention of chronic HBsAg carrier state in infants of surface antigen positive mothers by hepatitis B immunoglobulin. *Lancet*, **2**, 436.

230. Beasley, R.P., Hwang, Y.L., Stevens, C.E. *et al.* (1983) Efficacy of hepatitis B immune globulin (HBIG) for prevention of perinatal transmission of hepatitis B carrier state: final report of a randomised double-blind placebo controlled trial. *Hepatology*, **3**, 135–141.

231. Beasley, R.P. and Stevens, C.E. (1978) Vertical transmission of HBV and interruption with globulin. In: *Viral Hepatitis*, (eds G.N. Vyas, S.N. Cohen and R. Sched), Franklin Institute Press, Philadelphia, p. 333.

232. Beasley, R.P. and Hwant, L.Y. (1983) Postnatal infectivity of HBeAg carrier mothers. *J. Infect. Dis.*, **147**, 185.

233. Zuckerman, J.N., Cockcroft, A. and Zuckerman, A.J. (1992) Site of injection for vaccination. *Br. Med. J.*, **305**, 1158.

234. Beasley, R.P., Trepo, C., Stevens, C.E. *et al.* (1977) The e antigen and vertical transmission of the hepatitis B surface antigen. *Am. J. Epidemiol.*, **105**, 94–98.

235. Hadler, S.C. and Margolis, H.S. (1992) Hepatitis B immunization, vaccine types efficacy and indications for immunization. In: *Current Clinical Topics in Infectious Diseases*, (eds J.S. Remington and M.N. Swartz), Blackwell Scientific, Boston, pp. 282–308.

236. Tilzey, A.J., Laidler, P.W. and Banatvala, J.E. (1988) Reactogenicity and immunogenicity of a yeast derived recombinant DNA hepatitis B vaccine in healthy young adults. In: *Viral Hepatitis and Liver Disease*, (ed. A.J. Zuckerman), Alan R. Liss, New York, pp. 1047–1049.

237. Bernstein, S.R., Krieger, P., Puppala, B.L. and Costello, M. (1995) Incidence and duration of hepatitis B surface antigenaemia after neonatal hepatitis B immunization. *J. Paediatrics*, **125**, 621–622.

238. Kuhn, L. and Stein, Z.A. (1995) Mother to infant HIV transmission: timing, risk factors and prevention. *Paediatr. Perinatal Epidemiol.*, **9**, 1–29.

239. Stevens, C.E., Krugman, S., Szumness, W. *et al.* (1980) Viral hepatitis in pregnancy. Problems for the clinician dealing with the infant. *Paediatr. Rev.*, **2**, 121–125.

240. Tsen, Y.J., Chang, M.H., Hsu, H.Y. *et al.* (1991) Seroprevalence of hepatitis B infection in children in Taipei, 1989: five years after a mass hepatitis B vaccination programme. *J. Med. Virol.*, **34**, 96–99.

241. Ruff, T.A., Gertig, D.M., Otto, B.F. *et al.* (1995) Lombok hepatitis B model immunization project: toward universal infant hepatitis B immunization in Indonesia. *J. Infect. Dis.*, **171**, 290–296.

242. Wong, W.C and Tsang, K.K. (1994) A mass vaccination programme in Taiwan: its preparation, results and reasons for uncompleted vaccinations. *Vaccine*, **12**, 229–234.

243. Birnbaum, J.M. and Bromberg, R. (1992) Evaluation of prophylaxis against hepatitis B in a large municipal hospital. *Am. J. Infection Control*, **20**, 172–176.

244. Henning, K.J., Pollack, D.M. and Friedman, S.M. (1992) A neonatal hepatitis B surveillance and vaccination programme: New York city, 1987 to 1988. *Am. J. Public Health*, **82**, 885–888.

245. Centers for Disease Control (1996) Prevention of perinatal hepatitis B through enhanced case management – Connecticut, 1994–1995, and United States 1994. *MMWR*, **45**, 584–587.

246. Tilzey, A.J. (1995) Hepatitis B vaccine boosting: the debate continues. *Lancet*, **345**, 1000.

247. National Health and Medical Research Council (1997) *The Australian Immunization Handbook*, 6th edn, pp. 109–120.

248. Carman, W.F., Zanetti, A.R., Karayiannis, P. *et al.* (1990) Vaccine-induced escape mutant of hepatitis B virus. *Lancet*, **336**, 325–329.

249. Hoofnagle, J.H. and Lau, J. (1996) Chronic viral hepatitis: benefits of current therapies. *N. Engl. J. Med.*, **334**, 1470–1471.

250. Haria, M. and Barfield, P. (1995) Interferon alpha 2a. A review of its pharmacological properties and therapeutic use in the management of viral hepatitis. *Drugs*, **50**, 873–896.

251. Ruiz-Moreno, M., Rua, M.J., Molina, J. *et al.* (1991) Prospective randomised controlled trial of interferon alpha in children with chronic hepatitis B. *Hepatology*, **13**, 1035–1039.

252. Barbera, C., Bortolutti, F., Crivellaro, C. *et al.* (1994) Recombinant alpha interferon 2a hastens the rate of HBeAg clearance in children with chronic hepatitis B. *Hepatology*, **20**, 287–290.

253. Ruiz-Moreno, M., Campo, T., Jimenez, J. *et al.* (1995) Factors predictive of response to interferon therapy in children with chronic hepatitis B. *J. Hepatol.*, **22**, 540–544.

254. Lok, A.S.F. and Lai, C-L. (1990) Acute exacerbations in Chinese patients with chronic hepatitis B virus (HBV) infection. Incidence, predisposing factors and aetology. *J. Hepatol.*, **10**, 29–34.

255. Alexander, G. and Williams, R. (1988) Natural history and therapy of chronic hepatitis B infection. *Am. J. Med.*, **85**, 143–146.

256. Lok, A.S., Lai, C.L., Wu, P.C. *et al.* (1987) Spontaneous hepatitis B e antigen to antibody seroconversion and reversion in Chinese patients with chronic hepatitis B virus infection. *Gastroenterology*, **92**, 1839–1843.

257. Niederau, C., Heintges, T., Lange, S. *et al.* (1996) Long term follow up of HBeAg positive patients treated with interferon alpha for chronic hepatitis B. *N. Engl. J. Med.*, **334**, 1422–1427.

258. Ruiz-Moreno, M. (1995) Interferon treatment in children with chronic hepatitis B. *J. Hepatol.*, **22**(suppl 1), 49–51.

259. Utili, R., Sagnelli, E., Gaeta, G.B. *et al.* (1994) Treatment of chronic hepatitis B in children with prednisolone followed by alpha-interferon: a controlled randomized study. *J. Hepatol.*, **20**, 163–167.

260. Barbera, C., Calvo, P. Coslia, A. *et al.* (1994) Pre-core mutant hepatitis B virus and outcome of chronic infection and hepatitis in hepatitis e antigen positive children. *Paediatr. Res.*, **36**, 347–350.

261. Dienstag, J.L., Perrillo, R.P. and Schiff, E.R. (1995) A preliminary trial of lamivudine for chronic hepatitis B infection. *N. Engl. J. Med.*, **333**, 1657–1661.

262. Angus, P.W., Locarnini, S.A., McCaughan, G.W. *et al.* (1995) Hepatitis B precore mutant infection is associated with severe recurrent disease after liver transplantation. *Hepatology*, **21**, 14–18.

263. Price, J.S., France, A.J., Moaven, L.D. and Welsby, P.D. (1986) Foscarnet in fulminant hepatitis B. *Lancet*, **2**, 1273.

264. Brechot, C., Berneau, J., Theiro, V. *et al.* (1984) Multiplication of hepatitis B virus in fulminant hepatitis B. *Br. Med. J.*, **288**, 270–271.

265. Centers for Disease Control (1994) Recommendations of the US public health service task force on the use of zidovudine to reduce perinatal transmission of human immunodeficiency virus. *MMWR*, **43**(RR11), 1–20.

266. Matheson, P.B., Abrams, E.J., Thomas, P.A. *et al.* (1995) Efficacy of antenatal zidovudine in reducing perinatal transmission of human immunodeficiency virus type 1: the New York city perinatal HIV transmission collaborative study group. *J. Infect. Dis.*, **172**, 353–358.

267. Zuin, G., Principi, N., Tornaghi, R. *et al.* (1992) Impaired immune response to hepatitis B in HIV infected children. *Vaccine*, **10**, 857–860.

268. Roingeard, P., Sankale, J.L., Dubois, F. *et al.* (1992) Infection due to hepatitis delta virus in Africa: report from Senegal and review. *Clin. Infect. Dis.*, **14 (2)**, 510–514.

269. Rizzetto, M., Ponzetto, A. and Foranzi, I. (1991) Epidemiology of hepatitis delta virus: overview. In: *The Hepatitis Delta Virus*, (eds J.L. Gerin, R.H. Purcell and M. Rizzetto), Wiley-Liss, New York, pp. 1–20.

270. Lazinski, D.W. and Taylor, J.M. (1994) Recent developments in hepatitis delta virus research. *Adv. Virus Res.*, **43**, 187–231.

271. Zanetti, A.R., Ferroni, P., Magliano, E.M. *et al.* (1982) Perinatal transmission of the hepatitis B virus and of the HBV-associated delta agent from mothers to offspring in northern Italy. *J. Med. Virol.*, **9**, 139–148.

272. Lai, M.M. (1995) The molecular biology of hepatitis delta virus. *Annu. Rev. Biochem.*, **64**, 259–286.

273. Wang, K.S., Choo, Q-L. and Weiner, A.M. (1986) Structure, sequence of the hepatitis delta viral genome. *Nature*, **323**, 508–513.

274. Lee, C-Z., Lin, J-H., Chao, M. *et al.* (1993) RNA binding activity of hepatitis delta antigen involves two arginine rich motifs and is required for hepatitis delta virus RNA replication. *J. Virol.*, **67**, 2221–2227.

275. Wang, H-W., Cheu, P-J., Lee, C-Z. *et al.* (1994) Packaging of hepatitis delta virus RNA via the RNA-binding domain of hepatitis delta antigens: different roles for small and large delta antigens. *J. Virol.*, **68**, 6363–6371.

276. Chen, P.J., Chang, F-L., Wang, C-J. *et al.* (1992) Functional study of hepatitis delta virus large antigen in packaging and replication inhibition: role of the amino-terminal leucine zipper. *J. Virol.*, **66**, 2853–2859.

277. Xia, Y-P. and Lai, M.M.C. (1992) Oligomerization of hepatitis delta antigen is required for both the trans-activating and trans-dominant inhibitory activities of the delta antigen. *J. Virol.*, **66**, 6641–6648.

278. Wang, J-G. and Lemon, S.M. (1993) Hepatitis delta virus antigen forms dimers and multimeric complexes *in vivo*. *J. Virol.*, **67**, 446–454.

279. Xia, Y-P., Yeh, C-T., Ou, J-H. and Lai, M.M.C. (1992) Characterization of nuclear targeting signal of hepatitis delta antigen: nuclear transport as a protein complex. *J. Virol.*, **66**, 914–921.

280. Kuo, M-Y.P., Chao, M. and Taylor, J. (1989) Initiation of replication of the human hepatitis delta virus genome from cloned DNA: the role of delta antigen. *J. Virol.*, **63**, 1945–1950.

281. Chao, M., Hsieh, S.Y. and Taylor, J. (1990) Role of two forms of hepatitis delta antigen: evidence for a mechanism of self limiting genome replication. *J. Virol.*, **64**, 5066–5069.

282. Chang, F.L., Cheu, P.J. and Ts, S.J. (1991) The large form of hepatitis δ antigen is crucial for the assembly of hepatitis delta virus. *Proc. Natl Acad. Sci. USA*, **88**, 8490–8494.

283. Macnaughton, T.B., Gowans, E.J., McNamara, S.P. and Burrell, C.J. (1991) Hepatitis δ antigen is necessary for access of hepatitis δ virus RNA to the cell transcriptional machinery but is not part of the transcriptional complex. *Virology*, **184**, 381–390.

284. Fu, T-B. and Taylor, J. (1993) The RNAs of hepatitis delta virus are copied by RNA polymerase II in nuclear homogenates. *J. Virol.*, **67**, 6965–6972.

285. Hsieh, S.Y. and Taylor, J.M. (1991) Regulation of polyadenylation of hepatitis delta virus antigenomic RNA. *J. Virol.*, **65**, 6438–6446.

286. Chen, P.J., Kalpana, G., Goldberg, J. *et al.* (1986) Structure and replication of the genome of the hepatitis delta virus. *Proc. Natl Acad. Sci. USA*, **83**, 8774–8778.

287. Sharmeen, L., Kuo, M.Y.P. and Taylor, J. (1989) Self-ligating RNA sequences on the antigenome of human hepatitis delta virus. *J. Virol.*, **63**, 1428–1430.

288. Rizzetto, M., Hoyer, B., Canese, M.G. *et al.* (1980) Delta agent: association of delta antigen with hepatitis B surface antigen and RNA in the serum of delta infected chimpanzees. *Proc. Natl Acad. Sci. USA*, **77**, 6124–6128.

289. Casey, J.L., Grazia, A.N., Engle, R.E., *et al.* (1996) Hepatitis B virus (HBV)/hepatitis D virus (HDV) co-infection in outbreaks of acute hepatitis in the Peruvian Amazon basin. The roles of HDV genotype III and HBV genotype F. *J. Infect. Dis.*, **174**, 920–926.

290. Rizzetto, M., Verme, G., Recchia, S. *et al.* (1983) Chronic HBsAg hepatitis with intrahepatic expression of delta antigen: an active and progressive disease unresponsive to immunosuppressive treatment. *Ann. Intern. Med.*, **98**, 437–441.

291. Negro, F. and Rizzetto, M. (1995) Diagnosis of hepatitis delta virus infection. *J. Hepatol.*, **22**, (suppl 1), 136–139.

292. Negro, F., Baldi, M., Bonino, F. *et al.* (1988) Chronic HDV (hepatitis delta virus) hepatitis. Intrahepatic expression of delta antigen, histologic activity and outcome of liver disease. *J. Hepatol.*, **6**, 8–14.

293. Lai, M.M.C. (1995) Molecular biologic and pathogenic analysis of hepatitis delta virus. *J. Hepatol.*, **22**(suppl 1), 127–131.

294. Tang, J.R., Cova, L., Lamelin, J.P. *et al.* (1994) Clinical relevance of the detection of hepatitis

delta virus RNA in serum by RNA hybridization and polymerase chain reaction. *J. Hepatol.*, **21**, 953–960.

295. Aach, R.D., Stevens, C.E., Hollinger, F.B. *et al.* (1991) Hepatitis C virus infection in post-transfusion hepatitis. *N. Engl. J. Med.*, **325**, 1325–1329.

296. Moaven, L.D., Crofts, N. and Locarnini, S.A. (1993) Hepatitis C infection in Victorian injecting drug users in 1971. *Med. J. Aust.*, **158**, 574.

297. Chant, K., Kociuba, K., Munro, R. *et al.* (1994) Investigation of possible patient to patient transmission of hepatitis C in a hospital. *NSW Public Health Bull.*, **5**, 47.

298. Allander, T., Gruber, A., Naghuri, M. *et al.* (1995) Frequent patient to patient transmission of hepatitis C in a haematology ward. *Lancet*, **345**, 603.

299. Pereira, B.J.G., Milford, E.L., Kirkman, R.L. and Levey, A.S. (1991) Transmission of hepatitis C by organ transplantation. *N. Engl. J. Med.*, **325**, 454–460.

300. Yen-Hsuan, N., Mei-Hwei, C., Hung-Chi, L. *et al.* (1994) Post-transfusion hepatitis C in children. *J. Paediatrics*, **124**, 709–713.

301. Alter, M.J., Hadler, S.C., Judson, F.H. *et al.* (1990) Risk factors for acute nonA-nonB hepatitis in the United States and association with hepatitis C virus infection. *JAMA*, **264**, 2231–2235.

302. Brettler, D.B., Mannucci, P.M., Gringeri, A. *et al.* (1992) The low risk of hepatitis C virus among sexual partners of hepatitis C infected haemophiliac males: an international multicenter study. *Blood*, **80**, 540–543.

303. Wejstal, R., Widell, A., Mansson, H.S. *et al.* (1992) Mother to infant transmission of hepatitis C. *Ann. Intern. Med.*, **117**, 887–890.

304. Ohto, H., Terezawa, S., Sasaki, N. *et al.* (1994) Transmission of hepatitis C from mothers to infants. *N. Engl. J. Med.*, **330**, 744–750.

305. Lam, J.P.H., McOmish, F., Burns, S.M. *et al.* (1993) Infrequent transmission of hepatitis C. *J. Infect. Dis.*, **167**, 572–576.

306. Lin, H., Kao, J., Hsu, H. *et al.* (1994) Possible role for high titre maternal viraemia in perinatal transmission of hepatitis C virus. *J. Infect. Dis.*, **169**, 638–641.

307. Maccabruni, A., Bossi, G., Caselli, D. *et al.* (1995) High efficiency of vertical transmission of hepatitis C virus among babies born to human immunodeficiency virus-negative women. *Paediatr. Infect. Dis. J.*, **14**, 921–922.

308. Manzini, P., Salacco, G., Cerchier, A. *et al.* (1995) Human immunodeficiency virus infection as a risk factor for mother to child hepatitis C virus transmission: persistence of anti-hepatitis C virus in children is associated with the mother's anti-hepatitis C immunoblotting pattern. *Hepatology*, **21**, 328–332.

309. Meisel, H., Reip, A., Faltus, B. *et al.* (1995) Transmission of hepatitis C virus to children and husbands by women infected with contaminated anti-D immunoglobulin. *Lancet*, **345**, 1209–1211.

310. Resti, M., Azzar, C., Lega, L. *et al.* (1995) Mother to infant transmission of hepatitis C. *Acta Paediatrica*, 251–255.

311. Zanetti, A.R., Tanzi, E., Paccagnini, S. *et al.* (1995) Mother to infant transmission of hepatitis C virus. Lombardy study group on vertical HCV transmission. *Lancet*, **345**, 289–291.

312. Zuccotti, G.V., Ribero, M.L., Giovannini, M. *et al.* (1995) Effect of hepatitis C genotype on mother to infant transmission of virus. *J. Paediatrics*, **127**, 278–280.

313. Ogasawara, S., Kage, M., Kosai, K. *et al.* (1993) Hepatitis C virus RNA in saliva and breast milk of hepatitis C carrier mothers (letter). *Lancet*, **341**, 561.

314. Lin, H., Kao, J., Hsu, H. *et al.* (1995) Absence of infection in breast fed infants born to hepatitis C infected mothers. *J. Paediatrics*, **126**, 589–591.

315. Feinstone, S.M., Mihalik, K., Kamimura, T. *et al.* (1983) Inactivation of hepatitis B and non-A non-B hepatitis by chloroform. *Infection Immunity*, **41**, 816–821.

316. Bradley, D.W., Maynard, J.D., Popper, H. *et al.* (1983) Post-transfusion non-A non-B hepatitis: physicochemical properties of 2 distinct agents. *J. Infect. Dis.*, **148**, 254–265.

317. Bradley, D.W., McCaustland, K.A., Cook, E.H. *et al.* (1985) Post-transfusion non-A non-B hepatitis in chimpanzees: physicochemical evidence the tubule forming agent is a small, enveloped virus. *Gastroenterology*, **88**, 773–779.

318. Bradley, D.W. (1985) The agents of non-A non-B viral hepatitis. *J. Virolog. Methods*, **10**, 307–319.

319. Thomassen, R., Bonk, S. and Theile, A. (1993) Density heterogeneities of hepatitis C virus in human sera due to the binding of beta-lipoproteins and immunoglobulins. *Med. Microbiol. Immunol.*, **182**, 329–334.

320. Lohmann, V., Koch, J.O. and Bartenschlager, R. (1996) Processing pathways of the hepatitis C virus proteins. *J. Hepatol.*, **24**, (suppl 2), 11–19.

321. Wang, C., Sarnow, P. and Siddiqui, A. (1993) Translation of human hepatitis C RNA is mediated by an internal ribosome-binding mechanism. *J. Virol.*, **67**, 3338–3344.

322. Tanaka, T., Kato, N., Cho, M-J. *et al.* (1996) Structure of the 3' terminus of the hepatitis C virus genome. *J. Virol.*, **70**, 3307–3312.

323. Han, J.H. and Haighton, M. (1992) Group specific sequences and conserved secondary structures at the 3' end of HCV genome and its implication for viral replication. *Nucleic Acids Res.*, **20**, 3520.

324. Hijikata, M., Kato, N., Ootsuyama, Y. and Nakagawa, M. (1991) Gene mapping of the putative structural region of the hepatitis C virus genome by *in vitro* processing analysis. *Proc. Natl Acad. Sci. USA*, **88**, 5547–5551.

325. Santolini, E., Mihliaccio, G. and La Monica, N. (1994) Biosynthesis and biochemical properties of the hepatitis C core protein. *J. Virol.*, **68**, 3531–3541.

326. Hijikata, M., Mizushima, H., Akagi, T. *et al.* (1995) Two distinct proteinase activities required for the processing of a putative non-structural precursor protein of hepatitis C virus. *J. Virol.*, **67**, 4665–4675.

327. Chambers, T.J., Weir, R.C., Grakovi, A. *et al.* (1990) Evidence that the end terminal domain of non-structural protein NS3 from yellow fever virus is a serine protease responsible for site specific cleavages in the viral polyprotein. *Proc. Natl Acad. Sci. USA*, **87**, 8898–8902.

328. Tanj, Y., Hijikata, M., Satoh, S. *et al.* (1995) Hepatitis C virus encoded non-structural protein NS4A has versatile functions in viral protein processing. *J. Virol.*, **69**, 1575–1581.

329. Behrens, S-E., Tomei, L. and de Fracesco, R. (1996) Identification and properties of the RNA dependent RNA polymerase of hepatitis C virus. *EMBO J.*, **15**, 12–22.

330. Simmonds, P. (1995) Variability in hepatitis C virus. *Hepatology*, **21**, 571–583.

331. Bukh, J., Purcell, R.H. and Miller, R.H. (1993) At least 12 genotypes of hepatitis C predicted by sequence analysis of the putative E1 gene of isolates collected world-wide. *Proc. Natl Acad. Sci. USA*, **91**, 8239–8243.

332. Silim, E. and Modonelli, M.U. (1995) Significance of hepatitis C virus genotypes. *Viral Hepatitis Rev.*, **1**, 111–120.

333. Chu, P.W.G. and Westaway, E.G. (1992) Molecular and ultrastructural analysis of heavy membrane fractions associated with the replication of Kunjin virus RNA. *Arch. Virol.*, **125**, 177–191.

334. Bartholomeusz, A.I., Guo, K-J., Edwards, P.C. and Locarnini, S.A. (1996) Hepatitis C virus (HCV) RNA polymerase assay using cloned HCV non-structural proteins. *Antiviral Ther.*, **1**(suppl 4), 18–24.

335. Chu, P.W.G. and Westaway, E.G. (1987) Characterization of Kunjin virus RNA dependent RNA polymerase re-initiation of synthesis *in vitro*. *Virology*, **157**, 330–337.

336. Weiner, A.J., Brauer, M.J., Rosenblatt, J. *et al.* (1991) Variable and hypervariable domains are found in the regions of HCV corresponding to the flavivirus envelope and NS1 proteins and the pestivirus envelope glycoproteins. *Virology*, **180**, 842–848.

337. Nelson, D.R. and Lau, J.Y.N. (1996) Host immune response in hepatitis C virus infection. *Viral Hepatitis Rev.*, **2**, 37–48.

338. Martell, M., Esteban, J.I., Quer, J. *et al.* (1992) Hepatitis C virus (HCV) circulates as a population of different but closely related genomes: quasispecies nature of HCV genome distribution. *J. Virol.*, **66**, 3225–3229.

339. Selby, M.J., Choo, Q.L., Berger, K. *et al.* (1993) Expression, identification and subcellular localization of the protein encoded by the hepatitis C viral genome. *J. General Virol.*, **74**, 1103–1113.

340. Farci, P., Shimoda, A., Wong, D. *et al.* (1996) Prevention of HCV infection in chimpanzees by hyperimmune serum against the hypervariable region 1 of the envelope 2 protein. *Proc. Natl Acad. Sci. USA*, **93**, 15394–15399.

341. Weiner, A., Erikson, A.L., Kaasopen, J. *et al.* (1995) Persistent hepatitis C virus infection in a chimpanzee is associated with emergence of a cytotoxic T lymphocyte escape variant. *Proc. Natl Acad. Sci. USA*, **92**, 2655–2659.

342. Koziel, M.J., Dudley, D., Wong, J.T. *et al.* (1992) Intrahepatic cytotoxic T lymphocytes specific for hepatitis C virus in persons with chronic hepatitis. *J. Immunol.*, **149**, 3339–3344.

343. Cerny, A., McHutchinson, J.G., Pasquinelli, C. *et al.* (1995) Cytotoxic T lymphocyte response to hepatitis C virus-derived peptides containing the HLA.A2.1 binding motif. *J. Clin. Invest.*, **95**, 521–530.

344. Fong, T.L., Valinluck, B., Govindarajan, S. *et al.* (1993) Effect of short term prednisolone administration on aminotransferase (ALT) levels and HCV RNA in patients with chronic hepatitis C. *Hepatology*, **18**, 87A.

345. Onji, M., Kikuchi, Y., Kumon, I. *et al.* (1992) Intrahepatic lymphocyte subpopulations and HLA class 1 expression by hepatocytes in chronic hepatitis C. *Hepatol. Gastroenterol.*, **39**, 340–343.

346. Lohr, H.F., Schlaak, J.F., Kollmannsperger, S. *et al.* (1994) The role of cellular immune response in chronic HCV infection. *Hepatology*, **20**, A533.

347. Hellings, J.A., van der Veen du Prie, J., Snelting-van Deusen, R. and Stute, R. (1985) Preliminary results of transmission experiments of non-A non-B hepatitis by mononuclear leukocytes from a chronic patient. *J. Virol. Methods*, **10**, 321–326.

348. Younossi, Z.M. and Hutchison, J.G. (1996) Serological tests for HCV infection. *Viral Hepatitis Rev.*, **2**, 161–174.

349. Lau, J.Y.N., Davis, G.L., Kniffen, J. *et al.* (1993) Significance of hepatitis C virus RNA levels in chronic hepatitis C. *Lancet*, **341**, 1501–1504.

350. Nolte, F.S., Thurmond, C. and Fried, M.W. (1995) Preclinical evaluation of AMPLICOR hepatitis C virus test for detection of hepatitis C virus RNA. *J. Clin. Microbiol.*, **33**, 1775–1778.

351. Gretch, D.R., de la Rosa, C., Corey, L. and Carithers, R.J. (1996) Assessment of hepatitis C viraemia using molecular amplification technologies. *Viral Hepatitis Rev.*, **2**, 85–96.

352. Weiner, A.J., Kuo, G., Bradley, D.W. *et al.* (1990) Detection of hepatitis C viral sequences in nonA-nonB hepatitis. *Lancet*, **335**, 1–3.

353. Quiroga, J.A., Campillo, M.L., Catillo, I. *et al.* (1991) IgM antibody to hepatitis C virus in acute and chronic hepatitis C. *Hepatology*, **14**, 38–43.

354. Chayama, K., Sailoh, S., Arase, Y. *et al.* (1991) Effect of interferon administration on serum hepatitis C RNA in patients with chronic hepatitis C. *Hepatology*, **13**, 1040–1043.

355. Craske, J., Paver, W.K. and Farmer, D. (1993) An algorithm for confirming screen reactivity in blood donors in enzyme immunoassays for antibodies to hepatitis C virus. *J. Immunolog. Methods*, **160**, 227–235.

356. Zuckerman, A.J. and Zuckerman, J.N. (1995) Prospects for a hepatitis C vaccine. *J. Hepatol.*, **22**, (suppl 1), 97–100.

357. Zambon, M.C. and Lockwood, D.M. (1994) Hepatitis C seroconversion in pregnancy. *Br. J. Obstet. Gynaecol.*, **101**, 722–724.

358. Hoofnagle, J.H., Mullen, K.D., Jones, B. *et al.* (1987) Treatment of chronic non-A non-B hepatitis with recombinant human alpha interferon. A preliminary report. *N. Engl. J. Med.*, **315**, 1575–1578.

359. Van Thiel, D.H., Caraceni, P., Molloy, P.J. *et al.* (1995) Chronic hepatitis C in patients with normal or near normal alanine aminotransferase levels: the role of interferon alpha 2b therapy. *J. Hepatol.*, **23**, 503–508.

360. Kanai, K., Kako, M., Aikawa, T. *et al.* (1995) Clearance of serum hepatitis C virus RNA after interferon therapy in relation to virus genotype. *Liver*, **15**, 185–188.

361. Saracco, G. and Rizzetto, M. (1995) The long term efficacy of interferon alpha in chronic hepatitis C patients: a critical review. *J. Gastroenterol. Hepatol.*, **10**, 668–673.

362. Balisten, W.F. (1995) Treatment of chronic hepatitis C in children. *Viral Hepatitis Rev.*, **1**, 121–128.

363. Minohara, Y., Kato, T., Kanki, K. *et al.* (1995) Relationship between hepatitis C virus RNA levels and efficacy of interferon β therapy. *Acta Paediatr. Japon.*, **37**, 530–533.

364. Ruiz-Moreno, M., Rua, M.J., Castillo, I. *et al.* (1992) Treatment of children with chronic hepatitis C with recombinant interferon α: a pilot study. *Hepatology*, **16**, 882–885.

365. Bortolotti, F., Giacchino, R., Vajro, P. *et al.* (1995) Recombinant interferon alpha therapy in children with chronic hepatitis C. *Hepatology*, **22**, 1623–1627.

366. Fujisawa, T., Inui, A., Ohkowa, T. *et al.* (1995) Response to interferon therapy in children with chronic hepatitis C. *J. Paediatrics*, **127**, 660–662.

367. Terrault, N.A. (1996) Treatment of chronic hepatitis B and chronic hepatitis C. *Rev. Med. Virol.*, **6**, 215–228.

368. Sudo, K., Inoue, H., Shimiju, Y. *et al.* (1996) Establishment of an *in vitro* assay system for screening hepatitis C protease inhibitors using high performance liquid chromatography. *Antiviral Res.*, **32**, 9–18.

369. Devictor, D., Desplanques, L., Debray, D. *et al.* (1992) Emergency liver transplantation for fulminant liver failure in infants and children. *Hepatology*, **16**, 1156–1162.

370. Tan, K.C., Mondragon, R.S., Vougas, V. *et al.*

(1992) Liver transplantation for fulminant hepatic failure and late onset hepatic failure in children. *Br. J. Surg.*, **79**, 1192–1194.

371. Sato, S., Fujiama, S., Tanaha, M. *et al.* (1994) Co-infection of hepatitis C virus in patients with chronic hepatitis B infection. *J. Hepatol.*, **21**, 159–166.

372. Tsai, S.L., Liaw, Y.F., Yeh, C.T. *et al.* (1995) Cellular immune responses in patients with dual infections of hepatitis B and hepatitis C viruses: dominant role of hepatitis C virus. *Hepatology*, **21**, 908–912.

373. Weltman, M.D., Brotodihardjo, A., Crewe, E.B. *et al.* (1995) Co-infection with hepatitis B and C or B, C and delta viruses results in severe chronic liver disease and responds poorly to interferon-alpha treatment. *J. Viral Hepatitis*, **2**, 39–45.

374. Bowden, D.S., Moaven, L.D. and Locarnini, S.A. (1996) New hepatitis viruses: are there enough letters in the alphabet? *Med. J. Aust.*, **164**, 87–89.

375. Dawson, G.J., Schlauder, G.G., Coleman, P. *et al.* Prevalence and clinical significance of GBV-C. *Ninth Triennial International Symposium on Viral Hepatitis and Liver Disease*, Rome, Italy, abstract 33, p. 116.

376. Tacke, M., Kiyosawa, K., Stark, K. *et al.* (1997) Detection of antibodies to a putative hepatitis G virus envelope protein. *Lancet*, **349**, 318–320.

377. Pilot-Matias, T.J., Carrick, R.J., Coleman P.F. *et al.* (1996) Expression of the GB virus C E$_2$ glycoprotein using the Semliki Forest virus vector system and its utility as a serological marker. *Virology*, **225**, 282–292.

378. Moaven, L., Tennakoon, P.S., Bowden, D.S. and Locarnini, S.A. (1996) Mother to baby transmission of hepatitis G virus. *Med. J. Aust.*, **165**, 84–85.

379. Feucht, H.H., Zollner, B., Polyaka, S. and Laufs, R. (1996) Vertical transmission of hepatitis G (letter). *Lancet*, **347**, 1116.

380. Moaven, L., Locarnini, S.A., Bowden, D.S. *et al.* (1996) Hepatitis C, G and the GB agents. In: *Recent Advances in Microbiology, Volume 4*, (ed. V. Asche), Australian Society of Microbiology, Melbourne, pp. 119–160.

381. Leary, T.P., Muerhoff, A.S., Simons, J.N. *et al.* (1996) Novel member of the Flaviviridae associated with human non A-E hepatitis. *J. Med. Virol.*, **48**, 60–67.

382. Hsieh, S.Y., Yang, P-Y., Chen, H-C. and Lian, Y-F. (1997) Cloning and characterization of the extreme 5′-terminal sequences of the RNA genomes of GB virus-C/hepatitis G virus. *Proc. Natl Acad. Sci. USA*, **94**, 3206–3210.

383. McMahon, B.J., Beller, M., Williams, J. *et al.* (1996) A programme to control an outbreak of hepatitis A in Alaska using an inactivated hepatitis A vaccine. *Arch. Paediatr. Adolesc. Med.*, **150**, 733–739.

384. Margolis, H.S. and Shapiro, N. (1992) Who should receive hepatitis A vaccine? Considerations for the development of an immunization strategy. *Vaccine*, **10**, (suppl 1), 85–87.

385. Chang, M-H., Chen, C-J., Lai, M-S. *et al.* (1997) Universal hepatitis B vaccination in Taiwan and the incidence of hepatocellular carcinoma in children. *N. Engl. J. Med.*, **336**, 1855–1859.

J.E. Banatvala and I.L. Chrystie

INTRODUCTION

During the last decade the risks, frequency, sequelae and prevention of the nosocomial bloodborne virus (BBV) infections hepatitis B (HBV), hepatitis D (HDV) and human immunodeficiency viruses (HIVs) have become increasingly well recognized. There is, as yet, less information relating to the relatively newly recognized viruses, hepatitis C (HCV) and hepatitis G (HGV).

This chapter highlights some of the evidence linking transmission of these viruses, particularly HBV, HCV, and HIVs, from patient to health-care worker (HCW), HCW to patient, and patient to patient, emphasizing risks in obstetric and gynaecological practice. This evidence will be discussed in the context of UK recommendations and guidance for protecting HCWs against bloodborne virus infections and for preventing those who are infected from transmitting infection to their patients.

GENERAL FEATURES OF BLOODBORNE VIRUSES

VIRUSES CAUSING HEPATITIS

The hepatitis alphabet now extends from A to G. However, only HBV and HCV provide a significant nosocomial bloodborne problem (Table 11.1).

Both hepatitis A and hepatitis E are transmitted by the orofaecal route but, unlike HBV and HCV, do not induce either a prolonged viraemia or chronic infection (which may be associated with varying but sometimes high levels of viraemia) and, consequently, provide a very limited risk of virus transmission in a health-care setting. However, hepatitis E (which may cause endemics of acute hepatitis in many tropical countries) may result in maternal mortality of 20–30%, particularly if contracted in the last trimester (see Chapter 10).

Hepatitis B virus (HBV)

Figure 11.1 illustrates the morphological features of HBV. The virion is a spherical, 42 nm double-shelled particle comprising an internal partially single, partially double-stranded DNA within a 27 nm core surrounded by a lipoprotein envelope. The antigen associated with the viral envelope, hepatitis B surface antigen (HBsAg), is often present as 22 nm particles in large quantities in the serum of patients with acute infections as well as those developing a chronic carrier state. Hepatitis e antigen (HBeAg) is present in those with acute infection and among those carriers who are likely to transmit infection. In contrast, those developing antibodies to HBe antigen (anti-HBe) or who have no HBe markers are less likely to transmit infection (but see below).

Viral Infections in Obstetrics and Gynaecology. Edited by D.J. Jeffries and C.N. Hudson. Published in 1999 by Arnold, ISBN 0 340 74095 7.

Table 11.1 Characteristics of human hepatitis viruses and HIVs

Virus	Classification	Nucleic acid	Heterogenetic diversity	Nosocomial implications in O & G
Hepatitis A	Hepatovirus Picornaviridae	ss-RNA	No	None as BBV
Hepatitis B	Hepadnaviridae	ss/ds-DNA	Variation in surface, core and precore regions	Readily transmitted. HBeAg negative variants may occasionally be transmitted
Hepatitis C	Flaviviridae	ss-RNA	11 genotypes	Limited number of transmissions reported to date
Hepatitis D	Virusoid	ss-RNA	No	Co-infection or superinfection with HBV may cause severe disease
Hepatitis E	Caliciviridae	ss-RNA	No	None as BBV
Hepatitis G	Flaviviridae	ss-RNA	Probable	Not reported to date
Human immunodeficiency viruses	Lentivirinae	ss-RNA	Considerable	Transmissions are rare

It has been estimated that there are about 300–350 million carriers of HBV worldwide, with particularly high carrier rates occurring in parts of south east Asia (8–20%), sub-Saharan Africa (8–25%) and some Pacific islands (25–30%). However, the prevalence of antibodies to HBsAg (anti-HBs) indicates that, in these countries, a high proportion (70–95%) have been infected in the past, but recovered. The long-term carrier rate in south east Asia usually results from transmission from HBeAg-positive mothers to their infants whereas, in sub-Saharan Africa where fewer mothers are HBeAg-positive, infection is usually acquired during the first few years of life. Chronic liver disease and primary hepatocellular carcinoma (HCC) are common sequelae of chronic HBV infection in such parts of the world[1].

In Europe, about 1 million persons are estimated to be infected annually. About 90 000 become chronic carriers with approximately one-quarter eventually dying of cirrhosis or HCC[2]. Only about 20–25% of HBV infections among adults are symptomatic and those who develop symptoms usually clear their infection. About 2–10% of HBV-infected adults become carriers and, of these, 1–2% may clear the virus annually. In contrast with western Europe, where prevalence rates vary from 0.3% to 0.5%, some southern European countries, for example Italy, Greece and Spain, have prevalence rates of about 3%. However, higher carrier rates may also occur in some urban areas in western Europe, reflecting migration from HBV-endemic countries or such behavioural risk factors as injecting drug use or frequent change of sexual partners.

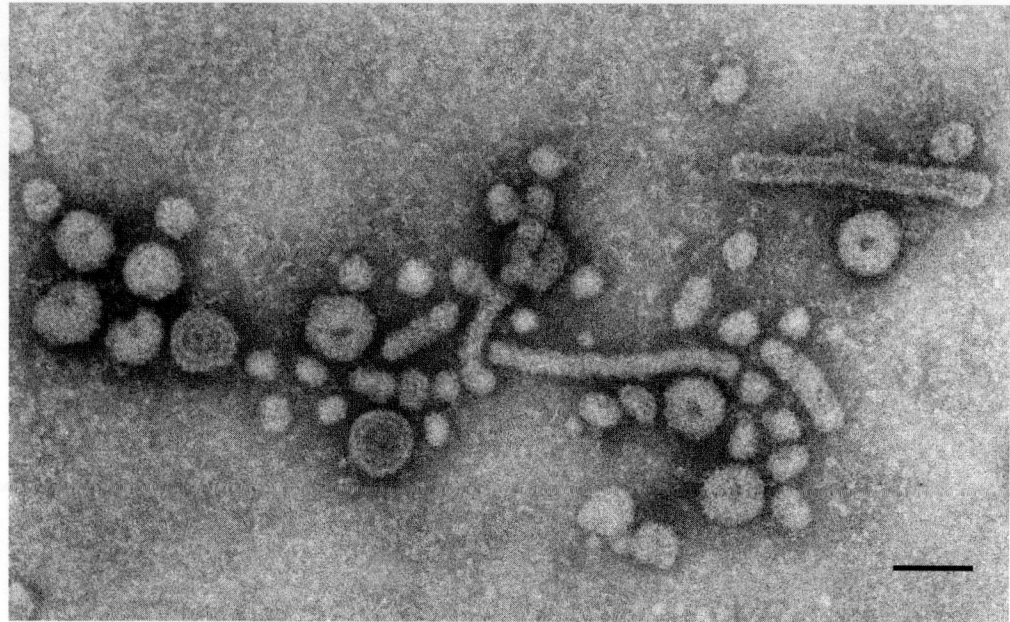

Figure 11.1 Electronmicrograph of hepatitis B virus showing the 42 nm, double-shelled Dane particle and 22 nm spheres and tubules of HBsAg. Negatively stained with 3% sodium phosphotungstate (pH 6.5). Bar = 50 nm.

Similar higher prevalence rates, e.g. up to 5% in Baltimore, have also been observed among adult patients attending emergency departments in inner-city hospitals in the USA[3].

Screening of pregnant women is an important factor in vaccination strategies. In parts of inner London about 1% of patients attending antenatal clinics (ANC) are HBV carriers[4]. However, attempts at selective screening proved unsuccessful with about 40% of HBsAg-positive women not being tested. Similar studies in the West Midlands, UK, have demonstrated that the dynamic nature of populations necessitates universal screening if at-risk patients are to be identified accurately[5].

Hepatitis C virus (HCV)

On the basis of molecular biological studies, HCV is a single-stranded RNA virus classified as a Flavivirus. However, there are no con-firmed reports relating to its fine structure. HCV is the primary cause of parenterally transmitted non-A non-B (NANB) hepatitis. Most infections are asymptomatic but a chronic carrier state may develop in up to 80% of persons; about 25–50% of these may eventually develop chronic liver disease, including cirrhosis and HCC, some 15–20 years after their initial infection[6].

About 1 in 2000 first-time British blood donors are HCV positive, many giving a history of injecting drug use prior to the introduction of routine blood donor screening in 1991. Worldwide, areas of relatively high seroprevalence (0.5–5%) are found in Japan, the Middle East, parts of Africa and some Mediterranean countries[7].

There is less information than for HBV relating to the prevalence of HCV among pregnant women in Britain. However, an extensive study of 3522 women attending ANC in the West Midlands showed that only

0.14% had anti-HCV antibody, although the prevalence of HBV infection was about four times greater. South east Asian and West Indian mothers had a higher prevalence of HBV infection whereas HCV infection was commoner in Caucasian women[8].

In addition to parenteral transmission, HCV may be transmitted sexually but much less frequently than HBV. Transmission from mother to baby is of the order of 5–10% but increases markedly if the mother is co-infected with HIV (up to 50%)[9].

Hepatitis G virus (HGV)

HGV is newly recognized and is also classified as a Flavivirus, being distantly related to HCV. HGV infection occurs frequently in multiply transfused patients (25%) and inject-ing drug users (~2%). In one study the prevalence among UK blood donors was reported to be 3.2%[10]. Co-infection with HCV is common and there have been reports of HGV being transmitted vertically[11]. Infection is usually asymptomatic. The role of HGV infection in chronic liver disease remains to be established.

HUMAN IMMUNODEFICIENCY VIRUSES (HIVs)

The HIVs are retroviruses belonging to the subfamily of lentiviruses. The 100–120 nm virus particle comprises a conical core, containing a single-stranded positive-sense RNA, surrounded by a fringed envelope formed of two major antigens, gp41 and gp120 (Figure 11.2), part of the latter being antigenically

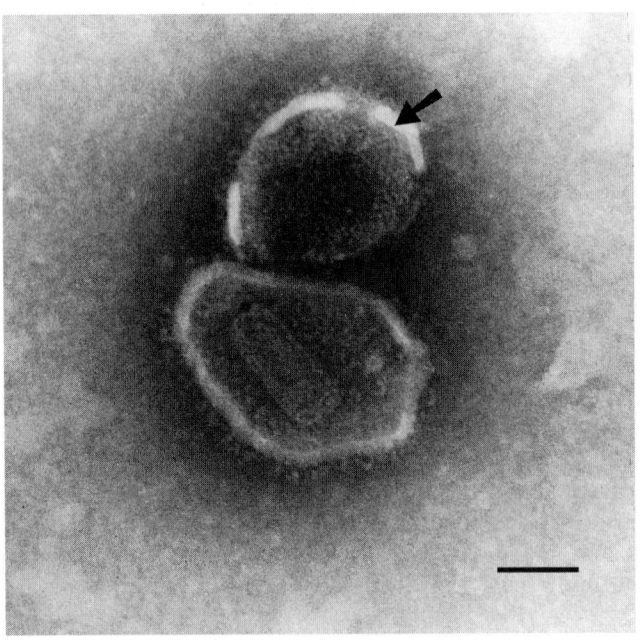

(a)

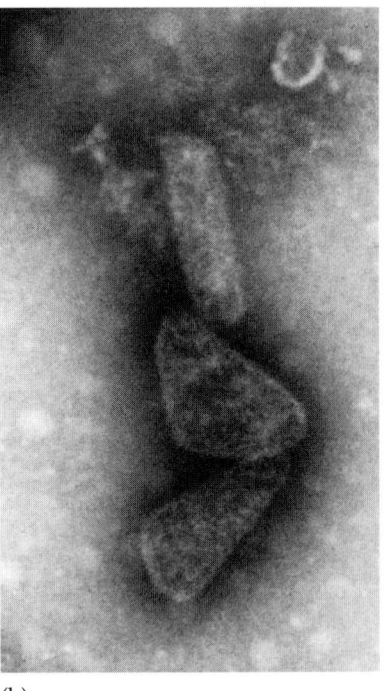

(b)

Figure 11.2 Electronmicrograph of human immunodeficiency virus negatively stained with sodium phosphotungstate pH 6.5. (a) Two virus particles from an HIV1 culture (H9/RF). The lipoprotein envelope with surface projections and geometric arrangement of the subunits (arrow), plus the core, are clearly resolved. (b) Three isolated HIV2 virus cores showing the characteristic wedge and rod shapes. Bar = 50 nm.

Table 11.2 Estimated adult HIV1 infections by continent or region from late 1970s to mid 1996 (based on reference[12])

Region	Cumulative total	Adults still alive
Western Europe	640 000	470 000
Eastern Europe/central Asia	31 000	30 000
North America	1.2 million	780 000
Latin America/Caribbean	1.9 million	1.6 million
North Africa/Middle East	220 000	200 000
Sub-Saharan Africa	19 million	14 million
Eastern Asia/Pacific	36 000	35 000
Australasia	23 000	13 000
South/south east Asia	5 million	4.8 million
Global total	27.9 million	21.8 million

hypervariable. Two distinct types of HIV are recognized: HIV1 is found worldwide whereas HIV2 is endemic in parts of west Africa, although it has now been imported to other parts of the world, including Britain. Although there is some antigenic homology between the core proteins of HIV1 and HIV2, their envelope-associated antigens are antigenically diverse. HIV1 is genomically diverse, comprising two types: type M, consisting of subtypes A–H, and type O. There are five subtypes of HIV2 (A–E).

HIV1 has a worldwide distribution (Tables 11.2 and 11.3) and only a few Asian countries and some Pacific Islands claim not to have any reported cases of AIDS. Although the burden of infection in sub-Saharan Africa is well established, with up to 20–30% of pregnant women being HIV1 positive, recent spread of infection in Asia and Latin America is giving rise to considerable concern. In developing countries, most HIV infection is acquired heterosexually. In many European countries and North America, although sex between men and injecting drug use represent major routes of infection, heterosexual acquisition of infection is rising. For example, in England and Wales, the number of heterosexually acquired HIV infections detected through voluntary confidential testing has been

increasing and, in 1994, made up 28% of new reports to the Communicable Diseases Surveillance Centre (CDSC)[13]. However, in most cases, infection was transmitted by persons in high-risk categories, particularly from partners having acquired infection in HIV endemic countries. During 1994–5 the prevalence of HIV infection among patients attending the A&E department of an inner London hospital was 1.8%. The majority were 26–45-year-old men presenting with major illnesses potentially requiring admission and not reporting their HIV status[14].

Studies among pregnant women conducted on an anonymized basis in England and Wales

Table 11.3 Total numbers of AIDS cases (adults and children) from late 1970s to mid 1996 (based on reference[12])

Region	Reported (%)	Estimated (%)
Africa	501 714 (36)	5 929 000 (77)
Americas (less USA)	181 174 (13)	462 000 (6)
USA	515 650 (37)	539 000 (7)
Asia	27 873 (2)	539 000 (7)
Europe	167 238 (12)	231 000 (3)
Oceania	<14 000 (1)	<77 000 (1)
Total	1 393 649	7.7 million

have shown that the prevalence increased significantly in inner London from 0.18% to 0.31% between 1990 and 1995 (0.2% to 0.59% among those aged 25–29)[15]. However, only 5% to ~25% of HIV-positive mothers have been identified by testing on a named patient basis: thus, the HIV status of the majority of HIV-positive women is known neither to the women themselves nor to those who care for them. In outer London, the prevalence among pregnant women has increased to that found in parts of inner London, but very little infection has been reported among those attending ANC in other parts of the country[15].

As expected, the prevalence of HIV among women delivering in some cities in the USA including Boston and New York is considerably higher, being about 2%[16,17].

NOSOCOMIAL INFECTIONS

GENERAL CONSIDERATIONS

HBV and HIV are present not only in blood but also in other body fluids, including semen, saliva, vaginal fluid, CSF, breast milk, amniotic fluid and serum exudates. However, as virus is usually present in much lower concentrations, the risk of transmitting infection via such body fluids in the health-care setting is generally much lower. Nevertheless, recent studies have demonstrated that HIV can be recovered from the cervico-vaginal fluid of most HIV-positive women and that the viral load is comparable with that detected in the patient's plasma[18]. There is much less information relating to the detection of HCV in body fluids other than blood although virus has been detected in saliva[19].

Transmission rates following percutaneous exposure to blood containing HBV, HCV and HIV are of the order of 30%, 3–10% and 0.3% respectively, possibly reflecting differences in viral load in these infections[53]. Exposure of mucosal surfaces to blood containing HBV and HIV may result in viral transmission, albeit extremely rarely. The relative risks of percutaneous and mucosal exposure to HIV are shown in Table 11.4.

Second- and third-generation serological assays for HCV antibodies are more specific than the earlier first-generation tests. Although markers of infectivity are not yet available, about 70–80% of serologically confirmed cases have detectable HCV RNA by PCR, indicating that their blood has the potential for transmitting infection. Persistent infection may, however, be characterized by fluctuating levels of HCV RNA and consideration should therefore be given to regular testing of those who are initially negative by PCR, not only because of the risk of nosocomial transmission but also as treatment may be indicated.

Virus can be recovered from virtually all HIV-positive patients and there is consequently little to be gained by detecting virus, whether by isolation or by nucleic acid amplification techniques. However, the latter are increasingly being used to assess prognosis

Table 11.4 Estimations of HIV transmission rate after single percutaneous and mucocutaneous exposures (from reference[20] with permission)

		Rate	*95% CI*
Estimate of HIV transmission rate after a single percutaneous exposure	6955 subjects in 25 studies	0.32%	0.18–0.45%
Estimate of HIV transmission rate after a single mucocutaneous exposure	2910 subjects in 21 studies	0.03%	0.006–0.19%

and response to antiviral chemotherapy. Furthermore, it is possible that such techniques may also be of value in assessing risks of viral transmission from patient to HCW.

PATIENT-TO-HCW TRANSMISSION

Considerable attention has been focused by the medical press and media on transmission of bloodborne virus infections from surgeons to patients during surgical practice. However, the risk to surgeons (including obstetricians/gynaecologists) and nurses (including midwives) of acquiring infection from their patients is far greater. Risks of percutaneous and mucosal exposure to blood are particularly high among obstetricians/gynaecologists, midwives and others attending delivery[21]. This reflects exposure, often heavy, to blood during delivery and the relatively high risks of sustaining injury during pelvic surgery. Risks are also related to the prevalence of bloodborne virus infections in the community (higher in inner-city areas), duration of practice and professional skills. Trainees are more likely to be at risk of sustaining percutaneous injuries than their more experienced seniors.

A study conducted among 1062 surgical and obstetric patients at a tertiary medical centre near New York showed that one in 15 had evidence of current HBV, HCV or HIV infection, this rate increasing to one in six among patients aged 25–44[22]. The high risks associated with gynaecological practice are illustrated by studies conducted by Tokars *et al.*[23] in New York and Chicago who, when observing a range of procedures in operating and delivery room settings, noticed that sharps injuries varied by specialty, ranging from 3.7% of 393 for orthopaedics to 10.1% of 307 for gynaecology. Particularly high injury rates were sustained during vaginal (21.3%) and abdominal hysterectomies (10.3%); other gynaecological procedures had an injury rate of 4.2%. Similar results were obtained during a study in an inner-London teaching hospital where sharps injuries were most frequent among cardiothoracic and obstetric and gynaecological surgeons. These surgeons were also least likely to report such incidents[24]. Percutaneous, mucosal or skin/blood contact rates per annum have also been reported as high among surgeons (81–135), obstetricians (77), midwives (188) and gynaecologists (124) [21].

Percutaneous exposure to HBsAg/HBeAg-positive blood carries a 30–40% risk of transmission of infection. Studies in the USA during the 1970s[25] showed that 0.8–4% of surgeons had chronic HBV infection (compared to 0.3% for the general population) and cohort studies during the late 1970s and early 1980s indicated that the infection rate per annum ranged from 0.5% to 5%, compared with an annual incidence of 0.1% in the general population in the USA. Risk factors included practising surgery for 10 years or more and not being vaccinated against HBV[26]. However, it is encouraging that there has recently been a significant decrease in the number of HCWs acquiring infection[27]. This probably reflects HBV vaccine uptake and improved standards of infection control, both in the operating theatre and elsewhere in the hospital.

The risks of acquiring HCV occupationally are considerably lower. Following needlestick exposure to patients who have serological evidence of HCV infection, it has been estimated that about 0–10% of HCWs are infected. Although Zuckerman *et al.*[28] have reported that the prevalence of infection is no higher than among blood donors, reports from the USA, Germany and the UK of significantly higher HCV seroprevalence among HCWs than among those in the general population who have no risk factors associated with the acquisition of bloodborne virus infections, suggest that transmission does occur[25].

Seroprevalence studies among surgeons suggest that HIV1 infection is uncommon and, when detected, may be associated with non-occupational risk factors. It is encouraging that only two orthopaedic surgeons, both with non-occupational risk factors, were found to be HIV positive among 3400 tested in the USA in 1991[23]. Another study showed that only one of 770 US surgeons working in an area of high HIV endemicity was HIV positive without non-occupational risk factors. This individual had been a general surgeon for 25 years[29]. Table 11.5 illustrates factors associated with high risks of acquiring infection and demonstrates that administration of zidovudine prophylactically is effective in reducing the risk of infection.

In an analysis of HIV infection acquired by HCWs, nurses and midwives were shown to be at high risk, with percutaneous exposures with blood-contaminated hollow needles being particularly hazardous. Almost 50% of reported seroconversions were among nurses, including phlebotomists and midwives, many injuries being sustained during or after venepuncture. This group included two nurses, both of whom had worked as midwives in Africa. Nine surgeons were infected occupationally, of whom four had worked in Africa. They had probably conducted a wide range of procedures including obstetrics and gynaecology. One had worked in Africa for three years and had undertaken emergency manual

Table 11.5 Risk factors for HIV infection in HCWs after percutaneous exposure to HIV-infected blood (from reference[30] with permission)

Risk factor	Adjusted odds ratio	95% CI
Deep injury	16.1	6.1–44.6
Visible blood on device	5.2	1.8–17.7
Procedure involving needle placed directly into a vein or artery	5.1	1.9–14.8
Terminal illness in source patient	6.4	2.2–18.9
Postexposure use of zidovudine	0.2	0.1–0.6

removal of the placenta without gloves on several occasions[20].

Consideration should also be given to the risks of medical students acquiring bloodborne virus infections while carrying out elective studies in areas of high HIV prevalence. Obstetrics should be regarded as a particularly high-risk procedure. Medical students are inexperienced and may be exposed to large volumes of blood. Furthermore, supervision (for example, in a missionary hospital) may be suboptimal. Some medical schools in Britain, although allowing students to conduct electives in HIV-endemic countries, prevent them from carrying out obstetrics.

HCW-TO-PATIENT TRANSMISSION

Since 1981 there has been a number of well-documented outbreaks of HBV infection in which patients have been infected by surgeons, including gynaecologists. However, this may be an underestimate since transmissions will not always be recognized, partly because a high proportion of HBV infections are subclinical and also because the incubation period may extend up to six months. Thus, acute hepatitis may not necessarily be attributable to recent surgery.

A particularly high risk is associated with surgical manipulation in which sharp instruments are guided by the surgeon's finger, for example during deep pelvic surgery. This increases the risk of percutaneous injury to the surgeon and consequently exposure of the patient to the surgeon's blood. It has also been shown experimentally that a surgeon who had transmitted HBV infection to 19 patients damaged his skin while participating in a one-hour simulation of repeatedly tying sutures, resulting in HBV leakage into his glove. As gloves provide only an imperfect barrier, particularly if only single gloving is employed, this suggests an alternative route by which infection may be transmitted from surgeon to patient[31].

The risks of gynaecological procedures are highlighted by a report of an extensive outbreak of HBV in which 22 patients were infected during gynaecological surgery[32]. Only five of these patients were icteric but all had been operated on by an HBeAg-positive HBV carrier in 1988. Initially, two women without HBV-associated risk factors were found to be positive for HBsAg (one was icteric). Both had been in the same gynaecological ward some months previously and a computer search of HBsAg-positive patients during the preceding months revealed yet another patient without risk factors; all three had been operated on by the same surgeon and none of the other members of the operating team were HBsAg positive. Two hundred and forty seven of 268 (92%) patients operated on by the gynaecologist were identified and screened for current or recent HBV infection, of whom 22 (9%) had positive markers. The operations carrying the greatest risk were hysterectomy (10 of 42–24%) and caesarean section (10 of 51–20%). There was no evidence of infection among 37 patients undergoing low-risk procedures such as D&C or termination of pregnancy but one medium-risk procedure, cone biopsy and D&C, was associated with viral transmission.

Until recently it was considered that lack of HBeAg correlated with low infectivity. However, four HBeAg-negative surgeons have recently been shown to have transmitted infection to patients during surgery. Subsequent analysis showed that all four had a particular form of precore mutant (premature stop codon 28)[33]. Two additional transmissions from HBeAg-negative surgeons with the same precore mutants have occurred (Sundkvist *et al.* unpublished). In five of these six cases, antibody to HBeAg was present. These findings have highlighted the importance of recognizing the role of such mutants in the occupational transmission of HBV.

Compared with HBV, the infectivity of HCV is much lower. There have been only two reports of HCV transmission during surgery, both HCWs involved being cardiothoracic surgeons. One surgeon in Spain infected 12 patients[34] and the other, in Britain, only one, despite an extensive lookback exercise involving 352 patients[35].

HCV infection has also been transmitted iatrogenically; 1150 of 1200 women in the Republic of Ireland given anti-D globulin from a single batch were infected. The preparation had been prepared from the plasma of a patient who had apparently recovered from acute Non-A, Non-B hepatitis in 1976, but had, in all probability, become an HCV carrier[36] since subsequent investigations showed that the HCV in the anti-D globulin and in the patients' sera were not only of the same genotype but also showed close sequence homology[37]. Contributing factors included the possibility of inadequate inactivation of the anti-D globulin and the fact that the preparation was given intravenously rather than intramuscularly. However, as a majority of acute HCV infections are subclinical and as HCWs involved in exposure-prone invasive procedures are not screened for evidence of HCV infection, further studies are required to assess the risks of transmission.

Despite the fears expressed in many articles in the lay press, transmission of HIV from HCW to patient is extremely rare. Thus, in a compilation of 42 look-back exercises in which an HIV-positive surgeon or dentist was identified, 16 357 of patients operated upon were followed up to determine whether they had been infected during surgery. Apart from a dental surgeon working in Florida who infected six of his patients via a route which remains to be established[38,39], none of the patients involved in these look-back exercises acquired infection as a result of surgery. Recently the French Ministry of Health and Social Security has announced that an HIV-infected French surgeon has probably transmitted the infection to one of nearly 1000 of his patients who were tested.

PATIENT-TO-PATIENT TRANSMISSION

Inadequate sterilization procedures, the re-use of disposable equipment (particularly needles and syringes) and the use of multidose vials have resulted in transmission of bloodborne viruses in hospital wards and clinics. Although such episodes have not as yet been reported in obstetric or gynaecological settings, vigilance is essential to ensure that high standards of infection control are practised in all wards and clinics, including those in the community.

Patient-to-patient transmission via environmental contamination may also provide risks. Depending on relative humidity and other factors, HBV and HIV may retain infectivity for prolonged periods. Thus, HBV may retain infectivity in dried blood for at least a week[40] and although HIV is more labile, if high concentrations are present, infectivity may be maintained for up to three weeks[41]. This emphasizes the importance of ensuring that good housekeeping practices, including handwashing and regular decontamination of environmental surfaces, are encouraged.

Shortcomings in hospital infection control procedures have resulted in patient-to-patient transmission of HCV to 17 patients in a haematology ward in Sweden[42], transmission of HIV to five patients in private surgical consulting rooms in Australia[43], and to an infant in a paediatric unit[44]. HIV1 has also been transmitted to an infant in the USA via unpasteurized breast milk from an infected donor[45]. This report has implications for hospital policy in developing countries with a high prevalence of HIV. The risk of patient-to-patient transmission of HBV, and more recently HCV, among patients undergoing haemodialysis is now well established[46]. A cluster of HIV cases in a Colombian haemodialysis unit resulting from inadequately reprocessed equipment, most probably access needles, was recently reported[46,47]. Those staffing such units are also at risk of being infected.

PREVENTION

GENERAL MEASURES TO PREVENT TRANSMISSION OF BLOODBORNE VIRUSES IN THE HEALTH-CARE SETTING

Basic precautions as listed in Table 11.6 should be routine practice in wards, clinics and primary care premises.

The precautions specific to maternity care and gynaecology are described in detail in the Third Report of the RCOG Scientific Advisory Committee's Working Party on HIV Infection in Maternity Care and Gynaecology[49]. General measures include the avoidance of sharps injuries, protection of hands by gloves and availability of suitable footwear to reduce the risk of percutaneous exposure by dropped syringes and needles. During labour, those in attendance should wear gloves and a plastic apron if there is a risk of contact with blood or amniotic fluid. Consideration should be given

Table 11.6 Infection control measures to prevent transmission of bloodborne viruses in the health-care setting (from reference[48] with permission)

Apply good basic hygiene practices with regular handwashing
Cover existing wounds or skin lesions with waterproof dressings
Avoid invasive procedures if suffering from chronic skin lesions on hands
Avoid contamination of person by appropriate use of protective clothing
Protect mucous membrane of eyes, mouth and nose from blood splashes
Prevent puncture wounds, cuts and abrasions in the presence of blood
Avoid sharps usage wherever possible
Institute safe procedures for handling and disposal of needles and other sharps
Institute approved procedures for sterilization and disinfection of instruments and equipment
Clear up spillages of blood and other body fluids promptly and disinfect surfaces
Institute a procedure for the safe disposal of contaminated waste

to double gloving in obstetric units in areas of high prevalence of bloodborne viruses.

Those conducting or assisting at delivery should wear full-length, long-sleeved, impermeable gowns. Spectacles or other eye protection and surgical masks should be worn to protect the face during delivery. Overshoes should be worn to minimize the risks of inadvertent dissemination of blood in health-care settings but boots are necessary for obstetric operations and other procedures carried out in the lithotomy position because the risk of exposure to blood and blood-contaminated body fluids is enhanced. In addition, repair of the perineum carries an increased risk of needlestick injury. For removal of the placenta, elbow-length gloves should be used if gowns with impermeable sleeves are unavailable. Immersion baths or birthing pools should be decontaminated after each use; a gravity drainage system is preferable.

Care must be taken in the resuscitation of newborn infants. Unprotected suction by mouth should not be carried out, mechanical suction being used wherever possible. If this is not available, protected mouth-operated suction devices with an appropriate barrier may be used. Gloves should be worn when handling all newborn infants until they have been cleansed of maternal blood and amniotic fluid. When sampling cord blood, the umbilical cord should not be bled directly into a tube. Needles and syringes should be used, taking care to avoid needlestick injury which is more likely to occur if the cord is held between finger and thumb rather than employing such instruments as sponge-holding forceps to isolate and steady the cord. When examining and handling the placenta, care must be taken to avoid splashing blood. Gloves, gown and face protection should be worn for this procedure.

IMMUNIZATION AGAINST HBV

In 1993, UK Health Department recommendations for protecting health-care workers and patients from HBV and HIV infections were published[48]. These recommendations emphasized the importance of ensuring that all HCWs carrying out exposure-prone procedures (EPPs) (see below), including surgeons, nurses and midwives, as well as students, should be vaccinated against HBV and their immunity checked. Those failing to respond to HBV vaccine should be further immunized. Consent should also be obtained for further testing to distinguish non-responders from HBV carriers.

EPPs are those where there is a risk that injury to the worker may result in the exposure of the patient's open tissue to the blood of the worker. These procedures include those where the worker's gloved hands may be in contact with sharp instruments, needle tips and sharp tissues (spicules of bone and teeth) inside a patient's open body cavity, wound or confined anatomical space where the hands or fingertips may not be completely visible at all times.

Procedures where the hands and fingertips are visible and outside the body at all times, and internal examinations or procedures that do not require the use of sharp instruments, are not considered to be exposure prone provided routine infection control procedures are adhered to at all times, including the wearing of gloves as appropriate and the covering of cuts or open skin lesions on the worker's hands. Examples of such procedures include the taking of blood, setting up and maintaining IV lines, minor surface suturing, the incision of abscesses or uncomplicated endoscopies.

A recent addendum to UK Department of Health guidelines[50] recommends that those involved in EPPs who have not been vaccinated, for example those who have recently arrived from HBV-endemic countries, should be tested for HBsAg and, if positive, for 'e' markers prior to being permitted to carry out EPPs. If negative, they may be given an accelerated course of hepatitis B vaccine (0, one and two months) with a booster at one year. It is also recommended that, as some HBeAg/anti-HBe assays are unreliable, those who are HBsAg positive should be tested for 'e' markers by two laboratories conducting different commercially available assays before deciding on the future work practices of HCWs involved in EPPs.

When the 1993 guidance was published, no outbreaks associated with HBsAg-positive HCWs who were not 'e' antigen positive had been reported. Consequently, those without 'e' markers were permitted to undertake EPPs unless they had been shown to transmit infection occupationally. However, six episodes of transmission from HBeAg-negative surgeons to patients have now occurred. Of the four that have been published [33], two cases involved obstetric or gynaecological procedures. Only one of the surgeons was positive for HBV DNA by liquid hybridization or dot-blot tests although all were positive by PCR. Subsequent investigations showed that all the surgeons carried a precore mutant with a premature precore stop codon mutation at position 28. These findings emphasize the importance of conducting further research, the results of which may be of value in identifying HCWs who are at risk of transmitting infection when performing EPPs, so that guidelines can be amended accordingly.

THE INFECTED HCW

HIV-infected HCWs must seek appropriate expert medical and occupational health advice. Those involved in the clinical care of patients should be under regular health supervision.

In the UK HCWs who are either HBeAg- or HIV-positive must not carry out EPPs.

The final decision about the type of work that may be undertaken by an infected HCW should be made on an individual basis, taking into account the specific working practices of the worker concerned.

Normal vaginal delivery in itself is not an EPP. However, when undertaking a vaginal delivery, infected HCWs must not perform procedures involving the use of sharp instruments such as infiltrating local anaesthetic or the suturing of a repair or episiotomy, nor can they perform an instrumental delivery requiring forceps or suction since these may need an episiotomy and subsequent repair. In practice, this means an infected HCW may only undertake a vaginal delivery if it is certain that a second midwife or doctor will also be present during the delivery and will be able to undertake all such operative interventions as might arise during the course of the delivery. This has important implications for the issue of confidentiality for an infected HCW.

A UK Advisory Panel for HCWs with bloodborne virus infection has been established to provide further advice to occupational or personal physicians about what activities the worker may or may not undertake. It is essential that the anonymity of the referred HCW is protected.

Look-back exercises may have to be carried out and attempts should be made to determine when HIV-infected HCWs were infected. If this information is not available, it is recommended that patients who have undergone EPPs during the last five years be informed. However, the decision as to how far back a look-back exercise should go should be taken in consultation with the Director of Public Health, taking into account individual circumstances and relevant epidemiological information [18].

In the USA there is no automatic prohibition of HIV- or HBeAg-positive HCWs performing EPPs. CDC guidelines put the onus on individuals and state that HCWs who carry out EPPs should determine their HIV and HBeAg status and, if infected, should not perform such procedures unless they have sought counsel from an expert review panel and been advised under what circumstances, if any, they may continue to perform these procedures. Such circumstances would include notifying prospective patients of the HCW's seropositivity before they undergo

EPPs[51]. Federal legislation requires that States adopt either the CDC recommendations or some equivalent measures. There is, however, considerable variability among States that have adopted their own guidelines, with some, for example New York and Michigan, not preventing HIV-positive workers from practising.

MANAGEMENT OF PERCUTANEOUS EXPOSURE OF HCWs EXPOSED TO BLOODBORNE VIRUS INFECTIONS

In the UK the risk of occupational exposure to and transmission of HBV should have been reduced considerably following the recommendations for immunization against the virus. All HCWs who perform EPPs should by now have been immunized and tested[50], although a report of a study conducted in 1994, one year after the UK recommendations were published, revealed that only 59% of surgeons in an inner-London teaching hospital had documented immunity to HBV[24]. Those who fail to respond to vaccination should not be prevented from carrying out EPPs but, following a high-risk incident, should be given passive protection with hepatitis B immunoglobulin, preferably within 48 h. New hepatitis B vaccines appear to be promising, producing responses in some of those who fail to respond to currently available vaccines[52].

Source patients should be tested following high-risk incidents and, if the source patient is HBsAg positive, a booster dose may be given to those who have been previously vaccinated successfully and active/passive immunization to HCWs who have not responded to vaccination.

No vaccine is available for hepatitis C and, in the event of a sharps injury, the source patient should be tested for evidence of HCV infection. If negative, the HCW should be tested at six months for HCV antibodies since there is a small risk that the source patient, although infected, may not as yet have developed an antibody response. In the event of the source patient being anti-HCV antibody positive the HCW should be tested for HCV antibodies at three and six months. If transmission has occurred, consideration should be given to treatment with α-interferon which has been shown to reduce HCV RNA levels in chronic HCV infection[54]. However, there is no evidence that interferon is of any value when used as post-exposure prophylaxis (PEP) and such use should be discouraged[55].

For HIV infections, it is important to provide reassurance that even percutaneous exposure carries a low risk of infection. No vaccine is as yet available but the findings of an American case control study indicate that if zidovudine is given as soon as possible after exposure, it reduces the risk of infection by 79%[30]. The UK Health Departments[56] now recommend that, after appropriate counselling relating to the risk of infection and the potential side effects of drugs, zidovudine together with two additional antiretroviral drugs (currently lamivudine and indinavir) should be recommended since not only may the source patient be infected with a zidovudine-resistant strain but the combined use of three drugs may be more effective in reducing viral load in the HCW, thereby improving prognosis should infection occur. To be most effective, PEP should be commenced as soon as possible after the incident and ideally within the hour (although a longer interval may not be a contraindication to starting treatment). Whenever possible, but only following consent, the source patient should be tested for HIV although it may be necessary to start chemotherapy prior to the result being available. In the event of the source patient being HIV-positive, at least six months should elapse after cessation of PEP before a negative antibody test is used to reassure the individual that infection has not occurred.

Note that UK guidelines do not say that any restriction should be placed on a HCW's work practices if the source patient of a needlestick incident is HIV positive. (This, of course, assumes that evidence of transmission to the HCW does not emerge.)

REFERENCES

1. Zuckerman, A.J. and Harrison, T.J. (1995) Hepatitis viruses. In: *Principles and Practices of Clinical Virology*, 3rd edn, (eds A.J. Zuckerman, J.E. Banatvala and J.R. Pattison), John Wiley, Chichester

2. Van Damme, P., Tormans, G., Beutels, P. and van Doorslaer, E. (1995) Hepatitis B prevention in Europe: a preliminary economic evaluation. *Vaccine*, **13**(suppl 1), S54–S57.

3. Kelen, G.D., Green, G.B., Purcell, R.H. *et al.* (1992) Hepatitis B and hepatitis C in emergency department patients. *N. Engl. J. Med.*, **326**, 1399–1404.

4. Chrystie, I.L., Sumner, D., Palmer, S.J. *et al.* (1992) Screening of pregnant women for evidence of current hepatitis B infection: selective or universal? *Health Trends*, **24**, 13–15.

5. Boxall, E. (1996) Vaccination of newborn at risk. In: *Prevention of Hepatitis B in the Newborn, Children and Adolescents*, (ed. A.J. Zuckerman), Royal College of Physicians of London, London.

6. Alter, M.J. (1993) The detection, transmission, and outcome of hepatitis C virus infection. *Infect. Agents Dis.*, **2**, 155–166.

7. Tibbs, C. (1995) Methods of transmission of hepatitis C. *J. Viral Hepatitis*, **2**, 113–119.

8. Boxall, E., Skidmore, S., Evans, S. *et al.* (1994) The prevalence of hepatitis B and C in an antenatal population of various ethnic origins. *Epidemiol. Infect.*, **113**, 523–528.

9. Zanetti, A.R., Tanzi, E., Paccagnini, S. *et al.* (1995) Mother-to-infant transmission of hepatitis C virus. Lombardy Study Group on Vertical HCV Transmission. *Lancet*, **345**, 289–291.

10. Jarvis, L.M., Davidson, F., Hanley, J.P. *et al.* (1996) Infection with hepatitis G virus among recipients of plasma products. *Lancet*, **348**, 1352–1355.

11. Feucht H.H., Zöllner, Polywka S. and Laufs R. (1996) Vertical transmission of hepatitis G. *Lancet*, **347**, 615–616.

12. World Health Organisation (1996) AIDS data as at 30th June 1996. *Wkly Epidemiol Record*, **71**, 205–208.

13. Unlinked Anonymous HIV Seroprevalence Monitoring Programme in England and Wales (1995) *Updated Report from the Unlinked Anonymous HIV Serosurveys Steering Group*, Department of Health, London.

14. Posnansky, M.C., Walters, J., Cruikshank, A. *et al.* (1996) The rising prevalence of HIV-1 infection in patients attending an inner city accident and emergency department. *J. A & E Med.*, **13**, 424–425.

15. Unlinked Anonymous HIV Seroprevalence Programme in England and Wales (1996) *Survey of Antenatal Clinic Attenders – Results to June 1995*. Department of Health, London.

16. Donegan, S.P., Steger, K.A., Recla, L. *et al.* (1992) Seroprevalence of human immunodeficiency virus in parturients at Boston City Hospital: implications for public health and obstetric practice. *Am. J. Obstet. Gynecol.*, **167**, 622–629.

17. Krasinski, K., Borkowsky, W., Bebenroth, D. and Moore T. (1988) Failure of voluntary testing for human immunodeficiency virus to identify infected parturient women in a high-risk population. *N. Engl. J. Med.*, **318**, 185.

18. O'Shea, A., de Ruiter, J., Muller, K. *et al.* (1997) Quantification of HIV-1 RNA in cervicovaginal secretions: an improved method of sample collection. *AIDS*, **11**, 1956–1958.

19. Abe, K. and Inchauspe, G. (1991) Transmission of hepatitis C by saliva. *Lancet*, **337**, 248.

20. Heptonstall, J., Porter, K. and Gill, N.O. (1995) *Occupational Transmission of HIV. Summary of Published Reports – December 1995*. Communicable Disease Surveillance Centre, UK

21. Chamberland, M.E., Ciesielski, C.A., Howard, R.J. *et al.* (1995) Occupational risk of infection with human immunodeficiency virus. *Surg. Clin. North Am.*, **75**, 1057–1070.

22. Montecalvo, M.A., Jorde U., Wuest D. *et al.* (1993) Seroprevalence of HIV-1, HBV and HCV among surgical patients. 33rd Interscience Conference on Antimicrobial Agents and Chemotherapy, New Orleans, abstract **622**, p. 232.

23. Tokars, J.L., Chamberland, M.E., Schable, C.A. *et al.* (1992) A survey of occupational blood contact and HIV infection among orthopedic surgeons. *JAMA*, **268**, 489–494.

24. Smith, E.R., Tilzey, A.J. and Banatvala, J.E. (1996) Hepatitis B vaccine uptake among surgeons at a London teaching hospital: how well are we doing? *Ann. Roy. Coll. Surg. England*, **78**, 447–449.

25. Shapiro, C.N. (1995) Occupational risks of infection with hepatitis B and hepatitis C virus. Prevention of transmission of blood borne pathogens. *Surg. Clin. North Am.*, **75**, 1047–1056.

26. Panlilio, A.L., Shapiro C.N., Schable C.A. *et al.* (1995) Serosurvey of human immunodeficiency virus, hepatitis B, and hepatitis C infection among hospital based surgeons. Serosurvey Study Group. *J. Am. Coll. Surg.*, **180**(1), 16–24.

27. Collins, M. and Heptonstall J. (1994) Occupational acquistion of acute hepatitis B infection by health care workers: England and Wales 1985–1993. *Commun. Dis. Rep.*, **4**(12), R153–155.

28. Zuckerman, J., Clewley, G., Griffiths, P. *et al.* (1994) Prevalence of hepatitis C antibodies in clinical health-care workers. *Lancet*, **343**, 1618–1620.

29. Panlilio, A.L., Foy D.R., Edwards J.R. *et al.* (1991) Blood contacts during surgical procedures. *JAMA*, **265**, 1533–1537.

30. Centers for Disease Control (1995) Case Control study of HIV seroconversion in health-care workers after percutaneous exposure to HIV-infected blood – France, United Kingdom, and United States, January 1988–August 1994. *MMWR* **44**, 929–933.

31. Harpaz, R., von Siedlen, L., Averhoff, E.M. *et al.* (1994) Transmission of hepatitis B virus from a thoracic surgeon to patients. *Infect. Control Hospital Epidemiol.*, **15**, 532 (abstract).

32. Welch, J., Webster, M., Tilzey, A.J. *et al.* (1989) Hepatitis B infections after gynaecological surgery. *Lancet*, **1**, 205–207.

33. Incident Investigation Team and others (1997) Transmission of hepatitis B to patients from four infected surgeons without hepatitis B e antigen. *N. Engl. J. Med.*, **336**, 178–184.

34. Esteban, J.L., Gomez, J., Martell, M. *et al.* (1996) Transmission of hepatitis C virus by a cardiac surgeon. *N. Engl. J. Med.*, **334**, 555–560.

35. Communicable Disease Surveillance Centre (1995) Hepatitis C virus transmission from health care worker to patient. *Commun. Dis. Rep.*, **5**(26), 1.

36. Centers for Disease Control (1995) *Report of the Expert Group on the Blood Transfusion Service.* Government of Ireland, Dublin.

37. Power, J.P., Lawlor, E., Davidson, F. *et al.* (1995) Molecular epidemiology of an outbreak of infection with hepatitis C virus in recipients of anti-D immunoglobulin. *Lancet*, **345**, 1211–1213.

38. Centers of Disease Control (1991) Update: transmission of HIV infection during an invasive dental procedure, Florida. *MMWR*, **40**, 21–27.

39. Ciesielski, C.A., Marianos, D.W., Schochetman, G. *et al.* (1994) The 1990 Florida dental investigation: the press and the science. *Ann. Intern. Med.*, **121**, 886–888.

40. Bond, W.W., Favero, M.S., Petersen, N.J. *et al.* (1981) Survival of hepatitis B virus after drying and storage for one week. *Lancet*, **1**, 550.

41. Report of the Working Party of the Royal College of Pathologists (1995) *HIV and the Practice of Pathology.* Royal College of Pathologists London.

42. Allander T., Gruber, A., Naghavi, M. *et al.* (1995) Frequent patient-to-patient transmission of hepatitis C virus in a haematology ward. *Lancet*, **345**, 603–607.

43. Chant, K., Lowe, D., Rubin, G. *et al.* (1993) Patient-to-patient transmission of HIV in private surgical consulting rooms. *Lancet*, **342**, 1548–1549.

44. Blank, S., Simonds, R.J., Weisfuse, I. *et al.* (1994) Possible nosocomial transmission of HIV. *Lancet*, **344**, 512–514.

45. Nduati, R.W., John, G.C. and Kreisi, J. (1994) Post natal transmission of HIV-1 through pooled breast milk. *Lancet*, **334**, 1432.

46. Corcoran, G.D., Brink, N.S., Millar, C.G.M. *et al.* (1994) Hepatitis C virus infection in haemodialysis patients: a clinical and virological study. *J. Infect.*, **28**, 279–285.

47. Velendia, M., Fridkin, S.K., Cardenas, V. *et al.* (1995) Transmission of HIV in a dialysis center. *Lancet*, **345**, 1417–1422.

48. Department of Health (1993) *HSG(93)40: Protecting Health Care Workers and Patients from Hepatitis B.* Department of Health, London.

49. RCOG Working Party (1997) *HIV Infection in Maternity Care and Gynaecology.* RCOG, London.

50. Department of Health (1996) *Addendum to HSG(93)40: Protecting Health Care Workers and Patients from Hepatitis B.* Department of Health, London.

51. Centers for Disease Control (1991). Recommendations for preventing transmission of human immunodeficiency virus and hepatitis B virus to patients during exposure-prone invasive procedures. *MMWR*, **40**(RR-8), 1–9.

52. Zuckerman, J.N., Sabin, C., Craig, F.M., Williams, A. and Zuckerman, A.J. (1997) Immune response to a new hepatitis B vaccine in health care workers who had not responded to standard vaccine: randomised double blind dose-response study. *Br. Med. J.*, **314**, 329–333.

53. Howard, R.J., Fry, D.E., Davis, J.M. *et al.* and the Surgical Infection Society (1997) Hepatitis C virus infection in healthcare workers. *J. Am. Coll. Surgeons*, **184**, 540–552.

54. Di Bisceglie, A.M. (1998) Hepatitis C. *Lancet*, **351**, 351–355.

55. Centers for Disease Control (1997) Recommendations for follow-up of health-care workers after occupational exposure to hepatitis C virus. *MMWR*, **46**, 603–606.

56. DoH (1997) *Guidelines on Post-exposure Prophylaxis for Health Care Workers Occupationally Exposed to HIV*. Stationery Office, London.

D.J. McCance

INTRODUCTION

Human papillomaviruses (HPV) are small double-stranded DNA viruses which cause both benign and malignant lesions mainly on stratified squamous epithelial or mucosal surfaces. Some types are associated with squamous cell carcinoma on cutaneous skin, but usually in individuals who are immunocompromised either through therapeutic means or because of some inherited genetic trait. There are numerous HPV types, of which over 20 infect the genital tract of both males and females. In fact, while most of the clinical research has been carried out on women, these viruses infect both sexes with equal frequency, although malignant disease in males is much less frequent.

This chapter will discuss the molecular biology of HPV in a simplified form, the evidence for the role of certain HPV types in the aetiology of lower genital tract cancers, in particular cancer of the cervix, and new and potentially exciting measures of prevention through vaccination.

Papillomavirus particles are 50–55 nm in diameter with an icosahedral capsid made of two proteins: L1, the major capsid protein, and L2, a minor component. Contained within the capsid is a double-stranded DNA molecule of approximately 8000 base pairs in length, which codes for eight proteins (Figure 12.1). Some of the functions of the proteins are known, but the complete picture of the pathogenetic pathways of the virus is far from clear. The virus infects and is confined to the epithelial layer of the skin and stratified epithelial surfaces. The fact that it replicates in apparently dead or dying keratinocytes is the antithesis of what one would expect since this virus relies, as do most viruses, on the cell's replicative machinery for its own propagation. Therefore the virus needs to alter the normal process of programmed differentiation observed in keratinocytes. The next few sections will deal with some ideas on how the virus achieves its ability to replicate and will describe known functions of the viral proteins involved. First, the mechanism of replication will be briefly described.

EARLY VIRAL PROTEINS: PROPERTIES AND FUNCTIONS

PROTEINS INVOLVED IN VIRAL DNA REPLICATION

It is only recently that propagation of the virus has been accomplished *in vitro* by transfection of human keratinocytes with the HPV-31b genome and subsequent differentiation of the cells using the raft culture system[1]. Briefly, in the raft culture method[2], keratinocytes are grown on a collagen gel and the gel and cells are placed on a support so that the cells

Viral Infections in Obstetrics and Gynaecology. Edited by D.J. Jeffries and C.N. Hudson. Published in 1999 by Arnold, ISBN 0 340 74095 7.

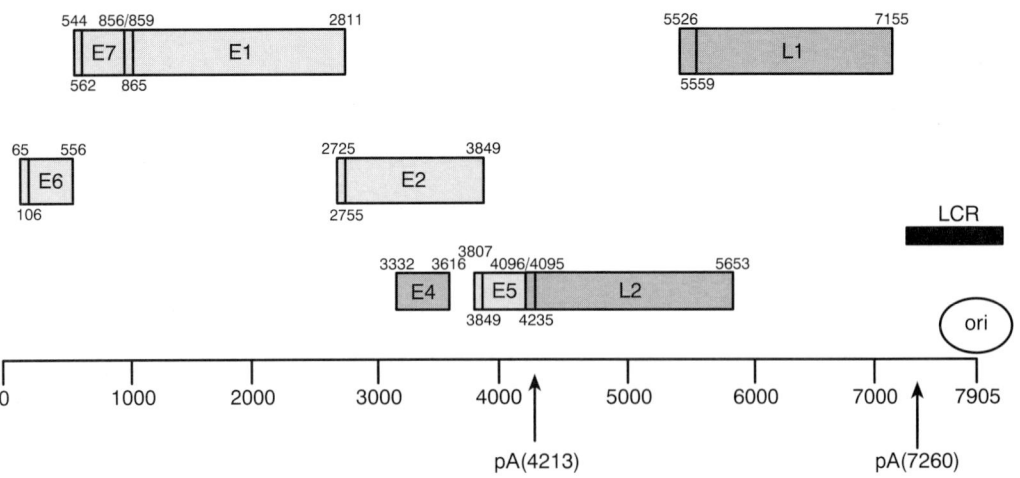

Figure 12.1 Genomic organization of HPV16 is shown and although it is represented as a linear genome for convenience, it should be remembered that the viral DNA is circular. The early genes are labelled E and the late capsid coding genes as L. The number below each of the reading frames is the position of the first ATG (start codon). LCR is long control region and it contains most of the major promoter for HPV16 at p97 and many different cellular transcription binding sites (see Figure 12.6), and also the origin of replication (ori).

are at an air–liquid interface and this allows stratification and differentiation of the cells. The differentiation observed is on a par with that seen *in vivo* as observed by various biochemical markers. The virus appears to need some components of the differentiating or partially differentiating cells to complete its replicative cycle, while at the same time requiring the host cell's replicative machinery, which would normally not be present in differentiating cells. While complete replication has been observed, the efficiency is low and few virus particles are produced[1].

All our knowledge of HPV DNA replication comes from studies in non-differentiating, dividing monolayer cells using a transient assay. This assay entails the transfection of cells with a plasmid carrying the viral origin of replication, plus plasmids carrying virally coded proteins which act in *trans* to replicate the origin-containing plasmid (Figure 12.2). Two viral proteins, E1 and E2 (Figure 12.1), are known to be involved in the replication of HPV[3,4,5]. Both are considered early pro-

teins, meaning that they are synthesized early in infection before viral replication begins. The E2 protein inhibits viral transcription from the viral promoter[6] and its function was initially unclear until it was shown to bind to E1 and be necessary for HPV genome replication[7,8]. E2 binds to a consensus sequence $ACCN_6GGT$, which occurs a number of times in the non-coding region of the HPV genome. This sequence is also found at the origin of replication and is an important *cis*-acting element (Figure 12.3). E1 is a 69 kDa protein which has at least two enzymatic activities, namely ATPase and helicase activity[9,10]. The helicase activity is necessary for unwinding the two DNA strands of the helix so that new complementary strands can be sequenced and the ATPase activity supplies the energy necessary. E1 also binds to the origin (Figure 12.3), although this interaction is weak in the absence of E2[5,10]. In the presence of E2, E1 binds more efficiently to the origin[11] and at present the main functional activity of the E2 protein is thought to be that

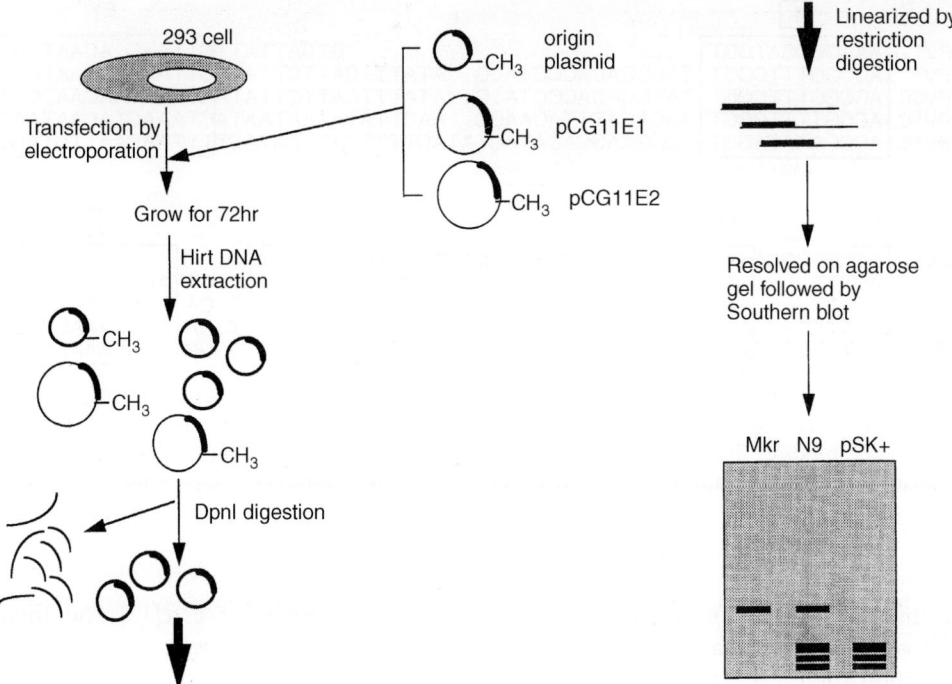

Figure 12.2 Schematic representation of the method used in the transient replication assay. 293 cells are transfected with three plasmids, one containing the origin of replication of HPV11 (N9) and two plasmids coding for HPV11 E1 (pCG11E1) and E2 (pCG11E2). After various times up to 4 days later, low molecular weight DNA is extracted by the Hirt method and the DNA digested with *Dpn*-1. This enzyme only cuts methylated DNA, i.e. bacteria-derived DNA and therefore any remaining in-put DNA. The rest of the DNA, i.e. that replicated in 293 cells and *Dpn*-1 resistant, is cut with a one-cut enzyme to produce linear molecules, which are then run on a gel, Southern blotted and hybridized with plasmid DNA to visualize the replicated origin N9.

E2 binding site	E1 binding site	Poly A tract	E2 binding site	E2 binding site

ACCGGTTTCGG TTACCCACACCCTACATATTTCCTTCTTAT ACTTAATAACAATCTTAG TTT AAAAAA GAGGAGGG ACCGAAAACGGT TCA ACCGAAAACGGT

Figure 12.3 Origin of replication of HPV11 indicating the important *cis*-acting elements, discussed more fully in the text.

of a facilitator to help the binding of E1. The fact that replication of HPV DNA *in vitro* is dependent only on the presence of E1 where there is an excess of the protein supports the notion that E2 is not directly involved in replication[12,13].

The origin of replication of all HPVs so far sequenced is very similar and contains binding sites for both E1 and E2 (Figure 12.4). In all HPVs sequenced to date, there are three E2-binding sites (E2BS), which are on either side of a stretch of DNA which contains the E1-binding site (E1BS), while bovine papillomavirus type 1 (BPV1) contains only two E2BS at each side of the E1BS (Figure 12.4). Other elements which are necessary for efficient replication but not essential are also found near the E1BS. One such element is the

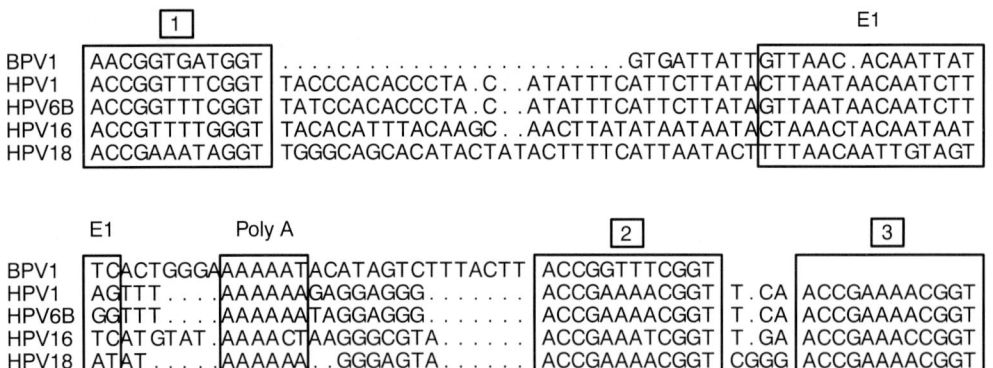

Figure 12.4 Comparison of the origins of replication of BPV1 and four HPV types 11, 6B 16 and 18. It is clear that there is conservation of the origin elements such as the three E2BS (1,2,3) in HPV. BPV1 has only two E2 binding sites. All viruses contain a poly A tract, which suggests that it has an important function, although it is not essential in experimental situations.

poly A tract (Figure 12.3) which, because of its relative instability, may be a convenient site of action for the E1 helicase to separate the two DNA strands. It should be remembered that while the poly A tract may not be essential in experimental assays, in natural infection its utility may be more obvious. The main *cis*-acting elements are the E2BS and the E1BS. The E2BS are absolutely essential for *in vivo* replication, while the E1BS is not necessary but greatly increases efficiency of replication[5]. Since both proteins are necessary for replication, why is the E1BS not essential? It appears that because E1 and E2 form a complex and that this can occur in the absence of the E1BS, this accounts for the observations. In naturally infected tissue it has not been possible to detect E1 by immunohistochemistry and so it is assumed to be produced in very small amounts. In addition, even in cells transfected with a vector containing E1, expression of E1 is difficult to detect. On the other hand, E2 has been detected *in vivo* and in cell culture. Therefore the present thinking is that E2 recruits E1 to the origin where it will bind to the E1BS and initiate replication with its helicase and ATPase activity. E1 has also been shown to bind DNA polymerase α[10] and therefore, as well as having enzymatic activities, will help recruit the cell's replicative machinery to the viral origin.

PROTEINS INVOLVED IN PROGRESSION THROUGH THE G1 PHASE OF THE CELL CYCLE

The three early proteins E6, E7 and E5 each have transforming properties observed in experimental situations, but their role *in vivo* is primarily to create an environment in which replication can proceed. As mentioned earlier, the virus replicates in the upper part of the stratified epithelium. The cells in this area would usually be terminally differentiated and would not possess the replicative machinery required by the virus. Therefore the virus has to stimulate the cells to move into the synthesis phase of the cell cycle and E6, E7 and E5 are instrumental in this process. While they will be discussed separately, they act together to stimulate keratinocytes and facilitate HPV DNA replication. These proteins act mainly in the G1 phase of the cell cycle to stimulate the cell's passage through G1 into S phase.

Activities of E6

The E6 protein is 158 amino acids long with a molecular weight of 18 kDa and is found in both the nucleus and cytoplasm of cells. It is a multifunctional protein with a number of biological properties which include the ability to transactivate certain promoters, bind to at least three cellular proteins (p53, E6AP and E6BP) and, in cooperation with E7, immortalize primary human keratinocytes. Structurally, E6 has two zinc fingers formed between four cys-x-x-cys (c-x-x-c) motifs (Figure 12.5a), which must be intact for full biological activity. Apart from the full-length E6 there are three forms of E6 which can be produced from the small reading frame by alternative splicing: E6*I, E6*II and E6*III. The biological relevance of these other forms is unclear but

the function of some of them, at least, may be to allow the more efficient translation of E7 from a polycistronic message which contains upstream E6, although a recent paper would suggest that this is not the case[14].

Unlike E7, E6 does not immortalize primary human keratinocytes on its own, but will cooperate with E7 to immortalize cells at a higher rate than E7 alone. E6 does, however, immortalize human primary mammary epithelial cells[15] although there is no suggestion that HPV types are involved in mammary cancers. E6 binds to p53 through its interaction with the cellular protein E6AP[16]. This latter protein is an ubiquitin ligase and is part of the ubiquitin proteolysis pathway in cells. The result of the complex formation is that p53 is targeted to this proteolytic pathway and degraded more readily in the presence of

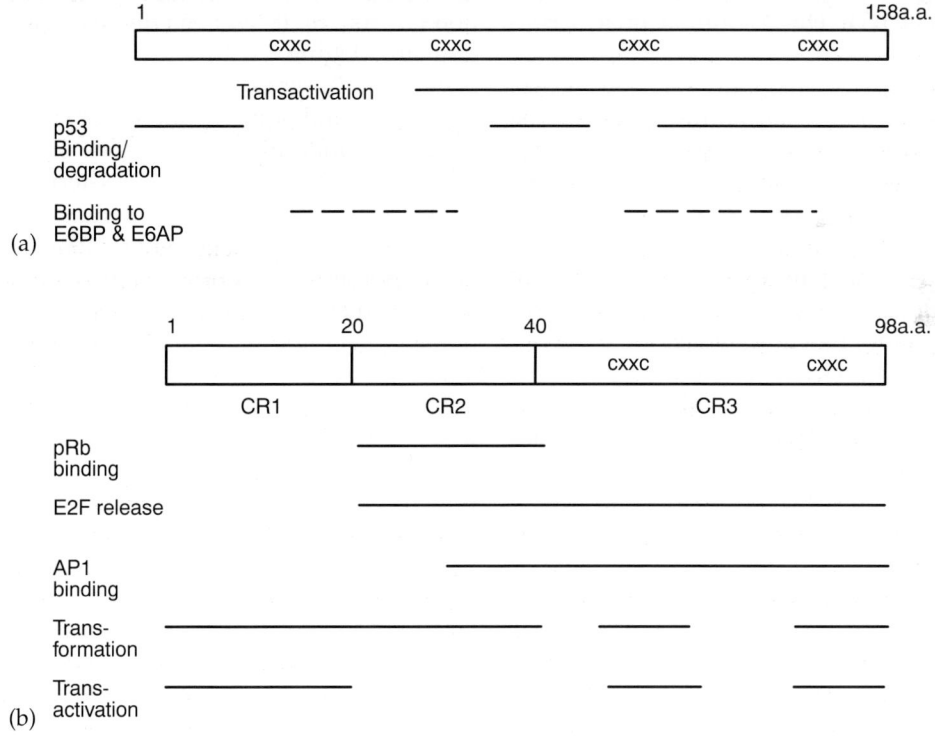

Figure 12.5 (a) Schematic representation of the domains of HPV16 E6. The lines next to each property indicate the region of E6 important for that function or where point mutations have disrupted that function. (b) Schematic representation of the domains of HPV16 E7.

E6[17]. It appears that only the E6 from oncogenic types causes degradation, although there is some controversy as to whether E6 from the non-oncogenic types can bind p53. In addition, there are discrepancies between the results of two research groups with regard to the regions of HPV16 E6 involved in degradation of p53. One holds that the C-terminal region between amino acids 106 and 110 is involved in binding and that an N-terminal domain (around amino acids 45–49) is important for degradation[18]. However, another study group[19] observes that the binding and degradation functions cannot be uncoupled and shows that several mutations and deletions throughout the protein inhibit binding and also degradation. Both groups used similar *in vitro* binding and immunoprecipitation assays to monitor binding and degradation, although Foster *et al.*[19] confirmed their findings with some *in vivo* assays for the amounts of p53. The resolution of this controversy is awaited.

p53 can transcriptionally activate genes whose promoters have binding sites for the protein. HPV16 E6 will suppress the transactivation ability of p53, and E6 mutations which allow binding of p53, but do not cause degradation, still retain the inhibitory function[20]. A similar result was observed with HPV18 E6[21]. E6 also has an independent transactivation function which is observed with the adenovirus E2 promoter[22]. The domain responsible for this function is thought to be between amino acids 123 and 137, which is downstream of the proposed p53 binding site and suggests that this transactivational function is not coupled to degradation of p53.

p53 is important for monitoring the cell as it passes through the G1 phase of the cell cycle, and molecular insults to the cell, such as chromosome damage through ionizing radiation, increase the level of p53, resulting in inhibition of the cell's progress towards S phase. It has been likened to a molecular policeman monitoring the health of a cell

during G1 and therefore anything that abrogates the activity of p53 is likely to result in inappropriate progression in the cell cycle.

Recently E6 was found to bind to a Ca^{2+}-binding protein designated E6BP, which is identical to the calcium-binding protein ERC-55, a member of the EF superfamily of calcium-binding proteins which act as regulators of epithelial differentiation. Nothing more concrete about the biological relevance is known at this time.

Activities of E7

E7 is a 98 amino acid protein and, like E6, has several functions which include the ability to transactivate certain promoters[23], transform rodent fibroblasts[24], immortalize human keratinocytes[2] and bind to cellular proteins including the retinoblastoma protein (pRb,[25]) and the AP-1 family of transcription factors[26]. It has been divided into three domains (Figure 12.5b) which are conserved between HPV types, both oncogenic and non-oncogenic, and some of these domains have sequence similarities with regions of the E1a protein of adenoviruses. The N-terminal 19 amino acids (called the CR1 domain to compare it with the E1a protein of adenoviruses) are important for transformation and transactivation[26,27], the amino acids 20–39 (CR2 domain) are important for binding to pRb[29] and responsible for the transformation properties of E7[30,31] and finally the C-terminal domain (CR3), which forms a zinc finger conformation important for dimerization[32], is involved in transactivation[33] and other functions described below.

E7 probably has multiple roles in stimulating cells to move into synthesis. Initially it was found to bind pRb, causing the latter to release a family of transcription factors called E2F. This cellular factor can activate a number of genes which are involved in the synthesis of cellular DNA and E7 has been shown to induce DNA synthesis in quiescent fibroblasts[34]. The release of E2F and transactivation of cellular genes is normally carried out in a controlled way by the cell through the phosphorylation of the pRb protein at the G1–S boundary. However, the binding of E7 to pRb releases E2F prematurely and may result in the movement of the cell into S phase when it is metabolically unready. The binding of pRb is through a LXCXE motif in E7 in the CR2 domain although the efficient release of E2F also requires the presence of the CR3 domain. E7, like E1a, binds to other retinoblastoma-related proteins, p107 and p130, but the biological outcome of these interactions is unclear.

Recently, E7 was shown to bind the AP-1 family of transcription factors[26]. Two members of this family, c-Jun and c-Fos, are important proteins active in G1 and are known also to activate genes whose products are important in DNA synthesis. E7 binds c-Jun and activates promoters which contain an AP-1 binding site. Mutations of the cys-x-x-cys motifs (c-x-x-c; Figure 12.5b), which are responsible for the zinc finger formation, inhibit the ability of E7 to bind AP-1 factors.

Therefore, from the results of a number of studies, it is becoming clear that E7 is involved in the stimulation of the cell's DNA replicative machinery by at least two pathways involving cellular factors controlling progression through the G1 phase of the cell cycle.

Activities of E5

While E5 is not well conserved between HPV types at the amino acid level, the physicochemical properties are conserved in that all E5 proteins are extremely hydrophobic and, as a consequence, are membrane bound. Both the bovine papillomavirus type 1 (BPV1) and HPV16 E5 proteins have been shown to bind to the 16 kDa subunit of the vacuolar ATPase[35,36], which is responsible for the acidification of endosomes. The epidermal growth factor receptor (EGFR) is the major growth factor receptor on keratinocytes and,

normally, when the the epidermal growth factor (EGF) binds to the receptor it results in dimerization and autophosphorylation of the latter, after which the receptor is internalized within a few minutes by an endosome-mediated pathway. Within the cytoplasm the endosomal contents become acidified due to proton transport into the lumen by the vacuolar ATPase and the receptor and ligand dissociate and are both eventually degraded. This results in a shortlived mitogenic signal. In the presence of E5, endosomal acidification is delayed by several hours[37] and the receptors remain undegraded but active, resulting in a prolonged mitogenic stimulus[38].

The BPV1 E5 protein has been shown to bind to the platelet-derived growth factor receptor (PDGFR[39]) and to activate it in the absence of the ligand, platelet-derived growth factor (PDGF). One study has shown that the HPV16 E5 protein binds the EGFR[40] while another has not been able to confirm such an interaction[41]. No matter how this resolves, it is clear that the increased activity of the EGFR in E5-expressing cells is dependent on the ligand and no activity is observed in its absence.

The E5 protein is the major oncoprotein of BPV1 and it is able to transform a number of different fibroblastic cells[42]. On the other hand, HPV16 E5 has a weak transforming activity for rodent fibroblasts and has been shown to extend the lifespan of human primary keratinocytes but, unlike E7, is unable to immortalize these cells[38]. Therefore a major activity of E5 is to stimulate cells through its indirect effect on the EGFR. Since stimulation by EGF is known to be needed for the passage of keratinocytes through the G1 phase of the cell cycle into the synthesis phase, any augmentation may increase the rate of progression through G1.

STRUCTURAL PROTEINS

There are two proteins, L1 and L2, which make up the icosahedral structure of the papillomavirus particle or virion. L1 is the major capsid protein while L2 is the minor component of the virion. L1 alone can form an icosahedral structure in eukaryotic cells using either a vaccinia virus or baculovirus expression system[43,44]. Viewed under the electron microscope, L1 forms particles approximately the size of a complete virion which are therefore called virus-like particles (VLPs). The L2 protein can also be expressed in cells and will form a similar capsid structure with L1. Co-expression of L1 and L2 leads to a four-fold increase in the amount of VLPs formed, suggesting that L2 helps to stabilize the capsid. L2 may also function in virions to bind the genome and facilitate folding into the virion.

The importance of the VLP system is that it has been shown for the first time that there are serological differences between HPV types, even between closely related types. For instance, the L1 protein of HPV16 and -31, which share 76% identity at the amino acid level, show very little cross-reactivity serologically and HPV6 and -11, which have 92% homology, exhibit a four-fold difference in reciprocal reactivity[45]. However, if the L1 protein is not folded into an icosahedral structure then there is extensive cross-reactivity between HPV types. Therefore, serological studies to detect specific HPV infections can only be carried out using VLPs. One consequence of this new finding is that if a vaccine were to be produced using VLPs, then a number of different virus types would have to be included, since one type would not induce cross-protection. The serological cross-reactivity will be discussed at greater length when vaccines and their potential are described (p. 250).

HPV TRANSCRIPTION

The long control region (LCR) or the upstream regulatory region (URR) contains major *cis*-acting control elements which regulate the transcription and replication of HPVs

(reviewed in[46]). This region, between the end of the L1 open reading frame (ORF) and the beginning of the the E6 ORF (Figure 12.1), contains a number of binding sites for cellular transcription factors and these factors appear to be the major regulatory elements in the expression of HPV mRNA[46]. While HPV replication is confined to human keratinocytes, and this cell specificity is thought to lie with transcription regulation rather than the failure of the virus to bind and be taken up by cells, there are as yet no known cell-specific factors which can explain keratinocyte specificity and all the cellular factor binding sites consistently found in the LCR are found in many cell types in which the virus cannot replicate (Figure 12.6).

Many of the transcription factor binding sites are conserved in their position in the LCR between different HPVs, but universal areas of conservation are the three E2BS and the E1BS around the origin of replication (Figures 12.4, 12.6). There is only one virally coded protein involved in the regulation of mRNA and this protein E2 appears to down-regulate the major promoter, p97 in the case of HPV16, and decrease the level of E6 and E7 mRNA. While E2 appears to inhibit transcription from the p97 promoter, it is essential for replication of the viral DNA. One scenario is that in early infection the Sp1 factor and the TFIID factors are bound to the DNA in this region and promote transcription of the early genes, E6, E7, E1, E2 and E5 (Figure 12.6). When a critical level of E2 is reached it displaces Sp1 and the basal transcription factor machinery and binds to the E2BS. The binding of the E2 to the sites at the origin inhibits further transcription, but E2 now acts to recruit E1 to the origin and subsequently the cell replicative machinery is assembled for the start of DNA replication. This situation is similar to the SV40 large T antigen, which is involved in the inhibition of its own transcription and at critical protein levels transcription is sequestered and DNA replication commences with the help of large T antigen.

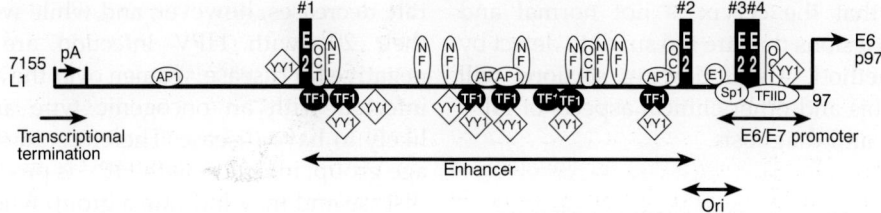

Figure 12.6 Cellular transcription factor binding sites in the LCR of HPV16, adapted from [47]. While the relative positions of some of the sites may vary between HPV types, one conserved region is the three E2BS and the one E1BS which make up the origin of replication.

However, since there are other transcription factor sites upstream of the origin, it would be a mistake to discount a role for these factors in transcription and even replication.

The major promoter is near the start of the E6 ORF, at p97 for HPV16 and -31 and at p90 for HPV11 [48,49,50]. There also appears to be a promoter in the E7 ORF for many of the mucosal viruses and this has been mapped to p674 for HPV11 and to p742 for HPV31. The exact coordinates of an E7 promoter for HPV16 have not been elucidated. In both HPV11 and -31 viruses, the E7 promoter transcribes mRNA potentially coding for both the L1 and L2 proteins. HPV transcripts are polycistronic and potentially code for up to five proteins. Two cell lines isolated from cervical lesions contain episomal copies of either HPV16 or -31 [50,51]. The major transcripts seen in undifferentiated, monolayer cultures code for E6 and E7 and also some of the spliced constructs of E6, although in one line very low levels of late transcripts capable of coding for L1 and L2 were observed [50]. When the keratinocytes were induced to differentiate using the raft system there were a number of other transcripts detected, suggesting differentiation-specific transcription [51]. Using the raft culture system, transcripts coding for early proteins were produced throughout the depth of the differentiated cells layer, while the L1 and L2 proteins were only found in the upper part of the epithelium, in a manner similar to that observed in cervical biopsies. Therefore there does appear

to be a change in the pattern of transcription on differentiation and alternative promoters utilized, but the signals and transcription factors involved are unknown.

CLINICAL DISEASES CAUSED BY GENITAL HPV

HPVs cause a variety of epithelial lesions from benign condyloma to carcinoma *in situ* and invasive cancer. The most common cancer is of the cervix, yet the virus infects many different parts of the genital tract equally well, in both males and females. The likely reason for this predilection for the cervix is the target cell. On the cervix the transformation zone is the area where intraepithelial neoplasia predominantly occurs and it is in this region where progressive disease and invasive cancers arise. This zone arises in puberty and disappears or becomes very small after the menopause and is made up of immature metaplastic cells. These cells are sensitive to external insults such as HPV infection, while in mature epithelium the infected cells are less prone to malignant conversion. The molecular reasons for this are unclear and difficult to investigate as reproducing the immature epithelium *in vitro* has not been achieved.

While HPV is readily detected in lesions, it has also been isolated from seemingly normal epithelium. Studies have shown that HPV DNA can be detected in cervical smears from a cervix that is cytologically and colposcopically normal. However, as discussed below, it is clear that the cervix is not normal and harbours lesions that are too small to detect by either method. The following sections will discuss this and other clinical aspects of HPV infection and diagnosis.

HPV INFECTION OF THE NORMAL CERVIX

HPV DNA can be detected in cervical cells from women with a normal cervix as observed by a normal smear and normal appearance of the cervix on colposcopy[52]. The rate of detection varies dramatically depending on the method used to detect the DNA, the age and demographics of the group studied. The most sensitive technique, the polymerase chain reaction (PCR), has recorded levels of 80% positivity for HPV16 in women with a normal cervix[53,54]. These results have subsequently been cast into doubt due to cross-contamination problems in the early days of PCR. It has been difficult to compare many of the studies on normal women because the subjects were of different ages, the method of testing for HPV infection was different, the women were of different socioeconomic status and the clinical definition of 'normal' varied, in that some studies have relied solely on the evidence of the cytology report and no colposcopy was carried out.

The highest detection rate is in young women and in one study of Berkeley students (mean age 22.9 years) 33% were positive for HPV DNA on the cervix, as detected by PCR[55]. The prevalence rate at both the cervix and vulva was 46%. This is one of the highest infection rates published to date. HPV types 16 and 18, which are commonly found in malignant disease, accounted for about one-third of the viruses detected, indicating that a large number of young women may be infected with HPV types which can cause malignant disease. It is clear that only a small number will ever develop disease, but recognizing those at risk is not possible at present. In older age groups (>35 years) the detection rate decreases, however, and while women in their 20s with HPV infection are mostly negative for disease, women over the age of 35 infected with an oncogenic type are more likely to have disease. Therefore, in the older age group, infection with HPV is predictive of disease and may indicate a group where HPV DNA testing would be of diagnostic value (see Diagnosis, below). It is becoming clear that there is a higher incidence of infection in the younger age groups, with up to 46% of women in their early 20s infected, but this drops to <10% in women over 40 and <5% in women over 55 years. It may be that if all women in the <25-year age group were screened by DNA testing at regular intervals over a five year period, all those who were sexually active would be HPV positive at some point, although infection and disease in the majority would be transitory.

Although the cervix is described as normal in these women by the criteria of 'no abnormal cells seen' on cytology and a normal appearance of the cervix when viewed by the colposcope, it is almost certain that the area in which the virus is replicating is histopathologically abnormal. So far, no one has shown by *in situ* hybridization the replication of HPV DNA in areas of normal tissue. Therefore, there are probably microlesions present on the cervix when someone is infected subclinically with HPV.

Serological studies, which have used nonconformational targets, have shown positive results in age groups not normally associated with sexually transmitted diseases. Using mostly bacterial fusion proteins containing various HPV-encoded proteins, groups have shown positive results for genital HPVs in various groups, including young children[56,57,58]. Because fusion proteins do not contain conformational epitopes it is not clear at present if these results represent infection with genital types such as HPV6 or 16 or cross-reactivities with cutaneous HPV types, since many proteins exhibit a high level of conservation, at least at the linear epitope level. Now that conformational epitopes are available in the form of VLPs it would be of interest to repeat such studies.

HPV AND THE ABNORMAL CERVIX

The most common genital lesion produced by HPV infection is the benign genital wart condyloma acuminatum, caused predominantly by HPV6 and 11. However, as discussed below, certain papillomaviruses also cause premalignant and malignant disease of the cervix. Warts are distributed throughout the female genital tract on the cervix, vaginal wall, vulva and perianal region. In males the lesions are found on the penis, in the perianal region, especially in homosexuals, and less often on the scrotum.

The premalignant lesions associated with HPV can arise on the same areas as described above for warts, although the cervix is where malignant conversion occurs most often. The premalignant lesions of the cervix, cervical intraepithelial neoplasia (CIN), are graded I to III in increasing order of severity with CIN III, including carcinoma *in situ*, preceding invasive cancer. Under the new Bethesda system, the nomenclature has been changed to low-grade squamous intraepithelial lesions (low SIL, previously atypias and CIN I) and high-grade SIL (previously CIN II and CIN III). HPV6 and 11 and newer isolates 42, 43 and 44 are found in low-grade SIL, while the onco-genic types, HPV16 and 18 and the less frequently found HPV 31, 33, 45 and 56, are found in all grades of SIL and, importantly, in malignant disease. Table 12.1 gives a list of viruses and their associated lesions. There are a number of additional HPV types but the full genomes have not been cloned, so they are not listed here.

As mentioned above, intraepithelial lesions of the cervix occur almost entirely on the transformation zone, which is an area of metaplastic epithelium between the mature exocervix and the columnar epithelium of the endocervical canal. Invasive cancer arises from these areas of SIL and malignant cells then migrate into the uterine stroma and out to local lymph nodes. HPV16 is the most common virus found worldwide in SIL and has been detected in 70% of cases of CIN III in Germany[60] and the United Kingdom[53] and isolated in 80% of cases of invasive cancer of the cervix. In the United States, HPV16 and 18 make up a total of 55% of high-grade SIL and over 70% of malignant disease of the cervix[61]. Epidemiology studies have shown that HPV detection is associated with a 10-fold or greater risk of CIN, while the relative risk of high-grade CIN is 40-fold[62,63].

While HPV6 and 11 have not been found in malignant disease of the cervix, they have been isolated from locally invading lesions of the vulva such as verrucous carcinoma and Buschke–Lowenstein tumours. Genomes from these lesions have been sequenced and found to have deletions and duplications in the upstream regulatory region (URR) leading to the suggestion that the rearrangements may have altered the pathogenesis[64]. However, recent evidence suggests that even HPV6 and 11 DNA from genital warts have a number of rearrangements in the URR, so it is unclear if the HPV6 and 11 DNA isolated from these locally invading lesions have an altered pathogenesis[65].

Malignant disease of the penis, while rare in industrialized countries, is much more common in resource-deprived parts of the world such as central and south America and parts of Africa. The viruses commonly associated with cervical cancer, such as HPV16 and 18, are also found in over 50% of penile cancers[65].

The incidence of HPV-negative cancers is between 5% and 10%. Interestingly, initial studies showed these cancers had mutations in pRB and p53, the two cellular proteins, which complex with the HPV proteins E7 and E6, respectively[66,67]. Therefore, it appeared that either inactivating the normal function of these two proteins by mutations or complexing with HPV proteins was an important step

Table 12.1 Genital Human Papillomavirus Types and the Site of Associated Lesions (adapted from reference[59] with help from Dr C. Wheeler)

HPV type	Associated lesion	Site
HPV6a-f	Condylomata acuminata	Vulva
		Vagina
		Cervix
		Penis:
		shaft, prepuce, urethral meatus
		Perianal
		Larynx
	CIN I–III*	Cervix
	VIN I–III†	Vulva
	PIN I–III‡	Penis
HPV11a, b	Condylomata acuminata	Vulva
		Cervix
		Perianal
		Larynx
	CIN I–III	Cervix
	PIN I–III	Penis
HPV16	Condylomata acuminata	Vulva, cervix and penis
	CIN I–III	Cervix
	VIN I–III	Vulva
	PIN I–III	Penis
	Bowenoid papulosis	Vulva and penis
	Invasive carcinoma	Cervix, vulva and penis
HPV18	CIN	
	Invasive carcinoma	Cervix and penis
HPV31	CIN	Cervix
	Invasive carcinoma	
HPV33	CIN	Cervix
	Invasive carcinoma	
HPV35	CIN	Cervix
	Invasive carcinoma	
HPV39	CIN	Cervix and penis
	PIN	
	Invasive carcinoma	
HPV40	CIN	Cervix
HPV42	CIN/VIN	Cervix and vulva
HPV43	CIN	Cervix
HPV44	CIN	Cervix
HPV45	CIN	Cervix
	Invasive carcinoma	
HPV51	CIN	Cervix
	Invasive carcinoma	
HPV52	CIN	Cervix
	Invasive carcinoma	
HPV53		Normal cervix
HPV54	Condyloma	Penis
HPV55	Bowenoid papulosis	Penis
	Condyloma	
HPV56	CIN	Cervix
	Invasive carcinoma	
HPV57	Intraepithelial neoplasia	Oral cavity, cervix
HPV58	CIN	Cervix
HPV59	VIN	Vulva
HPV61	VIN	Vulva
HPV62	VIN	Vulva
HPV64	VIN	Vulva
HPV66	Invasive carcinoma	Cervix
HPV67	CIN I	Cervix
HPV68	CIN	Cervix
	Invasive carcinoma	Cervix
HPV69	CIN	Cervix
HPV70	Condyloma	Cervix

*Cervical intraepithelial neoplasia; †Vulval intraepithelial neoplasia; ‡Penile intraepithelial neoplasia in oncogenesis. However, more extensive studies have shown that this inverse relationship was not found consistently [68,69], i.e. many HPV-negative cancers were found without mutations in p53 or pRb and a few HPV-positive cancers did have mutations in these cellular genes. Therefore, it is still not clear what other cellular factors affect disease progression and malignancy.

In both cervical and penile cancers, the HPV DNA is usually integrated into the host cell genome, whereas in premalignant lesions the viral DNA is free and unintegrated and able to produce infectious virus particles. The fact that most (90%) invasive cancers contain integrated sequences suggests that this may be a prerequisite for malignancy. While integration is random within the chromosomes the HPV DNA is integrated in the E1 and E2 regions of the genome. This particular integration state would appear to select cells for malignant conversion, since while HPVs integrate randomly, only those cells with the DNA integrated in E1 and E2 are observed in cancer tissue. There is evidence that integration in the E1 or E2 region of the genome causes an upregulation of E6 and E7 resulting from a greater stability in the mRNA coding for these proteins when a cellular rather than the viral poly A signal is used [70]. In addition, it is known that the continual expression of E6 and E7 is necessary *in vitro* to maintain the transformed phenotype, so upregulation may be one step in the malignant pathway. It has been established that integration can take place in a few cells at the premalignant phase of the disease and it is probably these cells that acquire the potential to invade [71]. However, other necessary cellular changes are unknown.

PERSISTENCE OF HPV DNA

HPVs may persist in squamous epithelial cells without producing clinically obvious lesions. Over 50% of allograft recipients develop cutaneous warts within a year of transplant-ation and it is now known that female transplant patients have a 10-fold increased risk of developing cervical cancer over age-matched controls. In addition, there is a high level of premalignant and malignant disease in individuals infected with the human immunodeficiency virus (HIV1). All this suggests that immunosuppressed patients either experience new infections or reactivate persistent virus. While both may be true, the latter is supported by the finding of HPV DNA sequences in biopsies of normal-appearing areas of larynx from individuals who have episodes of laryngeal papillomas [72] and in cells from an apparently normal cervix. Therefore if the viral DNA can persist, where is it harboured and is infectious virus produced? One consideration is the fact that the viral DNA is in a tissue which is constantly changing, with cells moving up through the stratified epithelium, differentiating and sloughing off into the vaginal vault. However, not all cells in the basal epithelium have the same capacity to divide, so the viral DNA may be sequestered in quiescent cells which, when they subsequently divide, may activate replication and produce lesions.

It is not clear whether viral persistence is a long-term situation, since in studies where individuals have been tested for the presence of HPV DNA over a period of time the isolation rate varied, with many being negative on subsequent testing, only for the viral DNA to reappear at the next testing time. This variability may depend more on the detection test used than on the levels of virus. For instance, the hybrid capture technique, which is less sensitive than PCR, gives more consistent results than those observed with PCR and because of its reduced sensitivity, is likely to detect only actively replicating virus. PCR, on the other hand, measures very low levels of DNA which may or may not indicate active infection. Therefore, the question is, do some women who have a cyclical DNA detection rate become reinfected or is the level of DNA found over a period variable? Recent evidence suggests that if the type detected is different from the original, this variation is related to the number of sexual partners of women over the testing period[63]. Those with the same sexual partner were found on subsequent testing to be negative or infected with the same HPV type. It is possible that results will show that, in most women, HPV persists for short periods of time, i.e. months, but in some, perhaps those destined to go on to develop disease, persistence may be long term, i.e. years. Whatever the case, persistence and reinfection may be due to an inadequate immune response.

The persistence of viral DNA and the nature of this persistence remains to be fully explained and does pose problems when DNA testing as a means of assessing risk of developing disease is discussed. One thing that can be said with confidence is that the least understood area of HPV biology is the natural history of infection, in particular the mechanism of persistence and some aspects of transmission, which will be considered next.

TRANSMISSION

It has been known since the early 1950s that genital warts are transmitted by sexual contact[73]. These results have been confirmed by many subsequent studies[74,75] while more recently, the sexual transmission of those viruses causing malignant disease has also been shown[76,77]. In addition, studies on the partners of women with CIN have shown that they have a high incidence of infection resulting in both benign and premalignant disease, depending on the HPV DNA type. Therefore, the sexual route of transmission is well established in adults.

Transmission to the neonate during vaginal delivery is thought to be the cause of laryngeal papillomas and may also contribute to some of the cases of genital infection seen in older children. Although children may be well into the latter part of their first decade when they first show clinical signs of HPV infection

either in the larynx or genital region, transmission at birth is a possibility since the viral DNA is known to persist. An alternative explanation for genital infections is that the child has had sexual contact. Serological studies have added to the confusion since they have indicated that children are positive for antibodies to genital HPV types. However, as stated earlier, all the studies used peptides or fusion proteins which do not have conformation epitopes as targets. These type of targets detect cross-reactive antibodies, which will interact with proteins from common non-genital HPV types such as HPV1 and 2, because of the conserved nature of the proteins. Therefore, these combined studies may not truly reflect the nature of the infecting virus. One finding which reduces non-intimate contact as a common means of transmission is that unlike lesions produced by cutaneous wart viruses, such as HPV2 which is commonly found in hand warts, the amount of infectious virus seen in genital lesions is small. Therefore, intimate and frequent contact may be necessary for infection to occur. However, we know very little about other modes of transmission, such as infection through fomites, so unless there are other suspicions of child abuse genital lesions should not automatically be assumed to be the result of sexual contact.

DIAGNOSIS

Now that the causal association between HPV infection and genital dysplasia has been confirmed, it is time to consider whether HPV DNA detection could be used as a diagnostic tool for detection of cervical lesions. Before a discussion of the type of HPV test to be used, it will be necessary to assess the need for such an approach and which group would benefit most.

The main problem with DNA testing as a diagnostic tool is the high rate of positivity in the younger age groups. Depending on the study design, the rate of infection of the cervix can be as high as 33%, with the oncogenic types accounting for one-third. In younger age groups, only 0.5 per 1000, who are HPV positive at one point in time, will have disease[78]. Therefore, DNA testing would not be cost-effective. However, at present young women are being needlessly treated, at great expense, by ablation therapy for lesions that are minor and probably transitory. This treatment can also result in psychological trauma for these young women[79]. One use of HPV testing would be to diagnose the infectious agent in those women with an abnormal smear. If they are infected with an oncogenic type this would indicate the need for treatment, but if a non-oncogenic type was found then they would be screened in a year's time. On many occasions they will be negative on subsequent testing, as it is clear that infection and disease are transitory in most cases. The aim would be to identify those we know are at risk, i.e. those infected with an oncogenic virus, even though not all will develop progressive disease.

Another situation where HPV testing may have a role is in women who are diagnosed, under the Bethesda system, as having atypical squamous cells of undetermined significance (ASCUS). Many of these women will harbour more serious disease and HPV testing may identify these women. If a non-oncogenic type was found then the women could be followed up with a smear in a year, but if an oncogenic type was identified, these women would be colposcoped, biopsied and treated if a significant lesion was present. The new cytologic technique called ThinPrep (Cytc, Boxborough, Massachusetts, USA) makes testing more convenient, because the cells from the cervix are transported to the laboratory in liquid medium and only a part is used to make a smear and the rest is stored. Therefore HPV testing can be carried out retrospectively on ambiguous cytology smears.

In older women i.e. >40 years, where the positivity rate is much lower (<5%) and where the disease rate associated with infection is higher, it may be that universal DNA testing would be cost effective[78]. Unlike the younger age groups, 10 per 1000 with HPV infection have significant disease, CIN 3 or cancer on single testing. HPV testing could be used as an adjunct to cervical screening. Therefore at present, when we know so little about other factors that act with HPV infection to promote disease, DNA testing should be limited in a way that is cost effective.

DNA HYBRIDIZATION TESTS

These tests detect specific HPV genomes in cells extracted from tissue biopsies or from cells taken as a cervical smear. At present, the most common methods used are the polymerase chain reaction (PCR) and hybrid capture but Southern blotting, considered the 'gold standard' by many, has been used, as has the dot-blot method. This chapter will cover only PCR and the hybrid capture method, because the former is the most sensitive and the latter is available in kit form.

Polymerase chain reaction

PCR is a powerful technique, which amplifies a specific piece of DNA from a small amount of template. In most cases the sequence of DNA to be amplified is known, so complementary primers can be synthesized, but it is possible to use consensus primers which will amplify all known HPV genomes, i.e. cloned and sequenced HPV DNA, as well as unknown HPV genomes. These consensus primers are made up of several different primers with nucleotide alterations in various sites along the primer. The amplified DNA fragment can then be assigned to a specific HPV type by hybridizing it with a piece of DNA that lies between the amplifying primers. Assignment to a particular type can only be done when the sequence of the HPV genome is known, while those not assigned are considered new HPV types. Therefore specific primers only amplify DNA from one particular HPV type, while consensus primers amplify all HPV types.

The great advantage of PCR is its sensitivity but this is also its major weakness. The great sensitivity means that if there is any cross-contamination of samples, the contaminating templates will be amplified as well as any DNA in the original sample. In addition, laboratories using this technique may also have bacterial cultures containing cloned HPV genomes and so aerosols containing HPV sequences will be created. Therefore, PCR should be carried out in separate rooms away from the main laboratory where no other molecular biology is being performed. Additionally, all solutions used should be made fresh and used only for PCR. Finally, positive displacement pipettes should be used for all solution manipulations. A reminder of the cross-contamination problem is provided by the first reports of the prevalence of HPV16 in cervical cells from normal individuals, when 70–80% were found to be infected. These results caused confusion in the field and led many to revise their view of the role of HPV in cervical cancer.

Another problem with PCR, related to its sensitivity, is the fact that since it can amplify from a small amount of template, it is not clear if a positive result indicates infection of cervical cells or if the cells are sloughed off from vaginal epithelium or are penile cells transferred from a partner during sexual intercourse. These problems are important if the test is intended to indicate women who are infected and, therefore, may have disease. Quantification of PCR is possible but difficult, so at present PCR does have limitations. For a review of PCR, see Innis *et al.*[80].

Hybrid capture

The hybrid capture method developed by Diagene is a sandwich capture method which detects 16 of the most common HPV types infecting the genital tract. The method detects HPV DNA in cells taken as cervical smears by hybridizing them with a cocktail of HPV RNAs supplied in the kit. The hybrids are captured by an antibody which is attached to the sides of a plastic multiwell dish and directed against DNA/RNA hybrids. The captured hybrids are then reacted with an antibody conjugated to alkaline phosphatase, the complex detected by a chemiluminescent substrate, and the intensity of light detected by a luminometer. Controls are supplied and the amount of light emitted is proportional to the amount of target DNA. This test kit is under multicentre trial by the National Cancer Institute in the USA.

TREATMENT AND PREVENTION

At present, the most effective treatment for cervical lesions is by ablation therapy. This will be discussed in the appendix to this chapter, so this section concentrates on potential vaccines, which could be used either prophylactically or therapeutically.

PROPHYLACTIC AND THERAPEUTIC VACCINES FOR HPV INFECTION

Animal studies have shown that immunization with papillomavirus-specific proteins results in protection from subsequent infection and that some of these proteins may also be used therapeutically to induce regression of existing lesions. In both cattle and rabbits, bacterial fusion proteins have been used to immunize the respective hosts prior to challenge with infectious virus[81,82]. In both cases L1 fusion proteins protected against infection. In addition, in cattle immunizations with L2 or E7 were also protective, although immunization with fusion proteins did allow lesions to develop transiently when they were challenged with live virus. Immunization with purified whole virus particles appeared to give better protection since no lesions were observed on any immunized animal on challenge[83]. The protection induced by the whole virus particle was type specific and so immunization with BPV2 did not protect against BPV4[84].

Recently, VLPs have been used to immunize rabbits and dogs against cottontail rabbit papillomavirus (CRPV)[85] and canine oral papillomavirus[86], respectively, with great success. Rabbits were immunized intramuscularly over a period of three months with monthly inoculations and then challenged two weeks to 12 months after the last dose. At two weeks there was complete protection which waned to 50% at 12 months, although the size of the lesions was greatly reduced. In a study using dogs, it was found that immunization with VLPs from canine oral papillomavirus protected dogs from oral challenge. The weekly immunizations into the footpad of the animals were carried out over a three-week period and the dogs were challenged in the mouth after abrasion with a wire brush. Only dogs immunized with either virions or VLPs were protected while those immunized with disrupted VLPs were not. This indicates that the conformational epitopes were important for protection against a virus infection. In addition, it was reassuring that parenteral inoculation protected against a local mucosal infection.

These initial results in animals, especially those with canine oral papillomavirus, bode well for studies in humans. However, it has to be remembered that using VLPs only protects against that particular virus type and so it will be necessary to use a cocktail of viruses to cover those that infect the genital region. Considering that HPV16 and -18 account for 70–80% of cervix disease in Europe and North America, the number of types to be used will be limited. Two groups of individuals could initially be studied: first, a population of individuals already infected with HPV and exhibiting disease, such as genital warts, to investigate if a vaccine made up of either the L1 protein or E7 would be therapeutic. Animal studies in cattle have shown both to induce regression. A second study would investigate a prophylactic vaccine composed of L1 to see if individuals are protected. The study group in this case would be more difficult to select, but one possible set of individuals could be college students, many of whom will be starting sexual activity on entry to university.

CONCLUSION

Epidemiological and laboratory research has shown certain HPV types to be an important component in the aetiology of genital cancers. However, there are a number of unanswered questions even on the basic natural history, such as how widespread infection is and what other modes of transmission exist, in addition to sexual contact. Also unknown are the mechanisms of action of the viral proteins and how they lead to abnormal growth of cells, resulting in inhibition of differentiation and eventually a malignant phenotype. However, the major aetiological agent is known and so, with the collaboration of epidemiologists, clinicians, basic scientists and grant-awarding bodies, these questions can be addressed.

REFERENCES

1. Frattini, M.G., Lim, H.B. and Laimins, L.A. (1996) *In vitro* synthesis of oncogenic human papillomavirus requires episomal genome for differentiation-dependent late expression. *Proc. Natl Acad. Sci. USA*, **93**, 3062–3067.
2. McCance, D.J., Kopan, R, Fuch, E. and Laimins, L.A. (1988) Human papillomavirus type 16 alters human epithelial cell differentiation *in vitro*. *Proc. Natl Acad. Sci. USA*, **85**, 7169–7173.
3. Ustav, M. and Stenlund, A. (1991) Transient replication of BPV-1 requires two viral polypeptides encoded by the E1 and E2 open reading frames. *EMBO J*, **10**, 449–457.
4. Chiang, C.-M., Ustav, M., Stenlund, A. *et al.* (1992) Viral E1 and E2 proteins support replication of homologous and heterologous papillomavirus origins. *Proc. Natl Acad. Sci. USA*, **89**, 5799–5803.
5. Lu, J, Z., Sun, Y-N., Rose, R.C., Bonnez, W. and McCance, D.J. (1993) Two E2 binding sites (E2BS) alone or one E2BS plus an A/T rich region are minimal requirements for the replication of the human papillomavirus type 11 origin. *J. Virol.*, **67**, 7131–7139.

6. Thierry, F. (1993) Proteins involved in the control of HPV transcription. *Papillomavirus Rep.*, **4**, 27–32.

7. Mohr, I.J., Clark, R, Sun, S. *et al.* (1990) Targeting the E1 replication protein to the papillomavirus origin of replication by complex formation with the E2 transactivator. *Science*, **250**, 1694–1699.

8. Blitz, I.L. and Laimins, L.A. (1991) The 68-kilodalton E1 protein of bovine papillomavirus is a DNA binding phosphoprotein which associates with the E2 transcriptional activator *in vitro*. *J. Virol.*, **65**, 649–656.

9. Yang, L., Mohr, I.J., Fouts, E. *et al.* (1993) The E1 protein of papillomavirus BPV-1 is an ATP dependent DNA helicase. *Proc. Natl Acad. Sci. USA*, **90**, 5086–5090.

10. Park, P., Copeland, W., Yang, L. *et al.* (1994) The cellular DNA polymerase α-primase is required for papillomavirus DNA replication and associates with the viral E1 helicase. *Proc. Natl Acad. Sci. USA*, **91**, 8700–8704.

11. Sun, Y-N., Lu, J-Z. and McCance, D.J. (1996) Mapping the HPV-11 E1 binding site and determination of other important cis-elements for replication of the origin. *Virology*, **216**, 219–222.

12. Yang, L., Rong, L., Mohr, I.J., Clark, R. and Botchan, M.R. (1991) Activation of BPV-1 replication *in vitro* by the transcription factor E2. *Nature*, **353**, 628–632.

13. Kuo, S-R., Liu, J-S., Broker, T.R. and Chow, L.T. (1994) Cell-free replication of the human papillomavirus DNA with homologous viral E1 and E2 proteins and human cell extracts. *J. Biol. Chem.*, **269**, 24058–24065.

14. Stacy, S.N., Jordan, D., Snijders, P.J.F. *et al.* (1995) Translation of the human papillomavirus type 16 E7 oncoprotein from bicistronic mRNA is independent of splicing events within the E6 open reading frame. *J. Virol.*, **69**, 7023–7031.

15. Band, V., Dalal, S., Delmolino, L. and Androphy, E.J. (1993) Enhanced degradation of p53 protein in HPV-6 and BPV-1 E6-immortalized human mammary epithelial cells. *EMBO J.*, **12**, 1847–1852.

16. Huibregtse, J.M., Scheffner, M. and Howley, P.M. (1993) Cloning and expression of the cDNA for E6AP, a protein that mediates the interaction of the human papillomavirus E6 oncoprotein with p53. *Mol. Cell. Biol.*, **13**, 775–784.

17. Scheffner, M., Werness, B.A., Huibregtse, J.M., Levine, A.J. and Howley, P.M. (1990) The E6 oncoprotein encoded by human papillomavirus types 16 and 18 promotes the degradation of p53. *Cell*, **63**, 1129–1136.

18. Crook, T., Tidy, J.A. and Vousden, K.H. (1991) Degradation of p53 can be targeted by HPV E6 sequences distinct from those required for p53 binding and transactivation. *Cell*, **67**, 547–556.

19. Foster, S.A., Demers, G.W., Etscheid, B.G. and Galloway, D.A. (1994) The ability of human papillomavirus E6 proteins to target p53 for degradation *in vivo* correlates with their ability to abrogate actinomycin D-induced growth arrest. *J. Virol.*, **68**, 5698–5705.

20. Lechner, M.S. and Laimins, L.A. (1994) Inhibition of p53 DNA binding by human papillomavirus E6 proteins. *J. Virol.*, **68**, 4262–4273.

21. Pim, D., Storey, A., Thomas, M., Massimi, P. and Banks, L. (1994) Mutational analysis of HPV-18 E6 identifies domains required for p53 degradation *in vitro*, abolition of p53 transactivation *in vivo* and immortalization of primary BMK cells. *Oncogene*, **9**, 1869–1876.

22. Desaintes, C., Hallez, S., van Alphen, P. and Burny, A. (1992) Transcriptional activation of several heterologous promoters by the E6 protein of human papillomavirus type 16. *J. Virol.*, **66**, 325–333.

23. Phelps, W.C., Yee, C.L., Munger, K. and Howley, P.M. (1988) The human papillomavirus type 16 E7 gene encodes transactivation and transformation functions similar to those of adenovirus E1A. *Cell*, **53**, 539–547.

24. Matlashewski, G., Schneider, J., Banks, L. *et al.* (1987) Human papillomavirus type 16 DNA cooperates with activated *ras* in transforming primary cells. *EMBO J.*, **6**, 1741–1746.

25. Dyson, N., Howley, P.M., Munger, K. and Harlow, E. (1989) The human papillomavirus-16 E7 oncoprotein is able to bind to the retinoblastoma gene product. *Science*, **243**, 934–937.

26. Antinore, M.J., Birrer, M.J., Patel, D., Nader, L. and McCance, D.J. (1996) The human papillomavirus type 16 E7 gene product interacts with and *trans*-activates the AP1 family of transcription factors. *EMBO J.*, **15**, 1950–1960.

27. Phelps, W.C., Munger, K., Yee, C.L., Barnes, J.A. and Howley, P.M. (1992) Structure–function analysis of the human papillomavirus type 16 E7 oncoprotein. *J. Virol.*, **66**, 2418–2427.

28. Brokaw, J.L., Yee, C.L. and Munger, K. (1994) A mutational analysis of the amino terminal domain of the human papillomavirus type 16 E7 oncoprotein. *Virology*, **205**, 603–607.

29. Jones, R.E., Wegrzyn, R.J., Patrick, D.R. *et al.* (1990) Identification of HPV-16 E7 peptides that are potent antagonists of E7 binding to the retinoblastoma suppressor protein. *J. Biol. Chem.*, **265**, 12782–12785.

30. Chesters, P.M., Vousden, K.H., Edmonds, C. and McCance, D.J. (1990) Analysis of human papillomavirus type 16 open reading frame E7 immortalizing function in rat embryo fibroblast cells. *J. Gen. Virol.*, **71**, 449–453.

31. Sang, B.C. and Barbosa, M.S. (1992) Single amino acid substitutions in 'low risk' human papillomavirus (HPV) type 6 E7 protein enhance features characteristic of the 'high risk' HPV E7 oncoproteins. *Proc. Natl Acad. Sci. USA*, **89**, 8063–8067.

32. McIntyre, M.C., Frattini, M.G., Grossman, S.R. and Laimins, L.A. (1993) Human papillomavirus type 18 E7 protein requires intact Cys-X-X-Cys motifs for zinc binding, dimerization, and transformation. *J. Virol.*, **67**, 3142–3150.

33. Watanabe, S., Kanda, T., Sato, H., Furuno, A. and Yoshiike, K. (1990) Mutational analysis of human papillomavirus type 16 E7 functions. *J. Virol.*, **64**, 207–214.

34. Banks, L., Edmonds, C. and Vousden, K.H. (1990) Ability of the HPV-16 E7 protein to bind RB and induce DNA synthesis is not sufficient for efficient transforming activity in NIH3T3 cells. *Oncogene*, **5**, 1383–1389.

35. Goldstein, D.J., Finbow, M.E., Andresson, T. *et al.* (1991) Bovine papillomavirus E5 oncoprotein binds to the 16K component of vacuolar H$^+$-ATPases. *Nature*, **352**, 347–349.

36. Conrad, M., Bubb, V.J. and Schlegel, R. (1993) The human papillomavirus type 6 and 16 E5 proteins are membrane-associated proteins which associate with the 16-kilodalton pore-forming protein. *J. Virol.*, **67**, 6170–6178.

37. Straight, S.W., Herman, B. and McCance, D.J. (1995) The E5 oncoprotein of human papillomavirus type 16 inhibits the acidification of endosomes in human keratinocytes. *J. Virol.*, **69**, 3185–3192.

38. Straight, S.W., Hinkle, P., Jewers, R.J. and McCance, D.J. (1993) The E5 oncoprotein of human papillomavirus type 16 transforms fibroblasts and effects the downregulation of the epidermal growth factor receptor in keratinocytes. *J. Virol.*, **67**, 4521–4532.

39. Petti, L., Nilson, L.A. and DiMaio, D. (1991) Activation of platelet derived growth factor by the bovine papillomavirus E5 transforming protein. *EMBO J.*, **10**, 845–855.

40. Hwang, E-S., Nottoli, T. and DiMaio, D. (1995) The HPV16 E5 protein: expression, detection and stable complex formation with transmembrane proteins in COS cells. *Virology*, **211**, 227–233.

41. Conrad, M., Goldstein, D., Andresson, T. and Schlegel, R. (1994) The E5 protein of HPV-6, but not HPV-16, associates efficiently with cellular growth factor receptors. *Virology*, **200**, 796–800.

42. DiMaio, D., Guralski, D. and Schiller, J.T. (1986) Translation of open reading frame E5 of bovine papillomavirus is required for its transforming activity. *Proc. Natl Acad. Sci. USA*, **83**, 1797–1801.

43. Zhou, J., Sun, X-Y., Stenzel, D.J. and Frazer, I.H. (1991) Expression of vaccinia recombinant HPV 16 Li and L2 ORF proteins in epithelial cells is sufficient for assembly of HPV virion-like particles. *Virology*, **185**, 251–257.

44. Kirnbauer, R., Taub, J., Greenstone, H. *et al.* (1993) Efficient self assembly of human papillomavirus type 16 L1 and L1-L2 into virus-like particles. *J. Virol.*, **67**, 6929–6936.

45. Rose, R.C. Personal communication.

46. Bernard, H.U. and Apt, D. (1994) Transcriptional control and cell type specificity of HPV gene expression. *Arch. Dermatol.*, **130**, 210–215.

47. O'Connor, M., Chan, S-Y. and Bernard, H-U. (1995) Transcription factor binding sites in the LCR control region of genital HPVs. In: *Human Papillomaviruses*, (eds G. Myers, H.U. Bernadt, H. Delius *et al.*), Los Alamos National Laboratory, New Mexico.

48. Smotkin, D. and Wettstein, F.O. (1986) Transcription of human papillomavirus type 16 early genes in a cervical cancer and a cancer-derived cell line and identification of the E7 protein. *Proc. Natl Acad. Sci. USA*, **83**, 4680–4694.

49. Chow, L.T., Nasseri, M., Wolinsky, S.M. and Broker, TR. (1987) Human papillomavirus types 6 and 11 mRNAs from genital condylomata acuminata. *J. Virol.*, **61**, 2581–2588.

50. Doorbar, J., Parton, A., Hartley, K. *et al.* (1990) Detection of novel splicing patterns in a HPV-16-containing cell line. *Virology*, **178**, 254–262.

51. Hummel, M., Hudson, J.B. and Laimins, L.A. (1992) Differentiation-induced and constitutive transcription of human papillomavirus type 31b in cell lines containing viral episomes. *J. Virol.*, **66**, 6070–6080.

52. McCance, D.J., Campion, M.J., Clarkson, P.K. *et al.* (1985) The prevalence of human papillomavirus type 16 DNA sequences in cervical intraepithelial neoplasia, and invasive carcinoma of the cervix. *Br. J. Obstet. Gynaecol.*, **92**, 1101–1105.

53. Young, L.S., Bevan, I.S., Johnson, M.A. *et al.* (1989) The polymerase chain reaction; a new epidemiological tool for investigating cervical human papillomavirus infection. *Br. Med. J.*, **298**, 16–18.

54. Tidy, J.A., Parry, G.C., Ward, P. *et al.* (1989) High rate of human papillomavirus type 16 infection in cytologically normal cervices. *Lancet*, **1**, 434.

55. Bauer, H.M., Ting, Y., Greer, C.E. *et al.* (1991) Genital human papillomavirus infection in female university students as determined by a PCR-based method. *JAMA*, **265**, 472–477.

56. Galloway, D.A. and Jenison, S.A. (1990) Characterization of the humoral immune response to genital papillomaviruses. *Mol. Biol. Med.*, **7**, 59–72.

57. Jenison, S.A., Yu, X., Valentine, J.M. *et al.* (1990) Evidence of prevalent genital type human papillomavirus infection in adults and children. *J. Infect. Dis.*, **162**, 60–69.

58. Cason, J., Kambo, P.K., Best, J.M. and McCance, D.J. (1992) Detection of antibodies to a linear epitope on the major coat protein (L1) of human papillomavirus type 16 (HPV-16) in sera from patients with cervical intraepithelial neoplasia and children. *Int. J. Cancer*, **50**, 349–355.

59. De Villier, E.M. (1989) Heterogeneity of the human papillomavirus group. *J. Virol.*, **63**, 4898–4903.

60. Wagner, D., Ikenberg, H., Boehm, N. and Gissmann, L. (1984) Identification of human papillomavirus in cervical swabs by deoxyribonucleic acid in situ hybridization. *Obstet. Gynecol.*, **64**, 767–772.

61. Lorincz, A.T., Reid, R., Jenson, A.B. *et al.* (1992) Human papillomavirus infection of the cervix: relative risk association of 15 common anogenital types. *Obstet. Gynecol.*, **79**, 328–337.

62. Morrison, E.A., Ho, G.Y., Vermund, S.H. *et al.* (1991) Human papillomavirus infection and other risk factors for cervical neoplasia: a case-control study. *Int. J. Cancer*, **49**, 6–13.

63. Schiffman, M. Personal communication.

64. Rando, R.F., Groff, D.E., Chirikjian, J.G. and Lancaster, W.D. (1986) Isolation and characterization of a novel human papillomavirus type 6 DNA from an invasive vulvar carcinoma. *J. Virol.*, **57**, 353–356.

65. Rubben, A., Beandenon, S., Favre, M. *et al.* (1992) Rearrangement of the upstream regulatory region of human papillomavirus type 6 can be found in both Buschke–Löwenstein tumors and in condylomata acuminata. *J. Gen. Virol.*, **73**, 3147–3153.

66. Scheffner, M., Munger, K., Byrne, J.C. and Howley, P.M. (1991) The state of p53 and retinoblastoma genes in human cervical carcinoma cell lines. *Proc. Natl Acad. Sci. USA*, **88**, 5523–5527.

67. Crook, T., Wrede, D. and Vousden, K.H. (1991) p53 point mutation in HPV negative human cervical carcinoma cell lines. *Oncogene*, **6**, 873–875.

68. Busby-Earle, R.M., Steel, C.M., Williams, A.R., Cohen, B. and Bird, C.C. (1994) p53 mutations in cervical carcinogenesis – low frequency and lack of correlation with human papillomavirus status. *Br. J. Cancer*, **69**, 732–737.

69. Park, D.J., Wilczynski, S.P., Paquette, R.L., Miller, C.W. and Koeffler, H.P. (1994) p53 mutations in HPV-negative cervical carcinomas. *Oncogene*, **9**, 205–210.

70. Jeon, S. and Lambert, P.F. (1995) Integration of human papillomavirus type 16 DNA into the human genome leads to increased stability of E6 and E7 mRNAs: implications for cervical carcinogenesis. *Proc. Natl Acad. Sci. USA*, **92**, 1654–1658.

71. Schneider-Maunoury, S., Croissant, O. and Orth, G. (1987) Integration of human papillomavirus type 16 DNA sequences: a possible early event in the progression of genital tumors. *J. Virol.*, **61**, 3295–3298.

72. Steinberg, B.M., Topp, W.C., Schneider, P.S. and Abramson, A.L. (1983) Laryngeal papillomavirus infection during clinical remission. *N. Engl. J. Med.*, **308**, 1261–1264.

73. Barrett, T.J., Silbar, J.D. and McGinley, J.P. (1954) Genital warts – a venereal disease. *JAMA*, **154**, 333–334.

74. Teokharov, B.A. (1969) Non-gonococcal infections of the female genitalia. *Br. J. Venereal Dis.*, **45**, 334–339.

75. Oriel, J.D. (1971) Natural history of genital warts. *Br. J. Venereal. Dis.*, **47**, 1–13.

76. Barrasso, R., de Brux, J., Croissant, O. and Orth, G. (1987) High prevalence of papillomavirus-associated penile intraepithelial neoplasia in sexual partners of women with cervical intra-epithelial neoplasia. *N. Engl. J. Med.*, **31**, 916–923.

77. Campion, M.J., McCance, D.J., Mitchell, M.S. *et al.* (1988) Subclinical penile human papillomavirus infection and dysplasia in consorts of women with cervical neoplasia. *Genitourin. Med.*, **64**, 90–99.

78. Schiffman, M.H. (1992) Recent progress in defining the epidemiology of human papillomavirus infection and cervical neoplasia. *J. Natl Cancer Inst.*, **84**, 394–398.

79. Campion, M.J., Brown, J.R., McCance, D.J. *et al.* (1988) Psychosexual trauma of an abnormal cervical smear. *Br. J. Obstet. Gynaecol.*, **95**, 175–181.

80. Innis, M.A., Gelfand, D.H., Sninsky, J.J. and White, T.J. (eds) (1990) *PCR Protocols: A Guide to Methods and Applications.* Academic Press, New York.

81. Jarrett, W.F.H., Smith, K.T., O'Neil, B.W. *et al.* (1991) Studies on vaccination against papillomaviruses: prophylactic and therapeutic vaccination with recombinant proteins. *Virology*, **184**, 33–42.

82. Lin, Y-L., Borenstain, L.A., Selvakumar, R., Ahmed, R. and Wettstein, F.O. (1992) Effective vaccination against papilloma development by immunization with L1 or L2 structural protein of cottontail rabbit papillomavirus. *Virology*, **187**, 612–619.

83. Jarrett, W.F.H., O'Neil, B.W., Gaukroger, J.M. *et al.* (1990) Studies on vaccination against papillomaviruses: a comparison of purified virus, tumor extract and transformed cells in prophylactic vaccination. *Veterin. Rec.*, **126**, 449–452.

84. Jarrett, W.F.H., O'Neil, B.W., Gaukroger, J.M. *et al.* (1990) Studies on vaccination against papillomaviruses: the immunity after infection and vaccination with bovine papillomaviruses of different types. *Veterin. Rec.*, **126**, 473–475.

85. Christensen, N.D., Reed, C.A., Cladel, N.C., Han, R. and Kreider, J.W. (1996) Immunization with virus like particles induces long-term protection of rabbits against challenge with cottontail rabbit papillomavirus. *J. Virol.*, **70**, 960–965.

86. Suzich, J.A., Ghim, S-J., Palmer-Hill, F.J. *et al.* (1995) Systemic immunization with papillomavirus L1 protein completely prevents the development of viral mucosal papillomavirus. *Proc. Natl Acad. Sci. USA*, **92**, 11553–11557.

Appendix: Clinical features

P. Walker

HISTORICAL BACKGROUND

Genital warts have been known since ancient times, Hippocrates (5th century BC) describes treatment for removing 'thymia' (warts) from the penis[1]. Bell[2] was the first to differentiate between the two conditions condylomata acuminata (plate K) and condylomata lata. Although vulval warts have long been recognized as a reasonably common condition, until recently cervical warts were thought to be rare. Describing a condyloma acuminatum of the cervix in 1921, Wharton wrote in a paper entitled 'Rare tumours of the cervix of the uterus of inflammatory origin – condyloma and granuloma', that 'Condyloma of the cervix is one of the rarest of gynaecological disorders . . . the cervical type is as rare as the vulval type is common'[3]. In 1952, Marsh[4] reviewed the world literature on papilloma of the cervix. He found that until that time there had been only 23 cases reported and that only eight of these could be considered condylomata acuminata.

The first real indication that cervical wart virus infection was more common came from two publications in the late 1970s. Meisels' group in Canada in 1976[5] described cytological patterns that were consistent with the diagnosis of condylomatous disease of the cervix, principally koilocytosis and dyskeratosis. In the following year[6] they reported that these changes were to be found in over 1% of a routinely screened population and in over 70% of cases that had previously been reported as mild dysplasia. The cytological findings were, in many cases, not due to exophytic condylomata acuminata but to a cervical lesion that they designated a 'flat wart', not visible to the naked eye but seen with the increased magnification available at colposcopy. Throughout the 1980s and 1990s increasing attention has been paid not only to the prevalence of human papillomavirus (HPV) infection of the female genital tract, but also the important link between HPV and cervical cancer and the possibility of a link between HPV and vulval cancer.

AETIOLOGY

Human papillomaviruses type 6 and 11 are those most frequently associated with benign condylomata acuminata of the vulva, vagina and perianal region. It is believed that minor epithelial abnormalities of the cervix (CIN I) are most usually associated with HPV6 and 11 and possibly HPV42, 43 and 44. It is the more oncogenic types HPV16 and 18 in particular and, less frequently, HPV31, 33, 45 and 56 that are found in significant disease (CIN II and CIN III and invasive cancer).

NATURAL HISTORY AND EPIDEMIOLOGY

The incubation period for this sexually transmitted disease is between three weeks and eight months with a mean of 2.8 months. Lesions first appear on areas that are subject to trauma during intercourse. In Oriel's definitive study[7] the distribution was as follows:

Urethra 8%
Vagina 15%
Perianal area 23%
Labia majora 31%
Labia minora and clitoris 32%
Fourchette 73%

Figures from the Statistical Bulletin provide information about sexually transmitted diseases reported from National Health Service genitourinary medicine clinics. In 1995 in the United Kingdom, the first attack of anogenital warts reported by females accounted for 25 047 cases. The peak age incidence was in the group aged 20–26 and accounted for 9160 cases. The total number of cases of anogenital wart virus infection in 1995, reported in both sexes, was 93 317 which represented an increase of 8% over the total for the previous year. Recurrent attacks in re-registered cases accounted for 45% of the total. Of the new cases in men, approximately 5% were reported as having been acquired through homosexual contact.

It should be remembered that many women with first-attack genital condylomata acuminata will present to general practitioners, gynaecological outpatients and, on occasions, dermatology clinics and be treated in those clinics. Such cases will not be registered within the NHS data collection system and therefore, new cases of female genital wart virus infection might reasonably be expected to be of the order of 50 000 to 75 000 new cases per annum.

Between 12% and 15% of women with vulval warts will have cervical condylomata acuminata which can be identified with the naked eye. Meisels and his group [5] described flat warts present on the cervix identifiable by colposcopy, but not visible with the naked eye. The group described fingerlike projections of epithelium, highlighted by the application of 5% acetic acid, each with a central capillary loop that they called asperites (Plates L, M). Laverty [8] described non-condylomatous wart virus infection. However, Walker *et al.*[9] demonstrated that it was not possible by colposcopy to make a distinction between those epithelial abnormalities of the cervix due to HPV infection and those due to CIN.

Clinical exophytic condylomata acuminata of the vagina are less common, but subclinical lesions can be identified at colposcopy. Perianal and anal condylomata acuminata are not infrequently found in normal women affected by HPV infection, but these areas are more frequently involved in women who are immunocompromised, either as a result of immunosuppressive drugs following transplantation or HIV infection. In the worst cases the lesions may extend up to and beyond the gluteal fold.

Subclinical HPV lesions may be identified on the vulva. The application of 5% acetic acid can reveal lesions not dissimilar to those that Meisels called asperites. However, the true significance of these vulval lesions is unclear. The subclinical lesions are rarely symptomatic and as long as a clear distinction is made between these lesions and vulval intraepithelial neoplasia, the subclinical lesions do not require treatment.

DIFFERENTIAL DIAGNOSIS

Vulval warts must be distinguished from other papular lesions of the vulva. Benign vulval tumours such as a fibroma, lipoma, hidradenoma, adenoma and endometrioma can be diagnosed if a histological biopsy specimen is taken. It is clearly important to distinguish the condyloma acuminatum of the vulval wart from the condylomata lata of syphilis. This will be made easier if a full screen for sexually transmitted diseases is carried out including serological tests for syphilis. In practical terms, in the vulva clinic an important differential diagnosis is that of vulval warts from vulval intraepithelial neoplasia (VIN). VIN is often associated with HPV infection, but VIN itself may consist of single or multiple lesions, papular or erosive, pigmented or non-pigmented. Although various terms have been used histologically to describe this condition over the years, a similar reporting system to cervical intraepithelial neoplasia is now in place, with VIN graded from 1 to 3. Studies have shown that HPV6 and 11 are frequently associated with condylomata acuminata but may also be found in VIN lesions. Indeed, high-risk viruses can be found within vulval intraepithelial neoplastic lesions. There is a hypothesis, so far unsubstantiated, that a young age of onset of a vulval carcinoma may arise from a group of women who have HPV-associated VIN lesions, whereas a different form of squamous carcinoma of the vulva may occur in an older age group associated with the background benign condition of lichen sclerosus et atrophicus.

On the cervix, condylomata acuminata that are visible to the naked eye may be better identified with the use of the colposcope and 5% acetic acid. The basic structure of the exophytic lesion is of single strands of epithelium, each with a central capillary loop coalesced into a larger mass. Subclinical asperite lesions may also be identified. An important differential diagnosis from exophytic condyloma acuminatum of the cervix is exophytic invasive cancer of the cervix. For this reason, as described later, no lesion on the cervix should be treated without prior satisfactory cervical cytology, preferably confirmed at the time by histology.

TREATMENT

VULVAL CONDYLOMATA ACUMINATA

The many therapeutic approaches to the treatment of vulval warts are testimony to the fact that no specific treatment is particularly effective.

Chemical agents

One of the most traditional treatments of vulval warts has been with the plant extract podophyllum. The agent is applied to the warts in concentrations up to 25% in compound tincture of benzoin. The patient is advised to wash the area after 6–8 hours. The clinician applying the treatment must be cautious only to treat the affected area and not the surrounding normal skin. Some patients may be fortunate enough to respond immediately to treatment, with the warts initially turning white and then falling off after a few days. However, many require recurrent treatments and even those women in whom the lesions have initially been completely eradicated may suffer later recurrences. Trichloracetic acid in a concentrated solution may be effective for small areas of warts but local damage to tissues may occur and recurrences have been reported in up to one-third of patients.

The antimetabolite 5-fluorouracil (5-FU), an agent which modifies DNA and RNA synthesis, has been used as a topical cream for the treatment of vulval warts. The agent may however cause quite severe local irritation and in some patients systemic side effects and it is not in widespread use today.

The understanding that vulval warts occur more frequently when cell-mediated immune response is diminished, as in Hodgkin's disease and during pregnancy, has led some to suggest that recombinant intralesional interferon might be an effective treatment. Initial encouraging results have been obtained in placebo-controlled trials[10,11] of interferon-α but long-term follow-up is incomplete and recurrence rates may rise over time. Another agent, imiquimod, which is a potent inducer of interferon-α and enhances cell-mediated cytolytic activity against viral targets, is undergoing trials. Initial studies suggest that there may be some advantage of imiquimod over other more traditional chemical agents[12].

Destructive treatments

Traditional treatments of vulval warts in genitourinary medicine clinics include the use of cryotherapy, either with a cryoprobe or a cotton ear bud modified to deliver liquid nitrogen to the wart. This procedure does not usually require local anaesthesia, although it may occasionally cause significant discomfort. It has the advantage of being a treatment that may be used in pregnancy.

Electrodessication by high-frequency sparking with a 'hyfrecator' is commonly used for the treatment of vulval warts. This treatment requires the insertion of a local anaesthetic, possibly after the area has been anaesthetized previously with an application of Emla cream. The advantage of this modality is that a biopsy specimen can be sent to the pathology laboratory. The majority of clinicians do not necessarily biopsy vulval warts prior to treatment if the clinical presentation is believed to be pathognomonic for the condition.

The carbon dioxide laser is an effective method of treating both clinical and subclinical wart virus infection of the vulva. Small areas may be treated with local anaesthesia and large areas can be treated under general anaesthesia. The lesions should be destroyed to the first surgical plane, the papillary dermis. The application of hydrocortisone cream to the area may reduce post-treatment inflammation. Postoperative pain may be most acutely felt on the third or fourth postoperative day. The advantage of the carbon dioxide laser is that not only clinically obvious lesions but new subclinical lesions can be destroyed, which will reduce the incidence of post-treatment recurrence or persistence. A disadvantage of the treatment is the cost associated with the purchase of the laser itself.

The use of equipment for large loop excision of the transformation zone (LLETZ) or loop electrosurgical excisional procedure (LEEP) can be effective when using local anaesthesia for removing small vulval warts and will allow for histological analysis. Standard surgical excision using scissors can be employed, particularly for perianal warts. Careful infiltration of the area with saline or local anaesthesia, even in the anaesthetized patient, will often allow the wart to be excised at the base with minimal removal of adjacent healthy tissue, thereby promoting better healing and less scarring as described by Thomson[13].

CERVICAL WART VIRUS INFECTION

Clinical exophytic condylomata acuminata of the cervix must be distinguished from exophytic carcinoma of the cervix, usually by cytology and almost certainly by colposcopy, but this requires biopsy prior to treatment of the cervical lesion. Chemical, electrophysical or laser therapy can be employed to destroy the lesion once it has been demonstrated as being benign.

Subclinical lesions associated with CIN are the most common manifestations of cervical HPV infection and are subject to the most controversy as to appropriate treatment. There is no doubt that CIN II and III are best treated because untreated, these lesions, particularly those associated with HPV16 and 18, have a 30–80% chance of progression subsequently to invasive cancer. However, the vast majority of women presenting, having been screened by cytology and in colposcopy clinics, have either borderline or mild abnormalities suggested by their smear. The majority of these women will have benign epithelial lesions often categorized as CIN I, which are usually associated with HPV6 and 11. Syrjanen[14] has demonstrated that conservative follow-up of such patients over a period of 10 years will result in only 14% of patients progressing to CIN III and requiring treatment. The majority of the lesions that progress to CIN III do so within the first 18 months. There is a steady recruitment over time to spontaneous regression of viral-associated CIN I lesions of the cervix. However, the resource implications of carrying out conservative management of minor grade cervical lesions within colposcopy clinics have resulted in the potential for over-treatment of women with such conditions, particularly in clinics which operate a 'see and treat' policy.

Providing a strict colposcopic protocol is observed, lesions on the cervix may be destroyed, once the biopsy has confirmed them as pre-invasive, by cryotherapy, radical electrocoagulation diathermy, cold coagulation or laser evaporation. Many practitioners prefer to use the laser to perform an excisional conization for significant CIN lesions allowing for further histological examination of material. The introduction of the large loop for the LLETZ procedure, which is a relatively cheap apparatus providing for simultaneous treatment and diagnosis of the lesion, has resulted in loop excision becoming the most common treatment modality for CIN in the United Kingdom. The loop, however, has limitations, particularly when a high-grade lesion, possibly a microinvasion, is being treated, and limited flexibility for use when lesions extend into the upper vagina. In these circumstances and when available, the carbon dioxide laser is preferable to knife conization of the transformation zone of the cervix.

As indicated earlier, extensive research carried out into the association between HPV16 and 18 and the development of high-grade cervical lesions and invasive cancer presents the future possibility of patients being triaged to treatment or non-treatment on the basis of their viral status. There is also the possibility that the condition itself could be prevented, or at least its natural history modified, by the use of vaccines. It is yet to be established whether there is a significant association between HPV types 16 and 18 and adenocarcinoma *in situ* of the cervix.

SPECIAL SITUATIONS

VERRUCOUS CARCINOMA

Verrucous carcinoma is a squamous cell carcinoma which can occur in the oral cavity, larynx or anogenital region. A slow-growing tumour with papillary fronds, the lesion has a well-defined deep margin which pushes on a broad front across the basement membrane. The cells within the tumour look relatively benign and the lesion is frequently covered with keratin.

The vulval lesions have been demonstrated to contain HPV6 and one variety of the tumour is the giant condyloma of Buschke and Löwenstein. Wide excision may be sufficient for treatment and traditionally it has been advised that radiotherapy should be avoided. On the cervix, because of the papillary nature of the tumour, it may be mistaken for an exophytic condyloma acuminatum.

A separate condition, condylomatous carcinoma, can occur on the cervix. The histological features suggest HPV infection but the invasion from the basement membrane demonstrates a different pattern from the verrucous carcinoma and the lesion is more aggressive.

CONDYLOMATOUS CARCINOMA

Occasionally an apparently simple exophytic lesion on the cervix, thought to be a condyloma acuminatum, may in fact be a condylomatous carcinoma. Plate N shows the colposcopic appearances of a patient referred at the age of 21 from a genitourinary medicine clinic with genital warts, a smear suggesting minor cytological change and an exophytic lesion on the cervix. Treated by loop excision, the histological diagnosis (Plates O–Q) represented a condylomatous carcinoma. The surface layers of the squamous epithelium contained koilocytes and appeared to differentiate normally. The lesion was invasive below the basement membrane and malignant cells were seen in endothelial spaces. This patient was treated by a further central conization to exclude persisting central disease and conservative expectant follow-up. She is alive and well five years after treatment.

PREGNANCY

Vulval warts occur more frequently in pregnancy because of modifications to the cell-mediated immune response associated with the physiology of pregnancy. Spontaneous resolution of condylomata acuminata of the vulva has been reported in the puerperium. If lesions of the vulva are treated during pregnancy then chemical methods such as podophyllum and interferon should not be used. The destructive methods of cryotherapy or laser ablation may be considered more appropriate. Vulval warts can proliferate to a degree where they cause patients great discomfort in pregnancy and it is under these circumstances that they may need to be treated. Large exophytic lesions may shed large quantities of virus and there is the theoretical risk of a neonate acquiring juvenile laryngeal papillomatosis (HPV6 and 11) as a result of passage through the birth canal. However, it has not been thought necessary or appropriate to recommend caesarean section for women with widespread lower genital tract papillomavirus disease unless the size of the lesions represents a physical bar to delivery or if it is felt that trauma to the vulva will be not only more severe as a result of the poor quality of the warty tissues but also represent an increased risk of infection and poor healing. This will be rare.

IMMUNOSUPPRESSED PATIENTS

Gynaecologists working in specialist clinics will be faced with a small group of women who are referred to them with multifocal multicentric lower genital tract intraepithelial neoplasia. The patients present with CIN, VAIN, VIN and AIN. The intraepithelial lesions are viral associated and frequently widespread and very resistant to treatment. These patients appear to have not only an increased prevalence of viral-associated disease and viral-associated intraepithelial neoplasia, but also a greater likelihood of progression to early invasive disease. Management in a specialist clinic is necessary with frequent resort to biopsy to exclude invasion, with symptomatic treatment as appropriate. It is usually advisable to consult with the clinicians supervising the active immunosuppression of women who have undergone transplantation, to see if any change in agent may improve the lower genital tract condition.

CONCLUSION

Although vulval warts have been recognized for a long time as a sexually transmitted disease that can be unaesthetic, occasionally produces symptoms and frequently requires treatment, in recent years the aetiological association between human papillomavirus and genital tract cancer and precancer has predominated. Important possibilities have arisen for enhancing the efficiency of the cervical screening programme by using viral tests in series, or in parallel, with the traditional Papanicolaou smear. The prevention of lower genital tract squamous cancers, or the modification of the natural history of those conditions, by the use of a specially designed vaccine represents a challenge for researchers in the years ahead.

REFERENCES

1. Hippocrates (1939) *The Genuine Works of Hippocrates*, (trans. F. Adams), Williams and Wilkins, Baltimore p. 331.
2. Bell, B. (1783) Treatise on gonorrhoea and Lues Venerea, Vol 1, pp. 411–421, Vol 2, p. 123 Edinburgh.
3. Wharton, L.R. (1921) Rare tumours of the cervix of the uterus – condyloma and granuloma. *Surg. Gynec. Obstet.*, **33**, 145.
4. Marsh, M.R. (1952) Papilloma of the cervix. *Am. J. Obstet. Gynecol.*, **64**, 281–291.
5. Meisels, A. and Fortin, R. (1976) Condylomatous lesions of the cervix and vagina I. Cytologic patterns. *Acta Cytol.*, **20**, 505–509.
6. Meisels, A., Fortin, R. and Roy, M. (1977) Condylomatous lesions of the cervix and vagina II. Cytologic, colposcopic and histopathologic criteria. *Acta Cytol.*, **21**, 379–389.
7. Oriel, J.D. (1971) Natural history of genital warts. *Br. J. Vener. Dis.*, **47**, 1–13.

8. Laverty, C. (1980) Noncondylomatous wart virus infection of the cervix: cytologic, histologic and electromicroscopic features. *Obstet. Gynecol. Surv.*, **34**, 820–822.

9. Walker, P.G., Singer, A., Dyson, J.L. *et al.* (1983) Colposcopy in the diagnosis of papillomavirus infection of the uterine cervix. *Br. J. Obstet. Gynaecol.*, **90**, 1082–1086.

10. Friedman-Kien, A.E., Eron, L.J., Conan, T.M. *et al.* (1988) Natural interferon alpha for treatment of condyloma acuminata. *JAMA*, **259**, 533–538.

11. Vance, J.C., Bart, B.J., Hansen, R.C. *et al.* (1986) Intralesional recombinant alpha-2 interferon for the treatment of patients with condyloma acu-minatum or verruca plantaris. *Arch. Dermatol.*, **122**, 272–277.

12. Beutner, K.R. and Ferenczy, A. (1997) Therapeutic approaches to genital warts. *Am. J. Med.*, **102**, 28–37.

13. Thomson, J.P.S. and Grace, R.H. (1978) The treatment of perianal and anal condylomata acuminata: a new operative technique. *J. Roy. Soc. Med.*, **71**, 180–185.

14. Syrjanen, K. (1994) Natural history of low grade SIL lesions. Screening of cervical cancer: for whom, why and how? 2nd International Congress of Papillomavirus in Human Pathology, Paris, pp. 10–17.

D. Casalaz and N. Marlow

INTRODUCTION

At birth a baby may show signs of early or recent fetal viral infection. Where infection has occurred in early pregnancy, the baby may have developmental abnormalities which reflect damage to those organ systems which were vulnerable at the time of infection (see earlier chapters). Despite a long time delay before delivery, active virus may still pose a further risk to its host in terms of progressive disease, for example hearing loss. Where fetal infection occurs close to delivery the baby may show signs of overwhelming infection, with disseminated disease, circulatory collapse and death. Alternatively, infection may be localized or even asymptomatic. Even in the latter cases, however, fetal infection may pose a significant long-term threat to the developing child.

Awareness of the possibility of maternal viral infection must always be communicated to the neonatal team, who may then initiate appropriate investigations and treatment if possible. Long-term follow-up is important for survivors of serious neonatal viral infection, who are at high risk of later disability, and for those with identified asymptomatic infection, who also may develop long-term effects of reactivated or progressive infection.

In the nursery, congenital infection must be suspected in a range of clinical situations. The infective agent may not be viral, as infection with *Toxoplasma gondii* or *Treponema pallidum*

may present with similar findings. The doctor should be alerted to the possibility of viral infection when faced with a baby with, for example, thrombocytopenia, anaemia, hepatosplenomegaly, a large or a small head, radiological evidence of heterotopic calcification or seizures, especially if the infant is small-for-gestational age.

When congenital viral infection is suspected, appropriate investigations should be instigated. These will depend upon the clinical indication and suspicion. It is not sufficient simply to request a 'TORCH' screen, as this reflects only a part of the spectrum of infective agents, and the term should now not be used[1]. Specific requests for culture of throat swabs, urine, stool, vesicle fluid or CSF and for serological testing are best discussed with a virologist if congenital infection is seriously contemplated. Specific features of infection with individual viruses and their diagnostic criteria are indicated below.

RUBELLA

Details of the epidemiology, virology and laboratory diagnosis of rubella virus infection were presented in Chapter 2.

CLINICAL MANIFESTATIONS

Rubella virus may infect all fetal organs, disruption to development may occur in many organs and the virus may persist for

Viral Infections in Obstetrics and Gynaecology. Edited by D.J. Jeffries and C.N. Hudson. Published in 1999 by Arnold, ISBN 0 340 74095 7.

long periods (Table 13.1)[2]. In its more severe form, congenital rubella causes fetal death and stillbirth. A wide spectrum of abnormalities may occur, ranging from severe multiple defects to the apparently normal newborn. Two-thirds of infected fetuses are asymptomatic at birth[3], but subsequent manifestations develop in over 70% of cases. Some presentations of congenital rubella may be transient (e.g. hepatitis) and others may manifest years later[4]. Congenital rubella should be considered in cases of sensorineural deafness and other developmental disorders, particularly if intrauterine growth restriction has been present.

Table 13.1 Common features of congenital rubella in the newborn

General
  Prematurity
  Growth retardation
Cutaneous
  Petechiae, purpura
  Rubelliform rash
  Jaundice
Neurological
  CNS – microcephaly
       – encephalitis
  Eye   – cataracts
       – salt and pepper retinitis
       – microphthalmia
       – cataracts
  Ear   – hearing loss (evident as auditory evoked responses)
Cardiac
  Patent ductus arteriosus
  Pulmonary stenosis/hypoplasia
Reticuloendothelial and haematological
  Hepatosplenomegaly
  Hepatitis
  Lymphadenopathy
  Thrombocytopenia
  Anaemia
  Lymphocytosis
Bone
  Radiolucencies on X-ray

Acute neonatal effects

Acute infection of liver and haemopoietic tissue results in hepatitis with jaundice, organomegaly and thrombocytopenia with petechiae and purpura. Haemolytic anaemia can occur and evidence of dermal erythropoiesis (the 'blueberry muffin' appearance) can be seen. A chronic rubelliform rash can be present with lymphadenopathy. Rubella may cause pneumonitis and myocarditis. Acute CNS involvement takes the form of an acute meningoencephalitis in around 10–20% of clinically affected infants with associated lymphocytosis in the CSF[5]. The CSF protein is generally elevated, even in the absence of acute encephalitis.

Chronic/early fetal infection

Classically, infants are small-for-gestational age, microcephalic and have evidence of leucocoria due to cataracts. Congenital heart defects (most commonly patent ductus arteriosus, pulmonary stenosis, aortic stenosis and tetralogy of Fallot) may be present[6]. Patent ductus is found in one-third of cases as the only lesion and is also commonly associated with pulmonary stenosis[6]. Late vascular manifestations, such as peripheral vascular disease and coronary artery disease, have also been documented[7]. Bone involvement is demonstrated on X-ray as striated bony translucencies. Long-term growth failure may occur in infancy[8].

Long-term outcomes

Severe learning disability, with or without microcephaly, is common, particularly following meningoencephalitis. In addition, behavioural and development disturbances occur[4,5] and 6% of infants with congenital infection may show features of autism. An illness similar to subacute sclerosing panencephalitis may occur towards the end of the first and into the second decade, associated with raised rubella antibody titres and elevated protein concentrations in CSF[9]. Rubella immune complexes have been found in both the serum and CSF in patients with this rubella-related SSPE and rubella virus has also been demonstrated in lymphocytes[10].

Rubella and the eye

Ocular involvement may be manifest as neonatal cataracts and microphthalmia in around one-third of cases (cataracts are bilateral in 50%)[11]. Retinal changes are seen as the classic 'salt and pepper' retinopathy which may progress to subretinal neovascularization[12]. In addition, during infancy glaucoma may occur in eyes without cataract, but presentation may be delayed by up to 22 years[13]. Other ocular manifestations include keratoconus, corneal hydrops and lens absorption[14].

Hearing loss

Deafness is one of the most important long-term sequelae of congenital rubella infection and occurs in over three-quarters of cases[15,16], affecting those both with and without neonatal features of infection. This is related to the protracted embryological development of the organ of Corti, making it susceptible to teratogenic effects of infection up to 20 weeks gestation.

Late endocrinological manifestations of congenital rubella

These are not infrequent and include insulin-dependent diabetes mellitus (IDDM) and thyroid dysfunction as the most common manifestations, seen in 20% and 5% respectively[15,17–19]. In both cases, autoantibodies can be demonstrated and coexistent IDDM and thyroid disease has been described. Other endocrinological disorders have been reported, including growth hormone deficiency, Addison's disease and precocious puberty[15,20,21].

Postnatal acquisition of rubella

This is usually a very mild illness and rarely results in serious problems. The incubation period is 2–3 weeks and a rash is usually the first manifestation and other features including fever, malaise, cough and coryza with conjunctivitis and lymphadenopathy can occur. Such infected infants pose a risk to unborn fetuses in susceptible pregnant women and if the illness is suspected, avoidance of contact is certainly advisable for two weeks after the onset of rash in the infant.

DIAGNOSIS

Where congenital rubella is suspected, a history of previous maternal vaccination and evidence of previous rubella antibody status should be sought. A history of vaccination does not exclude infection: case reports of vaccination failure and episodes of reinfection[22,23] have been reported. Congenital rubella has been reported despite protective levels of maternal antibody[24]. It is likely that the incidence of fetal damage following reinfection is much less than in primary infection, possibly less than 5%, even with reinfection in the first trimester[25] (see Chapter 2).

TREATMENT AND PREVENTION

There is no effective treatment for congenital rubella syndrome, although attempts using interferon, amantadine and isoprinosine have been reported[10,26,27]. The management of infected infants is thus supportive, based on appropriate prospective follow-up, detection of abnormality and family support.

Prevention of fetal infection is paramount and achieved mainly through vaccination programmes. Further preventive measures include avoidance of contact with pregnant women, although given the high rate of asymptomatic infection, this is difficult. If infection contact occurs, then the pregnant woman should be assessed and counselled appropriately.

CYTOMEGALOVIRUS

Details of the epidemiology, virology and laboratory diagnosis of cytomegalovirus were presented in Chapter 3.

Cytomegalovirus (CMV) is recognized as an important and almost universal human pathogen. Most CMV infections are subclinical but can have devastating effects, particularly in the fetus. The natural history of CMV infection is complex and viral shedding can last over long periods before latency occurs. Over time, episodes of reactivation occur and can also cause significant morbidity in the newborn infant. Furthermore, reinfection with antigenically diverse CMV strains can occur[28].

CLINICAL FEATURES

Acute perinatal infection

This can be acquired following maternal primary infection close to delivery, from direct contact during passage through the birth canal, breastfeeding, from transfusions and, uncommonly, through individual spread. The majority of infections are subclinical and, in most cases, maternally derived antibodies offer some protection following maternal viral shedding during a reactivated infection.

CMV pneumonitis is rarely seen in congenital infection but is a feature of postnatal disease, usually in very preterm infants with seronegative mothers, who can acquire CMV nosocomially or, more commonly, through transfusion with blood that has not been screened for CMV or is leucocyte depleted[29]. Such infants present 1–3 months post-transfusion with multisystem disease characterized by hepatosplenomegaly, thrombocytopenia, haemolysis, lymphocytosis and respiratory disease. Clinically, these babies may appear to have bacterial sepsis. Pneumonitis may be manifest as respiratory distress with an increased respiratory rate, cough and chest recession, but children are often afebrile.

Importantly, CMV pneumonitis has identical clinical and X-ray appearances to other viral agents and chlamydia. Histologically, cytomegalic inclusion cells may be recognized readily in the lungs and, in severe cases, there is marked lymphocytic infiltration. Although the infection runs a self-limiting course over 2–4 weeks, mortality in very preterm children is in the region of 20%[30]. Some survivors develop neurodevelopmental consequences, such as cerebral palsy, sensorineural deafness and choroidoretinitis. This is particularly so if CMV excretion develops within the first two months[31].

Rarely, normal term infants may develop pneumonitis. Of these, around 3–5% die; the remainder recover but almost half have some degree of respiratory morbidity in the longer term, having persisting wheeze with X-ray abnormalities at 12 months and abnormalities on pulmonary function testing at school age[32].

Acute infection acquired around birth may present with a hepatitic and haemolytic picture similar to that seen with rubella. Liver disease tends to improve both clinically and biochemically with time. Haemolytic anaemia can occur with resultant extramedullary haemopoiesis and hepatosplenomegaly, which again resolves with time. CMV infection frequently causes thrombocytopenia (by direct infection of megakaryocytes), presenting with petechial rash and bleeding[33,34]. Thrombocytopenia can persist for long periods, but generally resolves in the first few weeks.

Chronic/early fetal infection

CMV infection can have widespread multisystem effects in the fetus, which may be devastating, primarily by infection and teratogenesis in the CNS, eyes, ears and other systems. About 5% of infants with congenital infection have classic clinical features of CMV infection, including growth restriction, petechiae, hepatosplenomegaly, jaundice, thrombocytopenia with microcephaly, intracranial calcification, seizures, hypotonia, cataracts and choroidoretinitis. A further 5% have atypical presentations with some of these features. Premature delivery occurs in about a third of cases[33].

CNS involvement may be extensive with encephalitis which involves both white and grey matter. Severe seizures and neurological abnormality may occur but are not specific to CMV infection. Cytomegalic inclusions are found in neurones and glial supportive cells, choroid plexus, ventricular, meningeal and vascular tissue. Occasionally, cells with inclusions may be found in the CSF[35] and CMV may be cultured from CSF[36]. Associated with CNS infection, widespread calcification may develop, primarily involving the periventricular areas. Both microcephaly, secondary to cortical atrophy, and hydrocephalus, following ventricular obstruction, are associated with CMV infection.

CMV may be isolated from the eye[37,38] and is associated with a range of abnormalities, including microphthalmia, cataracts, choroidoretinitis, optic neuritis and colobomata. CMV may also be cultured from the inner ear[39]. Sensorineural deafness is the most common manifestation of congenital CMV infection and is a feature of subclinical infection[40]. Deafness tends to be more severe in symptomatic disease[33] and is bilateral in one-third of cases. Progressive hearing loss over the first few years is a feature of CMV infection.

Other organ systems are frequently involved. CMV hepatitis is well described and may be associated with calcification[41]. Renal infection occurs but is rarely clinically significant. Endocrine tissue may also show evidence of CMV infection and pancreatitis is described[42] but long-term endocrine disorders are not described. Dental enamel dysplasia, often with yellow discoloration, is common in symptomatic infants but does occur in subclinical infections[43].

DIAGNOSIS

Following perinatal infection, CMV cultures of urine or saliva become positive after three weeks of age; cultures taken before this will be negative[44]. CMV-specific IgG may be found where there is reactivated maternal infection, but if maternal CMV-specific IgG is negative and CMV-specific IgM develops in the baby, infection from a source other than maternal should be suspected. The diagnosis of congenital CMV is more complex but is supported by a clinical history of a CMV-like illness during the pregnancy. In the first two weeks after birth, neonatal viral isolation is diagnostic, but after this time CMV excretion may be the result of perinatal/postnatal infection.

TREATMENT AND PREVENTION

The antiviral agents ganciclovir and foscarnet have been used in treating CMV infection, particularly in AIDS-related CMV infections, in the last decade. While these medications have been shown to eradicate viral shedding for periods of time in congenital CMV[45,46], long-term neurodevelopmental outcome remains unaltered. Ganciclovir and foscarnet have been used successfully, in combination with intravenous immunoglobulin, in treating CMV pneumonitis in perinatally acquired infection[47] and there may be a role for antiviral agents in treating progressive choroidoretinitis[38].

Management is otherwise supportive, with appropriate community-based follow-up and monitoring of neurosensory function, including hearing, development and vision.

In the long term, prevention may be achieved though vaccination. CMV vaccines are currently under development but produce variable immunity[48]. However, the use of a live attenuated vaccine for seronegative women during pregnancy may put the fetus at risk. Likewise, there is a theoretical potential for reactivation of infection during pregnancy. CMV glycoprotein surface antigen subunit vaccines are being tested and may prove safer. In western countries, about half of the infants with congenital CMV are born to teenage, single mothers[48]. Targeting immunization of children may thus prevent, or significantly decrease, cases of congenital CMV.

A further approach to prevention is to screen pregnant (or pre-pregnant) women, advising those at risk about measures to minimize infection, such as handwashing after nappy changing. This may be particularly important for women working in childcare settings.

PROGNOSIS

The prognosis for symptomatic children with congenital CMV infection is poor. Up to 70% have psychomotor retardation, often with microcephaly and other neurological problems. Indeed, one or more impairment occurs in 90% of such children[49]. Poor progress is indicated by microcephaly, neurological dysfunction in the first year and ocular involvement. Recently neonatal cranial CT scanning has been evaluated as a predictor of adverse outcome[50]. In this study, 90% of children with an abnormal CT scan (most with intracerebral calcification) had at least one impairment, compared to 29% of those with normal scans. Neonatal clinical and laboratory findings did not predict either CT abnormalities or long-term outcome.

Although in the neonatal period 90% of congenital infections are subclinical, sensorineural deafness, microcephaly, learning difficulties, cerebral palsy, dental abnormalities and choroidoretinitis still develop later in around 10–15% of infected children[38,43,49]. Hearing loss can appear late, can be progressive, and is bilateral in around 40% of cases[33].

VARICELLA

Details of the epidemiology, virology and laboratory diagnosis of varicella virus were presented in Chapter 4.

The importance of varicella-zoster virus (VZV) as a cause of fetal damage was first noted by LaForet and Lynch in 1947[51] and subsequently a fetal varicella syndrome was described in 1974[52] (Table 13.2). Congenital chickenpox, occurring as a result of maternal primary VZV infection in the perinatal period, carries a significant mortality.

The potentially devastating effects to the fetus and newborn of primary VZV in pregnancy are fortunately rare. In general, over 90% of adult women have developed natural immunity to VZV before their reproductive years[53]. As a result, primary VZV infection is estimated to occur in less than one per 1000 pregnancies[53,54]. However, community outbreaks of infection are not uncommon and result in increased cases in susceptible pregnant women. VZV can be transmitted transplacentally, with the most important periods, in terms of fetal and neonatal consequences, being before 20 weeks' gestation and in the five days prior to birth. Primary VZV infection between these two periods tends to be

Table 13.2 Features of congenital varicella syndrome

General
   Low birthweight
   Skin scarring in dermatomes
Eye abnormalities
   Choroidoretinitis
   Horner's syndrome
   Microphthalmia
   Cataracts
   Nystagmus
Limb abnormalities
   Limb hypoplasia
   Abnormal/absent limbs
   Talipes equinovarus
Neural
   Cortical atrophy
   Microcephaly
   Mental retardation
   Poor sphincter control
   Seizures
   Bulbar palsy

self-limiting and not associated with major sequelae, although fetal multiorgan infection occurring with maternal infection at 23 weeks' gestation has been described[55]. Interestingly, fetuses exposed to maternal chickenpox between these two periods appear to have a higher frequency of and earlier onset of herpes zoster recurrences after primary infection compared to unexposed children[56].

CLINICAL FEATURES

Congenital varicella syndrome

The clinical manifestations of congenital varicella syndrome range from severe multiorgan involvement to dermatomal skin scarring and limb hypoplasia. It appears more frequent in females[55,57]. Diagnosis depends upon evidence of maternal varicella infection in pregnancy, with dermatomally distributed skin lesions and immunological evidence of *in utero* VZV infection[57].

Major clinical features are summarized in Table 13.2: skin, ocular, neurological and limb manifestations occur in at least 50% of affected babies and half are of low birthweight. Skin involvement is more frequent in the lower limb and generally appears as cicatricial, pigmented scarring, although other lesions have been described[58]. Many of these features can be attributed to spinal cord atrophy and consequent trophic limb abnormalities[59,60]. Colonic atresia associated with spinal cord atrophy has also been described[59]: histological specimens at laparotomy revealed segmental absence of ganglion cells at the level of the atretic area.

Perinatal chickenpox

This may be devastating, but the severity of illness is very dependent upon the timing of birth in relation to the onset of maternal disease. Between 25%[61] and 50%[62] of babies will be infected when maternal chickenpox develops in the three weeks preceding delivery. Acute neonatal VZV infection ranges from a mild illness with few cutaneous vesicles to a fulminant disease with pulmonary and hepatic involvement in addition to cutaneous vesicles, with mortality up to 30% in untreated babies[63]. Mortality is greatest when birth occurred within the period of four days after to two days before onset of maternal rash and correlates with absence of acquired antibodies in the infant[61]. In another review of 281 babies born to mothers with perinatal chickenpox, no antibodies were detectable in babies born within +/− 3 days of onset of the maternal rash, with progressively increasing levels from three to seven days before delivery[64].

Postnatal exposure to VZV may result in a slightly higher risk of severe infection when protective maternal antibodies are not present[65,66]. This has important nursing implications, particularly in very premature babies who normally have only low levels of maternal antibody. In term babies, in contrast, the presence of protective maternal antibodies makes the risk of infection low, but fatal VZV pneumonitis at 21 days of age in an infant with Turner's syndrome has been described, despite the presence of maternal antibodies[67]. It would seem prudent to take measures to prevent nosocomial infection.

Herpes zoster, with localized unilateral dermatomal distribution, may occur in babies who are infected with VZV in early gestation. However, it is rare in the neonatal period and reports of clinical zoster[68] may have been due to other viral infections[69].

PREVENTION AND TREATMENT

Prevention must be primarily by avoidance of contact. Mothers with no previous history of VZV infection should avoid potential contact, but if this is not possible, it is prudent to measure maternal anti-VZV IgG antibody titres and closely observe the pregnancy. It is not known whether passive immunization prevents fetal infection or whether antiviral chemotherapy with acyclovir has a role in preventing the uncommon occurrence of fetal varicella. Counselling and follow-up with ultrasound in cases of confirmed primary VZV infection in early pregnancy is mandatory.

Passive immunization of the baby with zoster immune globulin (ZIG), prepared from donor serum, has a role in preventing severe sequelae in at-risk children. Two studies[62,70] have reported no deaths where ZIG was used to treat a group of babies with a predicted mortality of 30% (babies whose mothers developed varicella within five days of birth). Initially it was recommended that 125 units ZIG be given to infants whose mothers developed VZV five days or less before delivery and in the 48 h after. However, there were reports of three fatalities in the UK over five years despite this dose[71] and 250 mg IM would appear more appropriate.

Babies receiving passive immunization need to be closely observed, and if symptoms develop acyclovir should be commenced (20 mg/kg 8-hourly), but it is not always successful in preventing mortality[71]. Some authors have recommended its routine prophylactic use in combination with ZIG as soon as possible after birth in at-risk babies[72] but evidence for moderation of disease or outcome in these groups is lacking.

Sick newborns, particularly very preterm or very low birthweight infants or following multiple exchange transfusions, must be considered for the passive immunization if they are in contact with VZV. These babies have low or undetectable levels of antibody due to lack of transplacental antibody transfer and are potentially at risk of severe infection.

In the hospital setting it would seem prudent to isolate mothers and babies with VZV infection and ideally arrange for discharge home as soon as possible when the condition of both allows. Certainly, when maternal rash occurs, delay of delivery by a few days, where possible, should decrease the subsequent risk to the newborn infant.

Vaccination with a live attenuated VZV vaccine is now possible and has been used for a number of years in Japan and some European centres. It has been licensed for use in the USA since 1995 and is recommended as part of the immunization programme in young children. Efficacy rates for VZV vaccine are between 65% and 100%[73] and in those who develop a modified vaccine-like syndrome, the illness is milder than following natural infection. Pregnant women who have evidence of lack of immunity to VZV, who receive or are in contact with varicella vaccine are at risk of fetal damage[74,75] and such women should receive passive immunization. The risk of congenital varicella syndrome related to varicella vaccine is likely to be small.

MEASLES

Details of the epidemiology, virology and laboratory diagnosis of measles virus were presented in Chapter 5.

CLINICAL FEATURES

No specific measles-associated embryopathy has been described, but measles acquired during gestation increases the risk of spontaneous abortion and premature delivery[76–79]. In most cases, the delivery occurs within the first week after onset of the exanthem. There are only isolated reports of infants with congenital defects following gestational measles[76,80,81].

Perinatal maternal infection may result in a serious fetal/infant infection, the rash being present at birth or appearing within the first 10 days. Symptoms are similar to infections at later ages, including the appearance of Koplik's spots. If the rash appears in the mother in the week before or after delivery less than one-third of fetuses develop symptomatic infection, implying some placental protection[82]. Historically such 'congenital measles' infections can be severe and carry a high mortality (about 33%), but advances in neonatal care and the use of immunoglobulin prophylaxis may have improved outcome[76]. Death is usually the result of measles pneumonitis.

In contrast, acute infection may be acquired by the baby after birth: in this situation the appearance of the rash is delayed beyond 14 days and the illness is milder, usually modified by passively acquired maternal antibody.

TREATMENT

Measles treatment is symptomatic and immunoglobulin has no role when the clinical infection has occurred. Close observation and attention to possible bacterial superinfection are needed and antibiotics administered when this occurs. In developing nations, vitamin A in two consecutive daily doses of 200 000 iu is advisable and has been shown to improve acute mortality and modify disease severity in children[83,84], including those in hospital[85]. However, in the infected newborn there are no data to support benefit from vitamin A. Infection with measles causes a fall in vitamin A levels, potentially reducing lymphocyte function, suggesting a possible effect in neonatal measles[86].

PREVENTION

All babies at risk of congenital measles should receive human normal immunoglobulin. Ideally, community vaccination programmes should protect the mother and newborn from exposure. Contacts do occur and immunoglobulin should be administered within the week after exposure. If given within 72 h, it is effective in preventing infection, but given subsequently it appears to modify the disease considerably.

There is a risk of spread of measles in maternity units. For individuals, the timing of exposure and history of vaccination are important and where doubt exists, measles antibody titres can be measured. If a suscepti-

ble mother is exposed to measles between 6 and 15 days antepartum, then both her and her newborn infant should receive immunoglobulin and be discharged home. Other mothers in contact should be tested and, if susceptible, they and their babies should receive immunoglobulin also. Where a mother develops measles in the five days before or after delivery, the baby should receive immunoglobulin. Likewise, other susceptible mothers in contact and their infants should also receive immunoglobulin. Naturally, isolation and discharge as early as possible are essential and health-care personnel should also be tested.

Even in the presence of maternal immunity, very preterm babies are at risk of measles, as antibody transfer occurs in the third trimester. Exposed babies born before 34 weeks gestation should also be given immunoglobulin.

PARVOVIRUS

Details of the epidemiology, virology and laboratory diagnosis of parvovirus virus were presented in Chapter 6.

Parvovirus B19 was first linked with fetal non-immune hydrops and intrauterine death in 1984[87,88]. Further suggestions that parvovirus B19 could have significant teratogenic effects[89,90] have not been supported by a specific pattern of abnormalities[91]. Parvovirus B19 infection may cause suppression of red cell production and aplastic crises, especially in patients with sickle cell and other red cell abnormalities, where red blood cell production is high[92]. During pregnancy, the fetus is similarly at risk and the resultant severe anaemia causes hydrops.

CLINICAL FEATURES AND DIAGNOSIS

Most cases of acute parvovirus infection in pregnancy have normal outcomes[92,93] and complete resolution can occur *in utero* without intervention[94]. Fetal infection may result in marrow suppression or occasionally myocarditis with subendocardial fibroelastosis, resulting in cardiac failure[95], which may explain certain cases of parvovirus-associated hydrops without severe anaemia[96].

Marrow suppression may also manifest as thrombocytopenia, which can be severe. Not only may this increase the risk of cordocentesis, but it may persist postnatally for many weeks: a self-limiting hepatitis, manifest as raised serum transaminases, may occur[94,95].

Neonatal morbidity relates to the direct consequences of marrow suppression as well as the increased tendency towards premature delivery and intrauterine growth restriction[97,98]. Transfusions may be required if anaemia persists, although usually this is only necessary in the first few months[99].

OUTCOME

The mortality rate is high for fetuses with documented hydrops and intervention in the form of fetal transfusion is not without risk. Controlled trials have not shown improved outcome, since it is well recognized that spontaneous resolution occurs. If the child is born and appears well, then it is likely that there will be no long-term consequences of maternal parvovirus infection confirmed in pregnancy. The presence of anaemia should, however, be sought and treated appropriately. Acquisition of parvovirus in the newborn period is likely to result in a non-specific self-limiting illness, but the incidence of neonatal infection is not known and is likely to be small.

HUMAN IMMUNODEFICIENCY VIRUS

Details of the epidemiology, virology and laboratory diagnosis of HIV were presented in Chapters 8, 9 and 11.

CLINICAL FEATURES

There is no evidence for an HIV-related embryopathy[100,101]. HIV infection may present in a variety of ways (Table 13.3) but

Table 13.3 Clinical features suggestive of possible HIV infection in infants

Failure to thrive
Hepatosplenomegaly, lymphadenopathy
Opportunistic infection (*Pneumocystis carinii* pneumonia, chronic candidiasis, *Mycobacterium avium/intracellulare* complex, herpes zoster)
Chronic parotitis (non-suppurative)
Recurrent, persistent infections
Thrombocytopenia and hypergammaglobulinaemia
Encephalopathy/developmental delay
Interstitial pneumonitis
Chronic diarrhoea
Nephrotic syndrome
Kaposi's sarcoma (rare in infants and children)

most newborns with HIV are asymptomatic, although 10–20% are born preterm[100,102]. The clinical spectrum of HIV-associated disease during infancy and childhood is very wide and outside the remit of this text. The reader is referred to recent reviews[103,104]. A wide range of immune abnormalities has been described (Table 13.4).

Neonatal HIV infection can present with severe manifestations, such as pneumocystis infection or bacterial sepsis, but this is

Table 13.4 Immune abnormalities in HIV-infected infants[167–169]

T-cell
    Decreased lymphocyte count
    Decreased CD4 count and proportion
    Decreased response to T-cell mitogens
        (e.g. phytohaemagglutinin)
    Decreased cytokine production
    Decreased natural killer cell activity
B-cell
    Immunoglobulins increased or decreased
    IgG subclass abnormalities
    Poor antibody response to vaccines
    Possible absent class switch from IgM to IgG
Monocyte/macrophage
    Decreased cytokine production
    Decreased numbers
    Decreased monocyte adherence

unusual. Some may present with hepatosple-nomegaly and lymphadenopathy with associated thrombocytopenia or anaemia and the combination of these features should encourage consideration of this diagnosis.

MANAGEMENT

The management of potential and overt HIV infection in newborn infants includes treatment of the HIV infection, management of and prophylaxis against illness resulting from HIV infection and, importantly, nutritional optimization and psychosocial support. Mothers and infants should be followed up by physicians experienced in the management of HIV infection.

Antiretroviral therapy

The decision to commence antiretroviral therapy is complex, but suggestions for starting criteria have been made[105]. Antiretroviral therapy should be initiated in symptomatic HIV-infected infants and children. In asymptomatic HIV-infected infants, the decision is less clear. Lymphocyte CD4 counts may be used as the basis for starting therapy, once infection has been confirmed (Table 13.5)[105].

Monotherapy, usually with zidovudine, is most frequently used in children but combinations with other drugs, including ddI (didanosine), ddC (dideoxcytidine) and 3TC, are under assessment at present. Combination therapy has a number of theoretical advantages, such as lower dosages, less resistance and possible synergistic actions.

It is essential that patients on antiretroviral therapy are regularly monitored clinically and blood tests done to assess full blood count, urea and electrolytes and liver function. Additionally, baseline CD4 cell counts and p24 antigen detection should be performed and other tests such as ECG, CXR and CT done as indicated after initial baseline assessment.

Prophylaxis

Prophylaxis in HIV-infected infants is directed against *Pneumocystis carinii* pneumonia (PCP), preventing bacterial disease and includes immunization.

PCP prophylaxis, with co-trimoxazole, should be instituted for all babies of HIV-infected mothers from one month of age. In contrast to adults, in whom a CD4 cell count of $<200/mm^3$ is indicative of high PCP risk, CD4 cell counts in infants give poor prediction[106]. In the first month, the risk of PCP is low and sulphonamides may exacerbate anaemia associated with zidovudine therapy or cause adverse reactions in the presence of immature hepatic metabolism. Prophylactic co-trimoxazole (150 mg trimethoprim and 750 mg sulphamethoxazole/m^2/day) is given for either three consecutive days or three alternate days per week. Alternatives are dapsone or pentamidine in nebulized or intravenous forms. Breakthrough infection, however, can occur with all forms of PCP prophylaxis and a low threshold of clinical suspicion should be maintained[107].

Prophylaxis should be continued until 12 months of age unless viral studies (culture, PCR, p24 antigen) are negative on at least two occasions. In infants older than 12 months of age, PCP prophylaxis should be continued if CD4 cell counts are <750 cells per mm^3 or a CD4 percentage of total lymphocytes is below 15%, and at 24 months if the CD4 cell count is <500 and/or CD4 percentage is $<15\%$[108]. In

Table 13.5 CD4 criteria for commencing antiretroviral therapy in HIV-infected asymptomatic children[105]

Age	CD4 count (cells per mm^3)	CD4 as % of lymphocytes
< 1 year	< 1750	< 30%
1–2 years	< 1000	< 25%
2–6 years	< 750	< 20%
6 years and over	< 500	< 20%

addition, if PCP occurs in the presence of 'normal' CD4 cell counts, subsequent prophylaxis should be considered. Careful consideration should be given to immunization in HIV-infected infants. These children should receive all routine childhood immunizations, excepting BCG and *live* polio vaccine[109]. This includes immunization against *Haemophilus influenzae* and *Streptococcus pneumoniae*. Measles, mumps and rubella vaccine (MMR) should be given despite containing live attenuated virus, due to the high risk of severe measles[109]. Live attenuated polio vaccine poses a risk of paralytic polio, not only to the infant but to other potentially immunodeficient household contacts. In industrialized countries, where the risk of tuberculosis is low, BCG should be avoided in HIV-positive patients. In areas where tuberculosis is still common, particularly now with the emergence of multiresistant organisms, the WHO recommends that BCG is given to HIV-infected babies, as the benefits outweigh the risks.

In some centres, monthly intravenous immunoglobulin is administered to HIV-infected children. However, some studies have failed to show benefit from immunoglobulin if the child is receiving antiretroviral therapy and PCP prophylaxis or if the CD4 cell count is <200 per mm^3[111]. It is recommended that immunoglobulin is given to children with hypogammaglobulinaemia or B-cell inertia with poor antibody responses to immunization, or in cases where recurrent significant bacterial infection occurs despite treatment[105]. Immunoglobulin should also be given following exposure to infective organisms, e.g. within 72 h of exposure to measles or varicella (hyperimmune globulin)[109]. Immunoglobulin may reverse thrombocytopenia which develops or persists despite antiretroviral therapy.

PROGNOSIS

Children with HIV infection tend to show more aggressive deterioration compared to adults. In perinatally acquired HIV infection, 10% will have symptoms in the first month[100,102] and up to 90% will be symptomatic by two years[112]. Survival has been improved by early recognition and appropriate management, but up to 50% may die in the first three years[113].

HERPES SIMPLEX VIRUS

Details of the epidemiology, virology and laboratory diagnosis of herpes simplex virus (HSV) infection were presented in Chapter 7.

Most neonatal infections are caused by HSV type 2 which is associated with genital herpes. The incidence of neonatal infection varies considerably from estimates of one in 50 000 newborns in the UK to as high as one in 1500 in North America[114]. The incidence may be increasing in some areas of the USA[115].

Only 5% of cases are acquired in early pregnancy following transplacental infection, whereas 85% of infections are acquired from the genital tract in the perinatal period[116,117]. The remainder arise as the result of postnatal infection[118].

CLINICAL FEATURES

Neonatal evidence of early intrauterine infection may be manifest by the presence of abnormal head size (micro- or hydrocephalus), eye involvement in the form of chorioidoretinitis and microphthalmia or cutaneous signs with vesicles and scarring evident at birth[116]. These features are not specific to HSV and thus accurate diagnosis is important.

Skin or eye lesions may be present at birth, particularly in the presence of prolonged membrane rupture, when early recognition, diagnosis and treatment are essential to prevent dissemination.

Neonatal HSV infection usually presents within the first 1–2 weeks after birth, although the onset may be delayed. Presentation can be divided into babies with localized skin, eye or mouth lesions and those with disseminated or severe disease, with or without associated or preceding localized disease.

Localized cutaneous infection

This is the most common initial presentation. Skin lesions range from isolated vesicles to crops of vesicles that can be large and bullous in nature[76]. More unusually, other skin lesions, including zoster-like eruptions, petechiae or erythema multiforme, can be seen. Eye involvement takes the form of keratoconjunctivitis with dendritic ulcers, with resultant choriodoretinitis. Cataracts can develop; optic atrophy and microphthalmia may occur as late sequelae.

Isolated oral and laryngeal vesicular lesions can develop as part of disseminated disease and have been noted in about 10% of infected infants[119].

Without treatment, over 70% of babies with evidence of localized cutaneous or ocular disease will develop disseminated infection[119–121]; vigilance is essential in preventing mortality and further morbidity[122]. More severe and disseminated disease usually follows the appearance of mucosal or skin lesions, but in 20% or more cases no cutaneous lesions are seen[120,122].

Disseminated infection

This presents usually in the first week, but can appear up to two weeks of age. It carries a poor prognosis and deterioration may be rapid, leading to death. Mortality, in the absence of treatment, may be 70% or more[119,123,124]. Presentation is often nonspecific with poor feeding, lethargy, fever, vomiting and irritability. Convulsions may occur with associated CNS involvement[76] and respiratory distress, apnoea and cyanosis along with hepatomegaly and jaundice are seen. Twenty five percent will develop evidence of disseminated intravascular coagulation (DIC) and shock with rapid progression, in most cases to death.

Herpes simplex pneumonitis

This may occur between three to seven days of age, presents with respiratory distress and can occur as a single system infection. Chest X-ray demonstrates diffuse, interstitial opacification and haemorrhagic pneumonitis can develop[119,124]. Early treatment is essential to prevent dissemination and despite its rarity, a low threshold of suspicion is needed.

Meningoencephalitis

This can occur in association with disseminated disease or as a localized CNS infection. Localized CNS infection tends to present in the second week with a mean age at presentation of 11 days (range 7–30 days)[76,119,124]. Signs of encephalitis are non-specific in the newborn, with fever, temperature, instability, poor feeding, irritability, lethargy and apnoeic episodes. Seizures are common and, when combined with an absent gag reflex, HSV meningoencephalitis is highly likely[76]. An EEG shows characteristic abnormalities: a temporal or parietotemporal focus, often with periodic slow and fast waves. The seizures tend to become intractable and generalized.

CNS imaging may be of value. CT scanning may demonstrate unilateral or bilateral temporal lobe changes in the form of loss of grey–white differentiation and decreased attenuation. Later, calcification and cerebral atrophy can develop.

PROGNOSIS

Infants with disease localized to cutaneous or mucosal sites have an excellent prognosis, providing the lesions are recognized and treatment started promptly. Infrequently, infants may develop long-term neurological impairment[76,120,125], possibly related to skin recurrences and dissemination early in life. Recent studies using retrospective PCR techniques have demonstrated the presence of HSV in CSF from 24% of infants with skin, eye or mouth involvement[126], which implies unrecognized dissemination.

Untreated, disseminated disease will develop in over 70% of cases. Both disseminated disease and localized CNS involvement carry a high mortality if untreated (74% and 50% respectively)[123]. Following treatment, mortality remains significant, at around 35–55% for disseminated disease and 10% for localized CNS disease[122,123,126]. Mortality is related to the presence of disseminated intravascular coagulation (DIC), prematurity, pneumonitis and the degree of CNS depression when therapy is commenced. Severe neurodevelopmental morbidity is very common in survivors: over 80% of those babies treated for disseminated disease and over 50% with meningoencephalitis have significant impairment[127]. Poor risk factors for severe neurodevelopmental morbidity are seizures, DIC, infection with HSV2 and presence of encephalitis in disseminated disease[125].

TREATMENT

Vidarabine (30 mg/kg per day infused over 12 h) was first shown to be effective in decreasing mortality and morbidity in neonatal HSV infection[123]. Subsequently, intravenous acyclovir therapy (10 mg/kg 8-hourly) has been shown to be equally effective[128]. Given the smaller administrative volume, acyclovir is preferred by most neonatologists and may be more effective in HSV encephalitis[129]. Both drugs should be given for 10–14 days.

In view of the concerns about dissemination and neurological morbidity, it may be prudent to treat localized disease for several months.

Both topical and systemic treatment with antiviral agents should be instituted for eye lesions and ophthalmological assessment sought urgently.

PREVENTION OF NEONATAL INFECTION

When a mother has active orolabial HSV lesions, babies may room in, as these infants usually have acquired maternal antibodies. Care must be taken to avoid contact with orolabial lesions present in visitors (including fathers), who often feel an overwhelming need to kiss newborn infants, as disseminated neonatal HSV infection can result from such contact.

HEPATITIS VIRUSES

Hepatitis viruses can be a significant problem to the newborn and many advances have been made in both the ability to diagnose the causative organism and in prevention and treatment. Many viruses, including CMV, rubella and enteroviruses, can cause hepatitis, and these are discussed elsewhere in this chapter. This section will deal with the 'hepatitis viruses' and specifically, hepatitis A and B will be discussed. Details of the epidemiology, virology and laboratory diagnosis of these viruses were presented in Chapter 10.

HEPATITIS A

Treatment and Prevention

The treatment is essentially supportive although, in rare cases, hepatic failure may occur and will need specialist intervention. Prevention of cross-infection is important, particularly in hospital. Strict attention to measures to prevent faecal–oral spread is needed. Where possible, the infant should be discharged home. When staff are the initial source of infection, passive immunization with human normal immunoglobulin should be administered to newborn infants in contact. Neonatal viral shedding in stool is prolonged compared with older children and virus has been isolated up to five months after disease onset.

Passive immunization also has a role when acute hepatitis occurs in the mother within 1–2 weeks before delivery and in the period afterwards. In this situation, the baby may become infected during birth and have little protective antibody. Active immunization is now possible.

Prognosis

Recovery is the rule but in the rare cases of fulminant disease with acute liver failure, mortality may be as high as 33%[130]. Liver transplantation in such cases may be the only option.

HEPATITIS B

Transmission of infection

Worldwide, transmission of HBV from carrier mothers to their infants is important and may be the result of *in utero* transplacental transmission or may occur around the time of delivery or shortly afterwards.

Clinical manifestations

Acute HBV infection in pregnancy is associated with an increased risk of premature delivery (up to 35%) and is not related to whether an infant shows evidence of infection[131]. There has been no documented embryopathy following acute HBV infection in pregnancy. Newborn infants who become infected with HBV may develop an acute, fulminant hepatitis but more usually are asymptomatic. Such babies have an 80% risk of developing the carrier state compared to 10% when infection is acquired after the first month.

Prevention

Passive immunization (HBIG) should be combined with vaccination for infants born to HBeAg-positive mothers. It may be considered for infants of HBeAg-negative and HBeAb-positive mothers in whom the risk of transmission is low but documented[132,133]. In high-risk areas, universal active and passive immunization or selective protection for children of HBsAg-positive mothers may decrease transmission by 90%[134,135].

Breastfeeding may carry a small risk of transmission of infection, although there is little evidence of this. Counselling should stress the benefits of breastfeeding which usually far outweigh the risk of hepatitis transmission.

ENTEROVIRUSES

INTRODUCTION

Enteroviruses are small RNA viruses (Picornavirus family) and comprise the polioviruses, echoviruses, coxsackie viruses and human enteroviruses 68–72. Primarily spread through the faecal–oral or respiratory routes, they can cause severe illness in newborn infants. All types of enterovirus have been associated with congenital and neonatal infection[136]. These viruses have a worldwide distribution and, particularly in temperate climates, can have seasonal peaks in summer and autumn. Transmission by hospital staff on paediatric wards has been documented[137].

TRANSMISSION

Transplacental spread may occur[138] but evidence tends to support perinatal transmission. Vertical transmission may result from contact with maternal blood and secretions at the time of delivery; enterovirus has been isolated in cervical secretions[76,139]. Given the rapid progression of enteroviral infection, neonatal illness occurring from the second to seventh day is almost certainly vertically acquired. Infection has been documented in babies born by caesarean section with intact membranes, suggesting that infection can be acquired from an ascending transmembrane route or alternatively from maternal blood[76].

Horizontal neonatal transmission also occurs: outbreaks in maternity wards and neonatal units have been recorded[140]. Horizontally acquired infection tends to cause less severe illness than vertically acquired infection[76,141], although this is not always so, particularly in coxsackie infections[142].

POLIOMYELITIS

Neonatal poliovirus infection is rare due to widespread vaccination programmes. Reversion of attenuated virus can cause infection and neonatal paralytic illness has been recorded from contact with a recently immunized older infant[143]. The virus can also be spread by visitors from regions where polio is still endemic and cause neonatal infection. This may develop even in the presence of protective maternal antibodies as inferred from the success of immunization in young infants.

Clinical features

Maternal polio may cause abortion and stillbirth[144], although this does not occur when vaccine virus is administered in the first trimester[76,145]. The severity of maternal illness increases the risk and premature delivery may be more common. There have also been suggestions of embryopathy due to wild or vaccine polio but the evidence is contradictory and a recent Finnish review failed to show any association[145].

Polio infection acquired postnatally presents similar features to those seen in adults and older children. The incubation period is from seven to 21 days and clinical symptoms initially are non-specific with early fever, malaise, diarrhoea and irritability. The illness rarely proceeds beyond the initial symptoms and less than 5% develop the typical aseptic lymphocyte-predominant meningitis or anterior horn cell destruction (paralytic polio)[109]. Where infection is acquired *in utero*, the infant can present with flaccid paralysis with respiratory compromise, with residual paralysis if the child survives.

ECHOVIRUSES

Neonatal infection with echoviruses can have devastating consequences. In contrast to polio, echovirus is not usually associated with abortion and prematurity, although intra-uterine death and stillbirth have been reported[138]. No embryopathy has been reported. Echoviral infections are most commonly caused by subtypes 6, 7 and 11[76].

Clinical features

Vertical transmission of echovirus infection tends to be associated with clinically significant disease in the majority of cases, which can be severe. In 50% of cases, maternal illness is apparent with fever, coryza or gastrointestinal upset and abdominal pain. The neonatal clinical pattern is variable, often a non-specific illness that is difficult to differentiate from bacterial disease, developing between days three to five. Occasionally there may be evidence of infection at birth.

Symptoms comprise fever, irritability and gastrointestinal upset with vomiting, diarrhoea and occasionally abdominal distension. There is often a mild respiratory tract illness with coryza and cough and an exanthem may be present. CSF examination reveals evidence of an aseptic meningitis in 5% of cases. Most babies with these non-specific features recover[141].

Occasionally, echovirus infection produces an overwhelming illness which begins with non-specific features and runs a rapid fulminant course leading to death[140,146]. The features noted above develop, with lethargy, hypotonia and poor feeding. Rapid progression occurs with hypotensive shock, metabolic acidosis, pallor, jaundice, hepatosplenomegaly and ascites. A severe coagulopathy ensues with widespread bleeding into all organs and fulminant hepatic necrosis. Death occurs in around 80%[76]. Further complications include pneumonitis, myocarditis and meningoencephalitis.

Occasionally, echovirus has been associated with isolated cases of pharyngitis, croup, coryza, herpangina, pneumonia and myocarditis[136]. A further clinical pattern, the 'cloud baby', has been associated with echovirus 20 in four term infants in the first postnatal week. Although well, these babies were colonized with *Staphylococcus aureus*, which they dispersed into the surrounding environment, until the echovirus infection had resolved. The mechanism for this synergistic effect is unknown[147].

In contrast, horizontally acquired neonatal echovirus infection tends to be mild and at least half are asymptomatic. These babies tend to present particularly after the second week and illness severity is not increased among preterm children[148]. Presentation may be with non-specific malaise, fever, irritability and apnoeic episodes. Aseptic meningitis may be present and pneumonitis, gastroenteritis and, rarely, myocarditis can develop[140,148] but death is unusual.

COXSACKIE VIRUSES

Coxsackie viruses can cause severe neonatal infection and, in contrast to echoviruses, horizontally acquired infection can cause as severe an illness as vertically transmitted disease[149,150]. Neonatal infection usually results from type B strains (B1-B5), although there are reports of infection with type A virus[151]. Coxsackie infections have a seasonally increased incidence with summer and spring peaks[152]. Coxsackie virus is a well-recognized cause of neonatal unit outbreaks[142,150,152]. The index case may have been vertically infected and acts as the source of infection, spreading to other babies via hospital staff. Occasionally hospital staff can be the initial source.

Clinical features

Coxsackie B infection in early pregnancy may be associated with increased risk of congenital malformation, particularly CNS[153] and cardiovascular[154], although the evidence for embryopathy is weak. Coxsackie infection may cause stillbirth[138] but the risk of premature delivery may not be increased. Transplacental infection may be more common in late pregnancy[76]. Intrauterine infection due to coxsackie virus B1 detected by amniotic fluid culture has been reported in 34 weeks' twins[155].

Neonatal coxsackie infection can be asymptomatic, a mild exanthematous illness with recovery over about three days, or a fulminant illness with significant mortality. Mild illness is seen in over 50% of clinically apparent neonatal infections[150].

The pattern of severe illness may be either rapidly fatal with sudden onset or an illness which runs a progressive, fatal course over 1–2 weeks, or there may be a biphasic pattern of illness, with an initial relatively mild non-specific febrile illness which goes through a recovery phase before an abrupt deterioration occurs up to a week later. Specifically, coxsackie virus infection may produce meningitis and myocarditis, either separately or together.

Myocarditis may be fatal and the clinical course is variable; examination may reveal a pale and sweaty infant, possibly with a rash, with cardiomegaly, hepatomegaly, poor peripheral perfusion and hypotension. No murmur is usually apparent. ECG and echocardiography reveal evidence of severe cardiac dysfunction[156]. Recovery with supportive treatment may occur, but some children have ongoing cardiac dysfunction requiring long-term management or possibly transplantation, although evidence for long-term cardiac dysfunction as a result of coxsackie virus myocarditis is scant.

Meningoencephalitis can occur, whether in isolation or in association with other features described above. The illness is difficult to distinguish from bacterial meningitis but the CSF tends to show lymphocytosis with a mildly raised protein and a relatively normal glucose content.

Other occasional manifestations of neonatal coxsackie virus infection have been noted, including pancreatitis, hepatitis, pneumonitis, paralysis, a necrotizing enterocolitis-like illness and pharyngitis. It has also been associated with a fulminant illness with hepatitis and coagulopathy indistinguishable from the 'sepsis-like' illness caused by echoviral infection[136].

PROGNOSIS FOLLOWING ENTEROVIRAL INFECTIONS

Neonatal polio carries a poor prognosis: around 50% die and 25% have residual paralysis[136]. Infection by one type of poliovirus does not prevent infection by the other two types, hence survivors of polio should be immunized.

The prognosis with echoviral and coxsackie virus disease depends upon the clinical presentation and illness severity. It is felt that the type of virus also impacts upon prognosis, with echovirus 11 and coxsackie B infection carrying an increased risk of neonatal mortality. Coxsackie virus myocarditis carries a high mortality.

In reports of babies following enteroviral meningitis, long-term neurodevelopmental disability may occur in 10–15% of cases[136,141] although one study reported no dysfunction in such infants[157].

TREATMENT AND PREVENTION OF ENTEROVIRAL INFECTIONS

Treatment in all cases of enteroviral infection is essentially supportive and intensive care may be necessary in many cases of vertically transmitted disease.

Immunoglobulin administration has been used, but there is no evidence of value in established illness[158]. If desired, high-dose intravenous immunoglobulin should be administered[159]. The use of interferon has been reported in neonatal coxsackie infection[150], but its role has not been established.

The use of passive immunization is important when trying to prevent spread in nursery outbreaks[160]. Where a mother has evidence of perinatal enteroviral disease, passive immunization of the newborn (400 mg/kg immunoglobulin by intravenous infusion) should be administered.

Finally, given the potential for hospital staff to spread enterovirus infection, effective infection control measures must be instituted. Strict handwashing, minimal handling of babies and isolation of suspected cases is essential. Where there is evidence of enteroviral infection, then no further admissions to that unit should occur until the infection has cleared.

MUMPS

The incidence in pregnancy is estimated at less than one per 1000 pregnancies in non-immunized populations[161,162]. It is associated with an increased risk of miscarriage in the first trimester[162]. The illness in pregnant women, in contrast to other viral illness, tends to run a similar course to infection in non-pregnant peers. Mumps infection in pregnancy does not appear to be associated with premature delivery.

CLINICAL FEATURES

There have been suggestions of a mumps-related embryopathy with endocardial fibroelastosis, intestinal atresia, cataracts or aqueduct stenosis, but the evidence is unclear[76,82,163]. There may be an increased risk of insulin-dependent diabetes mellitus in babies born to mothers who develop mumps in pregnancy[164]. Perinatal mumps causes little neonatal illness; parotitis is rarely reported. Postnatal neonatal exposure rarely results in illness, although pneumonitis has been reported[165,166].

TREATMENT AND PREVENTION

Symptomatic treatment and supportive care is all that is required in the majority of symptomatic cases and there is no role for passive immunization.

Prevention centres on widespread vaccination, which is part of the MMR vaccine administered at 12–15 months with a booster at 3–5 years recommended. It is highly effective and confers lifelong immunity.

Since neonatal illness is not a problem, mumps exposure in maternity units poses little threat to babies, but may cause problems for health-care staff and other mothers. Isolation and early discharge would seem advisable.

REFERENCES

1. Greenough, A. (1994) The TORCH screen and intrauterine infections. *Arch. Dis. Child.*, **70**(3), F163–F165.

2. Menser, M.A., Forrest, J., Slinn, R.F. *et al.* (1971) Rubella viruria in a 29 year old woman with congenital rubella. *Lancet*, **2**(728), 797–798.

3. Sever, J.L., Hardy, J.B., Nelson, K.B. *et al.* (1969) Rubella in the collaborative perinatal research study. II. Clinical and laboratory findings in children through 3 years of age. *Am. J. Dis. Child.*, **118**(1), 123–132.

4. Cooper, L.Z. (1985) The history and medical consequences of rubella. *Rev. Infect. Dis.*, **7**(suppl 1), S2–S10.

5. Cooper, L.Z., Prebuld, S.R., Alford, C.A. Jnr. (1995) *Infectious Diseases of the Fetus and Newborn Infant.*, W.B. Saunders, Philadelphia.

6. Hastreiter, A.R., Joorabchi, B., Pujatti, G. *et al.* (1967) Cardiovascular lesions associated with congenital rubella. *J. Pediatr.*, **71**(1), 59–65.

7. Fortuin, N.J., Morrow, A.G. and Roberts, W.C. (1971) Late vascular manifestations of the rubella syndrome. A roentgenographic-pathologic study. *Am. J. Med.*, **51**(1), 134–140.

8. Chiriboga-Klein, S., Oberfield, S.E., Casullo, A.M. *et al.* (1989) Growth in congenital rubella syndrome and correlation with clinical manifestations. *J. Pediatr.*, **115**(2), 251–255.

9. Wolinsky, J.S., Waxham, M.N., Hess, J.L. *et al.* (1982) Immunochemical features of a case of progressive rubella panencephalitis. *Clin. Exper. Immunol.*, **48**(2), 359–366.

10. Wolinsky, J.S., Dau, P.C., Buimovici-Klein, E. *et al.* (1979) Progressive rubella panencephalitis: immunovirological studies and results of isoprinosine therapy. *Clin. Exper. Immunol.*, **35**(3), 397–404.

11. Murphy, A.M., Reid, R.R., Pollard, I. *et al.* (1967) Rubella cataracts. Further clinical and virologic observations. *Am. J. Ophthalmol.*, **64**(6), 1109–1119.

12. Frank, K.E. and Purnell, E.W. (1978) Subretinal neovascularisation following rubella retinopathy. *Am. J. Ophthalmol.*, **86**(4), 462–466.

13. Boger, W.P. 3rd. (1980) Late ocular complications in congenital rubella syndrome. *Ophthalmology*, **87**(12), 1244–1252.

14. Givens, K.T., Lee, D.A., Jones, T. *et al.* (1993) Congenital rubella syndrome: ophthalmic manifestations and associated systemic disorders. *Br. J. Ophthalmol.*, **77**(6), 358–363.

15. Peckham C. (1985) Congenital rubella in the United Kingdom before 1970: the pre-vaccine era. *Rev. Infect. Dis.*, **7**(suppl), S11–S16.

16. Sever, J.L., South, M.A. and Shaver, K.A. (1985) Delayed manifestations of congenital rubella. *Rev. Infect. Dis.*, **7**(suppl), S164–S169.

17. Menser, M.A., Forrest, J.M. and Bransby R.D. (1978) Rubella infection and diabetes mellitus. *Lancet*, **1**(8055), 57–60.

18. Nieberg, P.I. and Gardner, L.I. (1976) Letter: thyroiditis and congenital rubella syndrome. *J. Pediatr.*, **89**(1), 156.

19. Ziring, P.R., Fedun, B.A. and Cooper, L.Z. (1975) Letter: thyrotoxicosis in congenital rubella. *J. Pediatr.*, **87**(6Pt1), 1002.

20. Preece, M.A., Kearney, P.J. and Marshall, W.C. (1977) Growth hormone deficiency in congenital rubella. *Lancet*, **2**(8043), 842–844.

21. Ziring, P.R. (1977) Congenital rubella: the teenage years. *Pediatr. Ann.*, **6**(12), 762–770.

22. Northrop, R.L., Gardner, W.M. and Geittmann, W.F. (1972) Rubella reinfection during early pregnancy: a case report. *Obstet. Gynecol.*, **39**(4), 524–526.

23. Braun, C., Kampa, D., Fressle, R. *et al.* (1994) Congenital rubella syndrome despite repeated vaccination of the mother: a coincidence of vaccine failure with failure to vaccinate. *Acta Paediatr.*, **83**(7), 674–677.

24. Plotkin, S.A. and Farquhar, J.D. (1972) Immunity to rubella: comparison between naturally and artificially induced resistance. *Postgrad. Med. J.*, **48**(suppl 3), 47–54.

25. Burgess, M.A. (1992) Rubella reinfection – what risk to the fetus? *Med. J. Aust.*, **156**(12), 824–825.

26. Arvin, A.M., Schmidt, M.J., Cantell, K. *et al.* (1982) Alpha interferon administration to infants with congenital rubella. *Antimicrob. Agents Chemother.*, **21**(2), 259–261.

27. Plotkin, S.A., Klaus, R.M. and Whitely, J.A. (1966) Hypogammaglobulinemia in an infant with congenital rubella syndrome; failure of 1-adamantanamine to stop virus excretion. *J. Pediatr.*, **69**(6), 1085–1091.

28. Huang, E.S., Alford, C.A., Reynolds, D.W. *et al.* (1980) Molecular epidemiology of cytomegalovirus infections in women and their infants. *N. Engl. J. Med.*, **303**(17), 958–962.

29. Adler, S.P., Chandrika, T., Lawrence, L. *et al.* (1983) Cytomegalovirus infections in neonates acquired by blood transfusions. *Pediatr. Infect. Dis.*, **2**(2), 114–118.

30. Ballard, R.A., Drew, W.L., Hufnagle, K.G. *et al.* (1979) Acquired cytomegalovirus infection in preterm infants. *Am. J. Dis. Child.*, **133**(5), 482–485.

31. Parayani, S.G., Yeager, A.S., Hosford-Dunn, H. *et al.* (1985) Sequelae of acquired cytomegalovirus infection in premature and sick term infants. *J. Pediatr.*, **107**(3), 451–456.

32. Brasfield, D.M., Stagno, S., Whitley, R.J. *et al.* (1987) Infant pneumonitis associated with cytomegalovirus, chlamydia, pneumocystis, and ureaplasmas: follow-up. *Pediatrics*, **79**(1), 76–83.

33. Boppano, S.B., Pass, R.F., Britt, W.J. *et al.* (1992) Symptomatic congenital cytomegalovirus infection: neonatal morbidity and mortality. *Pediatr. Infect. Dis. J.*, **11**(2), 93–99.

34. Almeida-Porada, G.D. and Ascensao, J.L. (1996) Cytomegalovirus as a cause of pancytopenia. *Leukemia Lymphoma*, **21**(3–4), 217–223.

35. Stagno, S. (1995) *Infectious Diseases of the Fetus and Newborn Infant*. W.B. Saunders, Philadelphia.

36. Jamison, R.M. and Hathorn, A.W. Jr. (1978) Isolation of cytomegalovirus from cerebrospinal fluid of a congenitally infected infant. *Am. J. Dis. Child.*, **132**(1), 63–64.

37. Troendle Atkins, J., Demmler, G.J., Williamson, W.D. *et al.* (1994) Polymerase chain reaction to detect cytomegalovirus DNA in the cerebrospinal fluid of neonates with congenital infection. *J. Infect. Dis.*, **169**(6), 1334–1337.

38. Hart, W.M. Jr, Reed, C.A., Freedman, H.L. *et al.* (1978) Cytomegalovirus in juvenile iridocyclitis. *Am. J. Ophthalmol.*, **86**(3), 329–331.

39. Anderson, K.S., Amos, C.S., Boppano, S. *et al.* (1996) Ocular abnormalities in congenital cytomegalovirus infection. *J. Am. Optometr. Assoc.*, **67**(5), 273–278.

40. Davis, L.E., Rarey, K.E., Stewart, J.A. *et al.* (1987) Recovery and probable persistence of cytomegalovirus in human inner ear fluid without cochlear damage. *Ann. Otol. Rhinol. Laryngol.*, **96**(4), 380–383.

41. Fowler, K.B., McCollister, F.P., Dahle, A.J. *et al.* (1997) Progressive and fluctuating sensorineural hearing loss in children with asymptomatic congenital cytomegalovirus infection. *J. Pediatr.*, **130**(4), 624–630.

42. Ansari, A.M., Davies D.B. and Jones M.R. (1977) Calcification in liver associated with congenital cytomegalic inclusion disease. *J. Pediatr.*, **90**(4), 661–663.

43. Pena-Alonso, R., Navarrete-Navarro, S., Ramon-Garcia, G. *et al.* (1996) Cytomegalovirus infection in children: frequency, anatomopathologic characteristics and underlying risk factor in 1618 autopsies. *Arch. Med. Res.*, **27**(1), 25–30.

44. Stagno, S., Pass, R.F., Reynolds, D.W. *et al.* (1980) Comparative study of diagnostic procedures for congenital cytomegalovirus infection. *Pediatrics*, **65**(2), 251–257.

45. Nigro, G., Scholz, H. and Bartmann, U. (1994) Ganciclovir therapy for symptomatic congenital cytomegalovirus infection in infants: a two regimen experience. *J. Pediatr.*, **124**(2), 318–322.

46. Attard-Montalto, S.P., English, M.C., Stimmler, L. *et al.* (1993) Ganciclovir treatment of congenital cytomegalovirus infection: a report of two cases. *Scand. J. Infect. Dis.*, **25**(3), 385–388.

47. Ljungman, P. (1995) Cytomegalovirus pneumonia: presentation, diagnosis and treatment. *Semin. Respir. Infect.*, **10**(4), 209–215.

48. Pass, R.F. (1996) Immunization strategy for prevention of congenital cytomegalovirus infection. *Infect. Agents Dis.*, **5**(4), 240–244.

49. Jones, C.A. and Isaacs, D. (1995) Predicting the outcome of symptomatic congenital cytomegalovirus infection. *J. Paediatr. Child Health*, **31**(2), 70–71.

50. Boppano, S., Fowler, K.B., Vaid, Y. *et al.* (1997) Neuroradiographic findings in the newborn period and long-term outcome in children with symptomatic congenital cytomegalovirus infection. *Pediatrics*, **99**(3), 409–414.

51. LaForet, E.G. and Lynch, C.L. Jr. (1947) Multiple congenital defects following maternal varicella. *N. Engl. J. Med.*, **236**, 534–537.

52. Srabstein, J.C., Morris, N, Larke, R.P. *et al.* (1974) Is there a congenital varicella syndrome? *J. Pediatr.*, **84**(2), 239–243.

53. Balducci, J., Rodis, J.F., Rosengren, J.F. *et al.* (1992) Pregnancy outcome following first-trimester varicella infection. *Obst. Gynecol.*, **79**(1), 5–6.

54. Gilbert, G.L. (1996) Congenital fetal infections. *Semin. Neonatol.*, **1**(2), 91–105.

55. Enders, G., Miller, E., Cradock-Watson, J.E. *et al.* (1994) Consequences of varicella and herpes zoster in pregnancy: prospective study of 1739 cases. *Lancet*, **343**(8912), 1548–1551.

56. Brunell, P.A. and Kotchmar, G.S. Jr. (1981) Zoster in infancy: failure to maintain virus latency following intrauterine infection. *J. Pediatr.*, **98**(1), 71–73.

57. Alkalay, A.L., Pomerance, J.J. and Rimoin, D.L. (1987) Fetal varicella syndrome. *J. Pediatr.*, **111**, 320–323.

58. Alexander, I. (1979) Congenital varicella. *Br. Med. J.*, **2**(6197), 1074.

59. Hitchcock, R., Birthistle, K., Carrington, D. *et al.* (1995) Colonic atresia and spinal cord atrophy associated with a case of fetal varicella syndrome. *J. Pediatr. Surg.*, **30**(9), 1344–1347.

60. Grose, C. (1989) Congenital varicella-zoster virus infection and the failure to establish virus-specific cell-mediated immunity. *Mol. Biol. Med.*, **6**(5), 453–462.

61. Myers, J.D. (1974) Congenital varicella in term infants: risk reconsidered. *J. Infect. Dis.*, **129**, 215–217.

62. Hanngren, K., Grandien, M. and Granstrom, G. (1985) Effect of zoster immunoglobulin for varicella prophylaxis in the newborn. *Scand. J. Infect. Dis.*, **17**(4), 343–347.

63. De Nicola, L.K. and Hanshaw, J.B. (1979) Congenital and neonatal varicella. *J. Pediatr.*, **94**(1), 175–176.

64. Miller, E., Cradock-Watson, J.E. and Ridehalgh, M.K.S. (1989) Outcome in newborn babies given anti-varicella-zoster immunoglobulin after perinatal maternal infection with varicella-zoster virus. *Lancet*, **2**(8689), 371–373.

65. Preblud, S.R. (1988) Nosocomial varicella: worth preventing, but how? *Am. J. Public Health*, **78**(1), 13–15.

66. Rubin, L., Leggiardro, R., Elie, M. *et al.* (1986) Disseminated varicella in a neonate: implications for immunoprophylaxis of neonates postnatally exposed to varicella. *Pediatr. Infect. Dis.*, **5**(1), 100–102.

67. Gustafon, T.L., Shebab, Z. and Brunell, P.A. (1984) Outbreak of varicella in a newborn intensive care nursery. *Am. J. Dis. Child.*, **138**(6), 548–550.

68. Querol, I., Bueno, M., Cebrian, A. *et al.* (1996) Connatal herpes zoster. *Cutis*, **58**(3), 231–234.

69. Music, S.I., Fine, E.M. and Togo, Y. (1971) Zoster-like disease in the newborn due to herpes-simplex virus. *N. Engl. J. Med.*, **284**(1), 24–26.

70. Gershon, A.A. (1995) Chickenpox, measles and mumps. In: *Infectious Diseases of the Fetus and Newborn Infant*, 4th edn, (eds J.S. Remington and J.O. Klein), W.B. Saunders, Philadelphia, p. 588.

71. Holland, P., Isaacs, D. and Moxon, E.R. (1986) Fatal neonatal varicella infection. *Lancet*, **2**(8516), 1156.

72. Haddad, J, Simeoni, U, Messner, J. *et al.* (1987) Acyclovir in prophylaxis and perinatal infection. *Lancet*, **1**(8575), 161.

73. White, C.J. (1996) Clinical trials of varicella vaccine in healthy children. *Infect. Dis. Clin. North Am.*, **10**(3), 595–608.

74. Irving, W.L. (1997) Varicella vaccine in pregnancy. Varicella zoster immunoglobulin should be given after exposure to the virus. *Br. Med. J.*, **314**(7075), 226–227.

75. Seidmann, D.S., Stevenson, D.K. and Arvin, A.M. (1996) Varicella vaccine in pregnancy. *Br. Med. J.*, **313**(7059), 701–702.

76. Isaacs, D. and Moxon, E.R. (1991) *Neonatal Infections*, Butterworth Heinemann Ltd, Oxford.

77. Seigel, M. and Fuerst, H.T. (1966) Low birth weight and maternal virus diseases. A prospective study of rubella, measles, mumps, chickenpox, and hepatitis. *JAMA*, **197**(9), 680–684.

78. Atmar, R.L., Englund, J.A. and Hammill, H. (1992) Complications of measles during pregnancy. *Clin. Infect. Dis.*, **14**(1), 217–226.

79. Eberhart-Phillips, J.E., Frederick, P.D., Baron, R.C. *et al.* (1993) Measles in pregnancy: a descriptive study of 58 cases. *Obstet. Gynecol.*, **82**(5), 797–801.

80. Jespersen, C.S., Litaauer, J. and Sagild, U. (1977) Measles as a cause of fetal defects. A retrospective study of the measles epidemics in Greenland. *Acta Paediatr. Scand.*, **66**(3), 367–372.

81. Gazala, E., Karplus, M, Liberman, J.R. *et al.* (1985) The effect of maternal measles on the fetus. *Pediatr. Infect. Dis.*, **4**(2), 203–204.

82. Gershon, A.A. (1995) Chickenpox, measles and mumps. In: *Infectious Diseases of the Fetus and Newborn Infant*, 4th edn, (Eds J.S. Remington and J.O. Klein), W.B. Saunders, Philadelphia.

83. Madhulika, Kabra, S.K. and Talati, A. (1994) Vitamin A supplementation in post-measles complications. *J. Trop. Pediatr.*, **40**(5), 305–307.

84. Hussey, G.D. and Klein, M. (1993) Routine high-dose vitamin A therapy for children hospitalised with measles. *J. Trop. Pediatr.*, **39**(6), 342–345.

85. Butler, J.C., Havens, P.L., Sowell, A.L. *et al.* (1993) Measles severity and serum retinol (vitamin A) concentration among children in the United States. *Pediatrics*, **91**(6), 1176–1181.

86. Rumore, M.M. (1993) Vitamin A as an immunomodulating agent. *Clin. Pharm.*, **12**(7), 506–514.

87. Brown, T., Anand, A., Ritchie, L.D. *et al.* (1984) Intrauterine parvovirus infection associated with hydrops fetalis. *Lancet*, **2**(8410), 1033–1034.

88. Knott, P.D., Welply, G.A. and Anderson, M.J. (1984) Serologically proved intrauterine infection with parvovirus. *Br. Med. J.* (clinical research edn), **289**(6459), 1660.

89. Tiessen, R.G., van Elsacker Niele, A.M., Vermeij Keers, C. *et al.* (1994) A fetus with a parvovirus infection and congenital anomalies. *Prenatal Diagn.*, **14**(3), 173–176.

90. Katz, V.L., McCoy, M.C., Kuller, J.A. *et al.* (1996) An association between fetal parvovirus B19 infection and fetal anomalies: a report of two cases. *Am. J. Perinatol.*, **13**(1), 43–45.

91. Public Health Laboratory Service Working Party on Fifth Disease (1990) Prospective study of human parvovirus (B19) infection in pregnancy. *Br. Med. J.*, **300**(6733), 1166–1170.

92. Kerr, J.R. (1996) Parvovirus B19 infection. *Eur. J. Clin. Microbiol. Infect. Dis.*, **15**(1), 10–29.

93. Kumar, M.L. (1991) Human parvovirus B19 and its associated diseases. *Clin. Perinatol.*, **18**(2), 209–225.

94. Pryde, P.G., Nugent, C.E., Pridjian, G. *et al.* (1992) Spontaneous resolution of nonimmune hydrops fetalis secondary to human parvovirus B19 infection. *Obstetr. Gynecol.*, **79**(5(Pt2)), 859–861.

95. Morey, A.L., Keeling, J.W., Porter, H.J. *et al.* (1992) Clinical and histopathological features of parvovirus B 19 infection in the human fetus. *Br. J. Obstetr. Gynaecol.*, **99**(7), 566–574.

96. Barton, L.L., Lax, D., Shehab, Z.M. *et al.* (1997) Congenital cardiomyopathy associated with human parvovirus B19 infection. *Am. Heart. J.*, **133**(1), 131–133.

97. Lynch, L. and Ghidini, A. (1993) Perinatal infections. *Curr. Opin. Obstetr. Gynecol.*, **5**(1), 24–32.

98. Dinsmoor, M.J. (1991) Obstetric and neonatal infection. *Curr. Opin. Obstetr. Gynecol.*, **3**(5), 707–714.

99. Sheikh, A.U., Ernest, J.M. and O'Shea, M. (1992) Long-term outcome in fetal hydrops from parvovirus B19 infection. *Am. J. Obstetr. & Gynecol.*, **167**(2), 337–341.

100. Blanche, S., Rouzioux, C., Guihard-Moscato, M.L. *et al.* (1989) A prospective study of infants born to women seropositive for human immunodeficiency virus type 1. HIV Infection in Newborns French Collaborative Study Group. *N. Eng. J. Med.*, **320**(25), 1643–1648.

101. European Collaborative Study (1994) Perinatal findings in children born to HIV-infected mothers. *Br. J. Obstetr. Gynaecol.*, **101**(2), 136–141.

102. European Collaborative Study (1991) Children born to women with HIV-1 infection: natural history and risk of transmission. *Lancet*, **337**(8736), 253–260.

103. Frenkel, L.D. and Gaur, S. (1994) Perinatal HIV infection and AIDS. *Clin. Perinatol.*, **21**(1), 98–107.

104. Chadwick, E.G. and Yogev, R. (1995) Pediatric AIDS. *Pediatr. Clin. North Am.*, **42**(4), 969–992.

105. Anon (1993) Antiretroviral therapy and medical management of the human immunodeficiency virus-infected child. Working Group in Anti-retroviral Therapy: National Pediatric HIV Resource Center. *Pediatr. Infect. Dis. J.*, **12**(6), 513–522.

106. Anon (1994) CD4 T cell count as predictor of *Pneumocystis carinii* pneumonia in children born to mothers infected with HIV. European Collaborative Study Group. *Br. Med. J.*, **308**(6926), 437–440.

107. Mueller, B.U., Butler, K.M., Husson, R.N. *et al.* (1991) *Pneumocystis carinii* pneumonia despite prophylaxis in children with human immunodeficiency virus infection. *J. Pediatr.*, **119**(6), 992–994.

108. Anon (1995) revised guidelines for prophylaxis against *Pneumocystis carinii* pneumonia for children infected with or perinatally exposed to human immunodeficiency virus. National Pediatric and Family HIV Resource Center and National Center for Infectious Disease, Center for Disease Control and Prevention. MMWR, **44**(RR-4), 1–11.

109. Davies, E.G., Elliman, D.A.C., Hart, C.A. *et al.* (1996) *Manual of Childhood Infections.* W.B. Saunders, London.

110. Anon (1996) Measles pneumonitis following measles-mumps-rubella vaccination of a patient with HIV infection, 1993. *MMWR,* **45**(28), 603–606.

111. Mofenson, L.M. and Moye, J. Jr. (1997) Intravenous immune globulin for the prevention of infections in children with symptomatic human immunodeficiency virus infection. *Pediatr. Res.,* **33**(1 suppl), S80–89.

112. Tovo, P.A., de Martino, M., Gabiano, C. *et al.* (1992) Prognostic factors and survival in children with perinatal HIV-1 infection. The Italian Register for HIV Infections in Children. *Lancet,* **339**(8804), 1249–1253.

113. Scott, G.B., Hutto, C., Makuch, R.W. *et al.* (1989) Survival in children with perinatally acquired human immunodeficiency virus type 1 infection. *N. Engl. J. Med.,* **321**(26), 1791–1796.

114. Hall, S.M. and Glickman, M. (1988) The British Paediatric Surveillance Unit. *Arch. Dis. Child.,* **63**(3), 344–346.

115. Sullivan-Bolyai, J., Hull, H.F., Wilson, C. *et al.* (1983) Neonatal herpes simplex virus in King County, Washington. Increasing incidence and epidemiologic correlates. *JAMA,* **250**(22), 3059–3062.

116. Hutto, C., Arvin, A., Jacobs, R. *et al.* (1987) Intrauterine herpes simplex virus infections. *J. Pediatr.,* **110**(1), 97–101.

117. Baldwin, S. and Whitley, R.J. (1989) Intrauterine HSV infection. *Teratology,* **39**(1), 1–10.

118. Yeager, A.S. and Arvin, A.M. (1984) Reasons for the absence of a history of recurrent genital infections in mothers of neonates infected with herpes simplex virus. *Pediatrics,* **73**(2), 188–193.

119. Whitley, R.J. and Arvin, A.M. (1995) Herpes simplex virus infections. In: *Infectious Diseases of the Fetus and Newborn Infant,* 4th edn. (Eds J.S. Remington and J.O. Klein), eds. W.B. Saunders, Philadelphia.

120. McIntosh, D. and Isaacs, D. (1992) Herpes simplex virus infection in pregnancy. *Arch. Dis. Child.,* **67**(10F), 1137–1138.

121. Whitley, R.J., Nahmias, A.J., Visintine, A.M. *et al.* (1980) The natural history of herpes simplex virus infection of mother and newborn. *Pediatrics,* **66**(4), 489–494.

122. Whitley, R.J., Corey, L., Arvin, A. *et al.* (1988) Changing presentation of herpes simplex virus infection in neonates. *J. Infect. Dis.,* **158**(1), 109–116.

123. Whitley, R.J., Nahmias, A.J., Soong, S.J. *et al.* (1980) Vidarabine therapy of neonatal herpes simplex virus infection. *Pediatrics,* **66**(4), 495–501.

124. Kohl, S. (1997) Neonatal herpes simplex virus infection. *Clin. Perinatol.,* **24**(1), 129–150.

125. Whitley, R.J., Arvin, A., Prober, C. *et al.* (1991) Predictors of morbidity and mortality in neonates with herpes simplex virus infections. The National Institute of Allergy and Infectious Diseases Collaborative Antiviral Study Group. *N. Engl. J. Med.,* **324**(7), 450–454.

126. Kimberlan, D.W., Lakeman, F.D., Arvin, A.M. *et al.* (1996) Application of the polymerase chain reaction to the diagnosis and management of neonatal herpes simplex virus disease. National Institute of Allergy and Infectious Diseases Collaborative Antiviral Study Group. *J. Infect. Dis.,* **174**(6), 1162–1167.

127. Whitley, R.J. (1993) Neonatal herpes simplex virus infections. *J. Med. Virol.,* (suppl 1), 13–21.

128. Whitley, R.J., Arvin, A., Prober, C. *et al.* (1991) A controlled trial comparing vidarabine with acyclovir in neonatal herpes simplex virus infection. Infectious Diseases Collaborative Antiviral Study Group. *N. Engl. J. Med.,* **324**(7), 444–449.

129. Whitley, R.J., Alford, C.A., Hirsch, M.S. *et al.* (1986) Vidarabine versus acyclovir therapy in herpes simplex encephalitis. *N. Engl. J. Med.,* **314**(3), 144–149.

130. O'Grady, J.G., Gimson, A.E., O'Brien, C.J. *et al.* (1988) Controlled trials of charcoal hemoperfusion and prognostic factors in fulminant hepatic failure. *Gastroenterology,* **94**(5 Pt1), 1186–1192.

131. Schweitzer, I.L., Dunn, A.E., Peters, R.L. *et al.* (1973) Viral hepatitis B in neonates and infants. *Am. J. Med.,* **55**, 762–771.

132. Shiraki, K., Yoshi, N., Shakurai, M. *et al.* (1980) Acute hepatitis B in infants born to carrier mothers with the antibody to hepatitis B e antigen. *J. Pediatr.,* **97**, 768–770.

133. Sinatra, F.R., Shah, P., Weissman, J.Y. *et al.* (1997) Perinatal transmitted acute icteric hepatitis B in infants born to hepatitis B surface antigen-positive and anti-hepatitis Be-positive carrier mothers. *Pediatrics,* **70**, 557–559.

134. Beasley, R.P., Hwang, L.Y., Lee, G.C.Y. *et al.* (1983) Prevention of perinatally transmitted hepatitis B virus infections with hepatitis B immune globulin and hepatitis B vaccine. *Lancet*, **2**(8359), 1099–1102.

135. Wong, V.C., Ip, H.M., Reesink, H.W. *et al.* (1984) Prevention of the HBsAg carrier state in newborn infants of mothers who are chronic carriers of HBsAg and HBeAg by administration of hepatitis-B vaccine and hepatitis-B immunoglobulin. Double-blind randomised placebo-controlled study. *Lancet*, **1**(8383), 921–926.

136. Cherry, J.D. (1995) Enteroviruses. In: *Infectious Diseases of the Fetus and Newborn Infant*, 4th edn, (Eds J.S. Remington and J.O. Klein), W.B. Saunders, Philadelphia, pp. 404–446.

137. Nagington, J., Wreghitt, T.G., Gandy, G. *et al.* (1978) Fatal echovirus 11 infections in an outbreak in special-care baby unit. *Lancet*, **2**(8092), 725–728.

138. Basso, N.G., Fonseca, M.E., Garcia, A.G. *et al.* (1990) Enterovirus isolation from fetal and placental tissues. *Acta Virologica*, **34**(1), 49–57.

139. Reyes, M.P., Zalenski, D., Smith, F. *et al.* (1986) Coxsackievirus-positive cervices in women with febrile illnesses during the third trimester in pregnancy. *Am. J. Obstetr. Gynecol.*, **155**(1), 159–161.

140. Modlin, J.F. (1986) Perinatal echovirus infection: insights from a literature review of 61 cases of serious infection and 16 outbreaks in nurseries. *Rev. Infect. Dis.*, **8**(6), 918–926.

141. Royle, J. (1996) Perinatal viral infections. *Semin. Neonatol.*, **1**(2), 107–118.

142. Anon (1986) Avoiding the danger of enteroviruses to newborn infants (editorial). *Lancet*, **1**(8474), 194–195.

143. Bergeisen, G.H., Bauman, R.J. and Gilmore, R.L. (1986) Neonatal paralytic poliomyelitis. A case report. *Arch. Neurol.*, **43**(2), 192–194.

144. Horn, P. (1955) Poliomyelitis in pregnancy. A twenty-year report from Los Angeles County, California. *Obstetr. Gynecol.*, **6**, 121.

145. Harjulehto-Mervaala, T., Aro, T., Hiilesmaa, V.K. *et al.* (1994) Oral polio vaccination during pregnancy: lack of impact on fetal development and perinatal outcome. *Clin. Infect. Dis.*, **18**(3), 414–420.

146. Morens, D.M. (1978) Enteroviral disease in early infancy. *J. Pediatr.*, **92**(3), 374–377.

147. Eichenwald, H.F., Kostelov, O. and Fasso, L.A. (1960) The 'cloud baby': an example of bacterial–viral interaction. *Am. J. Dis. Child.*, **100**, 161–163.

148. Isaacs, D., Dobson, S.R., Wilkinson, A.R. *et al.* (1989) Conservative management of an echovirus 11 outbreak in a neonatal unit. *Lancet*, **1**(8637), 543–545.

149. Kaplan, M.H., Klein, S.W., McPhee, J. *et al.* (1983) Group B coxsackievirus infections in infants younger than three months of age: a serious childhood illness. *Rev. Infect. Dis.*, **5**(6), 1019–1032.

150. Isacsohn, M., Eidelman, A.I., Kaplan, M. *et al.* (1994) Neonatal coxsackievirus group B infections: experience of a single department of neonatology. *Israel J. Med. Sci.*, **30**(5–6), 371–374.

151. Baker, D.A. and Phillips, C.A. (1980) Maternal and neonatal infection with coxsackievirus. *Obstetr. Gynecol.*, **55**(Suppl 3), 12S–15S.

152. Drutys-Voets, E., van Renterghem, L. and Gerniers, S. (1997) Coxsackie B virus epidemiology and neonatal infection in Belgium. *J. Infection*, **27**(3), 311–316.

153. Gauntt, C.J., Gudvangen, R.J., Brans, Y.W. *et al.* (1985) Coxsackievirus group B antibodies in the ventricular fluid of infants with severe anatomic defects in the central nervous system. *Pediatrics*, **76**(1), 64–68.

154. Brown, G.C. and Evans, T.N. (1967) Serologic evidence of Coxsackievirus etiology of congenital heart disease. *JAMA*, **199**(3), 183–187.

155. Strong, B.S. and Young, S.A. (1995) Intrauterine coxsackie virus, group B type 1 infection: viral cultivation from amniotic fluid in the third trimester. *Am. J. Perinatol.*, **12**(2), 78–79.

156. Krajden, S. and Middleton, P.J. (1983) Enterovirus infections in the neonate. *Clin. Pediatr.*, **22**(2), 87–92.

157. Bergman, I., Painter, M.J. Wald, E.R. *et al.* (1987) Outcome in children with enteroviral meningitis during the first year of life. *J. Pediatr.*, **110**(5), 705–709.

158. Abzug, M.J., Keyserling, H.L., Lee, M.L. *et al.* (1995) Neonatal enterovirus infection: virology, serology, and effects of intravenous immune globulin. *Clin. Infect. Dis.*, **20**(5), 1201–1206.

159. Hammond, G.W., Lukes, H., Wells, B. *et al.* (1985) Maternal and neonatal neutralizing antibody titers to selected enteroviruses. *Pediatr. Infect. Dis.*, **4**(1), 32–35.

160. Nagington, J., Gandy, G., Walker, J. *et al.* (1983) Use of normal immunoglobulin in an echovirus 11 outbreak in a special-care baby unit. *Lancet*, **2**(8347), 443–446.

161. Korones, S.B. (1988) Uncommon virus infections of the mother, fetus, and newborn: influenza, mumps, and measles. *Clin. Perinatol.*, **15**(2), 259–272.

162. Siegel, M., Fuerst, H.T. and Peress, M.S. (1966) Comparative fetal mortality in maternal virus diseases. A prospective study on rubella, measles, mumps, chickenpox and hepatitis. *N. Engl. J. Med.*, **274**, 768–771.

163. Siegel, M. (1973) Congenital malformations following chickenpox, measles, mumps and hepatitis. Results of a cohort study. *JAMA*, **226**(13), 1521–1524.

164. Fine, P.E., Adelstein, A.M., Snowman, J. *et al.* (1985) Long term effects of exposure to viral infections in utero. *Br. Med. J.* (clinical research edn), **290**(6467), 509–511.

165. Jones, J.F., Ray, C.G. and Fulginiti, V.A. (1980) Perinatal mumps infection. *J. Pediatr.*, **96**(5), 912–914.

166. Reman, O., Freymuth, F., Laloum, D. *et al.* (1986) Neonatal respiratory distress due to mumps. *Arch. Dis. Child.*, **61**(1), 80–81.

167. Shearer, G.M. and Clerici, M. (1993) Abnormalities of immune regulation in human immunodeficiency virus infection. *Pediatr. Res.*, **33**(suppl 1), S71–74.

168. Espanol, T., Garcia, X., Caragol, I. *et al.* (1991) Immunological abnormalities in pediatric AIDS. *Immunolog. Invest.*, **20**(2), 215–221.

169. Pahwa, S. (1990) Immune defects in pediatric AIDS, their pathogenesis, and role of immunotherapy. *Crit. Care Med.*, **18**(suppl 2), S138–143.

Viral infections with pathological consequences for reproduction in veterinary species

J. Brownlie and G.C.W. England

INTRODUCTION

An essential requirement for human civilization was the domestication of animals and the cultivation of crops. In a prescient essay, Francis Galton in 1865 concluded that six conditions were necessary for successful domestication of which his fifth, *they should breed freely*; was perhaps the most important. It was this ability to maintain and increase his domesticated 'prey', independent of the usual seasonal constraints, that transformed man into the supreme carnivore and prepared him for a population explosion that started some 8000 years ago and continues to run apace to the present day and to the foreseeable future. In a comprehensive review of the natural history of domesticated mammals, Clutton-Brock[1] examined the limited number of species that accord to the dictates of successful domestication. The central caveat has been the ability to breed in captivity and, from this has sprung the selection and development of breeds within a species that can range from the Shetland pony to the Shire horse, from the diminutive Dexter cow to Humped Zebu cattle and from the Dachshund to the Great Dane. Many of these breeds have been adapted over thousands of years to suit the conditions of their locality better, thereby extending the geographical range for mankind's establishment.

In a haunting comment about the future of non-domesticated species, Galton[2] stated that:

> It would appear that every wild animal has had its chance of being domesticated, that those few which fulfilled the above conditions were domesticated long ago, but that the large remainder, who fail sometimes in only one small particular, are destined to perpetual wildness so long as their race continues. As civilization extends they are doomed to be gradually destroyed off the face of the earth as useless consumers of cultivated produce.

It is an irony that many modern scientific techniques used for improved reproductive performance of domesticated species, e.g. artificial insemination and *in vitro* fertilization, are now a potential lifeline for endangered wildlife species.

COMPARATIVE ASPECTS OF REPRODUCTIVE PHYSIOLOGY AND PLACENTATION

Since earliest times, the differences in reproductive cycles of domesticated species has fascinated the human observer. For the herdsman, such information was critical for the breeding programme; for the early scientist, it was clearly an example of biological variation worthy of recording (Figure 14.1).

Viral Infections in Obstetrics and Gynaecology. Edited by D.J. Jeffries and C.N. Hudson. Published in 1999 by Arnold, ISBN 0 340 74095 7.

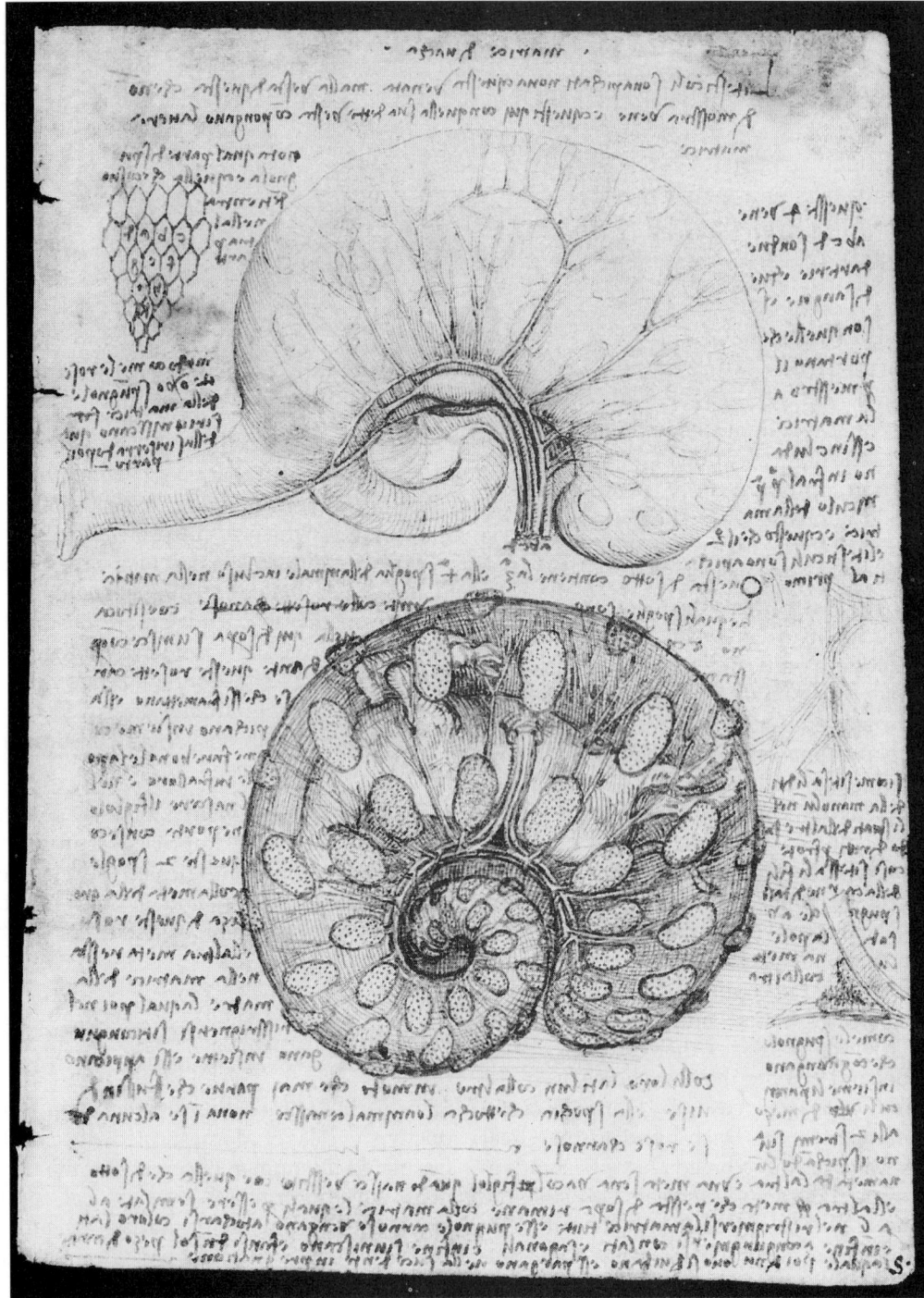

Figure 14.1 Bovine uterus containing an unborn fetus and revealing the typical caruncular placentation. Drawing by Leonardo da Vinci (1452–1519). (The Royal Collection © 1997. Her Majesty Queen Elizabeth II. Reproduced with permission.)

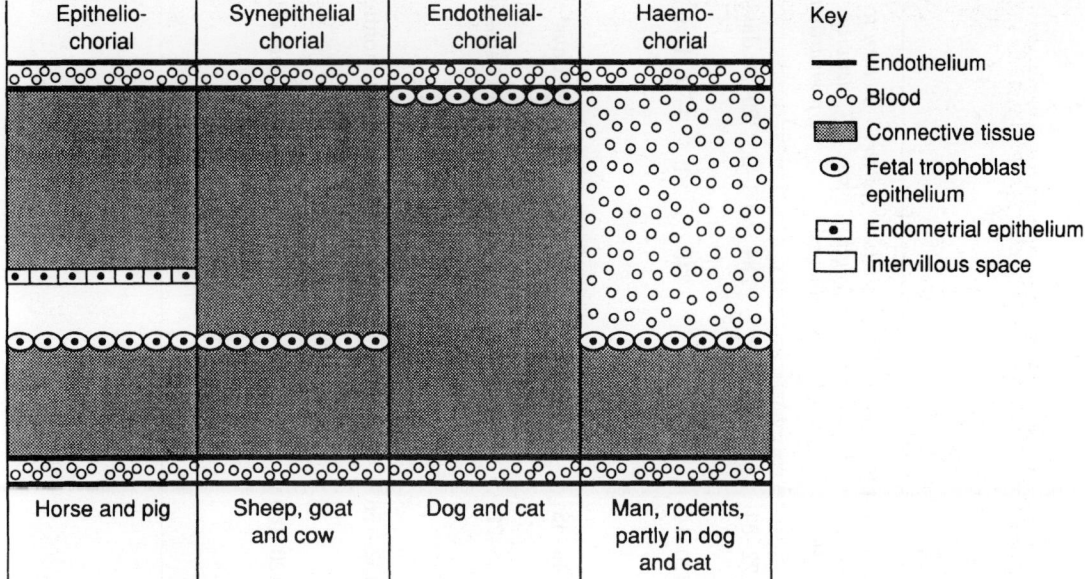

Epithelio-chorial	Synepithelial chorial	Endothelial-chorial	Haemo-chorial
Horse and pig	Sheep, goat and cow	Dog and cat	Man, rodents, partly in dog and cat

Key

━━ Endothelium
∘∘∘ Blood
▓ Connective tissue
⊙ Fetal trophoblast epithelium
▣ Endometrial epithelium
▢ Intervillous space

Figure 14.2 Diagrammatic representation of types of placenta found in domestic animals and man based on Grosser's original classification. (Reproduced by kind permission of Professor D.E. Noakes, Royal Veterinary College, from *Veterinary Reproduction and Obstetrics*, W.B. Saunders, London, 1996.)

The remarkable drawing by Leonardo da Vinci of the gravid bovine uterus illustrates the discrete but intimate apposition of fetal/maternal structures in the placental caruncles found in ruminants. There is, however, a variation in the type of placentation in the different species; a classification has been made dependent on the number and integrity of layers between fetal and maternal circulations (Figure 14.2). It can be seen from this scheme that human and rodents both have haemochorial placentation with a closer association of maternal/fetal circulation than that of ruminants, horses or pigs. The different 'placental barriers' in the species have consequences for certain diseases; haemolytic disease in the foal occurs after fetal antigens cross the placenta and prime the maternal immune system to produce antibodies and, because maternal antibodies cannot cross the equine placenta, the disease follows the uptake of colostral antibodies. In humans, where the transmission of maternal antibodies occurs directly across the fetal placenta, the same antibody–antigen disease may occur in the unborn fetus.

There are considerable variations in the ability of viruses to cause fetal pathology; the different viral tropisms and the different types of placentation both have implications for transmission to the fetus and potential pathology.

A composite review of normal values for reproduction cycles of the main veterinary species is shown in Table 14.1.

There is an extensive literature on normal and perturbed endocrine mechanisms in the reproduction of veterinary species[3].

Normal reproductive performance in veterinary species: substantial losses due to early fetal losses and to congenital abnormalities but often the cause is not known

The normal expectation of successful pregnancy in farm animals carries an implicit timing interval; maintenance of breeding

Table 14.1 Composite table of normal values for parameters of reproduction in domesticated species

Species	Chromosome number	Cyclicity	Interoestrous interval (days)	Duration of oestrus (h)	Time of ovulation	Time conceptus enters uterus (h)	Day of maternal recognition	Gestation length (days)	Litter size	Return to activity postpartum
Cow	60	Non-seasonal polyoestrus	21	18	12h after oestrus ends	72–84	16–17	284	1–2	20–30 days
Mare	64	Seasonal polyoestrus (long-day breeder)	21	120–150	1–2 days before end of oestrus	120–144	14–16	340	1	4–16 days
Sow	38	Non-seasonal polyoestrus	21	45	36h after oestrus begins	46–48	12	115	8–12	4–9 days*
Ewe	54	Seasonal polyoestrus (short-day breeder)	17	36	30h after oestrus begins	66–72	12–13	150	1–2	Next season
Bitch	78	Non-seasonal monoestrus	210–240	7–9 days	Approx. 1–2 days after oestrus begins	132–156	?	63	4–12	3–6 months
Queen	38	Seasonal polyoestrus (long-day breeder)	18	5–6 days	Induced 24–72 hours after coitus	120–160	?	62	3–6	1–6 weeks*

* Depends upon the length of lactation

animals beyond the predicted time for initiating pregnancy is an ecomonic loss for the farmer or the stud manager. As an example, it has been estimated that each day extension beyond the normal 365 days calving interval in cattle costs £3.35[4]. As the calving interval in the UK national herd is 395 days, the annual cost has been estimated to be over £300 million[3].

A consequence of breeding high-production animals, whether for meat or milk, is a significant perturbation of the normal physiology of reproduction and endocrine function; perhaps such demands may be likened to those experienced by top-class athletes or down-trodden academics. Reported figures for conception vary; the average conception rate for mares is 72.4%[5], for cattle 50–66%[3], for ewes 93%[6], for sows 90%[7] and for the bitch 70–80%[8].

The failure to maintain pregnancy is a further concern, the causes of which are controversial. The early elimination of 'unfit' embryos has been considered a natural selection mechanism for suitable offspring and the implication is that the failed embryos have genomic lesions[9]. In general, it is anticipated that, under normal farm conditions, 5–10% of pregnancies will not survive to full term. However, other causes of early embryonic losses can substantially increase this figure, such as poor nutrition of the dam (particularly important in hill sheep), twinning (a cause of 10–30% of abortions in mares), enviromental factors (e.g. temperatures and ingestion of toxic factors) and microbial infections (see below).

Of all reasons for culling in farm animals, infertility is a major cause. In dairy cattle, it is estimated to be about 33% in the UK[10] and, in the USA, up to 49.86%[11]. However, some caution may be needed in the veterinary use of the term *'infertility'*; it denotes failure to be fertile within the defined time for farming productivity whereas the more appropriate term may be 'subfertile'.

Major concerns for reproductive losses in veterinary species are considered to be infectious whereas similar human losses are considered to be genetic failures

The veterinary practitioner, when confronted with cases of reproductive failure, will consider the investigation of microbial causes as imperative. It is crucial for the control of infertility, abortion and congenital damage to be able to diagnose potential pathogens. Although a wide range of chromosomal abnormalities has been described in veterinary species, it is the first responsibility of the veterinary clinician to take samples (including fetal, where possible) to investigate viral, bacterial, mycoplasmal, protozoal or fungal causes of disease. Successful diagnosis of abortifacient pathogens is not easy and only from a percentage of abortions can a demonstration of potential causal organisms be shown, e.g. mares about 15%[5], cattle 4.3–7.4% (MAFF – VIDA II, years 1984–92), ewes 43.2–60.4% (MAFF – VIDA II, years 1984–92), sows 29.5–42.3% (MAFF – VIDA II, years 1984–92).

Within individual groups of animals, there can be devastating 'abortion storms' with up to 90% loss of pregnancies. For this reason, the veterinarian must be cognizant of potential microbial causes of reproductive loss and provide appropriate control, e.g. vaccination or isolation. The wide range of viral infections that can cause reproductive disease, both as explosive outbreaks and as low-grade debilitating infections, is detailed below.

COMPARATIVE ASPECTS OF HOST RANGE FOR REPRODUCTIVE DISEASE

In any investigation of reproductive disease the veterinarian will take account of the possibility of viral diseases that are species specific (e.g. equine viral arteritis), those that can be transmitted from one species to another (e.g. pestiviruses from sheep to cattle) and those that are vector borne (e.g. orbiviruses in ruminants and horses). Such epidemiological information is invaluable both for establishing a possible diagnosis and for designing control procedures. There is clearly a necessity for an awareness of potentially zoonotic infections; the intimacy of the veterinary approach to examinations of diseased animals requires a sound understanding of comparative microbiology. Many causes of reproductive diseases are both bacterial and zoonotic (e.g. brucella, salmonella and listeria) but viral zoonotic infections can also be a cause of concern to the practitioner (e.g. Rift valley fever, equine encephalitis viruses and Aujeszky's disease virus).

MECHANISMS OF REPRODUCTIVE FAILURE

The *in utero* environment provides both nutrient and microbial sterility for the secure development of the fetus. For much of this period, the fetus is immunologically incompetent and would be highly susceptible to viral infection. The fact that pregnancy is successful reflects the dam's ability to protect the fetus against such exposure. Damage to the placenta or depression of the dam's immune responsiveness can predispose to fetal damage; this can be seen with viruses that cause immune deficiencies (e.g. feline leukaemia virus, believed to be the single most common cause of infertility in the queen[12]).

Viruses can also cause vulvovaginitis, endometritis, salpingitis and oophoritis in all the veterinary species (e.g. bovine herpesvirus I and enteroviruses) but their direct action on fertility is variable. These viruses are often transmitted venereally after contact with infected males or following artificial insemination. Several viruses are demonstrable in semen and, due to the worldwide trade in frozen semen, there is real potential for rapid transmission of such infections. Most veterinary authorities are aware of these consequences and there are strict codes of conduct for the preparation and importation of semen.

In many virus diseases, the cause of fetal death is still poorly understood. Viruses can act indirectly by causing inflammation and sometimes necrosis to the placenta (e.g. Border disease virus of sheep[13]); such a placentitis can disrupt fetal nutrition, resulting in growth retardation or even death. The longer term consequences of placental insufficiency, proposed by the Barker hypothesis[14], have not, as yet, been identified in the veterinary species. Viruses can also act directly on the fetus providing they can traverse the placental barrier and establish infecion in the fetus. The outcome can be congenital damage, fetal death, abortion or persistent infection (e.g. bovine virus diarrhoea virus[15]). Mummification of the fetus is also not uncommon following virus infections of pregnant ruminants.

VERTICAL TRANSMISSION OF VIRAL INFECTIONS

The transmission of a virus from a female to an embryo, fetus or newborn animal, either during pregnancy or shortly after parturition, constitutes vertical transmission. This mechanism promotes survival of the virus within the population, particularly when the consequences of infection are persistent infection of the offspring. In certain cases there is specific transplacental infection (e.g. pestiviruses), whilst in other cases the fetus may be infected during passage through the birth canal (e.g. parvoviruses), and certain viruses are transmitted shortly after parturition via the colostrum or milk (e.g. ruminant lentiviruses). In many cases transplacental infection results in embryonic death and abortion (e.g. orbiviruses); in certain cases congenital disease may be produced (bunyaviruses).

The evidence for vertical transmission of infection is of considerable concern for the control and, ultimately, the eradication of disease. It is axiomatic that persisting viruses that can transmit vertically are virtually impossible to eliminate. That such viruses exist does present the veterinary clinical practitioner with real dilemmas for control. Such transmission can occur (a) *in utero* directly to the unborn fetus, (b) in the peripartum period or even (c) via the germline cells.

Evidence for *in utero* transmission is sometimes anecdotal but, for some examples of veterinary virus infections, remains irrefutable, e.g. pestiviruses in ruminants and pigs[15,16]. The immune capability of the dam is the most important mechanism by which transmission of virus to the fetus is typically thwarted. However, dams that are naive to an infection and support an initial viraemia during a primary infection provide a brief opportunity for viruses to travel to and cross the placental barrier. The consequence of this fetal infection appears to depend, amongst other factors, on fetal age. The early fetus, before the development of immunocompetence, is highly vulnerable to virus establishment. It provides a sterile environment with actively dividing cells in most organ systems without the protection of surveillant and effector immune cells. At the onset of immunotolerance, some established viruses appear to be accepted as 'self' with deletion of viral-reactive lymphocytes, thereby providing a means for their persistent infection (e.g. bovine virus diarrhoea virus).

Several viruses are said to cause *in utero* infections whereas evidence from controlled experimental infections has shown that vertical infections result from transmission during the peripartum period or from the ingestion of colostrum (e.g. the caprine lentivirus – caprine arthritis encephalitis virus). Such experimental studies on the target species are the province of veterinary scientists and may provide valuable comparative models for human viral infections. Recent advances in molecular techniques, particularly polymerase chain reaction (PCR) and *in situ* hybridization (ISH), have been of critical importance in defining non-culturable viruses (e.g. the virus causing bovine malignant catarrhal fever[17]) and in defining cell tropism[18].

Germline transmission of viruses is a major worry for veterinary scientists. Apart from the inaccessibility of viruses within germ cells and the inevitable vertical transmission from dam to offspring, there is a continuing awareness of the considerable international trade in germline cells, e.g. semen and fertilized embryos, and the potential they may pose for viral transmission. There are guidelines provided for the screening of semen for viral pathogens; whilst not an exhaustive list, it includes those pathogens that are notifiable, e.g. foot and mouth disease virus and blue tongue virus. For embryos, the International Embryo Transfer Society have provided a washing procedure that requires both saline and trypsin solution washes[19]. This is considered sufficient to remove all adherent virus from the zona pellucida, a contention that, under certain conditions, is questioned[20]. However, the washing procedures would have no influence on virus within blastomeres of the unhatched embryo. Good evidence for transmission of infectious viral pathogens is still awaited although there is preliminary evidence for the transmission of virus across the zona pellucida in mice[21] and for retroviral genes within chicken germline cells[22]. It has also been reported that sperm have the capacity to act as vectors for the introduction of foreign DNA into the female germ cells at fertilization[23]; the possible introduction of viral nucleic acid by the same route remains speculative. The presence of virus in high concentrations in semen has been reported for several animal infections (e.g. equine arteritis virus[24], blue tongue virus[25] and bovine virus diarrhoea virus[26]).

EMERGING DISEASES OF CONSEQUENCE FOR REPRODUCTION

The emergence of new diseases, particularly viral, is not exceptional; it has been calculated that, over the last 200 years, new epidemics of disease have occurred every 2–3 years of recorded history[27]. A review of veterinary publications over the last 50 years will confirm that this, if anything, is an underestimate. Some of these diseases are confined to veterinary species and may not attract widespread attention (e.g. porcine reproductive and respiratory syndrome and pigeon paramyxovirus) whereas some are of major political and public health significance (e.g. bovine spongiform encephalopathy (BSE) and the equine morbillivirus).

In presenting a review of viruses with potential pathology for the reproductive tissues, it must be understood that the list will be incomplete, not just for brevity but for our failure to anticipate the next plague.

SPECIES RESPONSE TO REPRODUCTIVE INFECTION

Although many viruses have the potential to infect the reproductive tissues, there is a limited repertoire of pathological responses available to the host. The responses are often characteristic of the species. Brief overviews of typical species responses are given below.

Bovine, ovine and caprine

The ruminant species are permissive to many viruses that cause considerable reproductive losses. Many of the viruses are outlined below but certain pathologies characterize their infection. Ruminant placentae do not permit maternal immune intervention to protect the fetus once there has been transplacental transmission. Infection of the early fetus during the first trimester, before immune competence has been established, leads to much congenital damage. Severe pathology can cause fetal death and abortion. In ruminants death often results in retention of the fetus and its subsequent mummification; such mummies can often give sufficient uterine signals for the apparent maintenance of pregnancy. This can

prevent a rapid return to oestrus. In multiparous pregnancy, as in sheep, it is not uncommon to have a live pregnancy with an associated mummified fetus.

Some virus infections can cause widespread 'abortion storms' when they infect a susceptible population. The nature of modern farming is that many ruminant animals will be at a similar stage of pregnancy and thereby present the virus with a concentration of high-risk hosts. Loss of the early fetus is sometimes difficult for the farmer to detect and the first indications may have to await obvious signs of a return to oestral cycling.

Equine

Reproductive failure in the mare is not uncommon and both viral and bacterial infections play an important role.

Early embryonic loss usually results in resorption which, if occurring after maternal recognition of pregnancy, is characterized by a muco-haemorrhagic discharge and a rapid return to oestrous behaviour. Rarely, there may be persistence of the corpora lutea. However, embryonic loss that occurs later than 40 days from ovulation results in a condition called pseudopregnancy type II. This is associated with persistence of the endometrial cups that secrete equine chorionic gonadotropin and thereby a failure to return to cyclical activity. For this reason, the mare must be carefully examined or the pregnancy loss may go unnoticed. Later, fetal loss usually results in abortion, unless there are multiple conceptuses with one remaining viable or some malpresentation and failure of expulsion; in either of these cases, mummification may result.

Porcine

The sow produces more offspring from each pregnancy than other domestic species – an average range of 8–12 piglets/litter. Some unevenness in piglet size is common, with one or two small 'runty' piglets being produced amongst otherwise normal-sized piglets. However, increased numbers of runts or small litter sizes can reflect microbial infection. There are several viruses that can cross transplacentally and that are permissive for fetal tissues. Some of these viruses cause congenital abnormalities whereas others cause fetal death and usually abortion (classic swine fever and swine infertility and respiratory syndrome virus). Reproductive failure is often followed by a return to oestrus within 4–9 days.

Canine

There are many causes of reproductive failure in the dog and bitch. For the owner, the most obvious sign is the absence of offspring despite a 'tied' mating during the fertile part of the reproductive cycle and an apparently normal pregnancy. However, these bitches may have never been pregnant, the confusion being caused by the clinical signs of pregnancy in the non-pregnant animal. Pseudopregnancy is a common and normal event in the bitch since the endocrine environment is almost identical in pregnancy and non-pregnancy. Non-pregnant bitches may have increased appetite, weight gain, mammary development and lactation and behavioural changes typical of late pregnancy. Pregnancy loss may also be considered when bitches sometimes exhibit a vulval discharge approximately one month after mating but this is not related to pregnancy or to loss of pregnancy.

In fact, the most common reason for conception failure is mating at an inappropriate time. However, viral infections do play a role in canine infertility although there are few data concerning their role in male infertility. In the female the principal effect is embryonic resorption, fetal abortion or neonatal death. Viral colpitis is rare and primary viral endometritis, salpingitis and oophoritis have not been reported. In many cases resorption may pass unnoticed by the owner, unless pregnancy has been diagnosed using diagnostic real-time ultrasound or measurement of acute-phase serum proteins. Resorption is sometimes characterized by the presence of a vulval discharge which is often haemorrhagic in nature. A rapid return to oestrus does not follow resorption, in contrast with many other domestic animals. After the end of the luteal phase, the bitch enters a variable period of anoestrus that may last between three and five months. In mid- and late pregnancy, fetal death is characterized by abortion since fetal mummification and retention is rare. These bitches usually have a dark red vulval discharge. Aborted material may be eaten by the bitch and not be available for inspection.

Feline

Reproductive failure is as common in the cat as it is in the dog and, while superficially the oestrous cycle of the queen appears similar to that of the bitch, there are marked differences. Most notably, the queen is an induced ovulator and ovulation failure is manifest by a rapid return to oestrus. Also, unlike the bitch, conception failure or very early embryonic death results in a short luteal phase. There is, therefore, a clearer distinction between pregnancy and non-pregnancy in the cat than in the bitch. Viral infection is not known to have a significant influence upon male fertility but, in the female, there is transplacental infection with either resorption or abortion. Fetal mummification is extremely rare. Following any pregnancy loss there is usually a return to cyclicity; in winter, however, the queen will often enter anoestrus.

Endometritis has been reported only following infection with feline leukaemia virus infection.

TOGAVIRUSES

Family: Togaviridae

HUMAN   *VETERINARY*
Genus: rubivirus
   Rubella
Genus: alphavirus   *Eastern equine encephalitis virus (EEEV)*
                                           Western equine encephalitis virus (WEEV)
                                           Venezuelan equine encephalitis virus (VEEV) plus more*

NB: plus more* *indicates that there are more members of this virus genus but, as they are not considered to be pathogenic for reproductive tissues, they are not listed.*

VIRUS AND ANTIGENIC CHARACTERISTICS

Alphaviruses have 70 nm icosahedral enveloped virions with two structural glycoproteins forming heterodimer spikes. They contain a genome of linear positive-sense ssRNA of about 9.7–11.8 kb in size. The non-structural proteins (nsP1, nsP2, nsP3 and nsP4) are encoded by the genomic RNA whereas the structural proteins (the capsid protein (C) and two enveloped glycoproteins (E1 and E2)) are encoded by a subgenomic 26S mRNA corresponding to the 3' third of the viral genome. The mRNA is polyadenylated and capped. Both genomic and subgenomic mRNA are translated into polyprotein and then cleaved post-translationally.

Alphaviruses are all antigenically related whereas rubella is distinct from them and is therefore classified in a separate genus. The major epitopes are found on the E2 protein.

EPIDEMIOLOGY AND TRANSMISSION

In general, alphaviruses are worldwide and have adapted to a wide range of hosts. Their lifecycle is complex and reflects their catholic taste in hosts, which includes infection of mosquitoes or haematophagous arthropods, often a persistent infection in reptilian, amphibian or avian species and then a further infection in mammalian species (including man) (Figure 14.3).

The distribution of the equine encephalitis viruses (EEE, WEE and VEE) is restricted to North and South America. There is a range in virulence with mortalities in horses of up to 20% with WEE but often as high as 80–100% with EEE and VEE.

CLINICAL ASPECTS

These viruses cause primarily an encephalomyelitis in horses with clinical signs of fever, depression, anorexia, incoordination, paralysis and death. Pathology in the reproductive tract is not a major feature following infection

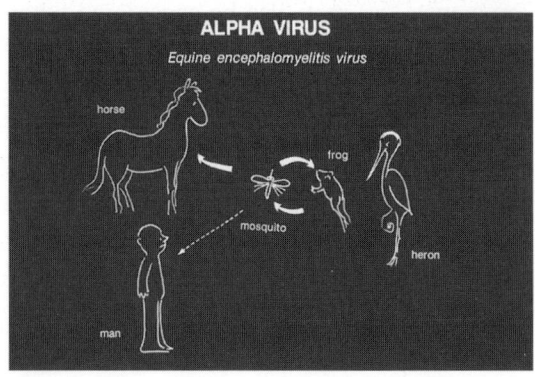

Figure 14.3 Cartoon of alphavirus life history.

although transplacental transmission of VEE has been reported in pregnant mares near full term[28]. There is a likelihood of human infection following epidemics of equine infection. A pregnant woman exposed to a live-attenuated VEE virus infection contracted hydrops fetalis with consequent death of the fetus[29].

CONTROL

Control depends on quarantine for sick horses, restriction of movement in infected areas and vaccination of all horses. There is an effective attenuated tissue culture vaccine, TC83, against VEE and also formalin-inactivated vaccines against WEE and EEE.

HERPESVIRUSES

Family: Herpesviridae

HUMAN   *VETERINARY*

Subfamily: alphaherpesvirinae

Genus: simple virus

Herpes simplex 1 and 2   *Bovine herpesvirus 2 (BoHV2)*
                                                 (bovine mamillitis virus/pseudo-lumpy skin disease virus)

                                                 plus more

Genus: varicellovirus   *Bovine herpesvirus 1 (BoHV1)* (infectious bovine rhinotracheitis virus
Human herpes 3   IBR, infectious pustular vulvovaginitis IPV)
(varicella-zoster virus)
                                                 Equid herpesvirus 1 (EHV1) (equine abortion herpesvirus)

                                                 Equid herpesvirus 3 (EHV3) (coital exanthema virus)

                                                 Equid herpesvirus 4 (EHV4) (equine rhinopneumonitis virus)

                                                 Pseudorabies virus (PRV) (Aujesky's disease virus)

                                                 Canid herpesvirus 1 (CaHV1)

                                                 Felid herpesvirus 1 (FeHV1)

                                                 plus more

Subfamily: betaherpesvirinae

Genus: cytomegalovirus virus

Human herpesvirus 5
(human cytomegalovirus)

Genus: roseolovirus   *Suid herpes 2 (SuHV2)* (swine cytomegalovirus)
Human herpesvirus 6   *Ovine herpes 1 (OvHV1)* (ovine cytomegalovirus)
Human herpesvirus 7
                                                 plus more

Subfamily: gammaherpesvirinae

Genus: lymphocryptovirus   **Genus: rhadinovirus**
Human herpesvirus 4
(Epstein–Barr virus)   *Equid herpesvirus 2 (EHV2)*

                                                 Bovine herpesvirus 4 (BoHV4)

                                                 Alcephine herpesvirus 1 (AIHV1) (malignant catarrhal fever virus)

                                                 Ovine herpes 2 (OvHV2 (sheep-associated malignant catarrhal fever)

                                                 plus more

This is a large and important group of viruses affecting veterinary species; many are capable of causing severe reproductive pathology, as well as other diseases. Most have a worldwide distribution and their control is dependent on vaccination, where available, and on serological screening within breeding programmes.

VIRUSES AND ANTIGENIC
CHARACTERISTICS

The virions of the various herpesviruses range between 90 and 200 nm in size with both glycosylated and non-glycosylated surface proteins projecting from the virus envelopes. The capsids are icosahedral and contain the linear ds DNA which can be 124–235 kb in size, containing a large number of open reading frames (ORF) from 70 to more than 200. However, the enveloped glycoproteins capable of inducing protection appear to be limited to two to three proteins, depending on the virus.

EPIDEMIOLOGY AND TRANSMISSION

Herpesviruses are generally adapted and restricted to their host. Typically, acute infections are not lethal but they become latent, thereby providing a reservoir for later recrudescence. An important exception to this general tenet is the immunocompromised animal or the immunologically immature fetus. It is for this latter reason that herpesviruses can cause such severe pathology within reproductive tissues.

Viruses are transmitted via aerosols and primary replication occurs in the epithelium of the nasal mucosa and conjunctiva. There may also be transmission by direct contact with infectious secretions, whether nasal or ocular secretions, urine and cervical or even seminal fluids from infected males (e.g. SuHV2). Virus can be recovered from nasal swabs for up to three weeks after infection. For some herpesviruses, there is subsequent viraemia (EHV1 infection) but this is not always the case (EHV4).

Early exposure to EHV1 is common in many young horses and the majority of mares have met several infections prior to breeding. Many abortigenic infections therefore develop from apparently clinically silent respiratory tract disease. Similar to other herpesvirus infections, there may be recrudescence of latent viral infection. The sites of latency are not unequivocally determined. Active infection may occur in these cases following transport, pregnancy, foaling or weaning. Experimentally, recrudescence has been induced following corticosteroid administration [30].

The reservoir for PRV of pigs is likely to be the latently infected pig that has recovered from the initial acute infection. Such animals can have recrudescence of infection and thereafter transmit virus by direct contact with oral/nasal discharges or milk or by airborne infection [31]. Urine, semen or preputial washings are considered unlikely sources of virus, in contrast to the other veterinary alpha-herpesviruses.

CaHV1 enters the body by oral or nasal routes and replicates principally within the tonsils, nasal turbinates and pharynx before entering the blood associated with white blood cells [32]. The excretion of the virus from infected animals can be via oral, nasal, vaginal or even preputial secretions. Secondary viral replication occurs in several sites including the spleen, liver, kidney and adrenal gland. Little is known about the role of latency and carrier animals in the aetiology of the disease. However, recrudescent virus shedding may be stimulated by the stress of pregnancy and parturition. Pups may be infected at parturition during passage through the birth canal.

FeHV transmission of virus occurs via the respiratory tract, with primary virus replication occurring within the nasal epithelium prior to dissemination throughout the bronchial tree. Viraemia results in the spread of virus to other sites including the reproductive tract in the pregnant female. Latency of the virus has been demonstrated[33]. Cats that recover from the disease may become carriers and virus tends to localize within the pharyngeal regions in these cases. Up to 80% of cats become chronic carriers, which spontaneously shed virus.

CLINICAL ASPECTS

Herpesviruses have a range of tropisms often reflecting their groupings, i.e. many alphaherpesviruses have a latency for sensory ganglia (e.g. BoHV1, BoHV3, PRV and FeHV), the betaherpesviruses for macrophages and salivary glands (e.g. SuHV2) and the gammaherpesviruses for B lymphocytes (e.g. AlHV1, BHV4, EHV2 and OvHV2). This tropism is relevant to the clinical signs of disease.

Alphaherpesviruses

BoHV2 infection causes vesicles on the skin, teats and perineum that ulcerate but typically heal within 2–4 weeks[34]. Generalized skin infection is recognized, as pseudo-lumpy skin disease, and can be produced experimentally by intravenous inoculation of BoHV2[35]. Latency is assumed but not proven.

BoHV1 causes not only the respiratory disease known as infectious bovine rhinotracheitis (IBR), but also severe pathology in the reproductive tissues[36]. It is responsible for infectious pustular vulvovaginitis (IPV) and for balanoposthitis of bulls. The strains producing IBR and IPV can be differentiated by molecular biological techniques. IPV-infected bulls can transmit infection during breeding and their semen is likely to contain infectious virus; this is a concern for artificial insemination (AI) programmes. Latency in caudal ganglia has been established and recrudescence occurs following undue stress such as long-distance transport, disease or even parturition. Infection of pregnant cattle with BoHV1 will cause a significant number

of abortions; these may be within a week of the initial febrile infection or up to 100 days later. Some fetuses may go to full term but be stillborn or not survive the neonatal period.

EHV1 and EHV4 were initially considered to be different subtypes of equine herpesvirus 1. Equine herpesvirus 1 causes abortion, respiratory disease (rhinopneumonitis) and neurological disorders and may cause significant illness in foals. Equine herpesvirus 4 is generally limited to causing respiratory tract disease. Both viruses cause upper respiratory tract disease, especially in the young horse. EHV1 produces a subsequent viraemia whereas EHV4 rarely does. The clinical signs of rhinopneumonitis include nasal discharge, depression, anorexia, lymphadenopathy and tracheobronchitis and there is often secondary bacterial infection. Certain virulent strains of EHV1 produce an inflammatory response within the spinal cord which results in hind leg ataxia. This may progress to quadriplegia. The neurological form of the disease can result in death, usually as a result of the prolonged recumbency. This form of the disease is associated with viral replication in nervous system endothelial cells, which results in the formation of microthrombi and focal infarcts.

In pregnant mares abortion may occur. This usually follows infection with an abortigenic strain of EHV1 during the last third of pregnancy; in these cases there may initially be minor clinical signs of respiratory tract infection. Following the viraemia there is transplacental spread and the interval between respiratory tract infection and abortion may vary from nine to 120 days[37]. Interestingly, pregnant mares that have neurological disease do not always abort. These two observations are noteworthy since EHV1 can infect endothelial cells six days after experimental infection. Often the aborted fetus is somewhat jaundiced and has increased volumes of both pleural and peritoneal fluid. There is usually a lymphocytic vasculitis which results in a focal thrombosis and infarction[38]. Whilst it is clear that the virus is transmitted to the fetus, in certain cases there may be extensive uterine disease that results in abortion of a virus-negative fetus[39]. Congenitally infected foals may be born alive, although they are usually weak and have respiratory distress and/or enteritis.

EHV3 causes equine coital exanthema in both mares and stallions. Approximately 4–7 days after sexual contact, multiple small circular raised nodules develop. In the mare these usually form in the perineal skin, on the ventral surface of the tail and within the mucosa of the vestibule and vagina. In the stallion, they develop on the shaft of the penis and the prepuce. The nodules become pustular in nature and ultimately burst to leave small ulcerated regions. In the absence of any secondary bacterial infection, the lesions usually heal within a few weeks. In the stallion there may be reduced libido and unwillingness to cover mares until the lesions have healed. Lesions may also occur on the teats of the mare and the muzzle of her foal[40]. It has been shown that the virus may persist in both mares and stallions from one year to the next. The condition is not associated with abortion.

Acute PRV infection of pigs (Aujesky's disease) can cause 100% morbidity and mortality in suckling piglets. The clinical signs are an initial febrile response followed by neurological signs of incoordination, tremors and recumbency. There is often respiratory distress, vomiting and diarrhoea. Death can occur within 12 h of the first clinical signs. Infection in growing and adult pigs is less severe but there is still respiratory and neurological disease and profound depression; this is dependent on the virulence of the virus isolate. The real problem for older pigs follows infection of the pregnant animal; in early pregnancy there is considerable early embryonic death and abortion and later in pregnancy there is further abortion, mummification of the fetus or the birth of stillborn piglets.

PRV has also been reported to infect cattle, goats, dogs and cats; it is equally pathogenic for these species and produces acute signs of respiratory and neurological disease with death often within 24 h. In cattle there is often an intense skin pruritis exciting an incessant licking. The losses from PRV, which can be considerable, are estimated to be mainly due to breeding losses.

CaHV1 infection generally produces only mild signs limited to the respiratory or genital tract in adult dogs. The uncomplicated disease may be unnoticed by the owner. The genital tract lesions are frequently raised red nodules that may be found along the length of the penis, most often on the inner surface of the sheath, the mucocutaneous junction and at the zone of reflection of the sheath onto the glans penis. Similar nodular lesions may, however, be found in normal dogs; these are lymphoid nodules which are pale in colour and are a normal finding. In the bitch, variable-sized vesicles, induced by CaHV1, are commonly observed in the vestibule[41]; frequently these lesions are evident at the onset of proestrus, suggesting that venereal transmission is probably important in adult dogs. Indeed, the virus has also been recovered from vesicular lesions on the genitalia of bitches[42].

Infection in the bitch with CaHV1 may be associated with infertility, abortion and stillbirths[43]. Infection of the pregnant bitch may result in the production of placental lesions and infection of the fetuses[44]. The infected placentae are macroscopically under-developed and possess small greyish-white foci which are characterized by focal degeneration, necrosis and the presence of eosinophilic intranuclear inclusion bodies. Experimental data suggest that infection during early pregnancy may result in fetal death and subsequent mummification, while infection during mid-pregnancy results in abortion and infection during late pregnancy results in premature birth[44]. Pups may become infected at birth, during passage through the vagina, and subsequently die with characteristic widespread histological necrotizing lesions[32]. The virus enters the body by oral or nasal routes, the source of the virus being oral, nasal, vaginal secretions or preputial excretions. The virus replicates principally within the tonsils, nasal turbinates and pharynx and is transported via the blood, associated with white blood cells. Secondary viral replication occurs in several sites including the spleen, liver, kidney and adrenal gland. Virus can be isolated readily from these tissues and pathological changes in affected pups, aborted fetuses and infected placentae are often characteristic of CaHV infection. There are often haemorrhagic and necrotic lesions in the liver, lungs and kidneys, with intranuclear inclusions. In adults, complement fixation or neutralization tests can be used to detect antibody.

Although pups which survive the illness may show persistent neurological disorders[45], little is known about the role of latency and carrier animals in the aetiology of the disease. Pups are only at risk while *in utero* and during the first three weeks of life; attempts to produce the generalized disease in older pups have failed[46]. In pups, the initial signs are soft faeces, anorexia, difficulty in breathing, and death within 24–48 h of the onset of the clinical signs.

FeHV1 (feline viral rhinotracheitis) is a common cause of respiratory tract disease in the cat. The virus is species-specific and exhibits haemagglutination with feline erythrocytes. There is a wide range of clinical effects in the adult cat, from mild respiratory tract disease to death in some cases. Mortality is usually due to a secondary bacterial bronchopneumonia and is more common in young or aged cats. The virus may also result in abortion during the fifth or sixth week of gestation and experimental infection during late pregnancy may result in the birth of stillborn kittens. Lesions may be found within the uterus but placental lesions have only been demonstrated following experimental infection[47]. In experimental studies vaginitis has also been reported, presumably due to effects of the virus on the vaginal mucosa

which are similar to those observed in the bitch infected with canine herpesvirus. In the naturally occurring disease, abortions are thought to be the result of a non-specific reaction to the infection[48].

Betaherpesviruses

The only cytomegalovirus of apparent veterinary significance that has been well described is SuHV2, originally designated porcine cytomegalovirus (PCMV). It is slow-growing and produces typical cytomegalic lesions in cell culture with distinctive intranuclear inclusions[49,50]. There are several simian cytomegaloviruses but few others, apart from SuHV2, are reported in the veterinary species. It is interesting that in the 6th Report of the International Committee on Taxonomy of Viruses, equid herpesvirus 2 (EHV2) has been classified as a cytomegalovirus but it has few characteristics of cytomegaloviruses and researchers have previously classified it within the gammaherpesviruses (as in this paper).

SuHV2 was first identified by its characteristic intranuclear inclusion bodies and cytomegaly in the nasal mucous glands of day-old piglets[51]; this clearly indicated transplacental infection. It has since been associated with field outbreaks of perinatal mortality[52,53] and later was proven experimentally to transmit transplacentally and cause fetal infection[54]. In a careful study of the tropism of SuHV2, viral localization was shown not in the placenta but within fetal tissues, most notably leptomeningeal cells, hepatic sinusoidal cells, peritoneal macrophages, periosteal cells and occasional alveolar cells[55]. Thus, it would appear that perinatal mortality is associated with the direct effect of SuHV2 on the fetus and not as a sequel to placentitis. This is in contrast to the placentitis observed with the pig alphaherpesvirus (PRV)[56], the porcine parvovirus[57] and the cytomegaloviruses of man[58], guinea-pigs[59] and mice[60].

Gammaherpesviruses

AIHV1 and OvHV2 have typical character-istics of gammaherpesviruses with a tropism for lymphoid tissue, particularly the B-cell lineage, and are not considered to be primary pathogens of reproductive or fetal tissues. They will not be considered further. However, EHV2 and BoHV4 infections have a tropism for reproductive tissues.

EHV2 has been recovered from a number of tissue sites including the respiratory tract in horses with respiratory disease, the con-junctiva and the genital tract. Its role in reproductive pathology is uncertain; it appears to be ubiquitous and avirulent.

BoHV4 has been proposed to be the bovine cytomegalovirus[61] but its ability to cause recognizable disease remains uncertain[62]. It has been associated with mild respiratory signs[63] and with genital disease in several countries including the USA[64], Italy[65] and Zaire[66]. It can cross the placenta and infect the fetus[67] and has been reported to cause abortion[68]. It appears not to be species-specific and can be recovered from American bison (*Bison bison*), African buffalo (*Syncerus caffer*) sheep and cat (it is considered that FHV2 is, in fact, a strain of BoHV4). As with all herpesviruses, it causes a persistent infection; the target cells are blood mononuclear cells.

CONTROL

Bovine herpesviruses

BoHV1 is present in the cattle population worldwide and control is by vaccination with either inactivated vaccine or modified live vaccination (temperature-sensitive mutant BoHV1). Eradication has been conducted with success in some herds, some areas and even some countries (Switzerland eradicated BoHV1 in 1987)[69].

Equine herpesviruses

An initial virus diagnosis is essential before mounting suitable control procedures. Unfor-tunately, EHV1 and EHV4 are not easy to differentiate on the basis of clinical signs of respiratory disease. As the viruses cross-react, they are also difficult to diagnose in ELISA antibody tests. Indirect immunofluorescence, with the use of monoclonal antibodies on frozen sections from the liver and lung of aborted fetuses is the most rapid means of diagnosis in an 'abortion storm' due to EHV1. Furthermore, EVH4 will grow only in equine cells whereas EHV1 will grow in a wide range of cells.

Mares should be stressed as little as possible during pregnancy to reduce the possibility of viral recrudescence. Animals should be iso-lated upon arrival at new premises and pregnant mares should be kept in small groups.

Advice on the control of equine herpesvirus is published by the Horse Race Betting Levy Board each year. This is a voluntary code of practice designed to help prevent and control venereal diseases during each breeding sea-son. If a mare aborts or a foal is born stillborn or ill, or if there is an outbreak of respiratory tract disease, the animals should be isolated, since close contact is required to allow virus transmission. Aborted material and congeni-tally infected foals should be removed. Infec-ted bedding should be destroyed and the area disinfected. It is recommended that animal movement is restricted for one month follow-ing the last case of an equine herpesvirus abortion.

The immunity following the respiratory tract infection is of short duration[70]. Although there may be an increased immune response following repeated infection, there is good evidence that infection may occur despite high antibody titres. Once latent infection is established within an individual there may be several episodes of viral recrudescence. It is for these reasons that vaccination has been so problematical. An inactivated EHV1 vaccine is available and vaccination of pregnant mares on three occasions during pregnancy has been shown to reduce the number of 'abortion storms'. It appears that such vaccination can reduce the level of viral excretion but, as it does not prevent viraemia [71], it is of limited use to prevent fetal infection.

EHV3 can be controlled by preventing animals with clinical disease from mating and also ensuring the use of sterile obstetric equipment when examining horses with suspected disease.

Porcine herpesviruses

The national impact of PRV infections can be considerable but control is made difficult by the ability of latently infected animals to shed virus several months after the initial infection. Different control measures have been utilized around the world: in the UK, an eradication policy was started in 1983 which, by 1985, had almost controlled the disease. Some countries are considered free of the virus, including Australia, Canada and Norway, whereas other countries, e.g. the USA, are taking active measures to enforce a vaccination and eradication programme. Several vaccines are available in those countries that permit vaccination, the most recent being a genetically engineered vaccine that, through deletion of a key glycoprotein, provides a marker to permit the differentiation of vaccine and infection immunity [72].

Canine herpesviruses

In pregnant bitches supportive therapy during the abortion is required. In the pups, the disease is rapidly fatal and treatment is often unrewarding; symptomatic therapy is all that is available since specific antiviral agents are not efficacious [73]. Resorbing and aborting bitches should be isolated from other pregnant bitches. Precautions should be taken to avoid contact with secretions or aborted material and infected bedding should be removed and the environment disinfected. The potential for viral transmission at coitus is uncertain but males with reproductive tract lesions should not be used for mating. Bitches which have previously given birth to infected pups may later deliver a normal litter. The duration of any immunity is not known.

Feline herpesviruses

Following infection with FeHV, a marked antibody response develops which persists for at least six months. However, 80% of infected animals become carriers with both latent periods and intermittent episodes of virus shedding. These animals may shed virus spontaneously or in response to various stresses. They need to be identified and isolated from breeding programmes. Maternally derived antibody may persist for up to 10 weeks, although the significance of this for protection from natural infection or interference with vaccination is uncertain.

Pregnant queens should not be allowed contact with aborted or stillborn fetuses and other cats with signs of respiratory tract infection. Queens which repeatedly produce infected litters should be removed from the breeding programme. Attenuated and inactivated virus vaccines are available for FeHV.

MORBILLIVIRUSES

Family: Paramyxoviridae

HUMAN   *VETERINARY*

Subfamily:paramyxovirinae

Genus:morbillivirus
   Measles   *Rinderpest virus (RPV)*
                                          Peste-des-petits ruminants virus (PPRV)
                                          Canine distemper virus (CDV)
                                          Phocine (seal) distemper virus (PDV)

                                          plus more

This group of viruses includes some members of apparent antiquity (e.g. rinderpest virus was a likely cause of the biblical cattle plague) but also newly emerging viruses (e.g. the phocine distemper virus, the cause of widespread harbour seal deaths in the North Sea in the 1980s). These viruses are the cause of fatal disease and also reproductive loss in ruminants, dogs and several wildlife species.

VIRUSES AND ANTIGENIC CHARACTERISTICS

Morbilliviruses are 150 nm, pleomorphic, enveloped virions with 2–3 transmembrane glycoproteins forming spike-like projections from the lipid envelope. The virions contain a single molecule of linear, non-infectious negative-sense ssRNA. The genome is transcribed into 6–10 subgenomic separate mRNAs. All mRNAs possess a 3′ poly (A) tract. Ten to 12 proteins are encoded within the RNA, mostly by unique mRNAs.

The major epitopes are found on the attachment (H or G) and fusion proteins (F). Morbilliviruses are distinguished by lacking neuraminidase and some species have no haemagglutinins. However, the viruses do crossreact in serological tests.

CDV possesses haemagglutination and fusion antigens. There are also M proteins lining the inner membrane of the virus and at least two nucleocapsid proteins. Isolation and culture are difficult, but the virus produces syncytia, intranuclear and cytoplasmic inclusion bodies and stellate cells. Most virus particles are between 150 and 300 nm in diameter, although some filamentous forms have been described.

EPIDEMIOLOGY AND TRANSMISSION

Morbilliviruses are highly infectious and primary infection occurs within the oropharynx and respiratory tissues. Most morbilliviruses have a limited but precise host range, with horizontal transmission between animals being dependent on airborne and direct contact. Initial disease is characterized by epizootics of disease, e.g. rinderpest, and recovered animals may become persistently infected. The last major outbreak of rinderpest in the UK was in the 1860s when the disease, imported from Europe, caused catastrophic losses. Simmonds, then Professor of Veterinary Pathology at the Royal Veterinary College in London, gave expert advice in 1865 to the politicians of his day and, in considering their arguments 'that the plague is a curable disease', stated that 'nothing can be more fallacious' and that their idea to collect all infected animals into sanatoria would 'convert England into one great pest house and . . . lead to the destruction of the whole of her cattle'[74]. Since that time, much effort has been put into the control of RPV and PPRV at the international level but both are still present in some African and Asian countries. Ever-watchful veterinary surveillance is necessary to ensure their epidemiological restriction.

CDV is transmitted principally by droplet infection, predominantly from dogs which have the respiratory form of the infection. However, the virus is also excreted in faeces and urine. The evidence for transplacental infection is limited to a single publication[75] but anecdotal evidence is abundant in demonstrating the role of the virus in producing abortion. Transplacental infection may result in fetal death and abortion, the birth of live pups which develop the disease or occasionally clinically silent excretors of the virus.

CLINICAL ASPECTS

All the morbilliviruses have the ability to cause severe, if not fatal, disease. Their tropism for reproductive tissues is not discrete although the outcome of rinderpest infection in pregnant cattle is often abortion[76] and, with peste-des-petits ruminants virus infections, superficial erosions of the vulva and prepuce can be observed[77].

CDV infection of susceptible dogs can produce a hyperacute form of disease with sudden onset of pyrexia and death although most infections, after an incubation of 3–7 days, result in primary respiratory tract or gastrointestinal tract disease. After either type of syndrome, some dogs may develop central nervous system lesions including behavioural changes, muscle spasm, epileptiform seizures and paresis. The early disease phase may have a mortality of between 30% and 80%. Death is usually the result of complications of secondary bacterial infection. Dogs which survive frequently have continual central nervous system signs and some may develop hyperkeratosis of the pads and nose, resulting in the term 'hard-pad' used by lay persons.

Experimental exposure of pregnant bitches to canine distemper virus was found to produce either clinical illness in the bitch, with subsequent abortion, or subclinical infection of the bitch and the birth of clinically affected pups[75]. This provides evidence for transplacental transmission, although the frequency of this under natural conditions is unknown. The virus has an affinity for lymphatic and epithelial cells including those within the reproductive tract of the male and female.

CONTROL

There are effective vaccines for the control of RPV and PPRV and their concerted use has eliminated the viruses from many parts of the world. However, with the breakdown of veterinary and agricultural systems in the various African and Asian war zones, the disease continues to exist and even to extend its range.

Interestingly, a human measles vaccine has been shown to protect calves against rinderpest[78], thereby confirming cross-reactivity between the morbilliviruses. A recombinant vaccine has been developed that expresses both the F and H genes in a vaccinia construct and has been shown experimentally to give protection against challenge[79].

Before widespread vaccination against CDV in dogs some 15 years ago, distemper could be diagnosed on the basis of clinical signs but the condition is now rare and often limited to stray city dogs or unvaccinated dogs in shelters. In the live animal, smears of conjunctival epithelium may shown intracytoplasmic inclusion bodies and may be positive with immunofluorescent antibody staining. At postmortem examination the inclusion bodies may be seen in the bronchial epithelium, lung macrophages or cells within the central nervous system. Both intracytoplasmic and intranuclear inclusion bodies may be found within the brain and demyelination of the cerebellar/pontine area is pathognomic. Virus isolation can be made from infected tissue in canine cell monolayers.

In immune dams there is significant colostral passage of antibody to the pup which prevents infection for up to 8–12 weeks after birth. Dogs that recover from an infection are usually immune for life; distemper virus produces an antibody and cell-mediated response. The antibody response appears to be inversely related to the severity of the disease, with recovered dogs having the largest titres and the lowest titres being observed in animals which die.

Vaccination for CDV was initially developed using inactivated virus, followed by virulent virus or by simultaneous administration of antiserum and virus. Interestingly, formalin inactivation destroys the immunogenicity of the F antigen. Immunization is now performed using attenuated live virus vaccines, which evoke antibody against both F and H antigens. Low levels of maternal antibody will neutralize live virus so vaccination should not commence until 12 weeks of age. However, measles virus has differing but cross-protective F antigens and maternal antibodies do not inactivate attenuated measles virus. This may allow early protection by administration of measles virus at six weeks of age.

PARVOVIRUSES

Family: Paravoviridae

HUMAN	*VETERINARY*

Subfamily: parvovirinae

Genus: erythrovirus
  B19

Genus: parvovirus

Aleutian mink disease virus (AMDV)
Bovine parvovirus (BPV)
Porcine parvovirus (PPV)
Canine parvovirus (CPV)
Feline panleucopenia virus (FPV)

plus more

VIRUSES AND ANTIGENIC CHARACTERISTICS

Parvoviruses are 18–26 nm in diameter, of icosahedral symmetry but without a surface envelope. They contain a linear ssDNA of about 4–6 kb in size. There are 2–4 virion protein species (VP 1–4) which are encoded by two major genes, the REP (or NS) and the CAP gene. The lack of viral enzymes encoded by its genome explains why parvoviruses require helper functions provided by helper viruses or host enzymes for their replication.

Canine parvovirus 1, CPV1, has not been confirmed as a major cause of disease and is said to produce a subclinical enteric infection. However, canine parvovirus 2, CPV2, appears to have arisen as a host range mutant of feline parvovirus.

EPIDEMIOLOGY AND TRANSMISSION

Aleutian mink disease virus (AMDV) can be transmitted by contact with faeces or urine of infected animals or by bite wounds[80]. There is also evidence of aerosol transmission. The virus may cross the placenta, resulting in congenitally infected kits which excrete virus. Interestingly, not all litters are born infected. In those that are not, there is usually, however, postnatal infection by direct contact with the dam. Viral replication occurs within the gastrointestinal tract and following a viraemia, there is persistent infection and the development of immune complex disease.

Bovine parvovirus (BPV) transmission in calves is likely to follow the ingestion of food contaminated with faecal material; virus is shed in high quantities within faeces. The route of transmission to the adult is likely to be similar.

Porcine parvovirus (PPV) has been recovered from aborted material and infected piglets, as well as semen and vaginal mucus. Infection is usually contracted from fomites or faeces. Virus replicates within the small intestine and this is followed by viraemia. Transplacental infection may occur at this stage. Some piglets in the litter may escape infection whereas others are congenitally infected and become persistent excretors of the virus. These piglets then become a reservoir of infection.

Canine parvovirus (CPV) in dogs is transmitted via the oropharyngeal route and the initial infection may occur in the tonsils. It then spreads via the lymphatics to produce a viraemia. The virus causes necrosis of the small intestinal epithelium resulting in the clinical signs. Faecal excretion of virus occurs within a few days of infection. Virus colonizes myocardial cells after the initial viraemia. The virus may persist in the environment for prolonged periods of time and, this together with its rapid transmission, results in endemic infection of a population.

Feline panleucopenia virus (FPV) of cats probably enters the body via the oropharyngeal route and replicates at this site. There is then a viraemia and spread of the virus to many areas of the body, particularly rapidly dividing cells of the intestine (resulting in enteritis) and the bone marrow (resulting in panleucopenia). There may be excretion of virus in some cats for many months after the acute phase of infection and these can be a reservoir of infection for other cats and for contamination of the environment. The virus is remarkably stable and is resistant to heat and to many disinfectants.

CLINICAL ASPECTS

Aleutian mink disease is caused by a persistent parvovirus infection in the mink that generates an uncontrollable B-cell response to the virus. The disease is characterized by initial anorexia, lethargy and weight loss. In some animals the condition is non-progressive, although the mink remains persistently infected. In others, the condition progresses over several months and results in polydipsia, haemorrhage and uveitis. There is a dramatic plasmocytosis, hypergammaglobulinaemia and immune complex formation. The latter results in hyaline degeneration of the kidney (resulting in polydipsia), arteritis (resulting in haemorrhage) and ocular lesions[81]. There may also be splenomegaly and focal hepatitis. Most animals become markedly emaciated before dying. The virus can cross the placenta and this usually results in the birth of infected kits that transmit the virus and subsequently succumb to the clinical disease. Not all mink are susceptible but in some strains (such as the blue or so-called Aleutian-coloured mink) there is an inherited immune dysfunction. These animals do not abrogate an infection but remain as carriers.

BPV is an ubiquitous parvovirus that produces no or mild enteric infection in calves. Infection is most common in susceptible calves, in which the virus causes pyrexia, lethargy and diarrhoea. In most cases there are no further effects and recovery is prompt.

The role of BPV in infertility is not clear, although the virus has been isolated in some cases of abortion, and it is known that experimental infection can produce abortion[82]. In addition, antibodies are found more frequently in cows with reproductive disease compared with normal cows[83]. The reproductive consequences of BPV infection are, however, rare.

PPV infection is usually subclinical in most pigs exposed to the virus but, unlike other parvoviruses, has limited effects upon the gastrointestinal tract. However, in breeding females the virus has been associated with stillbirths, mummification, embryonic death, infertility, abortion and neonatal death[84]. The clinical condition is often termed SMEDI as an abbreviation of the first four listed clinical signs. Developmental abnormalities, including intestinal atrophy and hare lip, may be present in piglets that are born alive. In young pigs, parvovirus infection may cause vesicular lesions of the snout and mouth.

CPV affects both the neonatal pup and the older dog, producing two clinical disease syndromes. In the susceptible neonate, viraemia is followed by localization of the virus in myocardial cells. This results either in sudden death of apparently healthy pups at less than eight weeks of age, or subacute heart failure weeks or months later. In older dogs there is usually an acute enteritis with vomiting, diarrhoea and rapid dehydration. There is often marked leucopenia. The morbidity is high; however, in adults the mortality is often as low as 1%, although it may be as high as 10% in puppies.

CPV has also been implicated by some breeders as a cause of infertility in their kennels. However, Meunier et al.[85] found that the conception rate, incidence of stillbirths, average litter size, or average number of pups weaned per litter, did not change after the introduction of CPV to a kennel of 2000 brood bitches. The reproductive consequences of CPV are related to the ability of the virus to cross the placenta and affect pups which then develop acute generalized infection and myocardial disease soon after birth[86]. Often, it is not clear whether infection occurred pre- or postpartum.

The severity of FPV disease may vary, although the worst clinical signs are observed in young kittens. Commonly, there is lethargy, pyrexia and vomiting. Profuse watery diarrhoea, often with some blood, may develop, resulting in electrolyte imbalance and death. The mortality rate may vary from 25% to 75%[87]. There is often secondary bacterial disease as the result of severe panleucopenia (the condition is referred to as feline panleucopenia by some workers). A subclinical form of the disease with no clinical signs has been reported.

FPV replicates within placental cells and infection during early pregnancy, with or without clinical signs in the queen, results in embryonic and fetal death, causing resorption and abortion[48]. There is occasional mummification. Kittens infected during mid- or late gestation or in the first few days after parturition may either die suddenly or become ataxic at approximately 2–3 weeks of age, when they attempt to walk[88]. This reflects the fact that the virus crosses the blood–brain barrier and this leads to cerebellar hypoplasia. Histologically, there is a marked reduction in the number of granular and Purkinje cells, which control motor function. The motor neurones that are destroyed by the virus are not replaced and kittens remain permanently ataxic. The entire litter is not necessarily affected. In some cases there is marked hydrocephalus.

CONTROL

AMDV of mink may be diagnosed on the basis of the clinical signs and the history of the breeding establishment. Postmortem examination usually reveals enlarged kidneys, liver and spleen. Histologically, there is extensive plasmocytosis of these organs as well as the lymph nodes. Often, there are vascular lesions and periodic acid-Schiff-positive inclusion bodies. Serum antibodies may be detected by a variety of methods, including immunofluorescence. There is presently no vaccine. Control is by removal of infected animals from the premises; all antibody-positive mink harbour the virus.

A diagnosis of BPV infection in cattle is not possible on the basis of the clinical signs. Virus may be detected within faecal material or can be isolated in tissue culture from aborted fetuses. Intranuclear inclusion bodies may be detected in infected cells and viral antigen can be demonstrated in infected tissue using immunofluorescence techniques. There is no vaccine available. Control of the disease involves general husbandry procedures aimed at reducing faecal contamination of the environment to reduce viral transmission.

For PPV, a presumptive diagnosis may be made on the basis of the clinical history of reproductive tract disease, usually in the absence of any abortions. Isolation of virus from stillborn fetuses and neonates is possible on porcine cell monolayers. The virus can be identified by immunofluorescence microscopy on tissues from dead fetuses. Paired serum samples may be useful for demonstrating an antibody response to infection; this can be detected using the haemagglutination-inhibition test.

Pigs infected with PPV usually develop solid immunity which lasts for life. However, while a response may occur within 10 days, faecal excretion of the virus may persist for several months. Passive immunity is usually present up to six months of age. Control of infection is difficult since the virus is resistant within the environment, subclinical infection is common and congenitally infected excretors of the virus are present. Mixing of non-pregnant sows with infected animals and the feeding of infected material to non-pregnant sows are often performed to induce immunity. When there is clinical disease, pregnant animals should be isolated and not allowed access to infected sows, vaginal discharges, infected piglets or bedding material.

Inactivated and modified live PPV vaccines are available in several countries to control the disease. There does not appear to be interference from passive immunity as there is with parvoviruses in other species. Vaccination should be performed prior to breeding.

A preliminary clinical diagnosis for CPV may be made on the basis of the clinical signs, supported by leucopenia (usually lymphopenia rather than neutropenia). However, a confirmatory diagnosis is usually made by identifying virus or viral proteins in the faeces. Antigen can be detected in clarified faeces by haemagglutination or commercial ELISA techniques. Intranuclear inclusion bodies can be detected histologically or by immunofluorescence in myocardial cells or ileal epithelial cells. Antibody in serum can be detected by haemagglutination inhibition but vaccination has now complicated the issue; these tests will not distinguish between active and passive immunity. Interestingly, fetal cerebellar hypoplasia, a sequel to feline parvovirus infection of cats during pregnancy, is not observed in the dog.

Dogs recovering from the infection are immune; a rapid humoral virus-neutralizing antibody response occurs within five days of infection. Antibodies appear to persist for a long period of time and certainly more than one year. Passive neutralizing antibody frequently persists until 16 weeks after birth and may therefore be present when pups are presented for vaccination at 12 weeks of age. Once breeding dogs become immune through exposure to the virus or vaccination, the incidence of cardiomyopathy decreases rapidly, since only neonates are susceptible to developing this condition, and passive immunity is generally protective. Inactivated feline parvovirus vaccine was used initially to control the disease. Subsequently inactivated canine parvovirus vaccine became available and more recently, live tissue culture attenuated vaccines have been produced.

For FPV, the reproductive consequences of infection, abortion and the birth of congenitally abnormal kittens are highly suggestive of infection with the virus. Gross pathological examination may reveal cerebellar hypoplasia in certain cases. In affected individuals there is a marked leucopenia. The diagnosis can be confirmed by viral isolation in swabs taken from the pharynx. Serological diagnosis can be made by virus neutralization or ELISA assay with paired serum samples. The immune response to FPV is somewhat dampened by the leucopenia, but in other respects the response is rapid and subsequent immunity is solid. After active infection, antibody titres persist for a long period of time and are probably boosted by repeated exposure to virus. Passive immunity persists for 2–3 months in kittens; thereafter, unvaccinated animals are extremely susceptible to the disease.

Infection is almost entirely preventable with suitable vaccination since the available vaccines produce solid and long-lasting immunity. Both live and inactivated vaccines are available and may be given to kittens after passive immunity wanes. Inactivated vaccines are safe and can be given to any cat, even if pregnant. The live vaccines replicate but are said not to be excreted.

RETROVIRUSES/LENTIVIRUSES

Family: Retroviridae

HUMAN	*VETERINARY*
Genus: BLV-HTLV retroviruses	
Human T-lymphotropic virus 1 (HTLV1)	*Bovine leukaemia virus (BLV)*
Human T-lymphotropic virus 2 (HTLV2)	*Feline leukaemia virus (FeLV)*
	plus more
Genus: lentivirus	
Human immunodeficiency virus 1 (HIV1)	*Equine lentivirus (EIAV)*
Human immunodeficiency virus 2 (HIV2)	(equine infectious anaemia virus)
	Bovine lentivirus (BIV)
	(bovine immunodeficiency virus)
	Ovine lentivirus (MVV)
	(maedi visna virus)
	Caprine lentivirus (CAEV)
	(caprine arthritis encephalitis virus)
	Feline lentivirus (FIV)
	(feline immunodeficiency virus)

VIRUSES AND ANTIGENIC CHARACTERISTICS

Retrovirus virions are enveloped, spherical and 80–100 nm in diameter and possess two surface proteins and 4–6 non-glycosylated structural proteins. They contain the unique reverse transcriptase enzyme which enables the transcription of infectious viral RNA into the proviral DNA. Each virion contains a dimer of linear positive-sense ssRNA with each monomer of about 7–11 kb in size. Typically, the genome organization is based on three main genes, 5′ -*gag-pol-env*-3′.

There are three subgroups of FeLV; their classification is based upon envelope interference and neutralization.

EPIDEMIOLOGY AND TRANSMISSION

Leukaemia viruses

Bovine leukosis, caused by BLV, is widespread throughout all continents and most countries but has been, over the past few years, eliminated from several countries (e.g. Denmark and UK) following active eradication schemes. It still remains active in north America and presents a considerable problem to herd health. Transmission is mainly by exchange of infected lymphocytes, either in natural secretions or by iatrogenic means. It is considered that congenital infection occurs in 4–8% of calves from BLV-infected dams.

The source of FeLV is likely to be the persistently viraemic cat, that is, either an apparently healthy carrier or one suffering from an FeLV-related disease. The virus is found in high concentrations in saliva and this appears to be the principal source of transmission. The infectivity of saliva rapidly reduces, especially upon drying, and it appears that relatively close contact of cats is required for transmission. In other cases the disease may be transmitted via the uterus to the developing embryo or fetus. Interestingly, it has been shown that considerable transmission occurs at the time of mating, although it is uncertain whether this is true venereal transmission or is related to contact with saliva.

Lentiviruses

Lentiviruses have been isolated from most of the main veterinary species, with the exception of pig and dog. Their distribution is widespread, although the number of isolated tissue-culturable strains of some lentiviruses is limited (e.g. BIV and FIV). A consistent feature of lentiviruses is that all animals, once infected, become persistently infected and are potential reservoirs of the virus. Any use of contaminated products, instruments, syringe needles or even rectal gloves has real potential for transmission. The main modes of transmission appear to vary between the viral species. EIAV is readily transmitted by biting flies and mosquitoes from infected animals to uninfected horses, a result of mechanical transmission. Although intrauterine infection is reported to occur with EIAV, another route that is important with EIAV, MVV and CAEV is through ingestion of colostrum and milk. FIV may also be transmitted by these routes but the most common transmission is by biting, particularly between old infected tomcats. The distribution and transmission of BIV is still uncertain [89] although similarities with the other lentiviruses will undoubtedly be shown.

CLINICAL ASPECTS

Leukaemia viruses

BLV becomes a persistent infection in cattle and causes a chronic B-cell proliferative disease. It is characterized by persistent lymphocytosis which often leads to malignant lymphosarcoma. This is a fatal disease but, unlike FeLV, has little defined reproductive pathology and will not be considered further.

Infection with FeLV may result in a number of clinical disease situations including the development of lymphosarcoma, fibrosarcoma, myeloproliferative disease, anaemia, immunosuppressive disease and other disease, including reproductive disorders. Most cats that are exposed to FeLV recover from the infection and develop immunity. Some become permanently infected and subsequently develop an FeLV-related disease. Queens infected with FeLV may demonstrate one or more reproductive disorders including embryonic resorption, fetal abortion, infertility, endometritis and the birth of infected kittens which rapidly die[90]. FeLV is believed to be the single most common cause of infertility in the queen[12]. Fetal resorption is seen frequently, although abortion and the birth of permanently infected kittens also occur. The aetiology of the reproductive disease is uncertain and while it is known that the virus may cross the placenta, one possibility is that secondary bacterial infections occur because of FeLV-induced immunosuppression[12]. Kittens born to persistently viraemic queens may be lethargic and wasted and have stunted growth and increased susceptibility to other diseases. These findings are often associated with atrophy of the thymus. In general, it appears that all kittens of viraemic queens are born persistently infected. These kittens will, if they survive until weaning, develop a FeLV-related disease within a short period of time after birth.

Lentiviruses

All lentiviruses, except BIV, have been shown to be responsible for progressive and fatal disease in their host species. However, there does not appear to be a specific tropism of lentiviruses for reproductive tissues and, although there is likely to be transmission of virus either *in utero* or, more likely, during the peripartum period, there is little evidence of pathology in this time. The clinical signs of pathology in non-reproductive tissues, e.g. encephalitis, respiratory disease, associated with these viruses will not be considered further.

CONTROL

BLV can, and has been, eradicated from several countries by programmes based on identifying and culling the infected carrier. Identification depends on either clinical evidence of lymphosarcoma, persistent lymphocytosis or detection of seropositive animals. Newborn calves should not be fed colostrum from seropositive animals and should be reared on 'clean' colostrum in isolation from BLV-carrier mothers. In some countries, e.g. USA and Canada, where the problem is widespread and the cost of eradication prohibitive, there is no attempt at national eradication. In the UK, the disease is notifiable and the country is considered free from infection.

FeLV may be suspected clinically on the basis of tumour development or signs of other FeLV-related disease, including a history of reproductive failure or deaths in young cats. FeLV can be diagnosed by virus isolation (virus detected in plasma), immunofluorescence (detection of virus protein p27 within neutrophils) and ELISA (detection of virus protein p27 in plasma). A cat that is positive by immunofluorescence for p27 is likely to be excreting FeLV; most of these cats remain positive for life. A cat that is negative by immunofluorescence for p27 has no detectable infected blood cells. As with a negative immunofluorescence result, a negative ELISA result demonstrates no detectable p27 but does not exclude the possibility that the virus is being incubated. Several studies have found some cats that are positive by ELISA but negative by immunofluorescence or by virus isolation[91]. It appears that these cats do not give birth to infected kittens and do not excrete the virus.

Following infection, cats may either remain persistently infected, in which case they lack both neutralizing antibody and feline oncovirus membrane-associated antigen (FOCMA) antibody, or they develop a self-limiting immunity, remain non-viraemic, and develop both neutralizing and FOCMA-related antibodies. It is the former cats that develop FeLV-related disease and the latter which do not. A final category of cats have a persistent viraemia together with an increase in FOCMA-related antibody; it appears that these either develop neutralizing antibody or the FOCMA-related antibody declines and the cat develops FeLV-related disease.

Control of FeLV is not simple and there is often a demand for routine screening of all cats. This, however, has several disadvantages, not the least being related to the high rate of false-positive diagnoses given by several testing methods [92]. It is clear, however, that breeding queens should not be allowed close contact with animals that have signs of any FeLV-related diseases. Consideration should be given to the euthanasia of persistently infected animals to reduce transmission of the disease. Persistently infected queens should be removed from the breeding programme since offspring are born infected and for this reason offspring are often better euthanized. Infected tom cats should not be used for breeding because of the high rate of transmission at this time.

Currently there are four vaccine types available within two vaccine groups, either subunit vaccines (envelope protein alone or multiple subunit components), or whole killed virus (adjuvanted or non-adjuvanted). The efficacy of vaccination is not 100% but vaccination is essential for the control of the disease in breeding animals.

FLAVIVIRUSES/PESTIVIRUSES

Family: Flaviviridae

HUMAN   *VETERINARY*

Genus: flavivirus
  Yellow fever virus   *Louping ill virus (LIV)*
  plus more   **plus more**

Genus: pestiviruses
                                                Bovine viral diarrhoea virus (BVDV)
                                                Swine fever virus (SFV)
                                                Border disease virus (BDV)

Genus: 'hepatitis C-like viruses'
  Hepatitis C virus

Louping ill is an acute encephalomyelitis affecting sheep and, on occasions, goats, deer, pigs, cattle and humans. It appears to have no tropism for reproductive tissues and will not be considered further.

Pestivirus infections, however, have major consequences for reproduction of cattle, sheep and pigs and will be considered below.

VIRUSES AND ANTIGENIC
CHARACTERISTICS

Pestiviruses are 40–60 nm in diameter, pleomorphic with a surface envelope. Each virion contains a single positive-sense molecule of ssRNA of about 10–12.5 kb size. There is no poly (A) tract at the 3' end. The pestiviruses exist in two biotypes, of which the cytopatho-genic biotype has additional integrated sequences derived from either host sequences or duplicated viral genomic RNA. There are four structural proteins: the nucleocapsid pro-tein (p14) and the three envelope glycopro-teins gp48, gp25 and the immunodominant glycoprotein (gp53).

EPIDEMIOLOGY AND TRANSMISSION

Pestiviruses have a worldwide distribution in both domesticated and free-living ruminant and porcine species. Classic swine fever has, however, been eliminated from Australasia, USA and some European countries, e.g. Scan-dinavia and the UK. BVDV and BDV remain worldwide although there are now campaigns in Scandinavia and the UK to have selected areas, if not whole countries, free of BVDV.

Transmission is by direct contact with infec-ted animals; the main reservoir for BVDV being the persistently infected animal. As these represent at least 1% of cattle in the UK national herd, the circulation of the virus is assured unless there are active procedures to identify and eliminate these carrier animals. The introduction of acutely infected or persis-tently infected (PI) animals is the main reason for outbreaks of pestivirus infection in naive herds. Meat products from infected animals have been incriminated in several outbreaks of classic swine fever virus (CSFV) as well. The widespread use of fetal calf serum in manufacturing processing, e.g. cell culture for vaccine production, has become another opportunity for dissemination of pestiviruses; many batches of fetal calf serum are contami-nated by BVDV and thereby introduce adven-titious pestivirus into vaccine preparations. Strict control on these processes is required. Semen from PI animals contains high concen-trations of virus; its use in artificial insemina-tion programmes can have serious conse-quences. The possibilities of passive transmission of virus by biting flies has been proposed. Wildlife reservoirs of virus (e.g.

deer, antelope and wild boar) are potential sources of infection for domesticated species.

CLINICAL ASPECTS

Pestivirus infections can cause a wide range of clinical syndromes from the inapparent to the fatal. The complexities of the overall patho-genesis have been reviewed elsewhere[15]. The relevance of pestivirus infections of repro-ductive tissues will now be considered.

All pestiviruses can establish infection and cause pathology in the urogenital tract. They can infect both ovarian[93] and testicular tissues and can be recovered from semen of acutely infected bulls[94,95]. The semen is often of poor quality[96] and has the potential to spread infection to seronegative heifers[26]. BVDV rarely infects the fetuses of seropositive cattle; the presence of maternal antibodies appears to correlate with prevention of viral transmission through the placentome to the fetus.

During acute infection in cattle, the virus invades the placentome, replicates and may cross to the fetus without producing lesions[97]. In sheep, BVDV has been shown to damage the maternal vascular endothelium within 10 days of infection and the resulting cellular debris is ingested by the fetal tropho-blast[13]. This could be a mechanism of virus transfer from dam to offspring but may also account for the placentitis that leads to the high level of abortion following BVDV infec-tion. It is well recorded that early embryonic death, infertility and 'repeat breeder' cows are often the sequel to pestivirus infection during pregnancy[16]. In a herd infected with BVDV, the conception rates were reduced from 78.6% in the immune cows to 22.2% in infected cattle[98].

In cattle that are persistently viraemic, there is less certainty about the pathway and timing of fetal invasion because all tissues, including the uterus, are continually infected. However most, if not all, fetuses born of viraemic dams become likewise persistently viraemic.

Whether infection of these fetuses occurs at the level of the germ cell or subsequent to the rupture of the zona pellucida upon implantation is still to be clarified. It has been reported that border disease virus antigen can be found in the germinal cells of the sheep ovary[99] and in the oviductal and granulosa cells of the cow[100].

Whether, following acute or persistent infection, the virus infects the fetus by either direct cell-to-cell transmission or systemic spread is not clear. The time taken for the passage of virus from dam to fetus is variable but it has been recorded that abortions due to BVDV can occur within 10–18 days after intramuscular injection[98]. Experimental experience has shown that abortions can also take place several months after fetal infection.

The outcome of fetal infection is dependent on two main variables: the age of the fetus at the time of infection and the biotype of the infecting virus. There is uncertainty about the pathogenesis of infection during the first 30 days of pregnancy. There is good evidence that BVDV will reduce the conception rate during this period[101] and that the virus will replicate freely in the maternal placenta[102]. However, there is also the view that limited transplacental infection occurs during this early stage[95] because the contact between maternal epithelium and fetal trophoblast is not sufficiently intimate for vertical transmission until the 'bridge' formation at around 30 days[13,103]. This has implications for the use of infected semen or even embryo transfer[26].

There is little doubt that fetal infection will occur after this 30-day period and the outcome depends on whether the virus establishes during the first (up to about 110–120 days), the second (to about 180–200 days) or third trimester (to full term, about 280 days). Infection during the first two trimesters can result in abortion[104] whereas infection during the first trimester can also produce calves that remain persistently viraemic for life (see below). Calves infected during the last trimester are able to mount an active immune response[105].

The outcome of infection with the non-cytopathogenic biotype during the first and second trimesters is frequently death, abortion or mummification of the fetus[97,106]. Fetal death can follow directly from viral invasion but damage of the maternal placenta may contribute by disrupting its vascular supply of nutrients. Experimental infections during this period have shown that more than 30% of fetuses are aborted[107] but recovery of virus from aborted tissues is poor. However, experimental infection of cattle during the first trimester of pregnancy with the cytopathogenic biotype does not give abortions and there is some doubt whether this biotype can even establish infection in the early fetus[108].

Viruses that establish in the early fetus during organogenesis can have the distinction of causing bizarre malformations that permanently affect the animal. BVDV has a well-documented teratogenic effect, in common with the other non-arboviral togaviruses[16]. When the lesions induced by BVDV infection are particularly severe, the fetus will die and be aborted. However, it is evident that the non-cytopathogenic biotype can replicate in the early fetus, often causing damage to selected tissues but not sufficient to cause death. Such calves are born with a variety of clinical signs that range from the apparently normal to the weakly, unthrifty calf or occasionally brain-damaged calf.

The pathogenesis of this wide range of lesions is unlikely to be due to a single defect. The virus appears catholic in its choice of cell in which to replicate. It has a preference for mitotically active cells, particularly those of the central nervous system (CNS) and lymphoid tissues[109–112]. Whether the pathogenetic event is an inhibition of normal cell division and differentiation or due to a direct lytic action of the virus is difficult to determine. Certainly, BVDV causes significant intrauterine growth retardation in many tissues of the fetus, particularly in the CNS and the thymus[111] and a direct cytolytic effect has been suggested for the hypoplasia in the germinal layer of the cerebellum[110] and other tissues[97]. Hypomyelination of the CNS, which is often associated with thymic hypoplasia, has also been observed[113,114]. A further consistent finding within the pestiviruses is the localization of the virus in the vascular endothelium and from the resulting vasculitis, there can be inflammation, oedema, hypoxia and cellular degeneration[16].

Persistent viraemia

Another outcome of fetal infection during the first trimester is the establishment of viraemia that persists for life[97,115]. The basis for this persistence is the bovine immune system which, before 110–120 days, has not developed sufficient immunocompetence to recognize the BVDV within the fetus as foreign. When 'self' antigens are recognized, soon after this 110–120 day period, the virus is accepted as a 'self' tissue and there is immunotolerance. This immunotolerance, reflected by the lack of specific antibody to the persisting virus, allows the virus to persist in the blood and tissues for the lifetime of the animal. It is worthy of mention that in all the recorded field and experimental data there is no evidence for persistence with the cytopathogenic biotypes, only with the non-cytopathogenic[108].

There is considerable variation in the signs and pathology described for these persistently viraemic cattle. Their identity is based on the recovery of non-cytopathogenic virus in high titre on successive occasions and the lack of antibody to the persisting virus. Their clinical appearance can range from normal to the grossly abnormal. Why some are more damaged than others can, at present, only be a speculation about the age, size, and timing of viral challenge of the early fetus. The pathogenesis of the grossly abnormal calf reflects the viral tropism for the CNS, lymphoid and epithelial cells. Within the CNS, the predilection sites for viral persistence are the cerebral cortex and the hippocampus[112]. Lesions in such tissues are often more severe when the fetus is infected during the second trimester[114,116] and account for the depression and incoordination seen in some newborn calves. Frequently these calves fail to survive and grossly abnormal brain lesions, such as cerebellar hypoplasia[110,111], can be seen at postmortem.

CONTROL

SFV has been eradicated from many industrialized countries and control in these countries depends on exacting importation restrictions of pigs only from SFV-free zones. It was eradicated from the UK by a process of widespread vaccination to lower the incidence of infection, and then by culling of infected and in-contact animals. The UK was declared free from swine fever in 1972.

BVDV is controlled by clinical surveillence and accurate diagnosis of persistently infected animals. Vaccination is used widely in some countries[117]; in the UK, a new inactivated BVDV vaccine has been developed that has proven protection for the fetus[118].

BDV infection of sheep, usually following mortalities in young lambs, is diagnosed by clinical assessment and confirmed by laboratory diagnosis. Control is by isolation and culling persistently infected animals.

PAPILLOMAVIRUSES

Family: Papovaviridae

HUMAN   *VETERINARY*

Genus: papillomavirus
  Human papillomavirus   *Bovine papillomavirus (BPV)*
                                 Sheep papillomavirus (SPV)

                                 plus more

VIRUSES AND ANTIGENIC CHARACTERISTICS

Papillomaviruses are non-enveloped, about 55 nm in diameter with an icosahedral capsid. Each virion contains a single molecule of circular ds DNA about 8 kb in length. There are two structural proteins, L1 and L2.

There are six viruses described, BPV1–BPV6, which are associated with either fibropapillomas (BPV1, BPV2 and BPV5) or with epitheliopapillomas (BPV3, BPV4 and BPV 6).

EPIDEMIOLOGY AND TRANSMISSION

Papillomas have a worldwide distribution and primarily affect cattle and horses. Transmission of virus is by direct contact or iatrogenically. Direct contact can occur venereally following mating.

CLINICAL ASPECTS

Papillomas (warts) are common in cattle and spontaneous recovery usually occurs within 6–18 months. They are not considered to be a clinical problem unless they are on the teats of milking animals or are genital. Genital warts on both vulva and penis can prevent mating and, if abraded, become infected. There are reports of congenital papillomatosis, recorded in horses only, which would indicate the potential for intrauterine transmission [119].

CONTROL

Control measures are usually not warranted as papillomas are self-limiting. However, it may be necessary to consider control, and for this purpose vaccines have been shown to be effective. Vaccines can either be autogenous vaccines made from formalinized homogenates of locally excised tumours or cell-cultured vaccines. Such vaccines have proven effective against experimental challenge [120]. It is important to realize that there are different virus serotypes before designing the correct vaccine strategy.

BUNYAVIRUSES

Family: Bunyaviridae

HUMAN   *VETERINARY*

Genus: bunyavirus   *Akabane virus (AKAV)*
  Bunyamwera virus
                                 plus more
plus more

Genus: nairovirus
  Crimean–Congo
  Haemorrhagic fever virus   *Nairobi sheep disease virus (NSDV)*

                                 plus more

Genus: phlebovirus
  Sand fly fever –Naples virus   *Rift valley fever virus (RVFV)*

                                 plus more

VIRUSES AND ANTIGENIC CHARACTERISTICS

Bunyaviruses comprise five genera and many species; the three genera of veterinary significance are the bunyaviruses, the nairoviruses and the phleboviruses. Virions are either spherical or pleomorphic, about 80–120 nm in diameter and enveloped. There are two surface glycoproteins (G1 and G2) that project from the lipid bilayer envelope as spikes and have haemagglutinating and neutralizing determinants. Each virion contains three molecules of negative or ambisense ssRNA of 11–20 kb size

Viruses in all three genera can replicate in both arthropods and vertebrates although they appear to cause little cytopathology in insect cells. The genetic reassortment that can occur between closely related viruses may account for the large and growing list of viruses identified within these genera.

EPIDEMIOLOGY AND TRANSMISSION

As with most arthropod-borne viruses, the consequent epidemiology of the vertebrate disease reflects the distribution and life cycles of the insect vector. Akabane disease was first isolated from mosquitoes in Japan[121] and then associated with congenital pathology in cattle in Australia[122]. Since that time, it has been reported in South east Asia, Africa and southern Europe (Israel and Turkey). Transmission to vertebrates (cattle sheep and goats) is by mosquitoes but transmission between them may be by direct contact or aerosol infection.

Nairobi sheep disease affects mainly sheep, goats and humans but rarely cattle. It is transmitted by ticks.

Rift valley fever has a wide host range affecting mainly sheep and cattle but also buffalo, camel and dogs. There are frequent outbreaks of disease in humans and it has been suggested that monkeys may even be a reservoir for the virus[123]. Transmission is largely by mosquitoes.

CLINICAL ASPECTS

Akabane virus infection usually produces no observable clinical signs but the outcome for pregnant cattle is a variety of congenital deformations of the fetus, the most characteristic being hydranencephaly and arthrogryphosis. Unborn calves are either aborted, cause dystocia because of their physical shape, or fail to survive postnatally. The condition can reach epidemic proportions in certain areas and causes considerable loss of reproductive performance.

Nairobi sheep disease is reported to be the most important pathogenic virus of sheep and goats in eastern Africa where it can cause up to 90% mortality. In humans it can give a mild febrile reaction but, in small ruminants, it causes fever, anorexia, dypsnoea and diarrhoea and it can also cause abortion in sheep.

Rift valley fever causes a range of clinical signs predominant among which is abortion in sheep, goats and cattle. It can cause 90% mortality in neonatal lambs and kids and, at postmortem examination, there is extensive focal hepatic necrosis. These outbreaks are often associated with influenza or dengue-type conditions in humans.

CONTROL

Control is difficult with these viruses; reduction and/or elimination of insect vectors is suggested. There are some effective vaccines available for RVFV but the mouse attenuated live RVFV vaccine should not be given to breeding ewes because it may be abortigenic or cause congenital defects.

REOVIRIDAE

Family: Reoviridae

HUMAN	*VETERINARY*
Genus: orbivirus	
Onungo virus	*Blue tongue viruses (types 1 to 24) (BTV 1–24)*
Kemerova virus	*Epizootic haemorrhagic disease virus (types 1–10) (EHDV 1–10)*
	plus more

VIRUSES AND ANTIGENIC CHARACTERISTICS

Orbiviruses are one of the nine recognized genera of the reoviruses. Their virions are icosahedral or spherical, about 60–80 nm in diameter and are not enveloped. There are seven viral proteins of which VP7 is the main serogroup-specific antigen and VP2 is the neutralizing antigen. Each virion contains 10 molecules of dsRNA which range from 3954 to 822 bp (with a total of 19.2 kb).

Orbiviruses can replicate in both arthropods and vertebrates although they appear to cause no pathology in insect cells. In vertebrates, they are responsible for haemorrhagic disease and fetal pathology which can be sufficiently severe to be fatal. The cyanotic lesion in the tongue gives the name 'blue tongue' to the group of viruses collectively called blue tongue viruses 1–24.

EPIDEMIOLOGY AND TRANSMISSION

Blue tongue viruses and EHD viruses are transmitted principally by *Culicoides* and are generally restricted to the vector geographical range, i.e. within the latitudes 40°N and 35°S, and this includes Africa, the Americas and Australia. Although BTV cause disease primarily in sheep, they also infect other ruminants[83] including free-living species, e.g. white-tail deer and elk. In contrast, EHD viruses infect primarily the free-living ruminant species but also infect sheep and cattle. EHD virus has been recorded regularly on all continents except Europe; interestingly the *Culicoides* vector is present in Europe but, as yet, has not been associated with virus transmission.

CLINICAL ASPECTS

Following infection with BTV, susceptible sheep are febrile, often showing respiratory distress and mucosal hyperaemia. This can advance to severe pneumonia, lacrimation, recumbency and death. The common sequel, however, is towards recovery, but infection of the pregnant animal is highly likely to lead to congenital damage of the lamb and its death. The most typical congenital pathology is hepatic necrosis, hydranencephaly and arthrogryphosis. Mortalities can reach 20–50% of the flock when it occurs for the first time.

EHD virus infections are characterized by fever, depression, mucosal haemorrhage and death. Fetal pathology has not been reported in free-living ruminants. EHD2 causes Ibaraki disease, characterized in cattle by vomiting copious clear fluids following the retention of inbibed water in a dilatation of the lower oesophagus. The prognosis is poor.

CONTROL

Control of insect vectors can be attempted. There are effective BTV vaccines but it is important to recognize serotypic differences and to ensure their inclusion in selected vaccines. It appears inadvisable to vaccinate pregnant sheep with live virus vaccines. International controls for importing livestock from BTV-infected areas to BTV-free areas should be sufficient to prevent introducing the virus to new areas.

ARTERIVIRUS

Family: ?? (similar genomically to Coronaviridae)

HUMAN   *VETERINARY*

Genus: arterivirus   *Equine arteritis virus (EAV)*
                                 Swine infertility and respiratory syndrome virus (SIRSV)
                                 (porcine respiratory and reproductive syndrome virus (PRRSV))

VIRUSES AND ANTIGENIC CHARACTERISTICS

Arteriviruses are pleomorphic or spherical in shape, about 60 nm in diameter and enveloped. There are four major viral proteins: nucleocapsid protein (N), a membrane protein (M) and two N-glycosylated surface proteins, G_s (small) and G_L (large). Each virion contains a single molecule of linear ssRNA of total length 13 kb).

EPIDEMIOLOGY AND TRANSMISSION

Equine arteritis virus is present in many countries with a high incidence recorded in USA standardbreds (over 50%). Although clinical disease is often unrecognized, the outcome of infection of pregnant mares can be severe with a 50% abortion rate. It is important to recognize that there are two modes of transmission of the virus. In most cases aerosol or oral infection results in replication of the virus in the lymphoid tissue of the nasopharynx, which is followed by viraemia. The second important mechanism is via the semen of an infected stallion. This may occur in any stallion during the acute phase of infection. However, approximately 34% of stallions remain chronically infected, such that they excrete the virus in their semen for prolonged periods of time after clinical recovery. Virus has also been transmitted in chilled and frozen-thawed semen. The tissues and fluid of aborted fetuses also contain virus and in some cases congenital infection can occur, with such animals remaining persistently infected.

Swine infertility and respiratory syndrome virus (SIRSV) (commonly called porcine respiratory and reproductive syndrome virus (PRRSV) or 'blue-ear' disease virus in Europe) is a new disease of swine, first described in 1987. It is a highly infectious disease and has rapidly become worldwide in distribution. It is transmitted by direct contact with infected pigs and via semen.

CLINICAL ASPECTS

The clinical signs of EAV infection vary considerably from one individual to another. There may be mild pyrexia and conjunctivitis or severe depression. In many horses there is pyrexia, mild anaemia, oedema of the limbs and swelling around the eyes. Most horses have nasal catarrh and coughing. This may progress to palpebral oedema ('pink eye') and marked ocular discharge, dyspnoea, abdominal pain and diarrhoea. In stallions the oedema may often be scrotal and preputial.

The common lesion involves necrosis of small arterial vessels, resulting in haemorrhage, oedema and, more rarely, thrombosis and infarction. Approximately 50% of pregnant mares will abort, usually 10–30 days after infection. Animals recover quickly from an infection, although asymptomatic chronic infection occurs in approximately one-third of stallions.

SIRSV causes signs of pyrexia, anorexia, lymphadenopathy and respiratory disease. In pregnant pigs, there is severe reproductive failure with abortions, stillborn piglets and weak piglets that fail to thrive. Affected piglets can have skin vascular lesions characterized by a blue discoloration of the ears, hence the descriptive term 'blue-ear disease'. There may also be some impairment of immune function, making infected pigs more susceptible to secondary infection[124].

CONTROL

With EAV, most horses recover spontaneously. In those with severe disease, supportive therapy combined with broad-spectrum antibiotic agents may help to control secondary bacterial disease. Horses that recover from infection have solid immunity. Passive immunity via the colostrum appears to persist up to six months of age. Passive immunity has been shown to interfere with the production of active immunity.

Horses should be quarantined for at least three weeks when entering a new environment since viral shedding can occur for this time after infection. Paired serology samples at arrival can be useful to confirm that recent exposure has not occurred. It is recommended that all stallions, teasers and preferably mares are vaccinated against EAV. A modified live virus vaccine has been investigated. Most frequently, a killed vaccine is used in the UK, although this is only available on the basis of an animal test certificate. The vaccine provides good immunity to viral challenge and has been suggested to prevent stallions from becoming persistent viral shedders.

Advice on the control of EAV is published by the Horserace Betting Levy Board each year. This is a voluntary code of practice designed to help prevent and control venereal diseases during each breeding season.

In the UK the disease is notifiable and therefore if an outbreak is suspected, the MAFF should be notified immediately. In this instance it is important to stop mating and semen collection, prevent movement of horses on to and off the premises and to isolate any animals with respiratory tract signs, and aborting mares. Aborted fetal material and any contaminated bedding should be destroyed and the area disinfected.

Control of SIRSV is complicated by the long-term persistence of the virus after acute infection; it has been recovered from oropharyngeal scrapings up to 157 days after infection[125]. There are no specific control measures other than rapid diagnosis on clinical, immunological (ELISA) and virological evidence. Presence of virus in semen can be detected by PCR techniques. Once SIRSV has been confirmed within a herd, isolation and culling procedures can be introduced.

CORONAVIRIDAE

Family: Coronaviridae

HUMAN   *VETERINARY*

Genus: coronavirus
  Human coronaviruses 229-E and OC43   *Feline infectious peritonitis virus (FIPV)*

plus more   **plus more**

VIRUSES AND ANTIGENIC CHARACTERISTICS

Coronaviruses are pleomorphic or spherical in shape, about 120–160 nm in diameter and enveloped. There are four viral proteins associated with the envelope: the large surface glycoprotein or spike protein (S), a nucleocapsid protein (N), an integral membrane protein (M) and a haemagglutinin-esterase protein (HE).

Each virion contains a single molecule of linear ssRNA about 30 kb in size.

EPIDEMIOLOGY AND TRANSMISSION

Feline coronavirus (also referred to as feline infectious peritonitis virus) occurs as two strains of varying virulence; one causes clinical infectious peritonitis whilst the other is less virulent and tends to cause only enteritis in young kittens.

Infection appears to enter the body via the oropharynx, probably by aerosol spread. The virus replicates within macrophages throughout the body as a cell-associated infection. There is a resultant vasculitis, disseminated intravascular coagulation and granuloma formation, each of which is the result of the immune response which inadequately controls the infection. Virus appears to be shed from the respiratory tract during the initial respiratory phase of the infection that may last for several weeks. The role of faecal excretion of the virus is uncertain. The virus is moderately labile in the environment.

CLINICAL ASPECTS

The virus causes a Coombs type III or Arthus type of immune complex vasculitis. In general, there are two clinical presentations, either effusive or non-effusive with respect to the peritoneal and pleural cavities. In both cases there is often pyrexia, anorexia and weight loss. There may be a preceding phase of a mild respiratory tract infection. Later, when other organs are involved, additional clinical signs may develop including CNS lesions such as ataxia, paresis, paralysis, nystagmus and fitting. In some cases there may be involvement of the eye resulting in hyphaemia and retinitis. Jaundice may occur in the late stages of the disease.

Feline infectious peritonitis virus has been implicated as a cause of endometritis, resorption and abortion, stillbirth and fading kitten syndrome[126]. Queens are not always ill and may suffer resorption or abortion which is unnoticed. Abortion generally occurs during the last two weeks of pregnancy[127]. Commonly, queens subsequently develop further clinical signs of infection with the virus.

CONTROL

Control depends on the rapid diagnosis and isolation of infected cats. Clinical examination combined with assessments of peritoneal and pleural fluid in effusive cases of infection can lead to a presumptive diagnosis being made. Virus isolation from peritoneal exudate can be attempted on feline cultures. In addition, antibody can be detected by indirect immunofluorescence or ELISA but while very high titres may be diagnostic, moderate titres may be present in some normal cats. In many cases a diagnosis is only confirmed at postmortem examination, when mesothelial hyperplasia and granulomatous infiltrates with focal necrosis are found.

There is no treatment for the reproductive consequences of infection. In generalized infections some response may follow the administration of immunosuppressant doses of corticosteroids but this effect is often only transient. Most cats die within a few months of diagnosis or are euthanased for humane reasons.

ADENOVIRIDAE

Family: Adenoviridae	
HUMAN	*VETERINARY*
Genus: mastadenovirus	
Human adenovirus 1–47	*Canine adenovirus 1 (CAdV1)*
	plus more

VIRUSES AND ANTIGENIC CHARACTERISTICS

Adenoviruses are icosahedral in shape, about 80–110 nm in diameter and are non-enveloped. There are some 40 viral proteins with about 12 associated with the structural proteins; the surface arrangement of the capsomeres is in repeated (240) hexons which have haemagglutination and neutralization activity.

Each virion contains a single molecule of linear dsDNA about 35 kb in size.

EPIDEMIOLOGY AND TRANSMISSION

Canine adenovirus 1 is a highly contagious disease known to produce infectious canine hepatitis. It is transmitted by direct contact, especially with contaminated urine. The virus is present within the urine during the acute phase of infection and may be secreted for many months after infection in some dogs. Virus may also be found in saliva and faeces. Ingestion is the most likely route of infection and initial viral replication occurs in the tonsil and retropharyngeal lymph nodes. In some cases initial viral replication may occur within the small intestine. A viraemia peaks at about 5–7 days after infection, when there is leucopenia and transport of the virus to the liver, vascular endothelium and lymphoid tissue. Immune-complex formation during the time of antibody production can result in renal and ocular lesions. Transplacental transmission may occur and pups are often born infected at term. The effect of infection earlier in pregnancy is uncertain.

CLINICAL ASPECTS

The virus produces a severe hepatitis and tonsillitis in young dogs. It is also associated with nephritis and ocular disease. There is often sudden onset and severe depression followed by sudden death. In dogs which survive this stage of infection, pyrexia and jaundice develop, often associated with massive abdominal effusion and oedema of the head and neck. Vomiting and diarrhoea are common. There is often a transitory oedema of the cornea which is the result of anterior uveitis.

The reproductive consequences of infection with this virus occur when the virus crosses the placenta during late pregnancy, resulting in the birth of pups which rapidly develop signs of systemic infection similar to those observed in older pups and adults. Some pups may be born dead whilst others are weak and die within a few days of parturition[128]. In other cases, pups are infected soon after birth

and this results in significant neonatal mortality[129]. The virus may be shed by bitches that have recovered from the clinical disease and therefore act as a source of infection for pups.

CONTROL

Infection may be diagnosed upon the basis of the clinical signs and certainly the development of corneal opacity may be used retrospectively to diagnose the condition. Virus can be isolated from blood or urine and infection can be confirmed in recovered animals by a rise in circulating antibody concentrations using the serum neutralization test. At postmortem examination there is often hepatomegaly and oedema of the gall bladder wall. Characteristic intranuclear inclusion bodies may be found, particularly within liver parenchymal cells.

Recovered animals have solid and permanent immunity to infection. Immune animals may, however, shed virus in their urine for prolonged periods of time. There is useful cross-immunity between canine adenovirus 1 and canine adenovirus 2 (infectious canine laryngotracheitis virus).

Adjuvanted inactivated vaccines are available and, in certain cases, their single administration can provide immunity for life. Live virus vaccines may produce corneal oedema and mild nephropathy, although new canine cell line passaged virus does not produce these adverse effects. Certain manufacturers rely upon the cross-immunity produced by canine adenovirus 2 to protect against hepatitis and respiratory tract infection.

TRANSMISSIBLE VENEREAL TUMOUR

Although a viral aetiology for canine transmissible venereal tumour has often been suggested, this disease appears to be spread by direct transfer of neoplastic cells. In male dogs the tumour may be found on the penis or within the sheath and in females it develops within the vestibule or vagina. The condition is transmitted by contact at coitus and infected dogs may develop secondary nasal lesions after licking their genitalia. The tumours may become excoriated and are painful and may prevent mating. Surgical excision can be useful although recurrence is common. Spontaneous tumour regression is observed in some dogs.

CONCLUSION

Reproductive failure can be a personal tragedy but, when epizootic within a population, it can become a threat to development or even survival. It is clear that a low level of embryonic loss occurs in all veterinary species and may represent a biological filter to remove 'unfit' offspring at the earliest moment of genotypic expression. However, increased reproductive failure beyond this background is attributable to several major causes, of which genetic infidelity, endocrine/metabolic dysfunction and microbial-induced pathology are best documented.

Genetic infidelity, usually visualized as chromosomal abnormalities by karyotyping, has been recorded in all major veterinary species and has been associated with congenital pathology. However, chromosomal abnormalities are not often implicated as a major cause of loss; this may reflect either a genuine low incidence or inconstancy in routine veterinary diagnostic procedures for genotyping. The potential for viruses to induce genetic damage in the early embryo of veterinary species has yet to be clarified.

Endocrine/metabolic dysfunction has many non-infectious causes; however, microbial damage to endocrine organs has also been shown to cause *in utero* growth retardation in late pregnancy and in the neonatal animal (e.g. pestiviruses in ruminants). Some microbial agents cause a placentitis and thereby promote degrees of placental insufficiency and metabolic dysfunction which may vary from mild to severe and life-theatening.

There is little doubt that the microbial causes of reproductive failure are of major importance. Establishing that a particular virus will cause pathology has depended greatly on experimental studies with the agent and the target species. Where possible, the experimental approach is essentially that outlined by Koch's postulates which demand that before ascribing causal pathogenicity, the presumptive pathogen must be associated with a defined clinical syndrome (e.g. reproductive failure), grown in pure culture, and inoculated into an appropriate host to reproduce the clinical disease with subsequent re-isolation of the pathogen. The question of 'appropriate animal' is an important and sensitive one. It is a restriction for medical research whereas, in veterinary sciences, studies can be directed in the target species. This advantage is reflected in the considerable advances in our understanding and control of veterinary virus diseases causing reproductive losses. However, it would be incautious to imply that all these diseases are under control; many continue to run amok in many parts of the world and cause pestilences of great severity and economic importance. Some of these have been described above.

The great strides made in recent years in *in vitro* fertilization and embryo cloning techniques, even to the point of producing a lamb successfully from the cloning of a somatic mammary cell[130], raise another problem that appears to have received little critical attention. This is the possibility that virus may be introduced into the culture conditions for embryo culture by use of biological supplements (e.g. fetal calf serum) or feeder cell lines (granulosa cell lines). If such viruses were non-cytopathogenic and able to infect the early blastocyst during the fertilization manipulations, then viral establishment would occur without immediate evidence of infection. It may be important to consider this risk and its implications for IVF programmes.

It is obvious from the descriptions of congenital damage given above that the fetus is highly susceptible to gross congenital defect, often resulting in death and abortion. These are the obvious consequences of viral infection. However, a more sinister legacy, which may not be so obvious and is presently underrated in veterinary medicine, is the potential for virally induced perturbation of the normal functioning of organ systems such as the immune, the endocrine and the reproductive systems. The changes in function may be subtle and not obvious at birth. Their appearance later in neonatal life would be difficult, on the one hand, to dissociate from either placental insufficiencies or, on the other hand, to associate with fetal infection unless the pathogen were to remain as a persistent infection. A similar concept for non-infectious causes has been put forward for the correlation between poor fetal nutrition and late-onset heart disease in humans (Barker hypothesis[14]).

An examination of the comparative virology of medical and veterinary reproductive diseases shows the involvement of several similar viral families (e.g. herpesviruses, retroviruses and flaviviruses) with, often, comparable pathogenesis. There are also several veterinary viruses which, at present, have no human equivalents in their reproductive system involvement (e.g. orbiviruses, arteriviruses and nairoviruses) but it would be unwise to consider that either list, medical or veterinary, is ever complete. The emergence of new viruses and new diseases is a continuum which has a malevolent pedigree over hundreds of years[27]. However, at this point, we might re-read the words of Hans Zinsser with interest:

Infectious disease is one of the few genuine adventures left. The dragons are all dead and the lance grows rusty in the chimney corner . . . about the only sporting proposition that remains unimpaired by the relentless domestication of a once free-living human species is the war against those ferocious little fellow creatures, which lurk in the dark corners and stalk us in the bodies of rats, mice and all kinds of domestic animals; which fly and crawl with insects, and waylay us in our food and drink and even in our love.

(Hans Zinsser (1934) *Rats, Lice and History*)

REFERENCES

1. Clutton-Brock, J. (1987) *A Natural History of Domesticated Mammals*. British Museum (Natural History) and Cambridge University Press, London.
2. Galton, F. (1865) *The First Steps towards the Domestication of Animals* (Trans. Ethnology Society, London). Reprinted in *Inquiries into Human Faculty*, J.M. Dent, London, 1907.
3. Arthur, G.H., Noakes, D.E., Pearson, H. and Pearson, T.J. (1996) *Veterinary Reproduction and Obstetrics*, 7th edn, W.B. Saunders, London.
4. Esselmont, R.J. (1992) *Daisy Dairy Information System Report. No 1*. University of Reading, Reading.
5. Ricketts, S.W. and Young, A. (1990) Thoroughbred mare fertility. *Vet. Record*, **126**, 68.
6. Smith (1991) Diploma in Sheep Health and Production. Dissertation. Royal College of Veterinary Surgeons.
7. Douglas, R.G.A., Mackinnon, J.D. and Hardy, B. (1993) Leg weakness in weaned first litter sows. *Pig Vet. J.*, **30**, 77–80.
8. England, G.C.W. (1992) Vaginal cytology and cervicovaginal mucus arborisation in the breeding management of bitches. *J. Small Animal Pract.*, **33**, 577–582.
9. Bishop, M.W.H. (1964) Paternal contribution to embryonic death. *J. Reprod. Fertil.*, **7**, 383–396.
10. Benyon, H. (1978) *The Disposal of Dairy Cows in England and Wales 1976–1977*. University of Exeter, Agricultural Economics Unit.
11. Kaneene, J.B. and Hurd, H.S. (1990) The National Animal Health Monitoring System in Michigan. 1. Design, data and frequencies of selected dairy cattle diseases. *Prevent. Vet. Med.*, **8**, 103–114.
12. Jarrett, O. (1985) Feline leukaemia virus. In: *Feline Medicine and Therapeutics*, (Eds E.A. Chandler, C.J. Gaskell and A.D.R. Hilbery), Blackwell Scientific Publications, Oxford, pp. 271–283.
13. Barlow, R.M. (1972) Experiments in border disease IV. Pathological changes in ewes. *J. Compar. Pathol.*, **72**, 151–157.

14. Barker, D.J.P. (1995) The fetal origins of adult disease. *Proc. Roy. Soc.*, Series B, **262**, 37–43.

15. Brownlie, J. (1991) The pathways for bovine virus diarrhoea virus biotypes in the pathogenesis of disease. *Arch. Virol.*, **S3**, 79–96.

16. Van Oirschot, J.T. (1983) Congenital infections with nonarbo togaviruses. *Vet. Microbiol.*, **12**, 14–18.

17. Brigden, A. and Reid, H.W. (1991) Derivation of a DNA clone corresponding to the viral agent of sheep-associated malignant catarrhal fever. *Res. Vet. Sci.*, **50**, 38–44.

18. Desport, M., Collins, M.E. and Brownlie, J. (1995) Detection of bovine viral diarrhoea virus RNA by *in situ* hybridisation with digoxigenin-labelled riboprobes. *Intervirology*, **37**, 269–276

19. Stringfellow, D.A. and Seidel, S.M. (eds) (1990) *Manual of the International Embryo Transfer Society*, 2nd edn. IETS, Champaign, Illinois.

20. Booth, P.J., Collins, M.E., Jenner, L. *et al.* (1994) Isolation of virus from IVS bovine embryos infected *in vitro* with non-cytopathogenic bovine viral diarrhoea virus following washing using IETS recommended procedures. 10th Symposium, of the European Embryo Transfer Association Lyon, France, p. 154.

21. Gwatkin, R.B.L. (1967) Passage of mengovirus through the zona pellucida of the mouse morula. *J. Reprod. Fertil.*, **13**, 577–578.

22. Crittenden, L.B. (1991) Retroviral elements in the genome of the chicken: implications for poultry genetics and breeding. *Crit. Rev. Poultry Biol.*, **3**, 73–109.

23. Lavitrano, M., Camaioni, A., Fazio, V.M. *et al.* (1989) Sperm cells as vectors for introducing foreign DNA into eggs: genetic transformation of mice. *Cell*, **57**, 717–723

24. Timoney, P.J., McCollum, W.H., Roberts, A.W. and Murphy, T.W. (1986) Demonstration of the carrier state in naturally acquired equine arteritis virus infection in the stallion. *Res. Vet. Sci.*, **41**, 279–280.

25. Gilbert, R.O., Coulbrough, R.I. and Weiss, K.E. (1987) The transmission of Bluetongue virus by embryo transfer in sheep. *Theriogenology*, **27**, 527–540.

26. Meyling, A. and Jensen, A.M. (1988) Transmission of bovine virus diarrhoea virus (BVDV) by artificial insemination (AI) with semen from a persistently-infected bull. *Vet. Microbiol.*, **17**, 97–105.

27. Scott, G.R. (1990) *To-morrow's animal plagues in perspective*. 25 Jahre seminar fur Tropenveterinarmedizin – Fachbereich Veterinarmedizin der Freien Universitat Berlin 1988.

28. Justines, G., Sucre, H. and Alvarez, O. (1980) Transplacental transmission of Venezuelan equine encephalitis virus in horses. *Am. J. Trop. Med. Hygiene*, **29**, 653–656.

29. Casamassima, A.C., Hess, L.W. and Marty, A. (1987) Venzuelan equine encephalitis vaccine exposure during pregnancy. *Teratology*, **36**, 287–289.

30. Edington, N., Bridges, C.G. and Huckles, A. (1985) Experimental reactivation of equid herpes virus I (RHV-I) following the administration of corticosteroids. *Equine Vet. J.*, **17**, 369–372.

31. Donaldson, A.I., Wardly, R.C., Martin S. and Ferris, N.P. (1983) Experimental Aujeszky's disease in pigs: excretion, survival and transmission of virus. *Vet. Record*, **113**, 490–494

32. Carmichael, L.E. (1970) Herpesvirus canis: aspects of pathogenesis and immune response. *JAVMA*, **156**, 1714–1725.

33. Gaskell, R.M., Dennis, P.E., Goddard, L.E., Cocker, F.M. and Willis, J.M. (1985) Isolation of felid herpesvirus I from the trigeminal ganglia of latently infected cats. *J. Gen. Virol.*, **66**, 391–394.

34. Gibbs, E.P.J. and Rweyemamu, M.M. (1977) Bovine herpesviruses II. Bovine herpesviruses 1 & 3. *Vet. Bull.*, **47**, 411–425.

35. Gigstad, D.C. and Stone, S.S. (1977) Clinical, serologic and cross-challenge response and virus isolation in cattle affected with three bovine dermatotropic herpes viruses. *Am. J. Vet. Res.*, **38**, 753–757.

36. Kahrs, R.F. (1977) Infectious bovine rhinotracheitis: a review and update. *JAVMA* **171**, 1055–1064.

37. Mumford, J.A., Rossdale, P.D., Jessett, D.M. *et al.* (1987) Serological and virological investigation of an equid herpesvirus abortion storm on a stud farm in 1985. *J. Reprod. Fertil.*, **35**(suppl), 509–518.

38. Edington, N., Smyth, B. and Griffiths, L. (1991) The role of endothelial cell infection in the endometrium, placenta and foetus of equid herpes virus I (EHV-I) abortions. *J. Comp. Pathol.*, **104**, 379–387.

39. Smith, K.C., Whitwell, K.E., Binns, M.M. *et al.* (1992) Abortion of virologically negative foetuses following experimental challenge of

pregnant pony mares with EHV-I. *Equine Vet. J.*, **24**, 256–259.

40. Crandell, R.A. and Davis, E.R. (1985) Isolation of equine coital exanthema virus (equine herpesvirus 3) from the nostril of a foal. *JAVMA*, **187**, 503–504.

41. Hashimoto, A., Hirai, K., Fukushi, H. and Fujimoto, Y. (1983) The vaginal lesions of a bitch with a history of canine herpesvirus infection. *Japan. J. Vet. Sci.*, **45**, 123–125.

42. Post, G. and King, N. (1971) Isolation of a herpesvirus from the canine genital tract: association with infertility, abortion and still-births. *Vet. Record*, **88**, 229–232.

43. Hashimoto, A. and Hirai, K. (1986) Canine herpesvirus infection. In: *Current Therapy in Theriogenology*, (ed. D.A. Morrow), W.B. Saunders, Philadelphia, pp. 516–520.

44. Hashimoto, A., Hirai, K., Okada, K. and Fujimoto, Y. (1979) Pathology of the placenta and newborn pups with suspected intra-uterine infection of canine herpesvirus. *Am. J. Vet. Res.*, **40**, 1236–1242.

45. Percy, D.H., Carmichael, L.E. and Albert, D.M. (1970) Lesions in puppies surviving infection with canine herpesvirus. *Vet. Pathol.*, **8**, 37–53.

46. Wright, N.G. and Cornwell, H.J.C. (1970) The susceptibility of six-week old puppies to canine herpesvirus. *J. Small Animal Pract.*, **10**, 669–674.

47. Hoover, E.A. and Griesemer, R.A. (1971) Comments: pathogenicity of feline viral rhinotracheitis virus and effect on germfree cats, growing bone, and the gravid uterus. *JAVMA*, **158**, 929–931.

48. Troy, G.C. and Herron, M.A. (1986) Infectious causes of abortion and stillbirth in cats. In: *Small Animal Reproduction and Infertility*, (ed. T.J. Burke), Lea and Fibiger, Philadelphia, pp. 258–269.

49. Weller, T.H., Hanshaw, J.B. and Scott, D.E. (1960) Serologic differentiation of viruses responsible for cytomegalic inclusion disease. *Virology*, **12**, 130–132.

50. Plummer G (1973) Cytomegalovirus of man and animals. *Prog. Med. Virol.*, **15**, 92–125.

51. Raq, R. (1961) Infectious rhinitis in pigs: laboratory aspects. *Aust. Vet. J.*, **37**, 91–93.

52. Cameron-Stephen, I.D. (1961) Inclusion body rhinitis of swine. *Aust. Vet. J.*, **37**, 87–91.

53. Corner, A.H., Mitchell, D.J., Julian, R.J. and Meads, A.B. (1964) A generalised disease of piglets associated with the presence of cytomegalic inclusions. *J. Comp. Pathol.*, **74**, 192–199.

54. Edington, N., Watt, R.G., Plowright, W., Wrathall, A.E. and Done, J.T. (1977) Experimental transplacental transmission of porcine cytomegalovirus. *J. Hygiene*, **78**, 243–290.

55. Edington, N., Wrathall, A.E. and Done, J.T. (1988) Porcine cytomegalovirus (PCMV) in early gestation. *Vet. Microbiol.*, **17**, 117–128.

56. Hsu, F.S., Chu, R.M., Lee, R.C.T. and Chu, S.H.J. (1980) Placental lesions caused by pseudorabies virus in pregnant sows. *JAVMA*, **177**, 636–641.

57. Cutlip, R.C. and Mengeling, W.L. (1975) Experimental induced infection of neonatal swine with porcine parvovirus. *Am. J. Vet. Res.*, **36**, 1179–1192

58. Monif, G.R. and Dische, R.M. (1972) Viral placentitis in congenital cytomegalovirus infection. *Am. J. Clin. Pathol.*, **58**, 445–449.

59. Griffith, B.P., McCormick S.R., Fong C.K.Y. *et al.* (1985) The placenta as a site of cytomegalovirus infection in guinea pigs. *J. Virol.*, **55**, 402–450.

60. Johnson, K.P. (1969) Mouse cytomegalovirus: placental infection. *J. Infect. Dis.*, **120**, 445–450.

61. Ehlers, B., Buhk, H.J., Ludwig, H. (1985) Analysis of bovine cytomegalovirus genome structure: cloning and mapping of the monomeric polyrepetitive DNA unit and comparison of European and American strains. *J. Gen. Virol.*, **66**, 55–68.

62. Thiry, E., Dubuisson, J., Bublot, M., Van Bressen, M.-F. and Pastoret, P.-P. (1990) The biology of bovine herpesvirus-4 infection of cattle. *Dtsche. Tierarztl. Wochenschr.*, **97**, 72–77.

63. Thiry, E., Bublot, M., Dubuisson, J. and Pastoret, P.-P. (1989) Bovine herpesvirus 4 (BHV-4) infections of cattle. In: *Herpesvirus Diseases of Cattle, Horses and Pigs. Developments in Veterinary Virology.* Kluwer Academic Boston, pp. 96–115.

64. Parks, J.B. and Kendrick, J.W. (1973) The isolation and partial characterisation of a herpesvirus from a case of bovine metritis. *Arch. Gesamt. Virusforsch.*, **46**, 238–247.

65. Castrucci, G., Frigeri, F., Cilli, V. *et al.* (1986) A study of herpes isolated from dairy cattle with a history of reproductive disorders. *Comp. Immunol. Microbiol. Infect. Dis.*, **9**, 13–21.

66. Eyanga, E., Jetteur, P., Thiry, E. *et al.* (1989) Recherche des anticorps diriges contre les BHV-1, BHV-2, BHV-4, le virus BVD-MD, les adenovirus A et B, le rotavirus et le coronavirus bovine chez des bovins de l'ouest du Zaire: resultats complementaires. *Revue d'Elevage et Medecine Veteinaire des Pays Tropicaux*, **19**, 305–315.

67. Kendrick, J.W., Osburn, B.I. and Kronlund, N. (1976) Pathogenic studies on a bovine herpesvirus. *Theriogenology*, **6**, 447–462.

68. Reed, D.R., Langpap, T.J. and Bergeland, M.E. (1979) Bovine abortion associated with mixed Movar 33/63 type herpesvirus and bovine viral diarrhea virus infection. *Cornell Veterinarian*, **69**, 54–66.

69. Ackerman, M., Weber, H.P. and Wyler, R. (1990) Aspects of infectious bovine rhinotracheitis eradication programmes in a fattening cattle farm. *Preventive Vet. Med.*, **9**, 121–130.

70. Hannant, D. (1991) Immune responses to common respiratory pathogens: problems and perspectives in equine immunology. *Equine Vet. J.*, **12**(suppl), 10–18.

71. Burrows, R., Goodridge, D. and Denyer, M.S. (1984) Trials of an inactivated equid herpesvirus I vaccine: challenge with a subtype I virus. *Vet. Record*, **114**, 369–374.

72. Van Oirschot, J.T., Wijsmuller, J.M., De Waal, C.A.H. and Van Lith, P.M. (1990) A novel concept for the control of Aujeszky's disease: experiences in two vaccinated pig herds. *Vet. Record*, **126**, 159–163.

73. Wright, N.G. and Cornwell, H.J.C. (1970) Further studies on experimental canine herpesvirus infection in young puppies. *Res. Vet. Sci.*, **11**, 221–226.

74. Pattison I. (1990) *A Great British Veterinarian Forgotten: James Beart Simonds 1810–1904.* J.A. Allen, London.

75. Krakowka, S., Hoover, E.A. and Koestner, A. (1977) Experimental and naturally occurring transplacental transmission of canine distemper virus. *Am. J. Vet. Res.*, **38**, 919–922.

76. Wafula, J.S., Rossiter, P.B., Wamwayi, H.M. and Scott, G.R. (1989) Preliminary observations on rinderpest in pregnant cattle. *Vet. Record*, **124**, 485–486.

77. Obi, T.U., Ojo, M.O. and Taylor, W.P. (1983) Studies on the epidemiology of peste des petits ruminants in Southern Nigeria. *Trop. Veterinarian*, **1**, 209–217.

78. Provost, A., Morris, Y. and Borredon, C. (1986) Protection against Rinderpest conferred in cattle by inoculation of measles virus: application to calves having passive immunity from maternal antibody. *Revue d'Elevage et Medecine Veterinaire des Pays Tropicaux*, **21**, 145–164.

79. Yilma, T.D. (1989) Prospects for the total eradication of rinderpest. *Vaccine*, **7**, 484–485.

80. Shen, D.T., Leendertsen, L.W. and Gorham, J.R. (1981) Evaluation of chemical disinfectants for Aleutian disease virus of mink. *Am. J. Vet. Res.*, **42**, 838–840.

81. Porter, D.D., Larsen, A.E. and Porter, H.G. (1980) Aleutian disease of mink. *Adv. Immunol.*, **29**, 261–286.

82. Storz, J., Young, S., Carroll, E.J. *et al.* (1978) Parvovirus infection in the bovine fetus: distribution of infection, antibody response, and age-related susceptibility. *Am. J. Vet. Res.*, **39**, 1099–1102.

83. Barnes, M.A., Wright, R.E., Bodine, A.B. and Alberty, C.F. (1982) Frequency of bluetongue and bovine parvovirus infection in cattle in South Carolina dairy herds. *Am. J. Vet. Res.*, **43**, 1078–1080.

84. Mengeling, W.L., Paul, P.S. and Brown, T.T. (1980) Transplacental infection and embryonic death following maternal exposure to porcine parvovirus near the time of conception. *Arch. Virol.*, **65**, 55–62.

85. Meunier, P.C., Glickman, L.T. and Appel, M.J.G. (1981) Canine parvovirus in a commercial kennel: epidemiologic and pathologic findings. *Cornell Veterinarian*, **71**, 96–101.

86. Guy, J.S. (1986) Diagnosis of canine viral infections. *Vet. Clin. North Am. Small Animal Pract.*, **16**, 1145–1156.

87. Gillespie, J.H. and Scott, F.W. (1973) Feline viral infections II. Feline panleucopaenia (FPL) infections. *Adv. Vet. Sci. Comp. Med.*, **17**, 164–179.

88. Gaskell, R.M. (1985) Feline panleucopenia (feline infectious enteritis). In: *Feline Medicine and Therapeutics*, (eds E.A. Chandler, C.J. Gaskell and A.D.R. Hilbery), Blackwell Scientific Publications, Oxford, p. 251–256.

89. Brownlie, J., Clarke, M.C. and Howard, C.J. (1984) Experimental production of fatal mucosal disease in cattle. *Vet. Record*, **114**, 535–536.

90. Hardy, W.D. (1981) Feline leukemia virus nonneoplastic diseases. *J. Am. Animal Hosp. Assoc.*, **17**, 941–947.

91. Jarrett, O., Golder, M.C. and Weijer, K. (1982) A comparison of three methods of feline leukaemia diagnosis. *Vet. Record*, **110**, 325–328.

92. Sturgess, C.P. (1996) Feline vaccination: an update. *Vet. Annual*, **36**, 202–216.

93. Ssentonga, Y.K., Johnson, R.H. and Smith, J.R. (1980) Association of bovine viral diarrhoea-mucosal disease virus with ovaritis in cattle. *Aust. Vet. J.*, **56**, 272–273.

94. Ramsey, F.K. and Chivers, W.H. (1953). Mucosal disease of cattle. *North Am. Veterinarian*, **34**, 629–633.

95. Whitmore, H.L., Gustafsson, B.K., Hauareshti, P., Duchateau, A.B. and Mather, E.C. (1978) Inoculation of bulls with bovine virus diarrhea virus: excretion of virus in semen and effects on semen quality. *Theriogenology*, **9**, 153–169.

96. Whitmore, H.L., Zemjanis, R. and Olson, J. (1981) Effect of bovine viral diarrhea virus on conception in cattle. *JAVMA*, **178**, 1065–1067.

97. Casaro, A.P.E., Kendrick, J.W. and Kennedy, J.W. (1971) Response of the bovine fetus to bovine viral diarrhea-mucosal disease virus. *Am. J. Vet. Res.*, **32**, 1543–1562.

98. Virakul, P., Fahning, M.L., Joo, H.S. and Zemjanis, R. (1988) Fertility of cows challenged with a cytopathic strain of bovine virus diarrhea virus during an outbreak of spontaneous infection with a noncytopathic strain. *Theriogenology*, **29**, 441–449.

99. Gardiner, A.C. (1980) The distribution and significance of border disease viral antigen in infected lambs and foetuses. *J. Comp. Pathol.*, **91**, 467–470.

100. Booth, P.J., Stevens, D.A., Collins, M.E. and Brownlie, J. (1996) Detection of bovine viral diarrhoea virus antigen and RNA in oviduct and granulosa cells of persistently infected cattle. *J. Reprod. Fertil.*, **105**, 17–24.

101. Kirkland, P.D., MacIntosh, S.G. and Moyle, A. (1994) The outcome and widespread use of semen from a bull persistently infected with pestivirus. *Vet. Record*, **135**, 527–529.

102. Parsonson, I.M., O'Halloran, M.L., Zee Y.C. and Snowdon, W.A. (1979) The effect of bovine viral diarrhoea-mucosal disease (BVD) virus on the ovine foetus. *Vet. Microbiol.*, **4**, 279–292.

103. Kendrick, J.W. (1976) Bovine viral diarrhea virus induced abortion. *Theriogenology*, **5**, 91–93.

104. Gillespie, J., Bartholomew, P., Thomson, R. and Mcentee, K. (1967) The isolation of non-cytopathic virus diarrhoea virus from two aborted fetuses. *Cornell Veterinarian*, **57**, 564–571.

105. Brown, T.T., Schultz, A.D., Duncan, J.R. and Bistner, S.I. (1979) Serological response of the bovine fetus to bovine viral diarrhea virus. *Infect. Immun.*, **25**, 93–97.

106. Kendrick, J.W. (1971) Bovine viral diarrhea-mucosal disease virus infection in pregnant cows. *Am. J. Vet. Res.*, **32**, 533–544.

107. Brownlie, J., Clarke, M.C., Howard, C.J. and Pocock, D.H. (1986) Mucosal disease: the dilemma of experimental disease. *Proceedings of the 14th World Congress of Cattle Diseases*, Dublin, Ireland, **1**, 199–203.

108. Brownlie, J., Clarke, M.C. and Howard, C.J. (1989) Experimental infection of cattle in early pregnancy with a cytopathic strain of bovine virus diarrhoea virus. *Res. Vet. Sci.*, **46**, 307–311.

109. Bielefeldt Ohmann, H. (1988) BVD virus antigens in tissues of persistently viraemic, clinically normal cattle: implications for the pathogenesis of clinically fatal disease. *Acta Veterin. Scand.*, **29**, 77–84.

110. Brown, T.T., De Lahunta, A., Scott, F.W. *et al.* (1973) Virus induced congenital anomalies of the bovine fetus. II Histopathology of cerebellar degeneration (hypoplasia) induced by the virus of the bovine viral diarrhea-mucosal disease. *Cornell Veterinarian*, **63**, 561–578.

111. Done, J.T., Terlecki, S., Richardson, C. *et al.* (1980) Bovine virus diarrhoea-mucosal disease virus: pathogenicity for the fetal calf following maternal infection. *Vet. Record*, **106**, 473–479.

112. Fernandez, A., Hewicker, M., Trautwein, G., Pohlenz, J. and Leiss, B. (1989) Viral antigen distribution in the central nervous system of cattle persistently infected with bovine viral diarrhoea virus. *Vet. Pathol.*, **26**, 26–32.

113. Anderson, C.A., Higgins, R.J., Smith, M.E. and Osburn, B.I. (1987) Border disease virus-induced decrease in thyroid hormone levels with associated hypomyelination. *Lab. Invest.*, **57**, 168–175.

114. Binkhorst, G.J., Journee, D.L.H., Wouda, W., Straver, P.J. and Vos, J.H. (1983) Neurological disorders, virus persistence and hypomyelination in calves due to intrauterine infections with bovine virus diarrhoea virus. *Vet. Quarterly*, **5**, 145–155.

115. Kahrs, R.F. (1973) Effects of bovine viral diarrhea on the developing fetus. *JAVMA*, **163**, 877–878.

116. Scott, F.W., Kahrs, R.F., De Lahunta, A. *et al.* (1973) Virus induced congenital abnormalities of the bovine foetus. I Cerebellar degeneration (hypoplasia), ocular lesions and fetal mummifications following experimental infection with bovine viral diarrhea-mucosal disease. *Cornell Veterinarian*, **63**, 536–540.

117. Bolin, S.R. (1990) Control of bovine virus diarrhoea virus. *Revue Scientifique et Technique de L'Office International des Epizooties*, **9**, 163–172.

118. Brownlie, J., Clarke, M.C., Hooper, L.B. and Bell, G.D. (1995) Protection of the bovine fetus from bovine virus diarrhoea virus by means of a new inactivated vaccine. *Vet. Record*, **137**, 58–62.

119. Radostits, O.M., Blood, D.C. and Gay, C.C. (1994) *Veterinary Medicine*, Baillière Tindall, London.

120. Jarrett, W.F.H., O'Neil, B.W., Gaukroger, J.M. *et al.* (1990) Studies on vaccination against papillomaviruses: a comparison of purified virus, tumour extract and transformed cells in prophylactic vaccination. *Vet. Record*, **126**, 449–452.

121. Oya, A., Okuna, T., Ogata, T., Kobayashi, T. and Matsuyama, T. (1961) Akabane virus: a new arbor virus isolated in Japan. *Japan. J. Med. Sci. Biol.*, **14**, 101–108.

122. Hartley, W.J., Wanner, R.A., Della-Porta, A.J. and Snowden, W.A. (1975) Serological evidence for the association of Akabane virus with epizootic bovine congenital arthrogryphosis and hydranencephaly syndromes in New South Wales. *Aust. Vet. J.*, **50**, 185–188

123. Kahrs, R.F. (1981) *Viral Diseases of Cattle*. Iowa State University Press, Iowa.

124. Collins, J.E. and Rossow, K.D. (1996) Porcine reproductive and respiratory syndrome in the boar and sow. Proceedings of Swine Reproduction Symposium, pp. 61–70.

125. Wills, R.W., Zimmerman, J.J. and Yoon, K.J. (1995) Porcine reproductive and respiratory syndrome virus – a persistent infection. *Proceedings of the International Symposium on PRRS*, **2**, 19.

126. Troy, G.C. and Herron, M.A. (1986) Infectious causes of infertility, abortion and stillbirths in cats. In: *Current Therapy in Theriogenology*, (ed. D.A. Morrow), W.B. Saunders, Philadelphia, pp. 834–837.

127. Norsworthy, G.D. (1979) Kitten mortality complex. *Feline Pract.*, **9**, 57–64.

128. Spalding, V.T., Rudd, H.K., Langman, B.A. and Rogers, S.E. (1964) Isolation of CVH from puppies showing the 'fading puppy' syndrome. *Vet. Record*, **76**, 1402–1403.

129. Cornwell, H.J.C. (1984) Specific infections. In: *Canine Medicine and Therapeutics*, (eds E.A. Chandler, J.B. Sutton and D.J. Thompson), Blackwell Scientific Publications, Oxford, pp. 340–366.

130. Wilmut, I., Schneck, A.F., McWhir, J., Kind, A.J. and Campbell, K.H.S. (1997) Viable offspring derived from fetal and adult mammalian cells. *Nature*, **385**, 810.

INDEX

Page numbers in *italics* refer to figures, those in **bold** refer to tables

Cytopathic effect (CPE), varicella-
zoster virus 62–3
Cytotoxic T-lymphocyte (CTL)
activity 3, 4

Dane particle *221*
Deafness, sensorineural 1–2, 17
CMV 35, 266, 268
rubella 264, 265
Delayed-type hypersensitivity
(DTH) 4, 95
Developing world
breastfeeding 2, 141–2
measles 95
see also HIV infection, African
women
Developmental abnormalities 1
Diabetes mellitus 18
Didanosine (ddI) 273
Didepoxytidine (ddC) 273
Disseminated intravascular
coagulation (DIC) 122, 275, 276
Dogs 297
canine adenovirus 325–7
canine distemper virus (CDV)
306, 307
canine parvovirus (CPV) 309, 310,
311
herpesvirus 300, 302–3, 305
Domestication of animals 289
Donor insemination, CMV
transmission 39–40
Drug abuse, hepatitis 168, 178

E1 and E2 proteins 236–8, 242, *243*
E2F protein 240–1
E5 protein 241, 242
E6 protein 239–40, 242, 243
E6BP calcium binding protein 240
E7 protein 239, 240–1, 242, 243
Echoviruses 278–9
Ectopic pregnancy 155
Electrodessication of vulval warts
259
Embryo
cloning techniques 327
screening veterinary species 295
veterinary species loss 293
Encephalitis 120, 122, 267
Enteroviruses 2, 277–80
prevention 280
prognosis 280
transmission 277
treatment 280
veterinary 294
Enzyme-linked immunosorbent
assays (EIA; ELISA) 22–3

Epidermal growth factor receptor
(EGFR) 241
Epizootic haemorrhagic disease
virus 321, 322
Epstein–Barr virus (EBV) 9, 40
Equine arteritis virus 322, 323–4
Equine encephalitis virus 298–9
Equine herpesvirus 300, 301–2,
304–5
Equine infectious anaemia virus
(EIAV) 312, 313
Erythema infectiosum 103, 105, 108
Erythroid hypoplasia of bone
marrow 109
Erythroid precursor cells 109
Erythroid progenitor cells 104
Erythrovirus 103
Exposure-prone procedures (EPPs)
229–30
Eye infections 120, 121–2, 265, 267

Famciclovir 123, 187
Feline coronavirus 324–5
Feline herpesvirus 303, 304, 305
Feline immunodeficiency virus
(FIV) 312, 313
Feline infectious peritonitis virus
324–5
Feline leukaemia virus (FeLV) 312,
313–14
Feline onco-virus membrane-
associated antigen (FOCMA)
314–15
Feline panleucopenia virus (FPV)
308, 309, 310, 312
Fetal varicella syndrome 71–4
acyclovir 74
clinical features 72–3
diagnosis 73
neurological abnormalities 72–3
ophthalmological abnormalities
73
pathogenesis 71
prevalence 71–2
skeletal abnormalities 73
skin lesions 72
varicella-zoster immune globulin
74
Fetus, host defences 2–7
Fifth disease, *see* Erythema
infectiosum
Flaviviruses, veterinary 315–18
5-Fluorouracil 258
Fomites, HPV transmission 248
Formula feeding, *see* Bottle feeding
Foscarnet 48, 188, 267
Fusion protein immunization 250

Gammaglobulin administration for
congenital varicella 76
Gammaglobulinemia 7
Gammaherpesvirus 304
Ganciclovir 48–9, 267
Gender inequity 152
Genetic infidelity 327
Genital dysplasia, HPV 248
Genital herpes
acyclovir suppressive therapy
125–6
caesarean section 125, 126
clinical manifestations in women
117–18
first episode 119, 122
prevention 124
primary 118, 119, 124
recurrent 118, 123, 125–7
risk identification 127
viral reactivation prevention
125–6
Genital infection 9–10
Genital tract, female 2
Genital ulcer disease 151, 152
Genital warts 256–61
benign 245
bovine papillomavirus (BPV) 319
HIV transmission 152
transmission 248
Germline transmission 295
Gestational age, congenital CMV
infection 46
Giant condyloma of Buschke and
Löwenstein 245, 260
Glaucoma 17, 265
Gloving 226, 229
Goats 296, 312
GpCMV model 45–6
Growth factors, pregnancy 8

Haemagglutination inhibition (HI)
22, 27
Haemolytic anaemia 266
Hassall's corpuscles 3
HBcAg 184
HBeAg 179, 181, 183, 219
chronic infection 184
health-care workers 230
infectivity 227
HBsAg 182, 219
antibody 183, 184, 220
marker 184
screening in pregnancy 201
testing in health-care workers
229
vaccines 185
HDAg 189